Annual Reports in Organic Synthesis—1982

Annual Reports in Organic Synthesis

ANNUAL REPORTS IN ORGANIC SYNTHESIS—1970
John McMurry and R. Bryan Miller, Eds.

ANNUAL REPORTS IN ORGANIC SYNTHESIS—1971
John McMurry and R. Bryan Miller, Eds.

ANNUAL REPORTS IN ORGANIC SYNTHESIS—1972
John McMurry and R. Bryan Miller, Eds.

ANNUAL REPORTS IN ORGANIC SYNTHESIS—1973
R. Bryan Miller and Louis S. Hegedus, Eds.
John McMurry, Series Editor

ANNUAL REPORTS IN ORGANIC SYNTHESIS—1974
Louis S. Hegedus and Stephen R. Wilson, Eds.
R. Bryan Miller, Series Editor

ANNUAL REPORTS IN ORGANIC SYNTHESIS—1975
R. Bryan Miller and L. G. Wade, Jr., Eds.

ANNUAL REPORTS IN ORGANIC SYNTHESIS—1976
R. Bryan Miller and L. G. Wade, Jr., Eds.

ANNUAL REPORTS IN ORGANIC SYNTHESIS—1977
R. Bryan Miller and L. G. Wade, Jr., Eds.

ANNUAL REPORTS IN ORGANIC SYNTHESIS—1978
L. G. Wade, Jr., and Martin J. O'Donnell, Eds.

ANNUAL REPORTS IN ORGANIC SYNTHESIS—1979
L. G. Wade, Jr., and Martin J. O'Donnell, Eds.

ANNUAL REPORTS IN ORGANIC SYNTHESIS—1980
L. G. Wade, Jr., and Martin J. O'Donnell, Eds.

ANNUAL REPORTS IN ORGANIC SYNTHESIS—1981
L. G. Wade, Jr., and Martin J. O'Donnell, Eds.

ANNUAL REPORTS IN ORGANIC SYNTHESIS—1982
L. G. Wade, Jr., and Martin J. O'Donnell, Eds.

Annual Reports in Organic Synthesis—1982

edited by
L. G. Wade, Jr.
Department of Chemistry, Colorado State University, Ft. Collins, Colorado
Martin J. O'Donnell
*Department of Chemistry, Indiana University–Purdue University at Indianapolis
Indianapolis, Indiana*

ACADEMIC PRESS   1983
A Subsidiary of Harcourt Brace Jovanovich, Publishers
NEW YORK   LONDON
PARIS   SAN DIEGO   SAN FRANCISCO   SÃO PAULO   SYDNEY   TOKYO   TORONTO

Academic Press Rapid Manuscript Reproduction

COPYRIGHT © 1983, BY ACADEMIC PRESS, INC.
ALL RIGHTS RESERVED.
NO PART OF THIS PUBLICATION MAY BE REPRODUCED OR
TRANSMITTED IN ANY FORM OR BY ANY MEANS, ELECTRONIC
OR MECHANICAL, INCLUDING PHOTOCOPY, RECORDING, OR ANY
INFORMATION STORAGE AND RETRIEVAL SYSTEM, WITHOUT
PERMISSION IN WRITING FROM THE PUBLISHER.

ACADEMIC PRESS, INC.
111 Fifth Avenue, New York, New York 10003

United Kingdom Edition published by
ACADEMIC PRESS, INC. (LONDON) LTD.
24/28 Oval Road, London NW1 7DX

LIBRARY OF CONGRESS CATALOG CARD NUMBER: 17-167779
ISBN 0-12-040813-9

PRINTED IN THE UNITED STATES OF AMERICA

83 84 85 86   9 8 7 6 5 4 3 2 1

CONTENTS

PREFACE ix
JOURNALS ABSTRACTED xi
GLOSSARY OF ABBREVIATIONS xiii

I. **CARBON–CARBON BOND FORMING REACTIONS** 1
  A. Carbon–Carbon Single Bonds (*see also:* I.E, I.F, I.G) 1
    1. Alkylation of Aldehydes, Ketones, and Their Derivatives ... 1
    2. Alkylations of Nitriles, Acids, and Acid Derivatives 6
    3. Alkylation of β-Dicarbonyl and β-Cyanocarbonyl Systems
       and Other Active Methylene Compounds 11
    4. Alkylation of N-, S-, and Se-Stabilized Carbanions 20
    5. Alkylation of Organometallic Reagents (*see also:* I.F, I.G) . 23
    6. Other Alkylation Procedures and Reviews 31
    7. Nucleophilic Addition to Electron-Deficient Carbon 37
       a. 1,2-Additions 37
           (1) Aldol-Type Condensations 37
              (a) Intermolecular 37
              (b) Intramolecular 49
           (2) Addition of N-, S-, or Se-Stabilized Carbanions 54
           (3) Grignard-Type Additions 58
       b. Conjugate Additions 70
           (1) Enolate-Type Carbanions 70
           (2) Organometallic Reagents 78
           (3) Other Conjugate Additions 85
    8. Other Carbon–Carbon Single Bond Forming Reactions 88
  B. Carbon–Carbon Double Bonds (*see also:* I.E.1, III.G,
    VI.A.16) 113
    1. Wittig-Type Olefination Reactions 113
    2. Eliminations 122
       a. Alcohols and Derivatives 122
       b. Halides 123
       c. Other Eliminations 125
    3. Other Carbon–Carbon Double Bond Forming Reactions ... 128
    4. Allene Forming Reactions 141
  C. Carbon–Carbon Triple Bonds (*see also:* VI.A.16) 145

D.	Cyclopropanations	153
	1. Carbene or Carbenoic Addition to Multiple Bonds (*see also:* VI.A.7)	153
	2. Other Cyclopropanations	157
E.	Thermal Reactions	165
	1. Cycloadditions	165
	2. Other Thermal Reactions	190
F.	Aromatic Substitutions Forming a New Carbon–Carbon Bond	205
	1. Friedel–Crafts-Type Reactions	205
	2. Coupling Reactions	212
	3. Other Aromatic Substitutions	215
G.	Synthesis via Organometallics	232
	1. Organoboranes	232
	2. Carbonylation Reactions	236
	3. Other Synthesis *via* Organometallics	241
	4. Reviews	244

II. OXIDATIONS 247
  A. C–O Oxidations 247
    1. Alcohol → Ketone, Aldehyde 247
    2. Alcohol, Aldehyde → Acid, Acid Derivative 250
  B. C–H Oxidations 253
    1. C–H → C–O 253
    2. C–H → C–Hal 255
    3. Other C–H Oxidations 258
  C. C–N Oxidations 258
  D. Amine Oxidations .... (1981, 259)
  E. Sulfur Oxidations 260
  F. Oxidative Additions to C–C Multiple Bonds 262
    1. Epoxidations 263
    2. Hydroxylation 264
    3. Other 265
  G. Phenol → Quinone Oxidation 265
  H. Oxidative Cleavages 266
  I. Photosensitized Oxygenations 270
  J. Dehydrogenation 270
  K. Other Oxidations and Reviews 272

III. REDUCTIONS 273
  A. C = O Reductions (*see also:* III.F.1) 273
  B. Nitrile Reductions 279
  C. Reduction of Sulfur Compounds 280
  D. N–O Reductions 280

	E.	C–C Multiple Bond Reductions 281
		1. C = C Reductions (*see also:* VI.A.6) 282
		2. C ≡ C Reductions 284
		3. Reduction of Aromatic Rings 285
	F.	Hydrogenolysis of Hetero Bonds 285
		1. C–O → C–H 286
		2. C–Hal → C–H 289
		3. C–S → C–H 291
		4. C–N → C–H .... (1981, 297)
	G.	Reductive Eliminations 293
	H.	Reductive Cleavages 296
	I.	Hydroboration (reduction only) 297
	J.	Other Reductions and Reviews 299
IV.	**SYNTHESIS OF HETEROCYCLES** 300	
	A.	Aziridines 300
	B.	Furans, etc. 301
	C.	Indoles 303
	D.	Lactams 306
	E.	Lactones 312
	F.	Pyridines, Quinolines, etc. 319
	G.	Pyrroles, etc. 325
	H.	Other Heterocycles with One Heteroatom (*see also:* II.F.1, VI.A.9) 327
	I.	Heterocycles with Two or More Heteroatoms 330
		1. Heterocycles with 2 Ns 331
		a. 5-Membered 331
		b. 6-Membered (*see also:* VI.A.15) 333
		c. Other 335
		2. Heterocycles with 1 N and 1 O 336
		3. Heterocycles with 1 N and 1 S 340
		4. Heterocycles with 1 S and 1 O 342
		5. Heterocycles with 3 Ns 343
		6. Other Heterocycles 343
	J.	General Reviews 346
V.	**PROTECTING GROUPS** 348	
	A.	Hydroxyl (*see also:* VI.A.10, VI.A.11) 348
	B.	Amine (*see also:* VI.A.4) 351
	C.	Sulfhydryl (*see also:* VI.A.19) 356
	D.	Carboxyl (*see also:* VI.A.4, VI.A.10) 357
	E.	Ketone, Aldehyde (*see also:* VI.A.18) 361
	F.	Phosphate 366
	G.	Pi Bond 367
	H.	Miscellaneous Protecting Groups 367

VI.	USEFUL SYNTHETIC PREPARATIONS	368
	A. Functional Group Preparations	368
	1. Acids, Acid Halides, etc. (*see also:* II.A.2)	368
	2. Alcohols, Phenols (*see also:* II.B.1, III.A., III.F.1)	371
	3. Alkyl, Aryl Halides (*see also:* II.B.2)	373
	4. Amides (*see also:* IV.D, VI.A.17)	376
	5. Amines (*see also:* III.D)	381
	6. Amino Acids and Derivatives (*see also:* VI.A.4, VI.A.10)	385
	7. Carbenes (*see also:* I.D)	389
	8. Enamines	390
	9. Epoxides (*see also:* II.F.1)	392
	10. Esters (*see also:* IV.E, V.D)	393
	11. Ethers (*see also:* V.A)	400
	12. Ketones and Aldehydes (*see also:* I.A.2, II.A.1)	402
	13. Nitriles	412
	14. Nitro	417
	15. Nucleotides, etc. (*see also:* IV.I.1a, b, V.F)	420
	16. Olefins, Acetylenes (*see also:* I.B, I.C, II.J, III.G)	422
	17. Peptides (*see also:* V.B, V.C, V.D, VI.A.4)	428
	18. Vinyl Halides, Vinyl Ethers, Vinyl Esters	433
	19. Sulfur Compounds (*see also:* II.E, III.C)	436
	B. Ring Enlargement and Contraction	445
	1. Enlargement	445
	2. Contraction	449
	C. Multistep Transformations	449
	1. Masked Carbonyl Systems	450
	2. Other Multistep Transformations	451
VII.	MISCELLANEOUS REVIEWS	452
	AUTHOR INDEX	471

PREFACE

One of the most difficult problems facing chemists today is that of "keeping up with the literature." For several reasons, the problem is particularly severe for the synthetic organic chemist. Bits of information of potential use are scattered throughout common chemistry journals and can be found in any paper, not just those dealing strictly with synthesis. Thus, synthetic chemists must read a large number of journals and must organize and index what they read to make the information available for future reference. All synthetic chemists do this; but the task is becoming more difficult each year as the flow of information increases.

The problem, however, is shared to some extent by all. Most organic chemists are at some time faced with the problem of synthesizing a desired material, and for many the problems are formidable. Nonspecialists faced with a synthetic problem are not likely to have kept pace with the developments in synthetic chemistry that may well solve their problems, and they will not have the necessary information in their files.

Thus, we felt that an organized annual review of synthetically useful information would prove beneficial to nearly all organic chemists, both specialist and nonspecialist in synthesis. It should help relieve some of the information-storage burden of the specialist and should enable the nonspecialist who is seeking help with a specific problem to become rapidly aware of recent synthetic advances. Ideally also, it should appear as promptly as possible after the close of the abstracting period. This year we have placed particular emphasis on keeping the abstracts as concise as possible, while indicating the generality of the reactions involved. We have tried to combine similar publications into inclusive abstracts, particularly in Chapter I. This practice has allowed us to include a larger number of references without a substantial increase in the book's length.

In producing *Annual Reports in Organic Synthesis—1982,* we have abstracted 48 primary chemistry journals, selecting useful synthetic advances. We have tried to present the information in an organized manner, emphasizing rapid visual retrieval. Only the common journals received by our libraries have been abstracted. Any journal received after March 1, 1983 will be covered in the next volume. We have also exercised selectivity in choosing which papers to abstract. Our general guidelines have been to include all reactions and methods that are new, synthetically useful, and reasonably general. Each entry is comprised primarily of structures, accompanied by very few comments. The purpose of this emphasis is to aid the reader in scanning the book. The mind is capable of absorbing a whole picture in an instant, but is considerably slowed by having to read sentences. If the pictures presented catch the reader's interest, he or she should then seek details from the original paper.

For the seventh year we have included a principal author index to aid the user. No subject index is included because to do so would greatly increase both the cost of the book and the lead time for publication. Instead, we have chosen to use an extensive table of contents. Chapters I–III are organized by reaction type and constitute a major part of the book. The organization of these sections is self-explanatory; thus, there should be no difficulty in locating a new method of oxidation or a new cyclo-propanation procedure. Chapter IV deals with methods of synthesizing heterocyclic systems and Chapter V covers the use of new protecting groups. Chapter VI is divided into three main parts and covers those synthetically useful transformations that do not fit easily into the first three chapters. The first part deals only with functional group synthesis; the second covers ring expansion and contraction; and the third involves useful multistep sequences, the individual steps of which may be well known. Future volumes of this series will maintain the present table of contents as much as possible. If no entry is found for a particular section, the last volume in which one appears will be cited in the table of contents.

Any undertaking of this type involves a series of compromises. We have chosen to emphasize reasonable cost, rapid publication, and rapid visual retrieval of information at the admitted expense of detail and beauty.

The arduous task of drawing the multitude of structures appearing in this review was carried out by Ms. Audrey Maakestad and Ms. Katy Krupa. We thank them very much for their efforts. We also thank Judi Brezausek, Dr. Jim McKearin, Lydia Milne, Dr. Forrest Sheffy, and Ron Wilde for aid in proofreading the manuscript.

L. G. WADE, JR.
MARTIN J. O'DONNELL

JOURNALS ABSTRACTED

Accounts of Chemical Research
Acta Chemica Scandinavica
Aldrichimica Acta
Angewandte Chemie International Edition in English
Australian Journal of Chemistry
Bulletin of the Chemical Society of Japan
Bulletin de Sociétés Chimiques Belges
Bulletin de la Société Chimique de France
Canadian Journal of Chemistry
Chemical Communications
Chemical and Pharmaceutical Bulletin
Chemical Reviews
Chemical Society Reviews
Chemische Berichte
Chemistry and Industry
Chemistry Letters
Collection of Czechoslovakian Chemical Communications
Comptes Rendus Hebdomadaires de Seances de l'Academie des Sciences (C)
Gazzetta Chimica Italiana
Helvetica Chimica Acta
Indian Journal of Chemistry
Journal of the American Chemical Society
Journal of Chemical Research
Journal of the Chemical Society (Perkin I)
Journal of the Chemical Society (Perkin II)
Journal of General Chemistry (USSR)
Journal of Heterocyclic Chemistry
Journal of Medicinal Chemistry
Journal of Organic Chemistry
Journal of Organic Chemistry (USSR)
Journal of Organometallic Chemistry
Journal für Praktische Chemie
Liebig's Annalen der Chemie
Monatshefte für Chemie
Nouveau Journal de Chimie
Organic Preparations and Procedures International
Organic Syntheses
Organometallics
Pure and Applied Chemistry
Recueil des Travaux Chimiques des Pays-bas
Russian Chemical Reviews
Steroids
Synthesis
Synthetic Communications
Tetrahedron
Tetrahedron Letters
Topics in Current Chemistry
Zeitschrift für Chemie

GLOSSARY OF ABBREVIATIONS

Ac	acetyl
AIBN	azobisisobutyronitrile
Ar	aryl
9-BBN	9-borabicyclo[3.3.1]nonane
BOC (t-Boc)	t-butyloxycarbonyl
Bu	butyl
Bz	benzyl
Cbz	benzyloxycarbonyl
COD	1,5-cyclooctadiene
Cp	cyclopentadienyl
CSA	camphorsulfonic acid
DABCO	1,4-diazabicyclo[2.2.2]octane
DBN	1,5-diazabicyclo[4.3.0]non-3-ene
DBU	1,5-diazabicyclo[5.4.0]undecene-5
DCC	dicyclohexylcarbodiimide
DDQ	2,3-dichloro-5,6-dicyanobenzoquinone
DEAD	diethyl azodicarboxylate
DIBAH (DIBAL)	diisobutylaluminum hydride
DMAD	dimethyl acetylenedicarboxylate
DMAP	4-N,N-dimethylaminopyridine
DME	1,2-dimethoxyethane
DMF	dimethylformamide
DMSO	dimethyl sulfoxide
E+	general electrophile
ee	enantiomeric excess
Et	ethyl
Fp	η^5-$C_5H_5Fe(CO)_2$
Hex	hexyl
HMPA, HMPT	hexamethyl phosphoramide (hexamethylphosphoric triamide)
hν	irradiation with light
KAPA	potassium 3-aminopropylamide
L	triphenylphosphine ligand
LAH	lithium aluminum hydride
LDA	lithium diisopropylamide
LICA	lithium isopropylcyclohexylamide
MCPBA	$meta$-chloroperbenzoic acid
Me	methyl
MEM	β-methoxyethoxymethyl
Ms	methanesulfonyl
MTM	methylthiomethyl
NBS	N-bromosuccinimide
NCS	N-chlorosuccinimide
Ni (R)	Raney Nickel
[O]	general oxidation
Ⓟ	polymeric backbone
PCC	pyridinium chlorochromate
Ph	phenyl
(Phen)	1,10-phenanthroline
Phth	phthaloyl
PPA	polyphosphoric acid
PPE	polyphosphate ester
Pr	propyl
Py, pyr	pyridine
PTC	phase-transfer catalysis
Q+	quaternary ammonium
RT	room temperature
Tf	trifluoromethane sulfonate
TFA	trifluoroacetic acid
TFAA	trifluoroacetic anhydride
THF	tetrahydrofuran
THP	tetrahydropyranyl
TMEDA	tetramethylethylenediamine
TMP	2,2,6,6-tetramethylpiperidine
TMS	trimethylsilyl
Tol	tolyl
Ts, Tos	p-toluenesulfonyl
Z	benzyloxycarbonyl; also used for electron-withdrawing groups such as -CN, -COOR, etc.
Δ	heat
ϕ	phenyl
18-C-6	18-crown-6

I
CARBON–CARBON BOND FORMING REACTIONS

I.A. Carbon-Carbon Single Bonds
(see also: I.E, I.F, I.G).

I.A.1. Alkylations of Aldehydes, Ketones and Their Derivatives

I.A.1-1 S. M. Makin et al., J. Org. Chem. (USSR), 18, 834, 1001 (1982); M. Suzuki, A. Yanagisawa and R. Noyori, Tetrahedron Lett., 23, 3595 (1982); O. Takazawa and T. Mukaiyama, Chem. Lett., 1307 (1982).

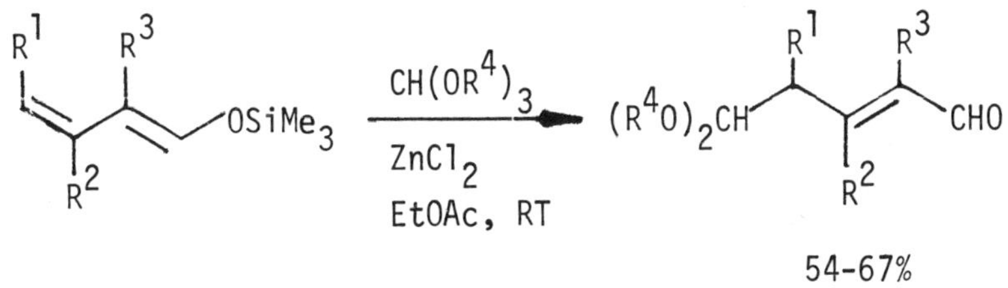

$$R^1R^2C=CR^3-CH=CH-OSiMe_3 \xrightarrow[\text{EtOAc, RT}]{\text{CH(OR}^4)_3, \text{ ZnCl}_2} (R^4O)_2CH-CR^1R^2-CR^3=CH-CHO$$

54-67%

I.A.1-2 A. S. Sarma and A. K. Gayen, Synth. Commun., 12, 151 (1982); J. A. Hirsch and X. L. Wang, ibid, 333; G. Sauer et al., Liebigs Ann. Chem., 459 (1982).

$$\text{substrate} \xrightarrow[\text{70°C}]{\text{KO}^t\text{Bu, }^t\text{BuOH, ClCH}_2\text{CO}_2\text{Et}} \text{product, 50\%}$$

I.A.1-3 D. Seebach et al., Helv. Chim. Acta, 65, 419 (1982).

$$\text{R-C(O}^-\text{)=CH-CH=CH}_2 \cdot \text{Li}^+\text{K}^+ \xrightarrow[\text{2) H}^+]{\text{1) E}^+} \text{R-C(O)-CH}_2\text{-CH=CH-E}$$

23-70%

E^+ = RX, RCO_2R, R_2CO, RCHO, Epoxides.

I.A.1-4 G. A. Russell et al., J. Org. Chem., 47, 1879 (1982).

$$\underset{\text{ArC=CHR}}{\overset{\text{OLi}}{|}} \xrightarrow[\text{THF}]{\text{Me}_2\text{C-Cl, NO}_2} \underset{\underset{\underset{\text{NO}_2}{|}}{\text{Me-C-Me}}}{\overset{\text{O}}{\underset{|}{\text{ArCCHR}}}} \quad \text{or} \quad \underset{\text{R}}{\overset{\text{O}}{\text{ArC-C=CMe}_2}}$$

I.A.1-5 E. Piers and B. Abeysekera, Can. J. Chem., 60, 1114 (1982); D. E. Dana and A. S. Hay, Synthesis, 164 (1982).

$$\text{cyclohexenyl-OLi} \xrightarrow[\text{2) H}_3\text{O}^+\text{; 3) NaH, DME}]{\text{1) BrCH}_2\text{-C(OEt)=CHP(O)(OEt)}_2, \text{THF, -78°C}} \text{bicyclic enone, 74\%}$$

I.A.1-6 D. R. Dimmel and D. Shepard, J. Org. Chem., **47**, 4799 (1982).

[Reaction scheme: 4-hydroxy-3-methoxyphenyl CO-CH₂-O-(2-methoxyphenyl) with 1) 4 LDA, THF, -78°C; 2) 4 MeI; 3) aq. NH₄Cl → corresponding α-methylated product, 50-65%]

I.A.1-7 P. W. Hickmott, Tetrahedron, **38**, 1975, 3363 (1982).

Review: "Enamines: Recent Advances in Synthetic, Spectroscopic, Mechanistic and Stereochemical Aspects." (Parts I and II).

I.A.1-8 A. Hosomi, Y. Araki and H. Sakurai, J. Amer. Chem. Soc., **104**, 2081 (1982); C. R. McArthur, C. C. Leznoff et al., Can. J. Chem., **60**, 1836 (1982); C. B. Kanner and U. K. Pandit, Tetrahedron, **38**, 3597 (1982).

[Reaction scheme: N-cyclohexyl imine of 2-methylcyclohexanone with 1) s-BuLi; 2) RX; 3) H₃O⁺ → 2-R-2-methylcyclohexanone, 53-76%]

(87-90% More Substituted α-Carbon Alkylation)

I.A.1-9   M. T. Reetz, Angew. Chem., Int. Ed. Engl., 21, 96 (1982).

Review: "Lewis Acid Induced α-Alkylation of Carbonyl Compounds."

I.A.1-10 C. Lion and J. E. Dubois, Bull. Soc. Chim Fr. II, 375 (1982); H. A. Khan and I. Paterson, Tetrahedron Lett., 23, 2399 (1982).

$$\text{R-C(=O)-CH(Me)}_2 \xrightarrow[\text{2) }^t\text{BuCl, TiCl}_4]{\text{1) KH, Me}_3\text{SiCl}} \text{R-C(=O)-C(Me)}_2{-}^t\text{Bu}$$

R = Me$_2$CH-, Me$_3$C-, Me$_2{}^t$BuC-

0-72%

I.A.1-11 S. Murata and R. Noyori, Tetrahedron Lett., 23, 2601 (1982); A. Hosomi, S. Iijima and H. Sakurai, ibid, 547.

$$\underset{\text{Me}_3\text{SiO}}{\text{PhC(=CH}_2\text{)}} \xrightarrow[\text{CH}_2\text{Cl}_2,\ -78°\text{C}]{\text{CH}_3\text{CO}_2\text{-(tetrahydrofuran-2-yl)}\ ,\ \text{TMSOTf}} \text{PhC(=O)CH}_2\text{-(tetrahydrofuran-2-yl)}$$

87%

I.A.1-12 T. Umemoto et al., Tetrahedron Lett., 23, 1169, 1471, 4101 (1982); T. Ishihara, T. Seki and T. Ando, Bull. Chem. Soc. Jpn., 55, 3345 (1982); I. Kuwajima, E. Nakamura and M. Shimizu, J. Amer. Chem. Soc., 104, 1025 (1982).

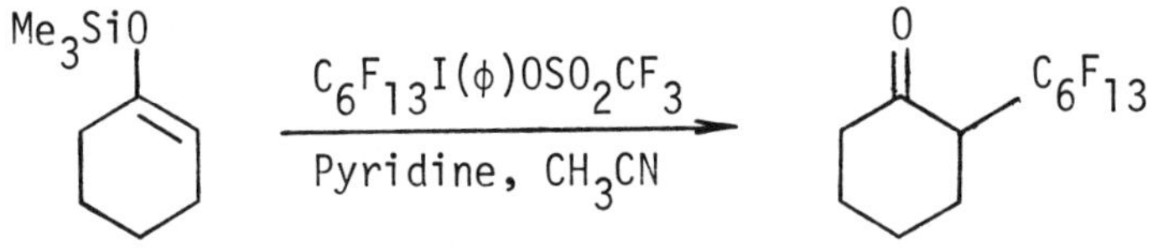

[cyclohexene with Me$_3$SiO] → [C$_6$F$_{13}$I(ϕ)OSO$_2$CF$_3$ / Pyridine, CH$_3$CN] → [cyclohexanone with C$_6$F$_{13}$]

71%

I.A.1-13 E. Negishi et al., J. Org. Chem., 47, 3188 (1982).

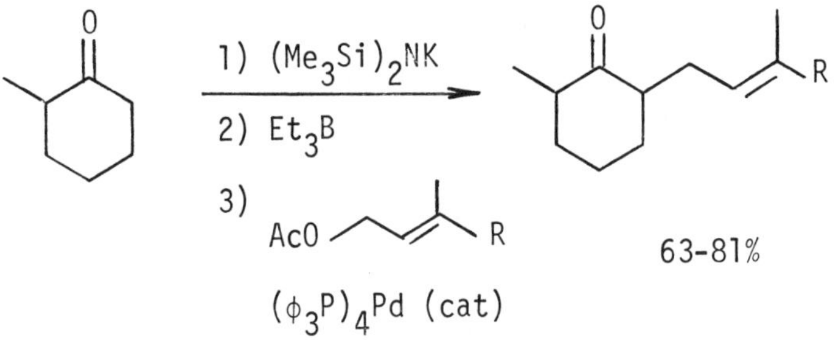

[2-methylcyclohexanone] → 1) (Me$_3$Si)$_2$NK 2) Et$_3$B 3) AcO–CH=C(CH$_3$)–R, (ϕ_3P)$_4$Pd (cat) → [alkylated product]

63-81%

I.A.1-14 P. J. Stang, M. Hanack and L. R. Subramanian, Synthesis, 85 (1982).

Review: "Perfluoroalkanesulfonic Esters: Methods of Preparation and Applications in Organic Chemistry."

I.A.2. Alkylations of Nitriles, Acids and Acid Derivatives

I.A.2-1 K. Takahashi et al., Chem. Lett., 1263 (1982); J. Chauffaille, E. Hebert and Z. Welvart, J. Chem. Soc., Perkin II, 1645 (1982); T. Wakamatsu et al., Heterocycles, 19, 481, 1395 (1982); J. Tsuji et al., Tetrahedron Lett., 23, 4361 (1982).

$$\underset{R^2}{\overset{R^1}{>}}C=CH-CH\underset{CN}{\overset{N\underset{}{\frown}O}{<}} \quad \xrightarrow[\substack{2) R^3X \\ 3) H_2O}]{1) LDA, THF} \quad \underset{R^2}{\overset{R^1}{>}}C=CH-\underset{\underset{CN}{|}}{\overset{R^3}{\underset{|}{C}}}-N\underset{}{\frown}O$$

30-100%

Products readily hydrolyzed to α,β-unsaturated ketones.

I.A.2-2 H. P. Husson et al., Tetrahedron Lett., 23, 3369 (1982); R. M. Coates, S. K. Shah and R. W. Mason, J. Amer. Chem. Soc., 104, 2198 (1982).

[piperidine with NC and Me substituents, N-CH$_2$-φ] $\xrightarrow[\substack{2) RX \\ 3) Na, NH_3}]{1) LDA}$ [piperidine with R and Me substituents, N-CH$_2$-φ] 60%

NaBH$_4$, CH$_3$OH Reductive Decyanation gives trans.

I.A.2-3 H. Stamm et al., Tetrahedron Lett., 23, 5021 (1982).

$$\text{Me}\underset{\text{Me}}{\overset{}{\triangle}}\text{N-G} \xrightarrow[\text{(G = Tosyl)}]{\phi_2\bar{C}\text{-CN}} \phi_2\underset{\text{CN}}{\overset{}{C}}\underset{\text{Me Me}}{\overset{}{\diagup\!\!\diagdown}}\text{NHTos} \quad \begin{array}{c} 70\% \\ (SN2) \end{array}$$

$$\xrightarrow[\text{(G = CO}_2\text{Et)}]{\phi_2\bar{C}\text{-CN}} \phi_2\underset{\text{CN}}{\overset{}{C}}\underset{}{\overset{\text{Me Me}}{\diagup\!\!\diagdown}}\text{NHCO}_2\text{Et} \quad \begin{array}{c} 40\% \\ (SET) \end{array}$$

I.A.2-4 N. Petragnani and M. Yonashiro, Synthesis, 521 (1982).

Review: "The Reactions of Dianions of Carboxylic Acids and Ester Enolates."

I.A.2-5 C. R. Johnson and T. R. Bade, Synthesis, 284 (1982); K. Tanaka, M. Terauchi and A. Kaji, Chem. Lett., 351 (1982).

$$\underset{Cl}{\overset{CH_3}{\diagdown}}CH\text{-}CO_2H \xrightarrow[\substack{-80°C \\ 2) \text{ RX}}]{1) \text{ 2 LDA, THF}} \underset{Cl}{\overset{CH_3}{\underset{|}{\overset{|}{R\text{-}C\text{-}CO_2H}}}} \quad 66\text{-}85\%$$

Other Electrophiles: RCOCl (Decarboxylates), Michael Acceptors (Cyclopropane Product).

I.A.2-6 C. R. Noe, Chem. Ber., 115, 1607 (1982).

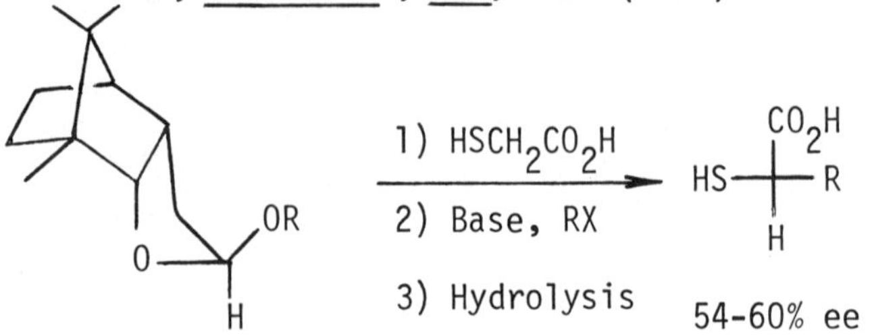

1) $HSCH_2CO_2H$
2) Base, RX
3) Hydrolysis

54-60% ee

I.A.2-7 D. Seebach et al., Chem. Ber., 115, 1705 (1982); Helv. Chem. Acta, 65, 385 (1982); M. Pohmakotr et al., Chem. Lett., 687 (1982); L. A. Paquette, G. D. Annis and H. Schostarez, J. Amer. Chem. Soc., 104, 6646 (1982).

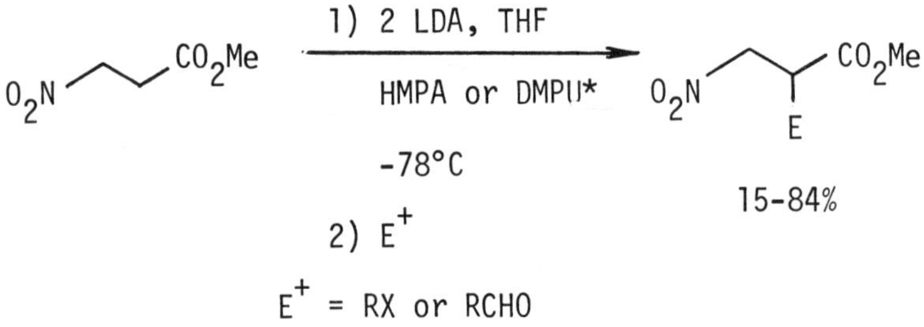

1) 2 LDA, THF
   HMPA or DMPU*
   -78°C
2) E^+

E^+ = RX or RCHO

15-84%

*DMPU = 3,4,5,6-Tetrahydro-1,3-Dimethyl-2(1H)Pyrimidinone (HMPA Substitute)

I.A.2-8 T. Severin and H. Lerche, Synthesis, 305 (1982).

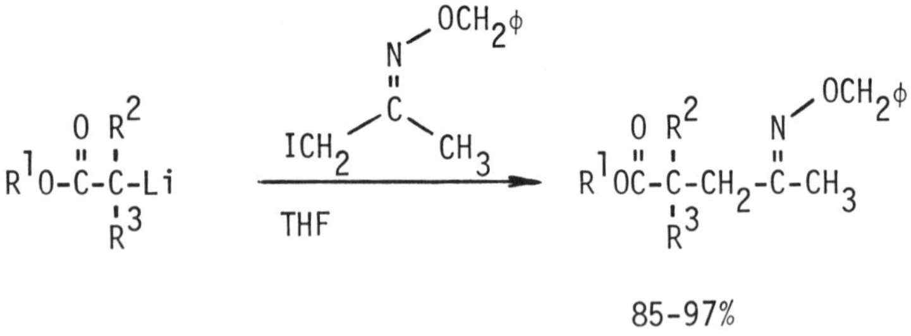

ICH_2, THF

85-97%

I.A.2-9 W. Ladner, Angew. Chem., Int. Ed. Engl., 21, 449 (1982).

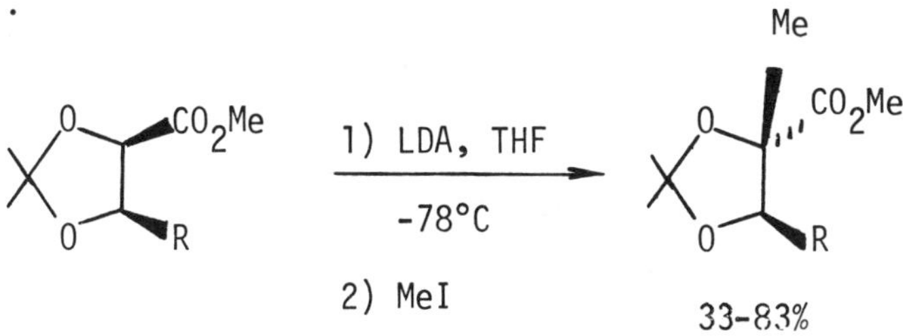

33-83%
(88- > 95% Diasteriosel.)

I.A.2-10 A. R. Chamberlin and M. Dezube, Tetrahedron Lett., 23, 3055 (1982); D. W. Brooks and R. P. Kellogg, ibid, 4991; A. Kramer and H. Pfander, Helv. Chim. Acta, 293 (1982); D. Wasmuth, D. Arigoni and D. Seebach, ibid, 344.

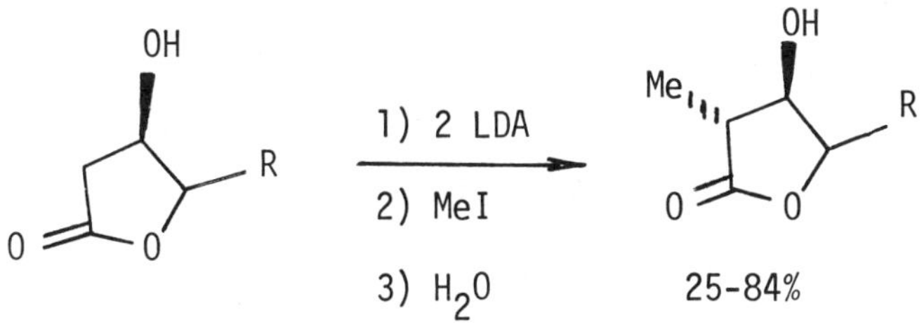

25-84%

I.A.2-11 P. D. Noire and R. W. Franck, Tetrahedron Lett., 23, 1031 (1982); C. Girard and R. Bloch, ibid, 3683; P. J. Garratt et al., J. Org. Chem., 47, 4731 (1982).

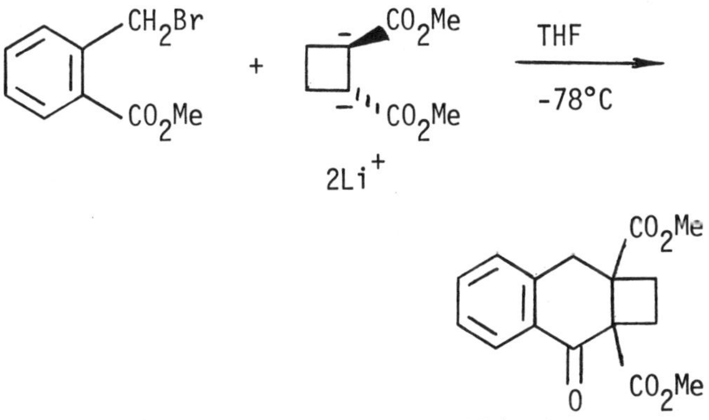

65%

I.A.2-12 A. S. Kende and B. H. Toder, J. Org. Chem., 47, 163 (1982); I. Hoppe and U. Schollkopf, Synthesis, 129 (1982); A. Pelter and R. Al-Bayati, Tetrahedron Lett., 23, 5229 (1982).

$$\text{(E)-alkene-CO}_2\text{Et} \xrightarrow[\text{THF, -78°C} \quad 2)\ E^+ \text{(RX or RCHO)}]{1)\ \text{LDA/HMPA}} \text{E-CH(CO}_2\text{Et)-CH=CH-CH}_3$$

$$\text{(Z)-alkene-CO}_2\text{Et} \xrightarrow{\text{Same Conditions}} \text{E-CH(CO}_2\text{Et)-CH=CH-CH}_3\ (Z)$$

Deconjugative Alkylation

I.A.2-13 S. Tanimoto et al., Synthesis, 723 (1982).

$$2\ \underset{R^2}{\overset{R^1}{>}}C=C\underset{OSiMe_3}{\overset{OR^3}{<}} \xrightarrow[\text{ZnCl}_2]{\text{Cl}_2\text{CH-OMe}} \begin{array}{c} R^1 \\ R^2-\overset{|}{\underset{|}{C}}-CO_2R^3 \\ CH-OMe \\ R^2-\overset{|}{\underset{|}{C}}-CO_2R^3 \\ R^1 \end{array}$$

78-98%

I.A.2-14 K. K. Mahalanabis, M. Mumtaz and V. Snieckus, Tetrahedron Lett., 23, 3971, 3975 (1982); P. J. Garratt and F. Hollowood, J. Org. Chem., 47, 68 (1982).

$$R_2\overset{O}{\overset{\|}{N}CCH_2CH_2\overset{O}{\overset{\|}{C}}NR_2} \xrightarrow[\substack{-78°C \\ 2)\ E_1^+ \\ 3)\ E_2^+}]{1)\ 2\ \text{LDA, THF}} R_2N-C(=O)-CH(E_1)-CH(E_2)-C(=O)-NR_2$$

30-91%

E^+ = RX, RCO$_2$Et, D$_2$O

I.A.2-15   D. A. Evans, Aldrichimica Acta, 15, 23 (1982).

Review: "Studies in Asymmetric Synthesis. The Development of Practical Chiral Enolate Synthons."

I.A.2-16   D. A. Evans, J. Amer. Chem. Soc., 104, 1737 (1982); Tetrahedron Lett., 23, 807 (1982).

[Oxazolidinone with N-acyl group containing R^1, isopropyl substituent]
1) LDA, THF, -78°C
2) ϕCH_2Br
3) R^2OLi, 0°C
→ R^2O_2C–CHR^1–$CH_2\phi$

Several transformations that nondestructively remove the chiral auxilaries from the desired chiral synthons.

I.A.3.   Alkylation of β-Dicarbonyl, β-Cyanocarbonyl Systems and Other Active Methylene Compounds

I.A.3-1   C. Reichardt and K. Y. Yun, Angew. Chem., Int. Ed. Engl., 21, 65 (1982); R. Ray and D. S. Matteson, J. Org. Chem., 47, 2479 (1982).

$NaCH(CHO)_2$
1) tropylium BF_4^-
2) NaOH
3) 150°C
4) HCl
5) ϕ_3C^+ $SbCl_6^-$
6) R_2N-CH_2-(P)

→ [cycloheptatriene with =C(CHO)₂ substituent]   38%

I.A.3-2 B. Costisella and H. Gross, Tetrahedron, 38, 139 (1982).

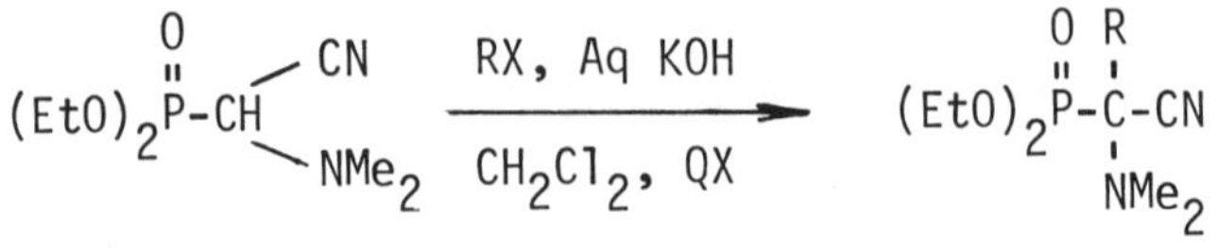

$$(EtO)_2\overset{O}{\overset{\|}{P}}-CH\overset{CN}{\underset{NMe_2}{\diagdown}} \xrightarrow[CH_2Cl_2, QX]{RX, Aq\ KOH} (EtO)_2\overset{O}{\overset{\|}{P}}-\overset{R}{\underset{NMe_2}{\overset{|}{C}}}-CN$$

8-37%

I.A.3-3 A. P. Krapcho, Synthesis, 805, 893 (1982).

Review: "Synthetic Applications of Dealkoxycarbonylations of Malonate Esters, β-Keto Esters, α-Cyano Esters and Related Compounds in Dipolar Aprotic Media."

I.A.3-4 S. E. Drewes and N. D. Emslie, J. Chem. Soc., Perkin I, 2079 (1982); K. Shankaran, D. G. Talekar and A. S. Rao, Ind. J. Chem., 21B, 408 (1982); Z. Welvart et al., J. Chem. Res. (S), 86 (1982).

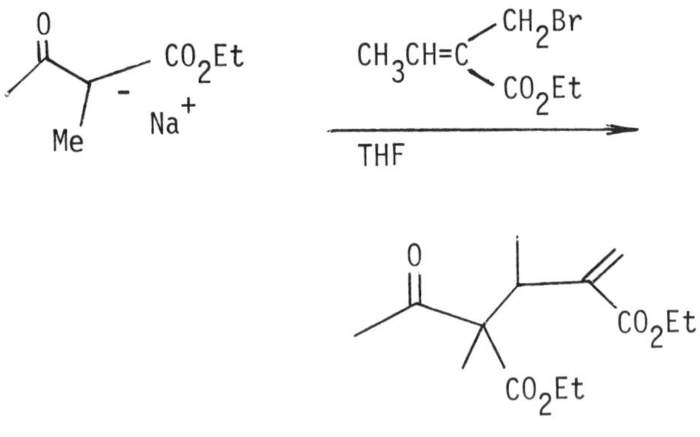

73%

(27% SN2 Product)

I.A.3-5 P. Lemmen, *Chem. Ber.*, **115**, 1902 (1982); H. Schick et al., *Tetrahedron*, **38**, 1279 (1982).

[Indanone with Me and CO_2Et substituents] $\xrightarrow[\phi CH_2Br]{NaOR, ROH}$ [Indanone with Me, CO_2Et, and $CH_2\phi$]

81%

I.A.3-6 P. G. Baraldi et al., *Chem. Commun.*, 1265 (1982); R. Tanikaga et al., *Synthesis*, 131 (1982); N. R. Ayyangar, R. J. Lahoti and T. Daniel, *Org. Prep. Proc. Int.*, **14**, 327 (1982).

[Thiolane with =O and CO_2Me] $\xrightarrow[\text{Acetone}]{\begin{array}{c}1) \text{ RX, } K_2CO_3\\ 2) \text{ 5% NaOH}\end{array}}$ [acrylate with CO_2Me and R]

25-77%

I.A.3-7 J. E. Hill and T. M. Harris, *Synth. Commun.*, **12**, 621 (1982).

[1,3-diketone dianion, $2 Li^+$] $\xrightarrow[\begin{array}{c}\text{IDA, THF}\\ 0°C\\ 2) \text{ Reflux}\\ 3) H_3O^+\end{array}]{1) LiCH(CO_2Me)_2}$ [R-CO-CH$_2$-CO-CH$_2$-CO-CH$_2$-CO_2Me]

60-66%

I.A.3-8 I. Rico, D. Cantacuzene and C. Wakselman, J. Chem. Soc., Perkin I, 1063 (1982).

$$\text{Et-CH(CO}_2\text{Et)}_2 \xrightarrow[\text{2) CF}_2\text{Br}_2,\ 0°\text{C}]{\text{1) NaH, THF}} \begin{array}{c} \text{CO}_2\text{Et} \\ | \\ \text{Et-C-CO}_2\text{Et} \\ | \\ \text{CF}_2\text{Br} \end{array}$$

45%

I.A.3-9 C. C. Chan and X. Huang, Synthesis, 452 (1982); D. G. Desai and R. B. Mane, Chem. Ind., 809 (1982); R. T. Jacobs, A. D. Wright and F. X. Smith, J. Org. Chem., 47, 3769 (1982); G. O. Torosyan, G. G. Gekchyan and A. T. Babayan, J. Org. Chem. (USSR), 18, 1423 (1982).

[Reaction scheme: R^1-substituted Meldrum's acid derivative reacts with R^2X, QX, K_2CO_3, $CHCl_3$, 50-60°C to give the R^1,R^2-disubstituted product in 81-97% yield.]

I.A.3-10 J. Tsuji, Pure Appl. Chem., 54, 197 (1982).

Review: "Catalytic Reactions via π-Allylpalladium Complexes."

I.A.3-11 B. Bosnich and P. B. Mackenzie, Pure Appl. Chem., 54, 189 (1982).

Review: "Asymmetric Catalytic Allylic Alkylation."

I.A.3-12 B. Akermark, J. E. Backvall and K. Zetterberg, Acta Chem. Scand., 36B, 577 (1982).

"Nucleophilic Addition to π-Olefin-, π-Allyl- and σ-Allyl-Palladium Complexes. Examples of "Umpolung" by the Use of Organometallic Reagents."

I.A.3-13 R. Lidor and S. Shatzmiller, Liebigs Ann. Chem., 226 (1982); P. A. Magriotis, W. V. Murray and F. Johnson, Tetrahedron Lett., 23, 1993 (1982).

$$\text{NaCH(CO}_2\text{R)}_2 \xrightarrow[\substack{\phi\text{H, 60°C} \\ 2)\ \text{H}_3\text{O}^+}]{1)\ \text{Cl-CH(CH}_3\text{)-CH=N}^+\text{(R)(O}^-\text{)}} (\text{EtO}_2\text{C})_2\text{CH-CH(CH}_3\text{)-CHO} \quad 40\%$$

I.A.3-14 M. Yamauchi, S. Katayama and T. Watanabe, Synthesis, 935 (1982).

$$R^1\text{-CO-CH}_2\text{-CO-}R^2 \xrightarrow[\text{Dioxane, }\Delta]{\text{piperidine-CH}_2\text{-S-Me}\cdot\text{HCl}} R^1\text{-CO-CH(CH}_2\text{-S-Me)-CO-}R^2 \quad 74\text{-}95\%$$

I.A.3-15 R. Tamura and L. S. Hegedus, J. Amer. Chem. Soc., 104, 3727 (1982); N. Ono, I. Hamamoto and A. Kaji, Chem. Commun., 821 (1982).

cyclopentenyl-CH$_2$-NO$_2$ $\xrightarrow[\substack{1\%\ (\phi_3\text{P})_4\text{Pd} \\ \text{DMF, 70°C}}]{\text{NaCH(CO}_2\text{Me)}_2}$ cyclopentenyl-CH(CO$_2$Me)$_2$ 70%

I.A.3-16 P. A. Wade, S. D. Morrow and S. A. Hardinger, J. Org. Chem., **47**, 365 (1982).

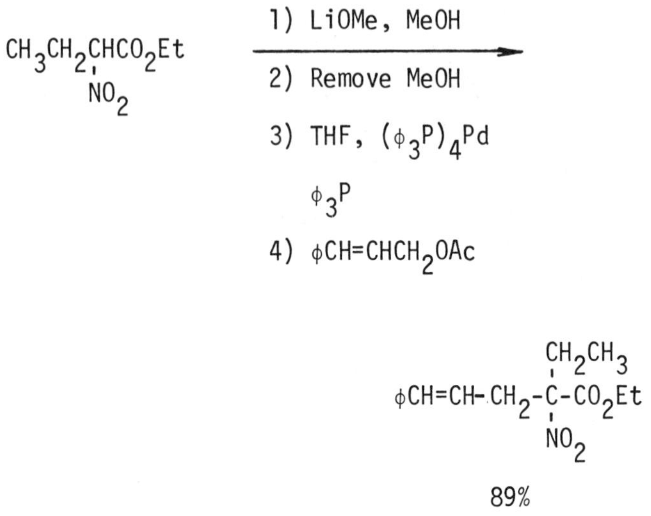

$$CH_3CH_2\underset{NO_2}{CH}CO_2Et \xrightarrow{\begin{array}{l}1)\ LiOMe,\ MeOH\\ 2)\ Remove\ MeOH\\ 3)\ THF,\ (\phi_3P)_4Pd\\ \quad \phi_3P\\ 4)\ \phi CH=CHCH_2OAc\end{array}}$$

$$\phi CH=CH-CH_2-\underset{NO_2}{\overset{CH_2CH_3}{\underset{|}{\overset{|}{C}}}}-CO_2Et$$

89%

I.A.3-17 T. Hirao et al., J. Organometal. Chem., **236**, 409 (1982); J. Tsuji et al., Tetrahedron Lett., **23**, 4809 (1982); M. Kumada et al., Chem. Commun., 1162 (1982); B. M. Trost and M. Lautens, J. Amer. Chem. Soc., **104**, 5543 (1982).

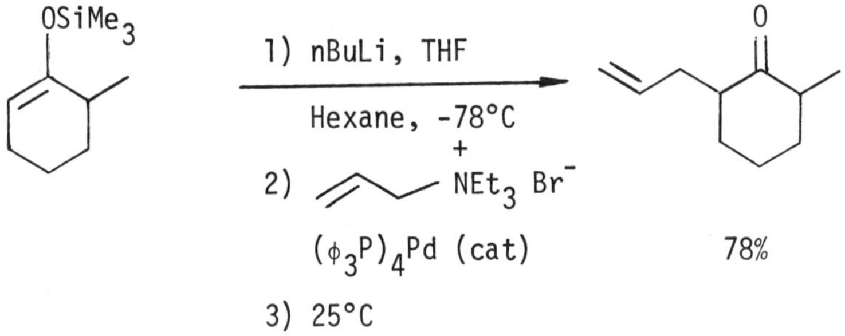

1) nBuLi, THF, Hexane, -78°C
2) $\diagup\!\!\!\diagdown\!\!\!\diagup$ NEt$_3$ Br$^-$
   $(\phi_3P)_4Pd$ (cat)
3) 25°C

78%

I.A.3-18 S. A. Godleski et al., J. Org. Chem., **47**, 4717 (1982); Y. Tanigawa, S. I. Murahashi et al., Tetrahedron Lett., **23**, 5549 (1982); J. P. Genet, M. Balabane and Y. Legras, ibid, 331.

$$\text{tBuCO(O)}\text{-cyclopentene-}\text{OCMe(O)} \xrightarrow[\text{NaCH(CO}_2\text{Me)}_2]{\text{cat }(\phi_3\text{P})_4\text{Pd}} \text{tBuCO(O)}\text{-cyclopentene-}\text{CH(CO}_2\text{Et)}_2$$

Trans substrate undergoes replacement of pivalate.

I.A.3-19 K. Yamamoto and J. Tsuji, Tetrahedron Lett., **23**, 3089 (1982); S. A. Godleski and R. S. Valpey, J. Org. Chem., **47**, 381 (1982); B. M. Trost and R. W. Warner, J. Amer. Chem. Soc., **104**, 6112 (1982).

$$\text{ketoester with }-\text{CH=CH-CH}_2\text{-O}\phi \xrightarrow[\substack{10\% \text{ Diphosphine} \\ \phi\text{H, Reflux}}]{5\% \text{ Pd(OAc)}_2} \text{2-vinylcyclohexanone with CO}_2\text{Me}$$

50-79%

(up to 48% ee)

I.A.3-20 A. J. Pearson, Chem. Ind., 741 (1982).

Review: "Organoiron Complexes as Intermediates for Natural Products Synthesis."

I.A.3-21 A. J. Pearson, et al., J. Org. Chem., 47, 3780 (1982); Chem. Commun., 807 (1982); J. Chem. Soc., Perkin I, 489, 1527, 2631, 2641 (1982); J. Organometal. Chem., 226, C39 (1982); L. F. Kelly, J. Org. Chem., 47, 3965 (1982).

$$\text{[cyclohexadienyl-Fe(CO)}_3\text{ cation with OMe, Me, CH}_2\text{CH}_2\text{OAc substituents]} \xrightarrow[\text{2) (NH}_4)_2\text{Ce(NO}_3)_6]{\text{1) NaCH(CO}_2\text{Me})_2}$$

[cyclohexenone product with Me, CH$_2$CH$_2$OAc, CH(CO$_2$Me)$_2$ substituents]

48%

I.A.3-22 M. Keil and F. Effenberger, Chem. Ber., 115, 1103, 1113 (1982); L. A. Paquette and R. G. Daniels, Organometallics, 1, 757 (1982); M. Franck-Neumann, D. Martina and M. P. Heitz, Tetrahedron Lett., 23, 3493 (1982); D. Martina and F. Brion, ibid, 857, 861, 865.

$$\text{[Me}_3\text{Si-cyclohexadiene-Fe(CO)}_3\text{]} \xrightarrow[\begin{array}{l}\text{2) Nu}^-\\\text{3) (NH}_4)_2\text{Ce(NO}_3)_6\text{, MeOH}\\\text{4) Me}_3\text{NO, }\phi\text{H}\end{array}]{\text{1) }\phi_3\text{C}^+\text{ BF}_4^-}$$

[Structure: cyclohexadiene with SiMe₃ and Nu substituents]

48-83%

Nu⁻ = BuLi, NaCH(CO₂Me)₂, NaCN, Enamines, Meldrum's Acid, φNMe₂.

I.A.3-23 L. Ghosez, M. J. O'Donnell et al., *Tetrahedron Lett.*, 23, 4255, 4259 (1982); P. Duhamel, J. Y. Valnot and J. J. Eddine, *ibid*, 2863; A. Mostamandi et al., *J. Org. Chem. (USSR)*, 18, 850 (1982); T. Yamashita et al., *Bull. Chem. Soc. Jpn.*, 55, 961 (1982).

$$R^1-\underset{\underset{CHAr}{N}}{CH}-CO_2Et \quad \xrightarrow[\text{cat QX}]{\substack{1)\ R^2X \\ KOH,\ CH_2Cl_2 \\ 2)\ \text{Hydrolysis}}} \quad R^1-\underset{NH_2}{\overset{R^2}{C}}-CO_2H$$

26-58%

Also, mono-alkylation of protected glycines by PTC.

I.A.3-24 U. Schollkopf et al., *Liebigs Ann. Chem.*, 1756, 1952 (1982); *Synthesis*, 861, 864, 866, 868 (1982).

[Structure: bis-lactim ether with φ, OMe, R¹ substituents] → [Structure: alkylated bis-lactim with R², φ, R¹ substituents]

1) Base
2) R²X

85-95%
Diast. Excess = 50->95%

I.A.3-25 K. I. Nunami, M. Suzuki and N. Yaneda, Chem. Pharm. Bull., 30, 4015 (1982).

1) MeI, NaH, THF
2) HCl, MeOH
3) NaOH

71%

I.A.4. Alkylation of N-, S- and Se- Stabilized Carbanions

I.A.4-1 H. Kurosawa, M. Sato and H. Okada, Tetrahedron Lett., 23, 2965 (1982); A. M. El-Khawaga, M. T. Ismail and A.M.A. Abdel-Wahab, Gazz. Chim. Ital., 112, 235 (1982).

$$R^1_2CNO_2^- \; Li^+ \xrightarrow[\text{MeOH or DMSO}]{R^2Tl(OAc)_2} R^1-\underset{R^2}{\overset{R^1}{\underset{|}{C}}}-NO_2$$

25°C   58-99%

R = Alkyl, Aryl, Vinyl.

I.A.4-2 P. Aleksandrowicz, H. Piotrowska and W. Sas, Monat. Chem., 113, 1221 (1982); Tetrahedron, 38, 1321 (1982).

$$R^1\text{—CH=C}(R^2)\text{—CH}(R^3)\text{—X} \xrightarrow[\text{MeOH}]{\underset{\text{Pd}(P\phi_3)_4 \text{ (cat)}}{=NO_2^- \; Na^+}} R^1\text{—CH=C}(R^2)\text{—C}(R^3)\text{—NO}_2$$

15-50%

I.A.4-3 G. A. Russell and F. Ros, J. Amer. Chem. Soc., 104, 7349 (1982).

$$\underset{\underset{Me}{|}}{\overset{\overset{O}{\|}}{Ar-C}}-\overset{Me}{\underset{|}{C}}-Cl \quad \xrightarrow[\substack{18-C-6,\ hv \\ Me_2SO \\ (Ar = 4NO_2C_6H_4-)}]{Me_2C=NO_2^- \ K^+} \quad \underset{\underset{Me}{|}}{\overset{\overset{O}{\|}}{Ar-C}}-\overset{Me}{\underset{|}{C}}-\overset{Me}{\underset{|}{C}}-NO_2 \qquad 77\%$$

Other Products: Oxiranes and α-Hydroxy Ketones.

I.A.4-**4** P. Beak and P. D. Becker, J. Org. Chem., 47, 3855 (1982); T. E. Goodwin et al., ibid, 815; M. Kodama, S. Ito et al., Tetrahedron Lett., 23, 3397 (1982).

[2,6-R-substituted aryl]—C(=O)—S—CHMe$_2$ $\xrightarrow[-98°C]{1)\ s\text{-BuLi, TMEDA}}$

2) E$^+$

[2,6-R-substituted aryl]—C(=O)—S—CMe$_2$—E

25-74%

E$^+$ = RX, RCHO, R$_2$CO, ArCO$_2$Me, EtOCOCl, CO$_2$, MeSiCl$_3$.

I.A.4-5 R. R. Regis and A. M. Doweyko, Tetrahedron Lett., 23, 2539 (1982); J. Otera et al., ibid, 4721; R. Block and J. Abecassis, ibid, 3277; C. G. M. Janssen and E. F. Godefroi, J. Org. Chem., 47, 3274 (1982).

$$Ar^1-CH_2-SO_2Ar^2 \xrightarrow[\text{NaOH, DMF}]{RX} Ar^1-\underset{R}{CH}-SO_2Ar^2$$

59-100%

Monohalogenation with CCl_4

I.A.4-6 L. A. Paquette and W. A. Kinney, Tetrahedron Lett., 23, 131 (1982); T. Cuvigny, C. Herve Du Penhoat and M. Julia, Bull. Soc. Chim. Fr. II, 43 (1982).

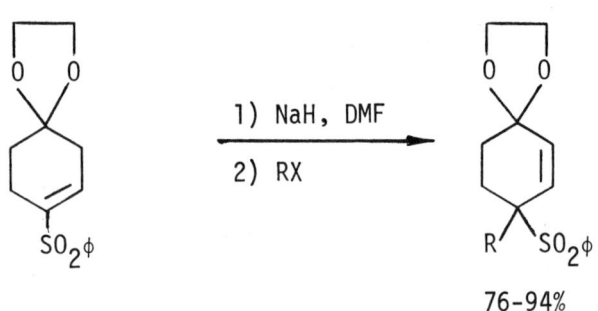

76-94%

I.A.4-7 K. Ogura et al., Chem. Lett., 813 (1982).

$$CH_2\underset{SO_2Me}{\overset{SMe}{\diagup}} \xrightarrow[\substack{50\% \text{ NaOH, } \phi CH_3 \\ QX, 60°C \\ 2) H_3O^+, MeOH, \Delta}]{1) Br(CH_2)_nBr} (CH_2)_n\diagup C=O$$

63-67%

(n = 3-5)

I.A.4-8 C. Lion, Compt. Rend. II, 294, 431 (1982); S.
Tanimoto et al., Bull. Chem. Soc. Jpn., 55, 339 (1982); N. H.
Andersen, A. D. Denniston and D. A. McCrae, J. Org. Chem., 47,
1145 (1982); M. Lissel, Liebigs Ann. Chem., 1589 (1982).

Ar—[S⟩ →(1) LDA, 2) RX)→ Ar,R—[S⟩

24-62%

2-Alkyl-1,3-Dithiolanes give Dithiocarbonic Ester Plus
Ethylene.

I.A.4-9 T. Cohen, R. H. Ritter and D. Ouellette, J. Amer.
Chem. Soc., 104, 7142 (1982).

HO~~~~SΦ (with SΦ below) →(1) 2 s-BuLi, THF, TMEDA, -78°C; 2) Aq NH₄Cl)→ cyclopentane with SΦ and OH

36%

I.A.5. Alkylations of Organometallic Reagents

(see also: I.F, I.G.).

I.A.5-1 M. Takamatsu, Y. Teras and M. Sekiya, Chem. Pharm.
Bull., 30, 2682 (1982); R. Menicagli et al., Tetrahedron
Lett., 23, 1937 (1982); C. G. Screttas and M. Micha-Screttas,
J. Org. Chem., 47, 3008 (1982).

Cl_3CCH_2N(morpholine) →(EtMgBr (3 eq.), Et_2O, 30°C)→ $CH_3CH=CHCH_2N$(morpholine)

42%

I.A.5-2 R. Goswami and D. E. Corcoran, Tetrahedron Lett., 23, 1463 (1982).

$$\phi NH-C(=O)-CH_2-CH_2-SnBu_3 \xrightarrow[\text{THF, } -78°C]{\substack{1) \; 2 \; n\text{-BuLi} \\ \text{DABCO}} \\ 2) \; E^+ \\ 3) \; H_2O} \phi NH-C(=O)-CH_2-CH_2-E \quad 66\text{-}90\%$$

E^+ = RX, R_2CO, MeOD, Me_3SiCl

I.A.5-3 E. Wenkert and T. W. Ferreira, Organometallics, 1, 1670 (1982).

$$\phi\text{-CH=CH-CH(OMe)-OMe} \xrightarrow[\text{cat. } (\phi_3P)NiCl_2]{\substack{1) \; \text{MeMgBr} \\ 2) \; \phi\text{MgBr}}} \phi\text{-CH=CH-CH(Me)-}\phi \quad 53\%$$

I.A.5-4 G. Schrumpf et al., J. Chem. Res. (S), 162 (1982); K. Itoh et al., Tetrahedron Lett., 23, 1267 (1982).

$$\text{RMgBr} \xrightarrow[\substack{\text{Et}_2O, \; 20°C \\ 2) \; H_2SO_4}]{1) \; 3.3 \; \text{epoxide}} RCH_2CH_2OH \quad 75\%$$

Maximized homologation

I.A.5-5 P. Knochel and D. Seebach, Tetrahedron Lett., 23, 3897 (1982).

(nitrocyclohexene with CH$_2$OC(O)– group) + RLi → (nitrocyclohexene with R group) 63-92%

I.A.5-6 W. F. Bailey and R. P. Gagnier, <u>Tetrahedron Lett.</u>, <u>23</u>, 5123 (1982); M. Tashiro and T. Yamato, <u>Chem. Lett.</u>, 61 (1982).

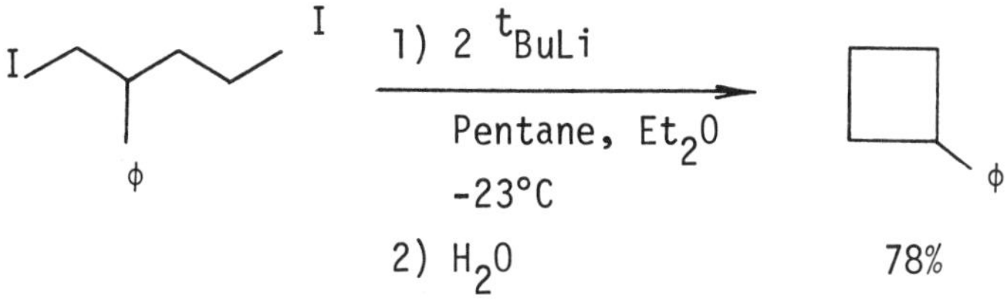
I
I
ϕ
1) 2 ^{t}BuLi
Pentane, Et_2O
-23°C
2) H_2O
ϕ
78%

I.A.5-7 T. Mukaiyama et al., <u>Chem. Lett.</u>, 1637 (1982); D. Hoppe and A. Bronneke, <u>Synthesis</u>, 1045 (1982).

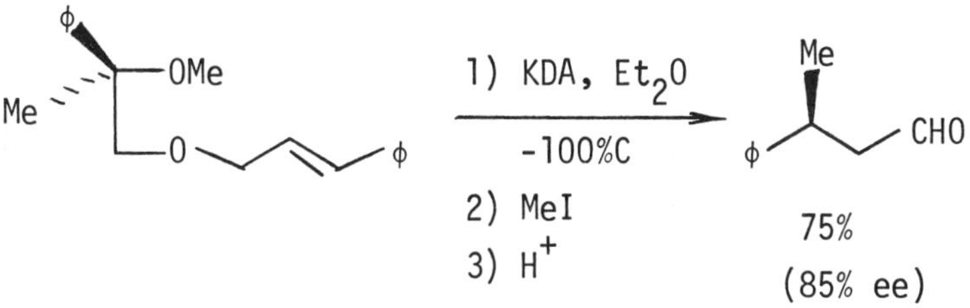
ϕ
OMe
Me
O
ϕ
1) KDA, Et_2O
-100%C
2) MeI
3) H^+
Me
CHO
ϕ
75%
(85% ee)

I.A.5-8 D. J. Kempf, K. D. Wilson and P. Beak, <u>J. Org. Chem.</u>, <u>47</u>, 1610 (1982).

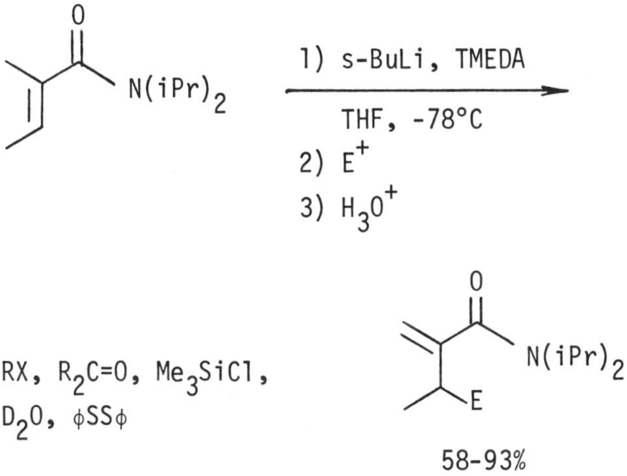
O
$N(iPr)_2$
1) s-BuLi, TMEDA
THF, -78°C
2) E^+
3) H_3O^+
O
$N(iPr)_2$
E
58-93%

E^+ = RX, $R_2C{=}O$, Me_3SiCl, D_2O, ϕSSϕ

I.A.5-9 D. A. Evans and C. H. Mitch, Tetrahedron Lett., 23, 285 (1982).

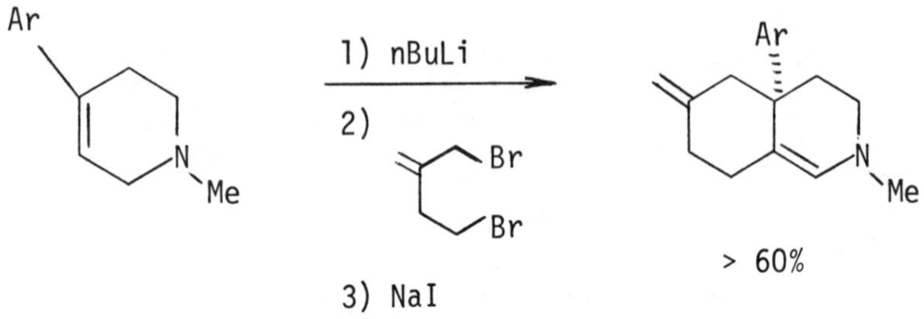
Ar
N
Me
1) nBuLi
2)
Br
Br
3) NaI
Ar
N
Me
> 60%

I.A.5-10 A. Mourino, W. H. Okamura et al., J. Org. Chem., 47, 1576 (1982).

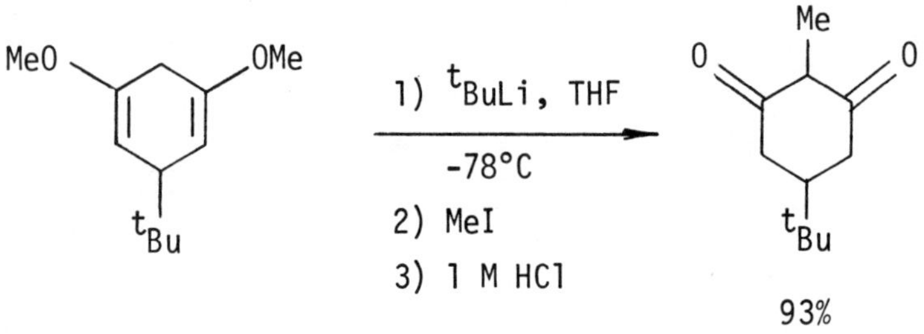
MeO
OMe
tBu
1) tBuLi, THF
-78°C
2) MeI
3) 1 M HCl
Me
O
O
tBu
93%

I.A.5-11 P. Schiess, S. Rutschmann and V. V. Toan, Tetrahedron Lett., 23, 3665, 3669 (1982); K. Ogura et al., Chem. Lett., 1697 (1982).

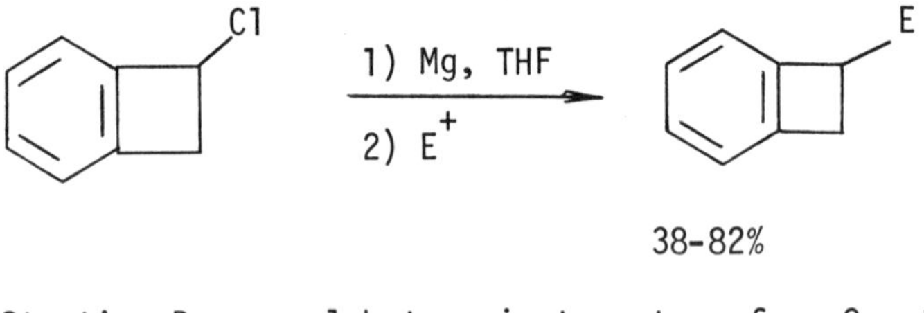
Cl
1) Mg, THF
2) E+
E
38-82%

Starting Benzocyclobutene in two steps from 2-methyl benzaldehydes.

I.A.5-12 H. Kropf and F. Angi, J. Chem. Res (S), 136 (1982); K. Schlogl and W. Weissensteiner, Synthesis, 50 (1982).

$$\phi_2C=N-NH_2 \xrightarrow[\substack{\text{2) } \Delta,\text{ THF} \\ \text{3) } E^+,\ -40°C \\ \text{4) } NH_4Cl}]{\text{1) } 2\ KNH_2,\ NH_3} \phi_2CH-E$$

15-67%

E^+ = RX, ϕCHO, RCOCl.

I.A.5-13 R. B. Bates and C. A. Ogle, J. Org. Chem., 47, 3949 (1982); D. Wilhelm, T. Clark and P. v. R. Schleyer, Tetrahedron Lett., 23, 4077 (1982).

p-xylene $\xrightarrow[\substack{\text{2) } Me_2SO_4 \\ \text{3) } nBuLi,\ KO^tBu \\ \text{4) } Et_2SO_4}]{\text{1) } nBuLi,\ KO^tBu}$ 1-ethyl-4-propylbenzene

74%

Also, reactions of dianions of xylenes.

I.A.5-14 K. Mori and T. Sugai, Synthesis, 752 (1982); U. Jensen-Korte and H. J. Schafer, Liebigs Ann. Chem., 1532 (1982).

$$\text{OTs-CH(CH}_3\text{)-CH}_2\text{CH}_2\text{-OCH}_2\phi \xrightarrow[Et_2O,\ -65°C]{R_2CuLi} \text{R-CH(CH}_3\text{)-CH}_2\text{CH}_2\text{-OCH}_2\phi$$

41-55%

I.A.5-15 B. H. Lipshutz and R. S. Wilhelm, *J. Amer. Chem. Soc.*, 104, 4696 (1982); E. Herbert, *Tetrahedron Lett.*, 23, 415 (1982).

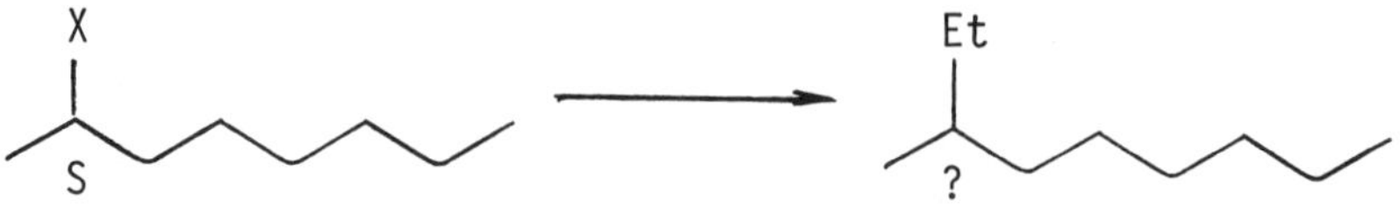

X	Reagent, Conditions	Stereochem.
I	Et$_2$CuLi, THF, -50°C	Racemization
Br	Et(Me)CuLi, THF, 0°C	Inversion

I.A.5-16 V. Calo, L. Lopez and G. Pesce, *J. Organometal. Chem.*, 231, 179 (1982).

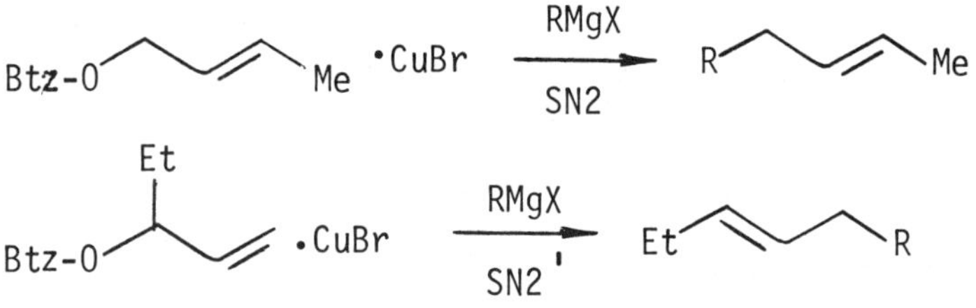

Btz = (2-benzothiazolyl)

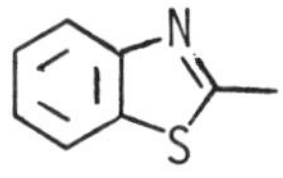

I.A.5-17 A. Carpita and R. Rossi, *Synthesis*, 469 (1982); C. Gallina, *Tetrahedron Lett.*, 23, 3093 (1982); V. Calo et al., *J. Org. Chem.*, 47, 4482 (1982).

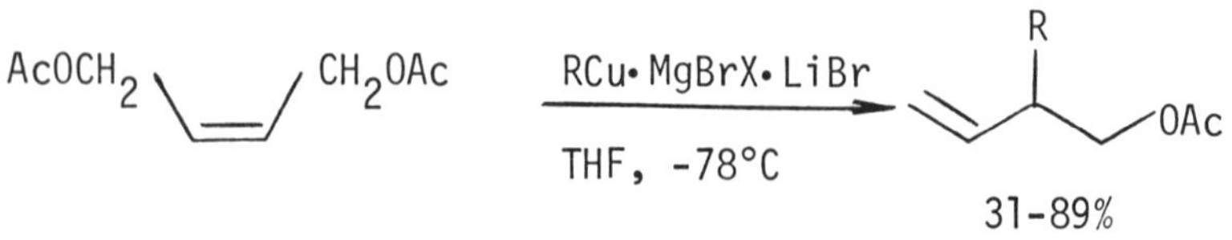

31-89%

I.A.5-18 Y. Butsugan et al., Chem. Lett., 177, 797 (1982); M. Schmid, F. Gerber and G. Hirth, Helv. Chim. Acta, 65, 684 (1982); S. P. Tanis, Tetrahedron Lett., 23, 3115 (1982).

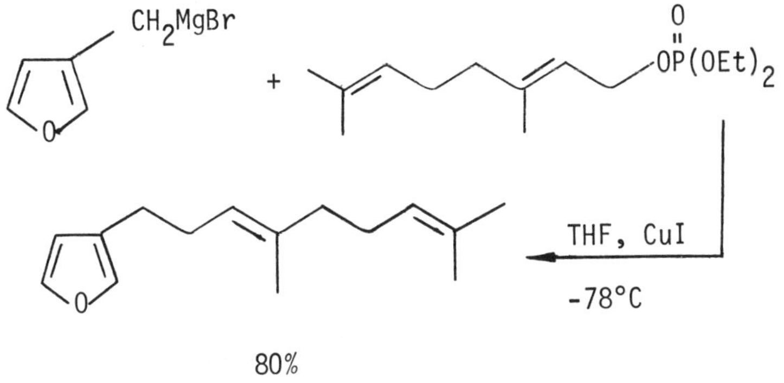

80%

I.A.5-19 Y. Tanigawa, Y. Fuse and S. I. Murahashi, Tetrahedron Lett., 23, 557 (1982); J. C. Fiaud and L. Aribi-Zouioueche, ibid, 5279.

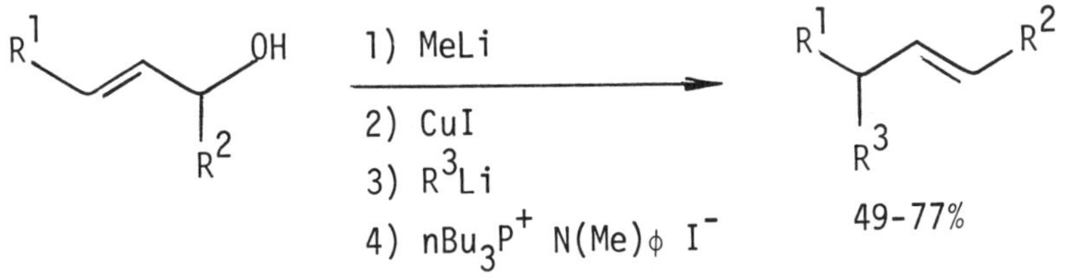

1) MeLi
2) CuI
3) R^3Li
4) $nBu_3P^+ N(Me)\phi\ I^-$

49-77%

I.A.5-20 B. H. Lipshutz, J. Kozlowski and R. S. Wilhelm, J. Amer. Chem. Soc., 104, 2305 (1982); H. M. Sirat, E. J. Thomas and J. D. Wallis, J. Chem. Soc., Perkin I, 2885 (1982); G. Teutsch, Tetrahedron Lett., 23, 4697 (1982).

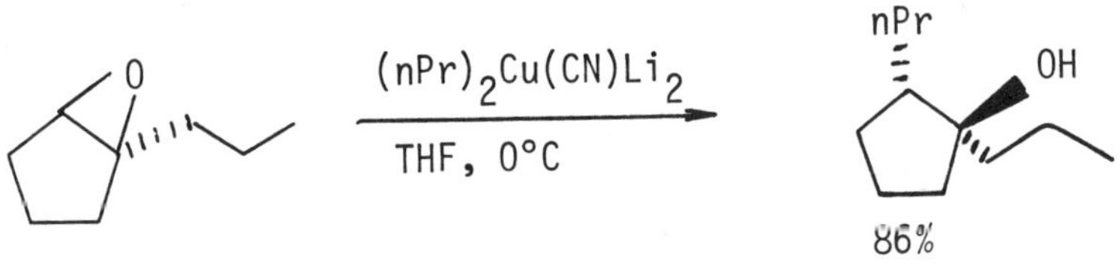

$(nPr)_2Cu(CN)Li_2$, THF, 0°C

86%

Milder reactions and better yields than with RCu(CN)Li.

I.A.5-21 A. Pfaltz and A. Mattenberger, Angew. Chem., Int. Ed. Engl., 21, 71 (1982); K. Oshima et al., Tetrahedron Lett., 23, 3597 (1982).

Me—[epoxide]—$(CH_2)_nOCH_2\phi$ $\xrightarrow[\phi CH_3, -20°C]{\text{2-3 Me}_3\text{Al} \atop \text{0.3 RLi}}$ $Me_2C(OH)$—$(CH_2)_nOCH_2\phi$

n = 1 or 2
cis or trans

76-87%
(95-> 99% Regioselective)

I.A.5-22 J. P. Marino and J. C. Jaen, J. Amer. Chem. Soc., 104, 3165 (1982); M. F. Schlecht, Chem. Commun., 1331 (1982).

[OTMS-Me epoxycyclohexene] $\xrightarrow[\text{2) Silica Chrom.}]{\text{1) (}^t\text{BuCuCN)Li}}$ [^{t}Bu-cyclohexenone-Me]

~ 100%

I.A.5-23 R. C. Larock and D. R. Leach, Organometallics, 1, 74 (1982); J. Barluenga et al., Chem. Commun., 355 (1982); J. Org. Chem., 47, 1560 (1982).

RHgBr $\xrightarrow[\text{3) MeI}]{\text{1) ICuPBu}_3 \atop \text{2) 3 }^t\text{BuLi}}$ R-CH$_3$

0-86%

R = Alkyl, Alkenyl or Aryl.

I.A.5-24 T. Kauffmann et al., Chem. Ber., 115, 645, 654, 659, 1810, 1818 (1982).

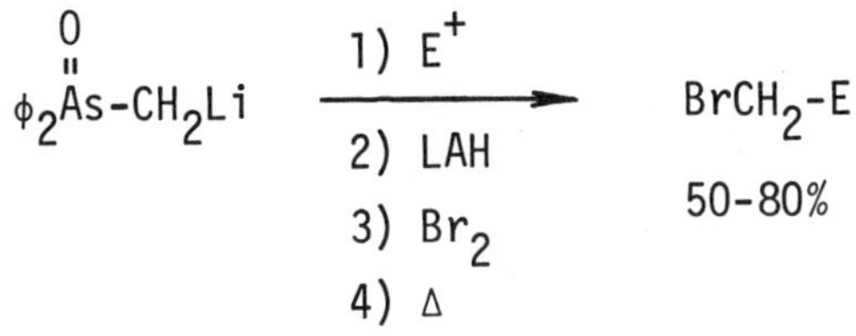

$$\phi_2\overset{O}{\underset{\|}{As}}-CH_2Li \xrightarrow[\begin{array}{l}2)\ LAH\\3)\ Br_2\\4)\ \Delta\end{array}]{1)\ E^+} BrCH_2-E \quad 50\text{-}80\%$$

E^+ = RX, RCHO, ArCHO, $R_2C=O$

I.A.6. Other Alkylation Procedures and Reviews

I.A.6-1 K. Oshima et al., Tetrahedron Lett., 23, 2953 (1982); G. A. Kraus and K. Neuenschwander, Chem. Commun., 134 (1982); S. Danishefsky and J. F. Kerwin, Jr., J. Org. Chem., 47, 3803 (1982).

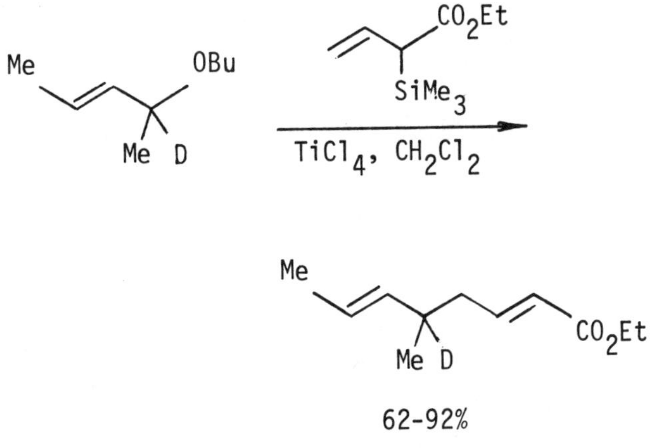

<chemical structures>

62-92%

I.A.6-2 A. J. Birch, L. F. Kelly and A. S. Narula, <u>Tetrahedron</u>, <u>38</u>, 1813 (1982); B. M. R. Bandara, A. J. Birch and W. D. Raverty, <u>J. Chem. Soc., Perkin I</u>, 1755, 1763 (1982).

[Structure: Me and CO_2Me substituted cyclohexadienyl cation complexed to $(CO)_3Fe$, PF_6^- counterion] + [isoprenyl-$SiMe_3$]

$\xrightarrow{CH_2Cl_2, \Delta}$

[Product: Me and CO_2Me substituted cyclohexadiene complexed to $(CO)_3Fe$, with pendant 1,1-dimethylallyl group]

95%

Also reactions with TMS enol ethers.

I.A.6-3 T. Sasaki, A. Nakanishi and M. Ohno, <u>J. Org. Chem.</u>, <u>47</u>, 3219 (1982); A. E. Sorochinskii, A. M. Aleksandrov and V. P. Kukhar, <u>J. Org. Chem. (USSR)</u>, <u>18</u>, 204 (1982).

[Adamantyl-OAc] $\xrightarrow[\text{allyl-}SiMe_3]{Me_3SiOTf}$ Ad-CH$_2$-CH=CH$_2$ 70%

(AdOAc)

I.A.6-4 C. Westerlund, Tetrahedron Lett., 23, 4835 (1982).

$$\underset{R^3}{\overset{R^2}{\underset{R^1}{\diagup\!\!\!\diagdown}}}\!\!\!\!\diagdown\!\text{SiMe}_3 \quad + \quad \underset{S}{\overset{S}{\bigcirc}}\!\!\!\!\!\!\diagup + BF_4^- \quad \xrightarrow{CH_2Cl_2}$$

$$\underset{S}{\overset{S}{\bigcirc}}\!\!\!\!\!\!\diagup\!\!-\!\!\underset{R^1}{\overset{R^2}{\text{C}}}\!\!-\!\!CH=CHR^3$$

60-79%

I.A.6-5 K. Itoh et al., Chem. Commun., 459 (1982); J. Org. Chem., 47, 2496 (1982).

$$RO-CH_2-SMe \quad \xrightarrow[SnCl_4,\ CH_2Cl_2]{\diagup\!\!\diagdown\!\!\diagup SiMe_3} \quad RO\diagdown\!\!\diagup\!\!\diagdown \quad 70\%$$

I.A.6-6 A. Ricci et al., Tetrahedron Lett., 23, 577 (1982); J. A. Cella, J. Org. Chem., 47, 2125 (1982).

$$ArCH_2SiMe_3 \quad \xrightarrow[\substack{KF/18\text{-}C\text{-}6 \text{ or} \\ Bu_4N^+ F^-/SiO_2}]{E^+} \quad ArCH_2\text{-}E \qquad 30\text{-}80\%$$

$E^+ = \phi CH_2Br,\ \phi CHO,\ CH_3\overset{O}{\overset{\diagup\diagdown}{CHCH_2}}$

I.A.6-7 G. E. Keck and J. B. Yates, J. Amer. Chem. Soc., 104, 5829 (1982).

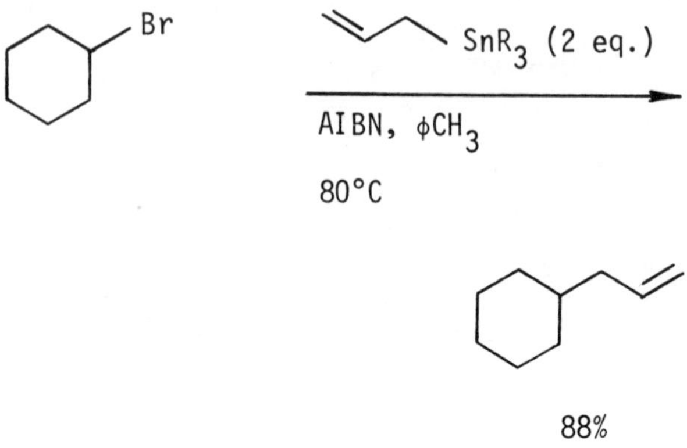

Cy-Br + CH$_2$=CHCH$_2$-SnR$_3$ (2 eq.) $\xrightarrow{\text{AIBN, }\phi\text{CH}_3, 80°\text{C}}$ Cy-CH$_2$CH=CH$_2$

88%

I.A.6-8 H. Klein, A. Erbe and H. Mayr, Angew. Chem., Int. Ed. Engl., 21, 82 (1982); S. M. Makin et al., J. Org. Chem. (USSR), 18, 651 (1982); Y. Nagai et al., Chem. Lett., 1255 (1982).

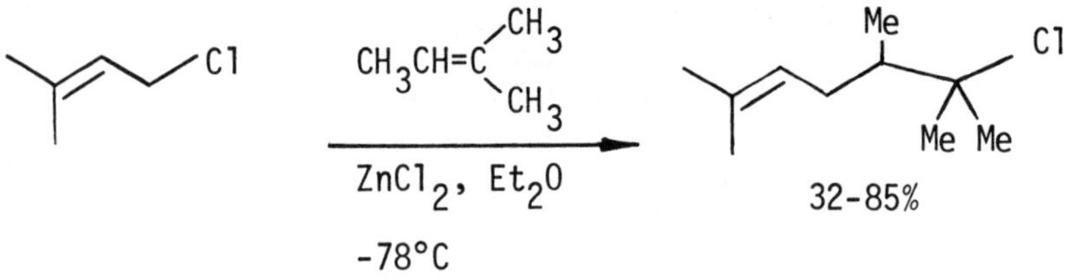

(CH$_3$)$_2$C=CHCH$_2$Cl + CH$_3$CH=C(CH$_3$)$_2$ $\xrightarrow{\text{ZnCl}_2\text{, Et}_2\text{O}, -78°\text{C}}$ (CH$_3$)$_2$C=CHCH$_2$CH(Me)C(Me)$_2$Cl

32-85%

I.A.6-9 L. S. Hegedus and S. Varaprath, Organometallics, 1, 259 (1982).

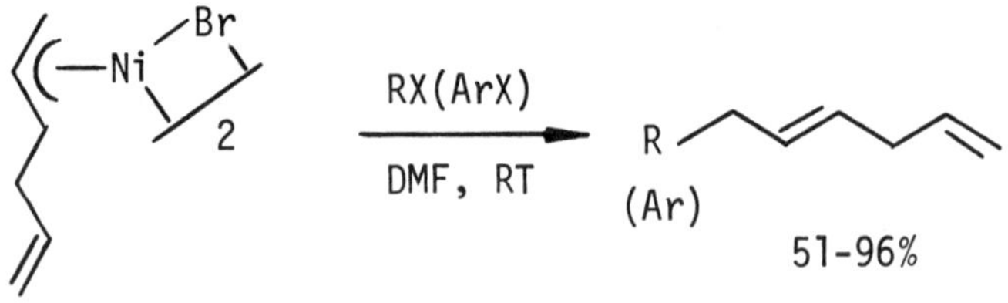

[(allyl)Ni-Br]$_2$ $\xrightarrow{\text{RX(ArX)}, \text{DMF, RT}}$ R(Ar)-CH$_2$CH=CHCH$_2$CH=CH$_2$

51-96%

I.A.6-10 J. D. McChesney and R. A. Swanson, J. Org. Chem., 47, 5201 (1982);   S. Bhattacharyya and D. Mukherjee, Tetrahedron, 38, 2961 (1982).

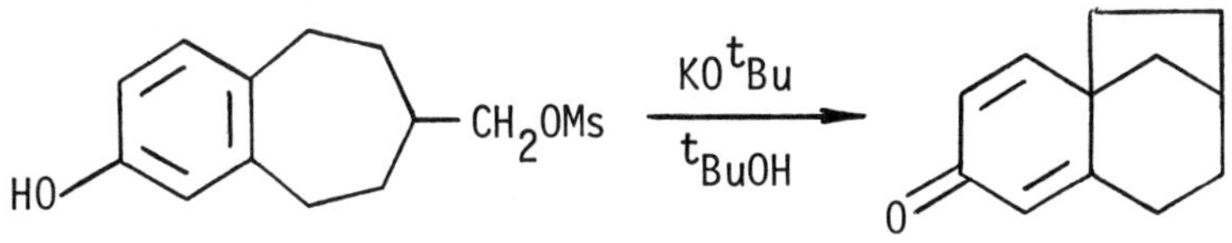

I.A.6-11 G. S. R. Subba Rao and N. S. Sundar, J. Chem. Soc., Perkin I, 875 (1982);   D. R. Dimmel and D. Shepard, J. Org. Chem., 47, 22 (1982);   S. Bhattacharyya and D. Mukherjee, Tetrahedron Lett., 23, 4175 (1982).

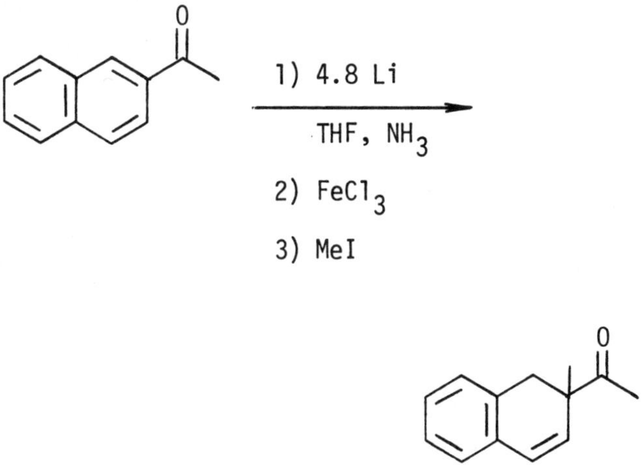

I.A.6-12 S. Chandrasekaran and J. V. Turner, Tetrahedron Lett., 23, 3799 (1982); J. M. Hook, L. N. Mander and M. Woolias, ibid, 1095; A. R. Murthy, N. S. Sundar and G. S. R. Subba Rao, Tetrahedron, 38, 2831 (1982).

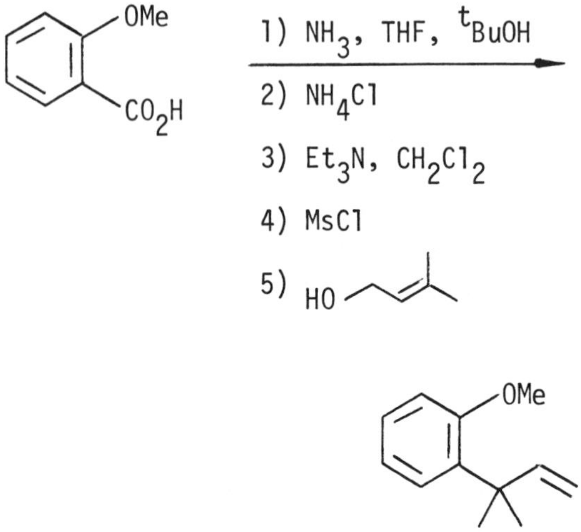

1) NH_3, THF, ^tBuOH
2) NH_4Cl
3) Et_3N, CH_2Cl_2
4) MsCl
5) HO~~~

61%

I.A.6-13 V. G. Granik, Russ. Chem. Rev., 51, 119 (1982); C. Galli and L. Mandolini, Chem. Commun., 251 (1982); C. J. M. Stirling et al., J. Chem. Soc., Perkin II, 579 (1982).

Review: "Influence of Ring Size on Properties and Reactivity of Cyclic Systems."

I.A.6-14 N. S. Zefirov and D. I. Makhon'kov, Chem. Rev., 615 (1982).

Review: "X-Philic Reactions."

I.A.6-15 G. Simchen et al., Synthesis, 1 (1982).

   Review: "Trialkylsilyl Perfluoroalkanesulfonates: Highly Reactive Silylating Agents and Lewis Acids in Organic Synthesis."

I.A.6-16 L. A. Paquette, Science, 217, 793 (1982).

   Review: "Silicon-Mediated Organic Synthesis."

I.A.6-17 J. P. Dunogues, CHEMTECH, 373 (1982).

   Review: "R_3Si: A Dandy Leaving Group."

I.A.6-18 H. Sakurai, Pure Appl. Chem., 54, 1 (1982).

   Review: "Reactions of Allylsilanes and Application to Organic Synthesis."

I.A.7. Nucleophilic Addition to Electron Deficient Carbon

I.A.7.a.1a. Intermolecular Aldol-Type 1,2-Additions

I.A.7.a.1a-1 S. Masamune and W. Choy, Aldrichimica Acta, 15, 47 (1982).

   Review: "Advances in Stereochemical Control: The 1,2- and 1,3-Diol Systems."

I.A.7.a.1a-2 S. Masamune et al., J. Amer. Chem. Soc., 104, 5521, 5523, 5526, 5528 (1982).

Aldol Methodology and Strategy.

I.A.7.a.1a-3 J. H. Clark and D. G. Cork, Chem. Commun., 635 (1982); C. Szantay et al., Liebigs Ann. Chem., 1173 (1982).

$$R^1\text{-CO-CH}_2\text{-}R^2 \xrightarrow{\begin{array}{l}1)\ R^3\text{CHO, Et}_2\overset{+}{\text{NH}}_2\ \text{Cl}^-\\ 2)\ \text{KF, 18-C-6}\\ 3)\ R^4\text{CH}_2\text{NO}_2\\ 4)\ \text{KMnO}_4,\ \text{SiO}_2\end{array}} R^1\text{-CO-CH}(R^2)\text{-CH}(R^3)\text{-CO-}R^4$$

71-91%

I.A.7.a.1a-4 T. Mukaiyama et al., Chem. Lett., 353, 1291, 1441, 1459, 1903 (1982); S. Shenvi and J. K. Stille, Tetrahedron Lett., 23, 627 (1982).

$$\phi\text{-CO-CH}_2\text{CH}_3 \xrightarrow{\begin{array}{l}1)\ \text{Sn(OTf)}_2,\ R_3N\\ 2)\ \text{RCHO}\\ 3)\ H_2O\end{array}} \phi\text{-CO-CH(Me)-CH(OH)-}R$$

41-86%

(86->95% Erythro)

I.A.7.a.1a-5 Y. Yamamoto, H. Yatagai and K. Maruyama, Tetrahedron Lett., 23, 2387 (1982); O Takazawa et al., Bull. Chem. Soc. Jpn., 55, 1907 (1982); D. L. J. Clive, C. G. Russell and S. C. Suri, J. Org. Chem., 47, 1632 (1982).

$$\text{Me}_3\text{SiO-cyclohexenyl} \xrightarrow[\substack{\text{2) Et}_3\text{B (1 eq.)} \\ \text{3) }\phi\text{CHO}}]{\text{1) nBuLi, THF}} \text{cyclohexanone-CH(OH)-}\phi$$

90%

(92% Threo)

I.A.7.a.1a-6 Y. Yamamoto and K. Maruyama, J. Amer. Chem. Soc., 104, 2323 (1982).

$$\underset{\underset{\text{HgX}}{|}}{\text{R}^2-\text{CH}}-\overset{\text{O}}{\underset{}{\text{C}}}-\text{R}^1 \xrightarrow[\text{BF}_3\cdot\text{Et}_2\text{O}]{\text{R}^3\text{CHO}} \text{R}^3\text{-CH(OH)-CH(R}^2\text{)-C(O)-R}^1$$

35-85% (GC)

(72->98% Erythro)

I.A.7.a.1a-7 J. Hooz and J. Oudenes, Synth. Commun., 12, 189 (1982); H. Hamana and T. Sugasawa, Chem. Lett., 1401 (1982); T. Mukaiyama and M. Yamaguchi, ibid, 509 (1982); M. Murakami and T. Mukaiyama, ibid, 241, 1271 (1982); H. Umezawa, M. Ohno et al., Tetrahedron Lett., 23, 521, 525, 529 (1982).

$$\underset{\text{R}^2}{\overset{\text{OBEt}_2}{\text{R}^1\text{-C=CH}}} \xrightarrow[\substack{\text{THF, 50°C} \\ \text{2) H}_3\text{O}^+}]{\text{1) CH}_3\text{CN}} \text{R}^1\text{-C(O)-CH(R}^2\text{)-C(O)-CH}_3$$

35-84%

I.A.7.a.1a-8 K. I. Watanabe and A. Imazawa, Bull. Chem. Soc. Jpn., 55, 3208, 3212 (1982); J. Muzart, Synthesis, 60 (1982); W. Reid and M. Vogl, Chem. Ber., 115, 403, 791 (1982).

$$Ar^1CHO + CH_3-\overset{O}{\underset{\|}{C}}-Ar^2 \xrightarrow[\text{of Pyridine Containing Copolymer, DMF}]{\text{Co(II) Complex}} Ar^1CH=CH\overset{O}{\underset{\|}{C}}Ar^2 \quad 44\text{-}98\%$$

Also, Michael Additions

I.A.7.a.1a-9 K. H. Theopold, P. N. Becker and R. G. Bergman, J. Amer. Chem. Soc., 104, 5250 (1982).

[Structure: Me/φ-N(Me)-CH(Me)-P(φ)(φ)-Co(Cp)(lactone)]
1) LDA
2) ^{t}BuCHO
3) $FeCl_3$, 0°C
→ [methylenecyclobutane with CH(OH)^{t}Bu substituent]
69%

(Optically Pure, NMR)

I.A.7.a.1a-10 S. Miyano, et al., Bull. Chem. Soc. Jpn., 55, 534, 1331 (1982); K. Matsumoto, Angew. Chem., Int. Ed. Engl., 21, 922 (1982); S. Danishefsky, M. Kahn and M. Silvestri, Tetrahedron Lett., 23, 703, 1419 (1982); P. T. Lansbury and J. P. Vacca, Tetrahedron, 38, 2797 (1982); K. Annen et al., Synthesis, 34 (1982).

$$R^1-C(OSiMe_3)=C(R^2)(R^3) \xrightarrow[\text{2) }H_2O]{\text{1) }CH_2ClI,\ Me_2NCH_2NMe_2,\ DMSO,\ RT} R^1-\overset{O}{\underset{\|}{C}}-\underset{CH_2NMe_2}{\overset{R^2}{\underset{|}{C}}}-R^3$$

18-71%

I.A.7.a.1a-11 R. E. Tirpak and M. W. Rathke, J. Org. Chem., 47, 5099 (1982); E. Vedejs and B. Nader, ibid, 47, 3193 (1982); W. Ando and H. Tsumaki, Tetrahedron Lett., 23, 3073 (1982); M. V. Rangaishenvi, S. V. Hiremath and S. N. Kulkarni, Ind. J. Chem., 21B, 56 (1982); N. N. Sidorov et al., J. Org. Chem. (USSR), 18, 499 (1982); W. Krasuski, D. Nikolaus and M. Regitz, Liebigs Ann. Chem., 1451 (1982).

Cyclohexenyl-OSiMe$_3$ + CH$_3$COCl $\xrightarrow[\text{CH}_2\text{Cl}_2,\ 0°C]{\text{ZnCl}_2\ \text{or}\ \text{SbCl}_3}$ 2-acetylcyclohexanone

4-94% (GC)
(Some O-Acylation)

I.A.7.a.1a-12 P. Plath and W. Rohr, Synthesis, 318 (1982); S. E. Tolchinskii, A. A. Petrov et al., J. Org. Chem. (USSR), 18, 973 (1982); K. Grohe and H. Heitzer, Liebigs Ann. Chem., 884 (1982); T. Shono et al., Tetrahedron Lett., 23, 1201 (1982).

$$\underset{\underset{Me\diagup \ \diagdown NHMe}{\overset{\|}{C}}}{R^2O_2C\diagdown CH} \xrightarrow[\text{Et}_3\text{N},\ \phi\text{CH}_3]{R^1COCl} \underset{\underset{Me\diagup \ \diagdown NHMe}{}}{R^2O_2C\diagdown\!\!=\!\!\diagup\overset{O}{\overset{\|}{CR^1}}}$$

52-76%

Products used for Pyrazole Synthesis.

I.A.7.a.1a-13 F. Effenberger et al., Chem. Ber., 115, 2766 (1982); R. Brehme and H. E. Nikoliewski, Tetrahedron Lett., 23, 1131 (1982).

$$\text{Cl}_3\text{C}-\overset{\overset{O}{\|}}{\text{C}}-\text{Cl} \xrightarrow[\text{2) Distillation}]{\text{1) CH}_2=\text{CH-OEt},\ 25°\text{C}} \text{Cl}_3\text{C}\diagdown\!\!\overset{O}{\overset{\|}{C}}\!\!\diagup\!\!=\!\!\diagdown\text{OEt}$$

I.A.7.a.1a-14   R. Knorr and A. Weiss, Chem. Ber., 115, 139
(1982);   M. T. Reetz, R. Steinbach and K. Kesseler, Angew.
Chem., Int. Ed. Engl., 21, 864 (1982).

$$R^1N=C(R^2)CH_2R^3 \quad \xrightarrow[\substack{2) \; R^4(EtO)C=NR^1 \\ 3) \; H_3O^+}]{1) \; LDA} \quad R^2C(R^1NH)=C(R^3)-C(R^4)=NR^1 \quad 42\text{-}91\%$$

I.A.7.a.1a-15   J. A. Virgilio and E. Heilweil, Org. Prep. Proc.
Int., 14, 9 (1982);   C. Reichardt and K. Schagerer, Liebigs
Ann. Chem., 530 (1982);   C. Petrier, A. L. Gemal and J. L.
Luche, Tetrahedron Lett., 23, 3361 (1982);   M. Pulst, L. Beyer
and M. Weissenfels, J. Prakt. Chem., 324, 292 (1982);   M.
Muraoka, Y. Yamamoto and T. Takeshima, Chem. Lett., 101 (1982).

$$ArCOCH_2R \quad \xrightarrow[\substack{DMF \\ 2) \; H_2, \; Base \\ 5\% \; Pd/C}]{1) \; POCl_3} \quad ArCH_2CHR(CHO) \quad 57\text{-}84\%$$

I.A.7.a.1a-16   A. S. Kende and D. A. Becker, Synth. Commun.,
12, 829 (1982);   H. Ila, H. Junjappa et al., Synthesis, 693
(1982);   J. Vebrel and R. R. Carrie, Bull. Soc. Chim. Fr. II,
116, 161 (1982).

$$\text{MeCOCH(Me)}_2 \quad \xrightarrow[\substack{CS_2, \; 25°C \\ 2) \; MeI \\ 3) \; HgO, \; BF_3 \cdot Et_2O \\ THF, \; MeOH}]{1) \; NaO^tAm, \; \phi H} \quad \text{MeCOC(Me)}_2\text{CO}_2\text{Me} \quad 70\%$$

I.A.7.a.1a-17   L. Oshry and S. M. Rosenfeld, <u>Org. Prep. Proc. Int.</u>, <u>14</u>, 249 (1982).

Review: "Synthesis and Uses of B-Keto Acids."

I.A.7.a.1a-18   N. Matsumura, T. Ohba and H. Inoue, <u>Bull. Chem. Soc. Jpn.</u>, <u>55</u>, 3949 (1982).

$$R^1N=C(R^2)(NR^1)C(OMgBr)=O \xrightarrow[2)\ H^+]{1)\ \phi CCH_3,\ DMF} \phi\text{-}C(=O)\text{-}CH_2CO_2H$$

45%

I.A.7.a.1a-19   C. Cativiela, J. I. Garcia and E. Melendez, <u>Synthesis</u>, 763 (1982); H. Thies, W. Franke and H. Schwarz, <u>ibid</u>, 587 (1982); T. Maier and F. Cavagna, <u>Angew. Chem., Int. Ed. Engl.</u>, <u>21</u>, 546 (1982); W. Bauer and J. Daub, <u>Tetrahedron Lett.</u>, <u>23</u>, 4773 (1982).

$$\phi CNHCH_2CO_2H \xrightarrow[2)\ R^3NH_2,\ \phi H,\ \Delta]{1)\ R^1C(=O)R^2,\ Ac_2O,\ Pb(OAc)_2,\ \Delta} R^1R^2C=C(CNHR^3)(NHC\phi)$$

41-98%

I.A.7.a.1a-20   J. L. Moreau and R. Couffignal, <u>Tetrahedron Lett.</u>, <u>23</u>, 5271 (1982); R. R. Schmidt and R. Klager, <u>Angew. Chem., Int. Ed. Engl.</u>, <u>21</u>, 210 (1982).

dioxolane-CH$_2$CO$_2$SiMe$_3$ $\xrightarrow{\text{1) LDA, Et}_2\text{O, -60°C; 2) R}^1\text{R}^2\text{C=O; 3) H}_3\text{O}^+}$

R1
R2
OH
O
O
CO2H

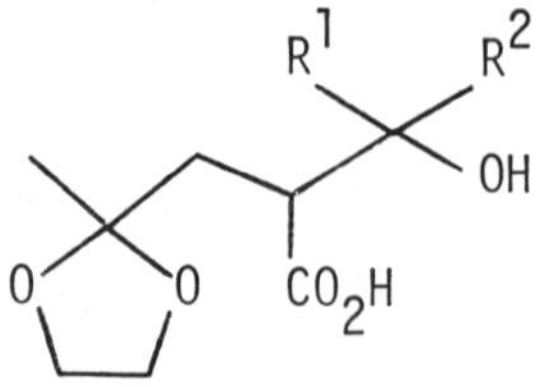

86-90%

Product Thermolysis Give B-Ethylenic Ketones.

I.A.7.a.1a-21 B. Rague, Y. Chapleur and B. Castro, J. Chem. Soc., Perkin I, 2063 (1982); T. Mukaiyama, et al., Chem. Lett., 145, 929 (1982); M. F. El-Newaihy et al., J. Prakt. Chem., 324, 379 (1982).

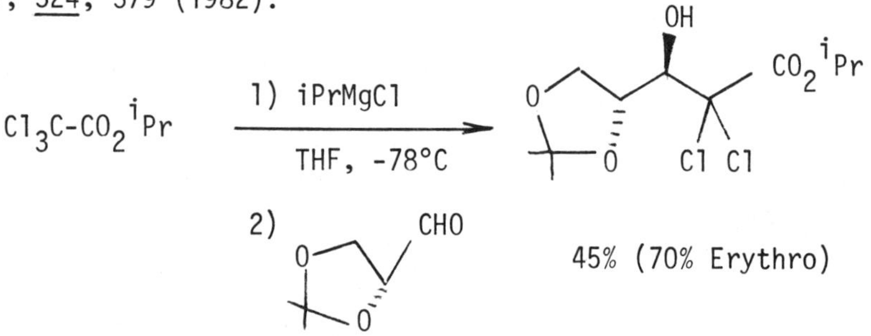

Cl3C-CO2iPr
1) iPrMgCl
THF, -78°C
2)
CHO
O
O
OH
CO2iPr
O
O
Cl Cl

45% (70% Erythro)

I.A.7.a.1a-22 R. H. Schlessinger and M. S. Poss, J. Amer. Chem. Soc., 104, 357 (1982); T. H. Chan and G. J. Kang, Tetrahedron Lett., 23, 3011 (1982); P. Albaugh-Robertson and J. A. Katzenellenbogen, ibid, 23, 723 (1982); Y. Naruta, H. Uno and K. Maruyama, Chem. Lett., 961 (1982).

CO2Me
N
1) LDA, THF
2) iPr-CHO, -78°C
3) Standard Transforms.
OH
HO2C

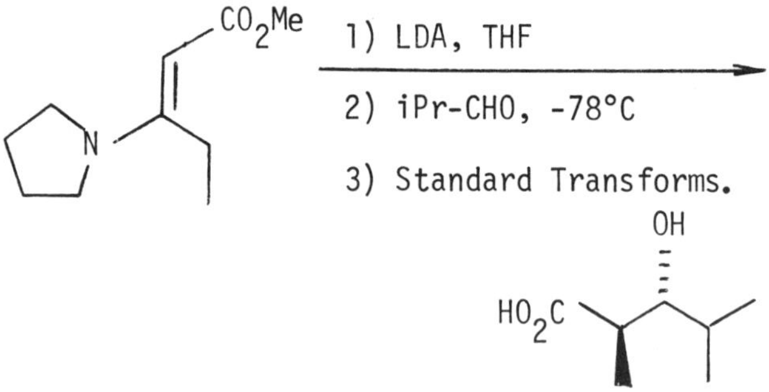

I.A.7.a.1a-23 T. Mukaiyama et al., *Chem. Lett.*, 161, 467, 1601 (1982).

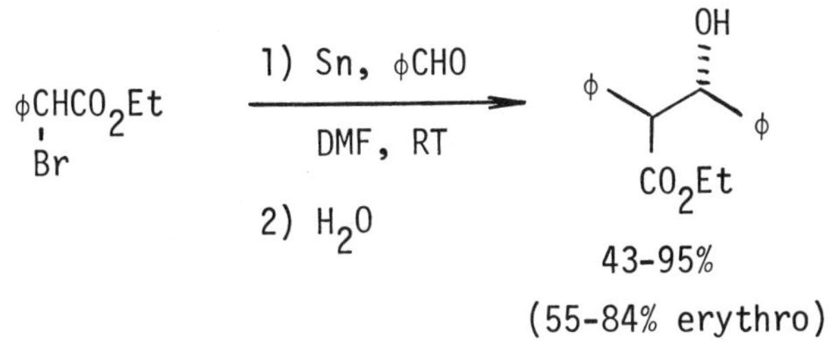

ϕCHCO$_2$Et → (1) Sn, ϕCHO, DMF, RT; 2) H$_2$O) → ϕ-CH(OH)-CH(ϕ)-CO$_2$Et
  |
  Br

43-95%
(55-84% erythro)

I.A.7.a.1a-24 D. A. Widdowson, G. H. Wiebecke and D. J. Williams, *Tetrahedron Lett.*, 23, 4285 (1982); J. Mulzer and A. Chucholowski, *Angew. Chem., Int. Ed. Engl.*, 21, 777 (1982).

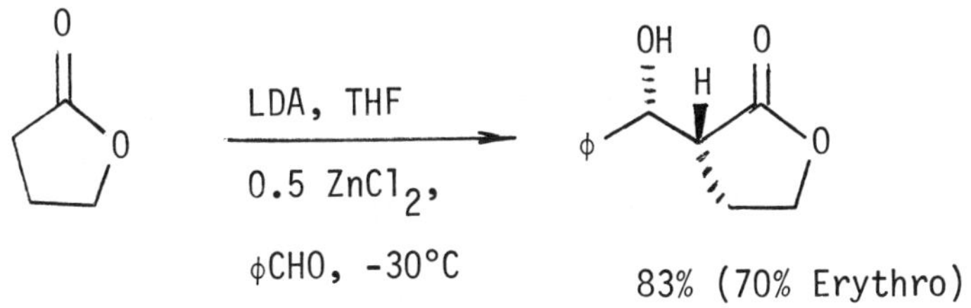

γ-butyrolactone + LDA, THF, 0.5 ZnCl$_2$, ϕCHO, -30°C → α-(ϕ-CH(OH))-γ-butyrolactone

83% (70% Erythro)

Stereoselectivity reversed with lithium cation.

I.A.7.a.1a-25 G. Solladie et al., *Helv. Chim. Acta*, 65, 1602 (1982).

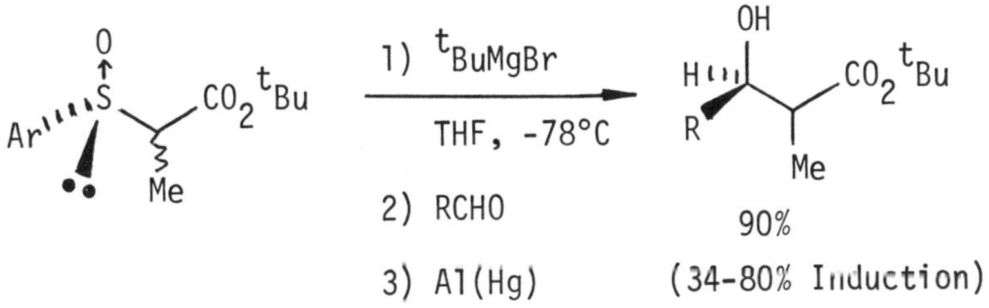

Ar-S(O)-CH(Me)-CO$_2$^{t}Bu → (1) ^{t}BuMgBr, THF, -78°C; 2) RCHO; 3) Al(Hg)) → R-CH(OH)-CH(Me)-CO$_2$^{t}Bu

90%
(34-80% Induction)

I.A.7.a.1a-26 S. H. Bertz, G. Dabbagh and P. Cotte, J. Org. Chem., 47, 2216 (1982); A. I. Meyers and D. G. Walker, ibid, 47, 2999 (1982).

$$\begin{array}{c} CO_2Et \\ | \\ C \\ ||| \\ C \\ | \\ H \end{array} \quad \xrightarrow[\text{2) NaH, HCO}_2\text{Et}]{\text{1) Cu(I), EtOH}} \quad \begin{array}{c} CO_2Et \\ \diagup \diagdown \\ OHC \quad CHO \end{array}$$

65%

I.A.7.a.1a-27 Z. Yoshida et al., J. Amer. Chem. Soc., 104, 4018 (1982); J. Liebscher and B. Abegaz, Synthesis, 769 (1982); S. Florio et al., Tetrahedron, 38, 557 (1982).

$$CH_3CH_2\overset{S}{\overset{||}{C}}NH\phi \quad \xrightarrow[\substack{\text{3) (CH}_3)_2\text{CHCHO,} \\ -78°C}]{\substack{\text{1) 2 nBuLi, THF} \\ \text{2) Me}_3\text{SiCl (1 eq)}}}$$

[product: iPr–CH(OH)–CH(Me)–C(=S)–NHφ]

97%

(94% Erythro)

I.A.7.a.1a-28 D. Enders and H. Lotter, Tetrahedron Lett., 23, 639 (1982).

$$CH_3CN \xrightarrow[\substack{\text{2) LDA, THF} \\ \text{3) RCHO} \\ \text{4) }\Delta}]{\substack{\text{1) Me}_2\text{NH} \\ \text{KCN, H}_2\text{O}}} \underset{\underset{\text{Me}_2\text{N}}{|}}{CH_3-CH}-\overset{O}{\overset{\|}{C}}-R$$

44-81%

I.A.7.a.1a-29 T. Hiyama and K. Kobayashi, Tetrahedron Lett., 23, 1597 (1982).

$$R^1CH_2CO_2{}^tBu \xrightarrow[\substack{\text{Et}_2\text{O, 0 °C} \\ \text{2) R}^2\text{CN} \\ \text{3) aq. NH}_4\text{Cl}}]{\substack{\text{1) 2 iPr}_2\text{NH} \\ \text{1 EtMgBr}}} \underset{H_2N}{\overset{R^2}{\diagdown}}C=C\underset{CO_2{}^tBu}{\overset{R^1}{\diagup}}$$

25-86%

I.A.7.a.1a-30 S. Tomoda, Y. Takeuchi and Y. Nomura, Chem. Lett., 1787, 1733 (1982).

$$\underset{R^1}{\overset{H}{\diagdown}}C=\underset{\overset{+}{N}-O^-}{\overset{R^2}{\diagup}} \quad \underset{CH_3CN, 25°C}{\xrightarrow{R^3CH=C(OSiMe_2{}^tBu)(OR^4)}} \quad R^1-\underset{OSiMe_2{}^tBu}{\overset{R^2}{N}}-\overset{R^2}{\underset{}{C}H}-\overset{R^3}{\underset{CO_2R^4}{C}H}$$

63-94%

Also, Ketene Silyl Acetals + φSeCN.

I.A.7.a.1a-31 M. J. Bourgeois et al., Bull. Soc. Chim. Belg., 91, 871 (1982); J. Obaza and F. X. Smith, Synth. Commun., 12, 19 (1982); R. P. Houghton and D. J. Lapham, Synthesis, 451 (1982).

$$\underset{\underset{Li}{Me'}}{\overset{Me}{\diagdown}}C\text{-}CO_2Me \quad \xrightarrow[\text{THF}]{(\text{Im})_2C=O} \quad MeO_2C\text{-}\underset{Me}{\overset{Me}{\underset{|}{C}}}\text{-}\overset{O}{\underset{\|}{C}}\text{-}\underset{Me}{\overset{Me}{\underset{|}{C}}}\text{-}CO_2Me$$

60%

I.A.7.a.1a-32 H. J. Liu and H. Wynn, Tetrahedron Lett., 23, 3151 (1982); F. Texier-Boullet and A. Foucaud, ibid, 23, 4927 (1982); F. Bonadies, M. L. Scarpati and F. Savagnone, Gazz. Chim. Ital., 112, 1 (1982); R. W. Holder et al., J. Org. Chem., 47, 1445 (1982); M. Havel et al., Coll. Czech. Chem. Commun., 47, 1240 (1982).

$$NC\text{-}CH_2\text{-}\overset{O}{\underset{\|}{C}}S^tBu \quad \xrightarrow[\text{2) NaBH}_4, \text{EtOH}]{1) \text{ cyclohexanone, DABCO, THF}} \quad NC\text{-}CH\text{-}\overset{O}{\underset{\|}{C}}\text{-}S^tBu \text{ (cyclohexyl)}$$

84%

I.A.7.a.1a-33 R. Gompper, E. Kujath and H. U. Wagner, Angew. Chem., Int. Ed. Engl., 21, 543 (1982); H. Bohme and G. Ahrens, Liebigs Ann. Chem., 1022, 1030 (1982); Z. Arnold, et al., Tetrahedron Lett., 23, 1725 (1982); Synthesis, 823 (1982).

$$Me_2N\diagdown\diagup\overset{\phi_3P^+}{\diagup}\diagdown NMe_2 \quad 2ClO_4^- \quad + \quad MeO_2C\text{-}CH_2\text{-}CN \quad \xrightarrow{KOH, MeOH}$$

$$MeO_2C\diagdown\diagup\overset{NC}{\diagup}\diagdown\diagup\overset{P\phi_3}{\diagup}\diagdown\diagup\overset{CN}{\diagup}\diagdown CO_2Me$$

90%

I.A.7.a.1a-34 J. T. Gupton, Synth. Commun., 12, 35, 939 (1982); W. Reid and H. E. Erle, Liebigs Ann. Chem., 201 (1982).

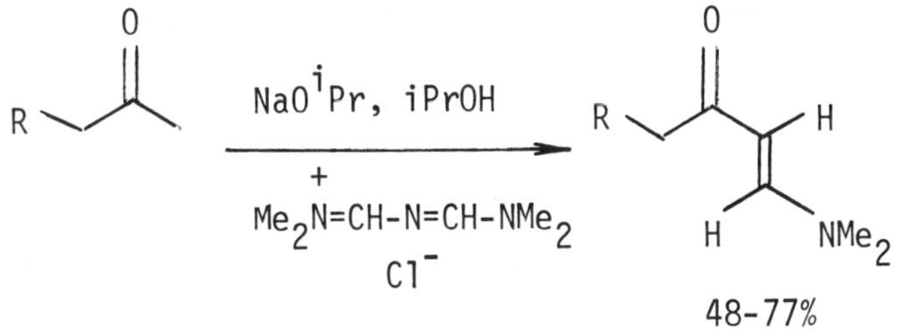

R−C(=O)−CH₃ + Me₂N−CH=N−CH−NMe₂ Cl⁻ →(NaO^iPr, iPrOH)→ R−C(=O)−C(=CH−NMe₂)−H

48-77%

I.A.7.a.1b. Intramolecular Aldol-Type 1,2-Additions

I.A.7.a.1b-1 J. E. Baldwin and M. J. Lusch, Tetrahedron, 38, 2939 (1982).

Rules for Ring Closure: Intramolecular Aldol Condensations

I.A.7.a.1b-2 H. Shick, B. Pogoda and S. Schwarz, Zeit. Chem., 22, 185 (1982); G. M. Strunz and G. S. Lal, Can. J. Chem., 60, 2528 (1982); M. Fetizon, M. T. Montaufier and J. Rens, J. Chem. Res. (S), 9 (1982); J. M. Cook, U. Weiss, J. V. Silverton et al., J. Amer. Chem. Soc., 104, 318 (1982).

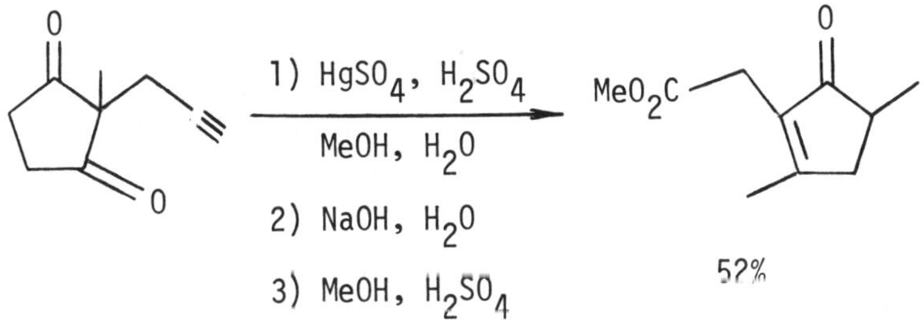

1) $HgSO_4$, H_2SO_4, MeOH, H_2O
2) NaOH, H_2O
3) MeOH, H_2SO_4

52%

I.A.7.a.1b-3 M. Karpf, Tetrahedron Lett., 23, 4923 (1982); G. M. Strunz and G. S. Lal, Can. J. Chem., 60, 572 (1982); C. G. M. Janssen, L. H. J. G. Simons and E. F. Godefroi, Synthesis, 389 (1982); J. Drouin and J. M. Conia, Synth. Commun., 12, 81 (1982).

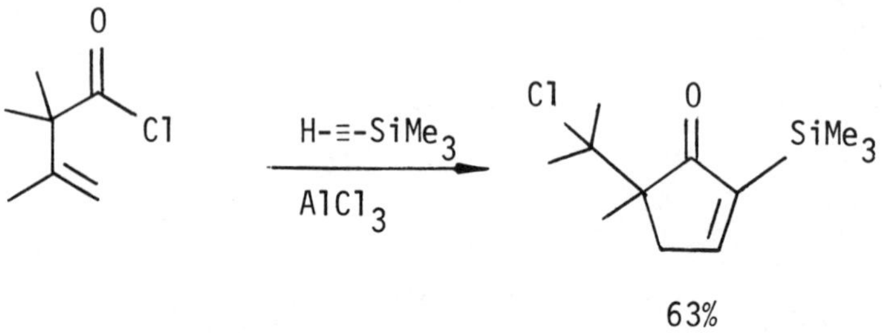

I.A.7.a.1b-4 F. Johnson et al., J. Amer. Chem. Soc., 104, 2190 (1982); J. Org. Chem., 47, 4254 (1982).

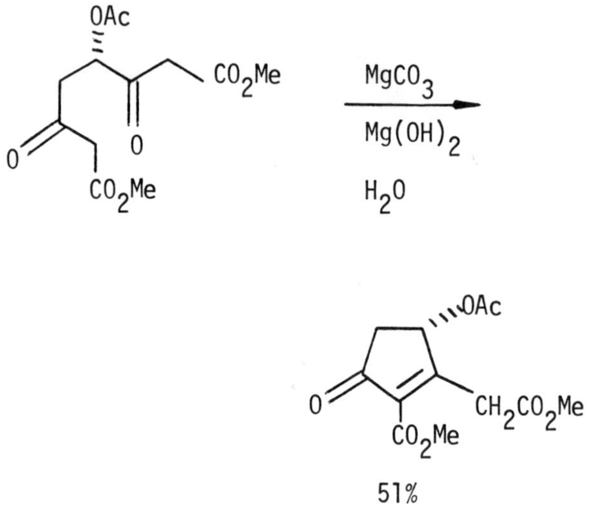

I.A.7.a.1b-5 S. D. Burke et al., J. Amer. Chem. Soc., 104, 872 (1982); J. Org. Chem., 47, 1349 (1982).

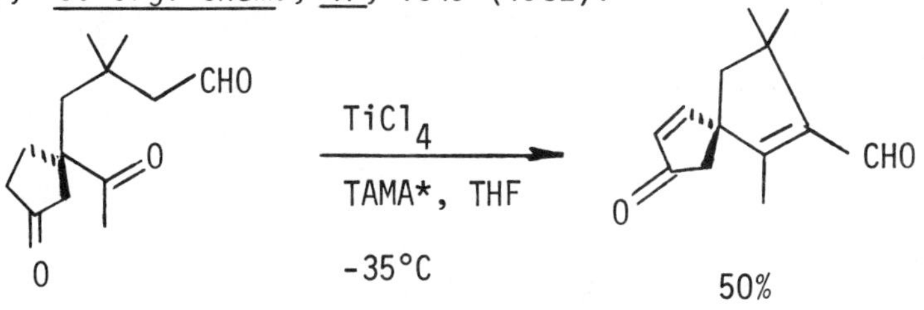

$$\xrightarrow[-35°C]{TiCl_4, TAMA^*, THF}$$

50%

TAMA = N-Methylanilinium Trifluoroacetate.

I.A.7.a.1b-6 M. E. Vandewalle et al., Tetrahedron, 38, 2279 (1982); T. Yoshida and S. Saito, Bull. Chem. Soc. Jpn., 55, 3931 (1982).

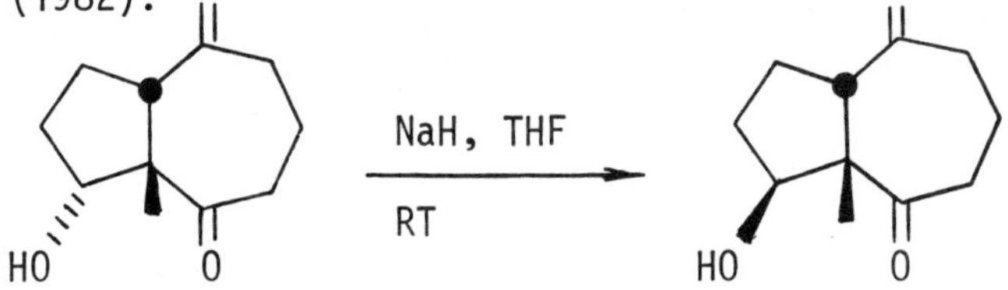

$$\xrightarrow[RT]{NaH, THF}$$

73% (Retroaldol-Aldol)

I.A.7.a.1b-7 D. Kontonassios and C. Sandris, Steroids, 39, 411 (1982); T. Fujinami et al., Chem. Lett., 123 (1982); E. Piers et al., Chem. Commun., 404 (1982).

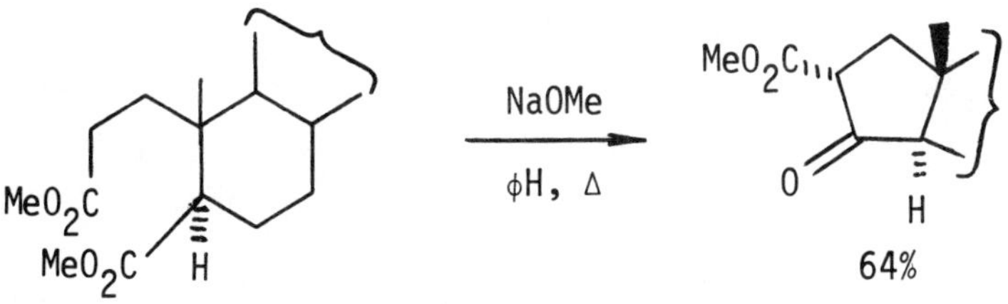

$$\xrightarrow[\phi H, \Delta]{NaOMe}$$

64%

I.A.7.a.1b-8 Y. Tamai, H. Hagiwara, H. Uda, Chem. Commun., 502 (1982); T. R. Kasturi, S. M. Reddy and P. S. Murphy, J. Chem. Soc., Perkin I, 2791 (1982); E. Y. Belyaev et al., J. Org. Chem. (USSR), 18, 1299 (1982).

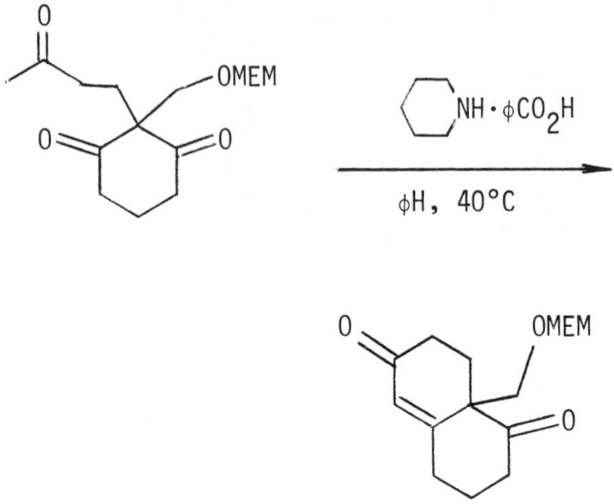

75%

I.A.7.a.1b-9 H. Tomioka, K. Oshima and H. Nozaki, Tetrahedron Lett., 23, 99 (1982); M. Scotton et al., Can. J. Chem., 60, 1327 (1982).

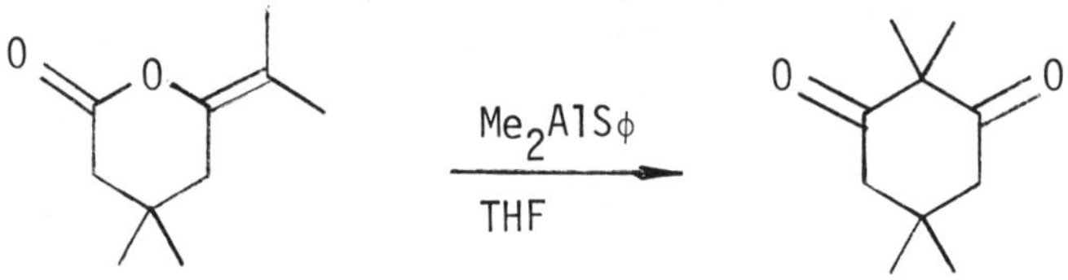

91%

I.A.7.a.1b-10 R. K. Boeckman, Jr. and F. W. Sum, J. Amer. Chem. Soc., 104, 4604 (1982); Y. Kishi et al., J. Amer. Chem. Soc., 104, 7371, 7372 (1982).

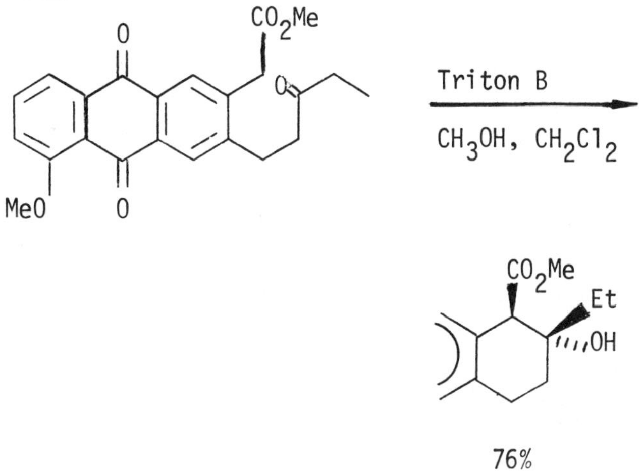
CO2Me
O
O
O
MeO
Triton B
CH3OH, CH2Cl2
CO2Me
Et
OH
76%

I.A.7.a.1b-11 S. H. Bertz, G. Rihs and R. B. Woodward, Tetrahedron, 38, 63 (1982); S. H. Bertz and G. Dabbagh, Angew. Chem., Int. Ed. Engl., 21, 306 (1982).

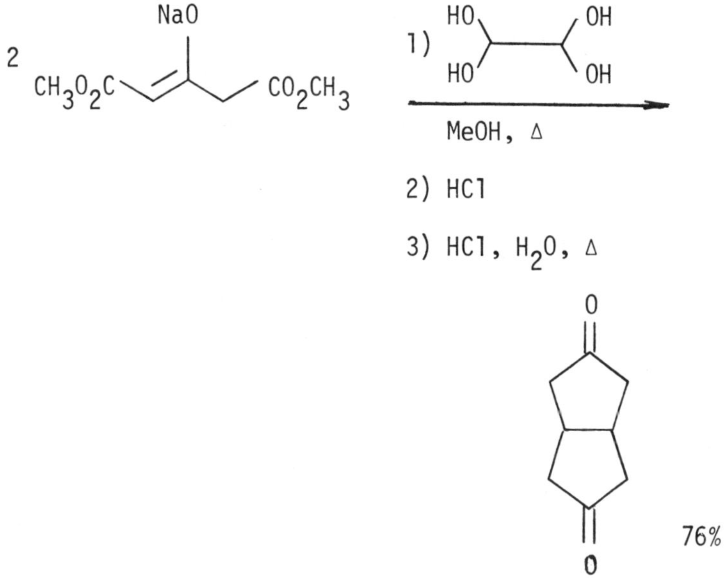
2
NaO
CH3O2C
CO2CH3
1)
HO
OH
HO
OH
MeOH, Δ
2) HCl
3) HCl, H2O, Δ
O
O
76%

I.A.7.a.1b-12 S. A. Monti and T. R. Dean, J. Org. Chem., 47, 2679 (1982); A. B. Smith, III, B. A. Wexler and J. Slade, Tetrahedron Lett., 23, 1631 (1982); T. Momose et al., Synth. Commun., 12, 1039 (1982).

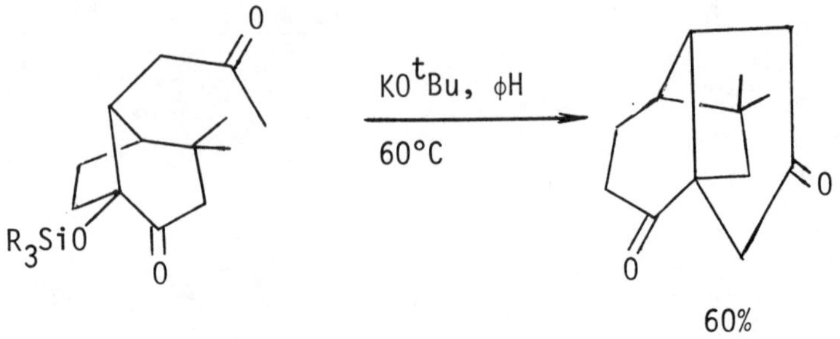

$$\text{substrate} \xrightarrow[60°C]{KO^tBu, \phi H} \text{product} \quad 60\%$$

Tandem Aldol-Pinacol.

I.A.7.a.2. 1,2-Additions of N-, S- or Se- Stabilized Carbanions

I.A.7.a.2-1 M. V. Prostenik and I. Butula, Angew. Chem., Int. Ed. Engl., 21, 139 (1982); I. M. Bazavova and R. G. Dubenko, J. Org. Chem. (USSR), 18, 584 (1982); D. Seebach et al., Helv. Chim. Acta, 65, 1101 (1982).

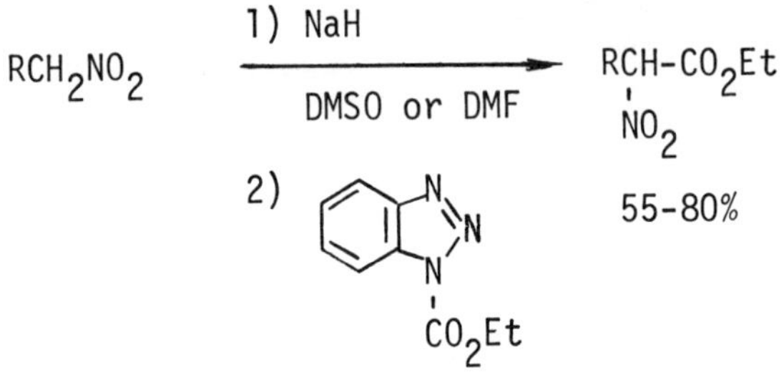

$$RCH_2NO_2 \xrightarrow[\text{DMSO or DMF}]{1)\ NaH,\ 2)\ \text{benzotriazole-CO}_2Et} \underset{NO_2}{RCH-CO_2Et} \quad 55\text{-}80\%$$

I.A.7.a.2-2 T. Takeda, H. Furukawa and T. Fujiwara, <u>Chem. Lett.</u>, 593 (1982); D. Morgans, Jr. and G. B. Feigelson, <u>J. Org. Chem.</u>, <u>47</u>, 1131 (1982).

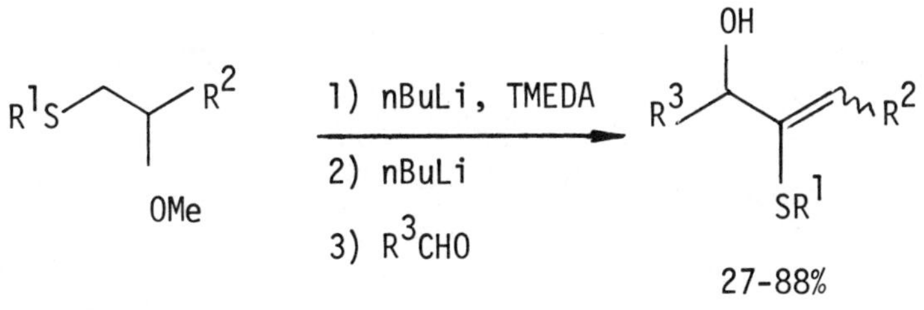

R^1S
R^2
OMe
1) nBuLi, TMEDA
2) nBuLi
3) R^3CHO
OH
R^3
R^2
SR^1
27-88%

I.A.7.a.2-3 H. Yamamoto et al., <u>J. Amer. Chem. Soc.</u>, <u>104</u>, 7663 (1982); H. Kotake, T. Yamamoto and H. Kinoshita, <u>Chem. Lett.</u>, 1331 (1982); H. Baba, T. Hayashi and T. Oishi, <u>Chem. Pharm. Bull.</u>, <u>30</u>, 3852 (1982).

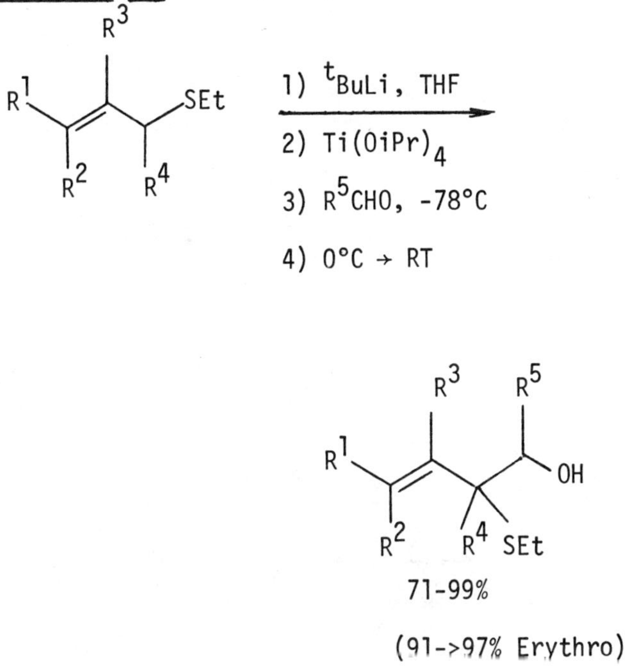

R^3
R^1
SEt
R^2
R^4
1) ^tBuLi, THF
2) $Ti(OiPr)_4$
3) R^5CHO, -78°C
4) 0°C → RT
R^3
R^5
R^1
OH
R^2
R^4
SEt
71-99%
(91->97% Erythro)

I.A.7.a.2-4 A. Kumar, R. Singh and A. K. Mandal, Synth. Commun., 12, 613 (1982); S. Schwarz et al., Tetrahedron, 38, 1261 (1982).

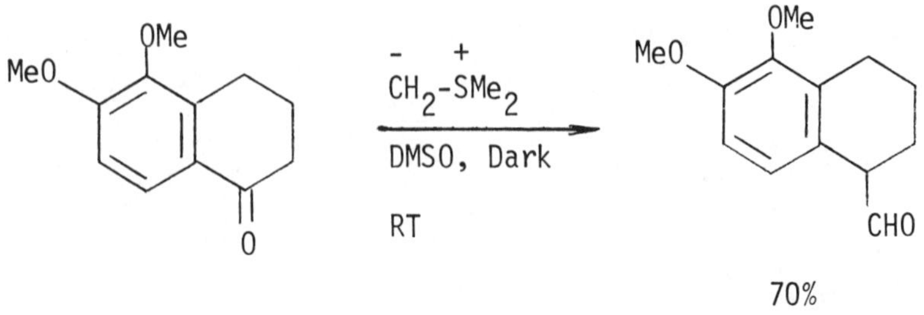

$$CH_2\text{-}SMe_2^{+-} \xrightarrow{\text{DMSO, Dark, RT}}$$

70%

I.A.7.a.2-5 W. Ried et al., Liebigs Ann. Chem., 355, 360, 396 (1982).

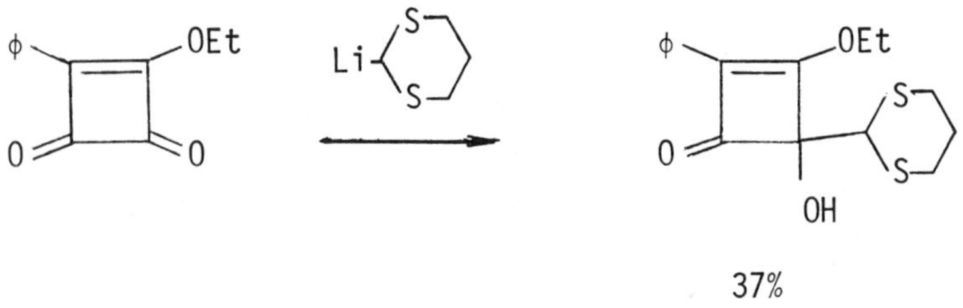

37%

I.A.7.a.2-6 R. Annunziata, M. Cinquini and F. Cozzi, Synthesis, 929 (1982); E. J. Corey and D. J. Hoover, Tetrahedron Lett., 23, 3463 (1982); M. Yokoyama, M. Hayashi and T. Imamoto, Chem. Lett., 953 (1982).

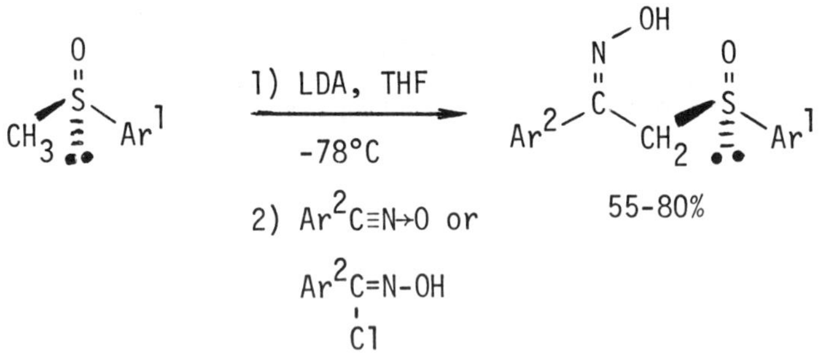

1) LDA, THF, -78°C

2) $Ar^2C{\equiv}N{\rightarrow}O$ or $Ar^2C{=}N{-}OH$ with Cl

55-80%

I.A.7.a.2-7 C. N. Hsiao and H. Shechter, Tetrahedron Lett., 23, 1963 (1982); M. Ochiai, K. Sumi and E. Fujita, ibid, 23, 5419 (1982); D. Savoia, C. Trombini and A. Umani-Ronchi, J. Org. Chem., 47, 564 (1982).

$Me_3Si\sim\sim SO_2\phi$ $\xrightarrow[\substack{1)\ nBuLi,\ Et_2O \\ -70°C \\ 2)\ R^1COR^2 \\ 3)\ MeSO_2Cl \\ 4)\ Na,\ Hg}]{}$ $Me_3Si\sim\sim C(R^1)=CR^2$ 85-95%

I.A.7.a.2-8 H. J. Reich and M. J. Kelly, J. Amer. Chem. Soc., 104, 1119 (1982).

$\xrightarrow[\text{THF, -78°C}]{\phi SO_2CR_2^-\ Li^+}$ 69-71%

Silyl Ketone Chemistry.

I.A.7.a.2-9 A. Krief et al., Chem. Commun., 564 (1982); Tetrahedron Lett., 23, 983, 4385 (1982); Y. Yamamoto, K. Maruyama et al., ibid, 23, 4597, 4959 (1982).

$\xrightarrow[\substack{Me \\ | \\ RSe-C-Li \\ | \\ Me}]{}$

Product to Hindered Epoxides or Olefins. 48-85%

I.A.7.a.2-10 K. Itoh et al., Tetrahedron Lett., 23, 4103 (1982); T. Sakakibara, S. I. Ikuta and R. Sudoh, Synthesis, 261 (1982).

$$\phi Se\underset{R^1}{\overset{R^2}{\diagup\!\!\diagdown}}\!\!=\!\!O \xrightarrow[\substack{Et_2O,\ -78°C \\ 2)\ H_2O \\ 3)\ Cat.\ SnCl_2}]{1)\ Me_3SiCH_2Li} R^1\!\!\diagup\!\!\overset{R^2}{\diagdown}\!\!\diagup\!\!Se\phi \quad 33\text{-}87\%$$

I.A.7.a.2-11 T. Hata et al., Bull. Chem. Soc. Jpn., 55, 218, 224 (1982); M. Obayashi, K. Kondo et al., Tetrahedron Lett., 23, 2323, 2327 (1982); Y. A. Zhdanov, L. A. Uzlova and L. M. Maksimushkina, J. Gen. Chem. (USSR), 52, 818 (1982).

$$\underset{OSiMe_3}{\phi CH\text{-}\overset{O}{\overset{\|}{P}}(OEt)_2} \xrightarrow[\substack{2)\ RCOCl\ or \\ (RCO)_2O}]{1)\ LDA} \underset{OSiMe_3}{\overset{\overset{O}{\overset{\|}{P}}(OEt)_2}{\phi\text{-}C\text{-}\overset{O}{\overset{\|}{C}}\text{-}R}} \quad 39\text{-}88\%$$

Cleavage of Product with NaOH, EtOH Gives α-Hydroxy Ketones.

I.A.7.a.3. 1,2-Additions of Grignard-type Carbanions

I.A.7.a.3-1 R. W. Hoffmann, Angew. Chem., Int. Ed. Engl., 21, 555 (1982).

Review: "Diastereogenic Addition of Crotylmetal Compounds to Aldehydes."

I.A.7.a.3-2   M. Tramontini, Synthesis, 605 (1982).

Review: "Stereoselective Synthesis of Diasteriomeric Amino Alcohols from Chiral Aminocarbonyl Compounds by Reduction or by Addition of Organometallic Reagents."

I.A.7.a.3-3   F. Pietra et al., J. Chem. Soc., Perkin I, 979 (1982);   G. Di Maio, E. Vecchi and E. Zeuli, Tetrahedron Lett., 23, 5211 (1982).

$$\text{bicyclic ketone} \xrightarrow[\text{Et}_2\text{O}]{\text{MeMgI}} \text{bicyclic alcohol with Me, HO}$$

90%

Axial : Equatorial Attack = 19 : 1

I.A.7.a.3-4   R. Perez-Ossorio et al., Chem. Commun., 452 (1982) H. Takahashi et al., Chem. Pharm. Bull., 30, 922, 3160 (1982); C. Scolastico et al., Tetrahedron, 38, 2725 (1982);   Y. Sakito and G. Suzukamo, Tetrahedron Lett., 23, 4953 (1982);   N. Baggett. and R. J. Simmonds, J. Chem. Soc., Perkin I, 197 (1982).

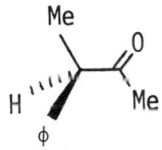

Stereochemistry of Addition Based on Nucleophilicity of φM (φMgBr, φ$_2$Mg, φLi, φ$_3$Al).

I.A.7.a.3-5 A. J. Guildford and R. W. Turner, Synthesis, 46 (1982).

[Reaction: 4-(trimethylsilyloxy)-4-cyano-cyclohexa-2,5-dienone treated with 1) R^1R^2CHLi, THF, -70°C; 2) $\phi COCl$; 3) NaF, H_2O, THF → 4-(ϕCO-O)-4-(CHR^1R^2)-cyclohexa-2,5-dienone, 20-75%]

I.A.7.a.3-6 W. Oppolzer et al., Tetrahedron Lett., 23, 3901 (1982); R. L. Snowden, B. L. Muller and K. H. Schulte-Elte, ibid, 23, 335 (1982); T. Hiyama, M. Obayashi and A. Nakamura, Organometallics, 1, 1249 (1982); A. Doucoure, B. Mauze and L. Miginiac, J. Organometal. Chem., 236, 139 (1982).

[Reaction: Me-CH=CH-CH$_2$-Cl + Mg, THF, CO_2 → HO_2C-CH(Me)-CH=CH$_2$, 94%]

Special Apparatus Avoids Usual Coupling Side Reactions.

I.A.7.a.3-7 F. Sato, Y. Suzuki and M. Sato, Tetrahedron Lett., 23, 4589 (1982); S. I. Pennanen, Synth. Commun., 12, 209 (1982).

[Reaction: $CH_2=CH-CH_2-SiMe_3$ treated with 1) nBuLi, HMPA; 2) $(\eta^5-C_5H_5)_2TiCl$; 3) RCHO; 4) H_3O^+; 5) Air → R-CH(OH)-CH(SiMe$_3$)-CH=CH$_2$, 86-98%]

I.A.7.a.3-8 M. L. Mancini and J. F. Honek, Tetrahedron Lett., 23, 3249 (1982); M. Kumada et al., Tetrahedron, 38, 3347 (1982); G. Courtois and P. Miginiac, Bull. Soc. Chim. Fr. II, 395 (1982); L. Birkofer and D. Wundram, Chem. Ber., 115, 1132 (1982).

$$Me_3SiCH_2Cl \xrightarrow[\substack{2)\ Paraformaldehyde \\ 3)\ Aq.\ NH_4Cl}]{1)\ Mg,\ Et_2O} Me_3SiCH_2CH_2OH \quad 97\%$$

I.A.7.a.3-9 P. Magnus et al., Organometallics, 1, 553, 893 (1982).

$$Me_3SiCH_2OMe \xrightarrow[\substack{2)\ -30°C \\ 3)\ R^1R^2C=O}]{1)\ s\text{-BuLi},\ THF,\ -78°C} R^1R^2C(OH)\text{-}CH(OMe)\text{-}SiMe_3 \quad 55\text{-}89\%$$

Adducts easily converted to aldehydes, enol ethers, methoxymethyl alcohols and methoxymethyl ketones.

I.A.7.a.3-10 A. I. Meyers and G. E. Jagdmann, Jr., J. Amer. Chem. Soc., 104, 877 (1982).

$$\underset{\substack{\text{Me-N-CH}_2SiMe_3 \\ \| \\ \text{N-}t\text{Bu}}}{} \xrightarrow[\substack{2)\ R^1R^2C=O \\ 3)\ NaBH_4 \\ 4)\ H^+\ (pH\ 6)}]{1)\ nBuLi} MeNH\text{-}CH(R^1)(R^2) \quad 52\text{-}70\%$$

I.A.7.a.3-11 S. R. Wilson and A. Shedrinsky, J. Org. Chem., 47, 1983 (1982).

$$R^1-\overset{O}{\underset{\|}{C}}-R^2 \xrightarrow[\text{2) BF}_3\cdot\text{AcOH}]{\text{1) Me}_3\text{SiCH}_2\text{CH}_2\text{Li}, \text{Et}_2\text{O, -78°C}} R^1-\underset{R^2}{\overset{CH}{\underset{|}{C}}}-CH=CH_2$$

38-97%

I.A.7.a.3-12 C. J. Kowalski and K. W. Fields, J. Amer. Chem. Soc., 104, 1777 (1982); R. R. Schmidt, J. Talbiersky and R. Betz, Chem. Ber., 115, 2674 (1982).

58%

I.A.7.a.3-13 J. Barluenga, J. Florez and M. Yus, Chem. Commun. 1153 (1982); Y. F. Zhou and N. Z. Huang, Synth. Commun., 12, 795 (1982); S. Masson and A. Thuillier, Tetrahedron Lett., 23, 4087 (1982); C. Kashima and Y. Yamamoto, Heterocycles, 19, 1211 (1982).

$$\xrightarrow[\text{2) Li}^+ \text{C}_{10}\text{H}_8^-, \text{-100°C}]{\text{1) nBuLi, -78°C}}$$

47%

I.A.7.a.3-14 S. Nakahama et al., Synthesis, 461 (1982); K. Hattori, K. Maruoka and H. Yamamoto, Tetrahedron Lett., 23, 3395 (1982); D. Lenoir, H. R. Seikaly and T. T. Tidwell, ibid, 23, 4987 (1982).

$$R^1_{}\!\!\diagup\!\!\underset{R^1}{C}=N-SiMe_3 \quad \xrightarrow[\text{2) } H_2O]{\text{1) } R^2Li} \quad R^1-\underset{R^2}{\overset{\phi}{\underset{|}{\overset{|}{C}}}}-NH_2$$

50-100%

I.A.7.a.3-15 R. Kober, W. Hammes and W. Steglich, Angew. Chem. Int. Ed. Engl., 21, 203 (1982); M. W. Anderson, R. C. F. Jones and J. Saunders, Chem. Commun., 282 (1982).

$$R^1\overset{O}{\overset{\|}{C}}NH-C\underset{Br}{\diagdown}\!\!\overset{CO_2Et}{\diagup}\!\!{CO_2Et} \quad \xrightarrow[\text{2) } H_3O^+]{\text{1) } 2\ R^2MgBr} \quad R^1\overset{O}{\overset{\|}{C}}NH-C\underset{R^2}{\diagdown}\!\!\overset{CO_2Et}{\diagup}\!\!{CO_2Et}$$

50-98%

I.A.7.a.3-16 M. G. Constantino, P. M. Donate and N. Petragnani, Tetrahedron Lett., 23, 1051 (1982); G. Pattenden and S. J. Teague, ibid, 23, 5471 (1982).

1) Na-≡-≡-H (3 eq.)
2) HCO_2H
3) H_3O^+

31%

I.A.7.a.3-17 L. M. Fuentes and G. L. Larson, Tetrahedron Lett., 23, 271 (1982); T. Fujisawa et al., ibid, 23, 3193, 5059 (1982); T. Fujisawa et al., Chem. Lett., 569 (1982).

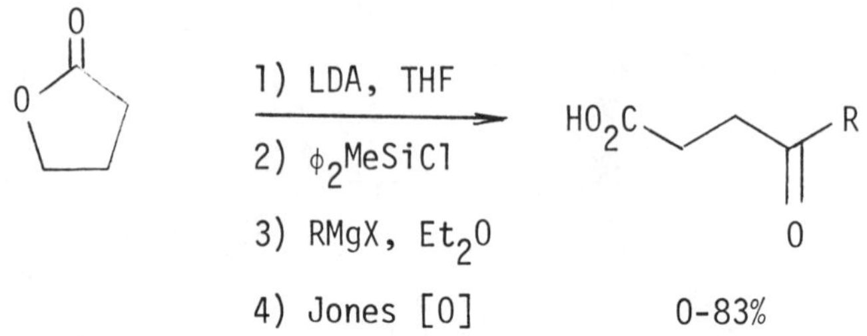

butyrolactone
1) LDA, THF
2) ϕ_2MeSiCl
3) RMgX, Et_2O
4) Jones [O]

→ $HO_2C-CH_2CH_2-C(=O)-R$

0-83%

I.A.7.a.3-18 G. W. J. Fleet and C. R. C. Spensley, Tetrahedron Lett., 23, 109 (1982); C. Jennings-White and R. G. Almquist, ibid, 23, 2533 (1982); S. R. Wilson, M. S. Hague and R. N. Misra, J. Org. Chem., 47, 747 (1982).

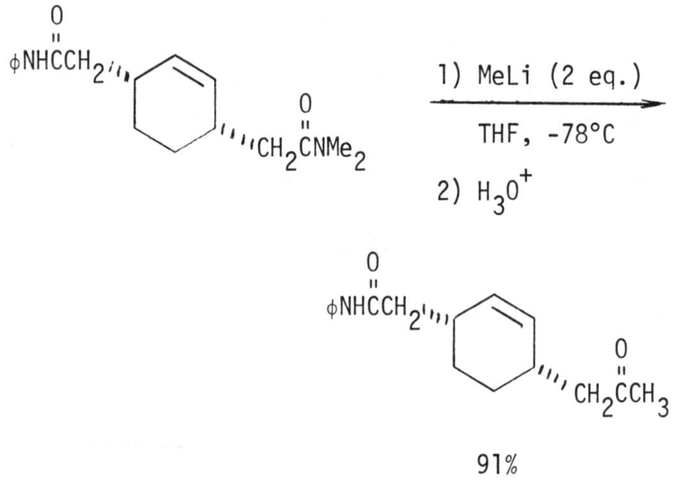

cyclohexene with $\phi NHCCH_2$— and —CH_2CNMe_2 substituents

1) MeLi (2 eq.)
   THF, -78°C
2) H_3O^+

cyclohexene with $\phi NHCCH_2$— and —CH_2CCH_3 (ketone) substituents

91%

I.A.7.a.3-19 J. E. Dubois, I. Saumtally and C. Lion, Bull. Soc. Chim. Fr. II, 318 (1982); D. W. Walba and M. D. Wand, Tetrahedron Lett., 23, 4995 (1982).

$$iPr_3C-\underset{O}{\underset{\|}{C}}-Cl \xrightarrow[\substack{2) \text{ MeI, NaNH}_2 \\ \text{DME}}]{1) \text{ RCH}_2\text{MgX} \\ \text{CuCl}} iPr_3C-\underset{O}{\underset{\|}{C}}-\underset{Me}{\underset{|}{C}}-R$$

Highly Hindered Ketones

I.A.7.a.3-20 S. W. Baldwin and H. R. Blomquist, Jr., J. Amer. Chem. Soc., 104, 4990 (1982); Tetrahedron Lett., 23, 3883 (1982); S. Watanabe et al., Aust. J. Chem., 35, 1739 (1982).

1) CH_3Li
2) NOCl
3) hv
4) pTsOH, φH

89%

I.A.7.a.3-21 C. J. Kowalski and K. W. Fields, J. Amer. Chem. Soc., 104, 321 (1982).

$$RCO_2Et \xrightarrow[\substack{2) ^t\text{BuLi} \\ 3) \text{EtOH}}]{1) \text{LiCHBr}_2} RCH_2CO_2Et$$

63%

Carbon Analogue of Hofmann Reaction.

I.A.7.a.3-22 J. Lebibi, J. Brocard and D. Couturier, Bull. Soc. Chim. Fr. II, 357 (1982).

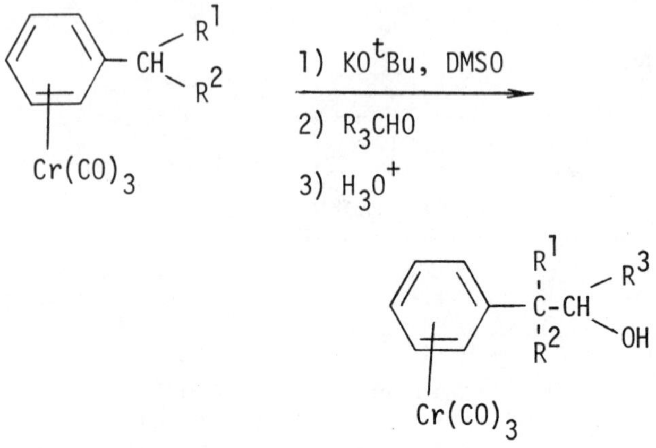

ArCH(R^1)(R^2) [Cr(CO)$_3$]
1) KO^{t}Bu, DMSO
2) R_3CHO
3) H_3O^+
→ ArC(R^1)(R^2)-CH(R^3)(OH) [Cr(CO)$_3$]

15-86%

I.A.7.a.3-23 B. H. Han and P. Boudjouk, J. Org. Chem., 47, 5030 (1982); S. G. Hegde and J. Wolinsky, J. Org. Chem., 47, 3148 (1982).

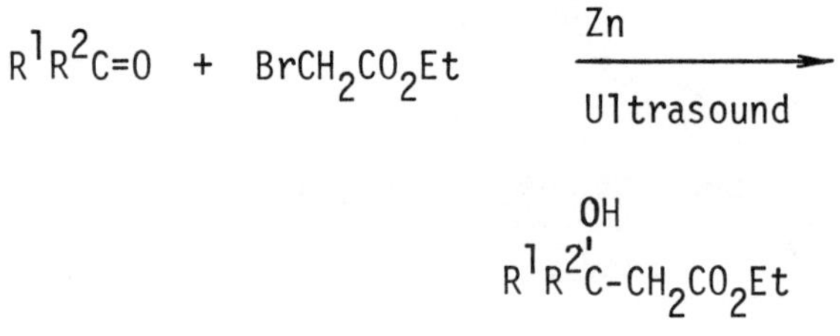

$$R^1R^2C=O + BrCH_2CO_2Et \xrightarrow[\text{Ultrasound}]{Zn} R^1R^2\underset{}{\overset{OH}{C}}-CH_2CO_2Et$$

High yields and very short reaction times in Reformatsky reaction.

I.A.7.a.3-24 D. J. Burton, T. Ishihara and M. Maruta, Chem. Lett., 755 (1982); T. Sato, T. Itoh and T. Fujisawa, ibid, 1559 (1982).

$$(nBuO)_2\overset{O}{\overset{\|}{P}}CF_2ZnBr \quad \xrightarrow[\text{Triglyme, RT}]{R-\overset{O}{\overset{\|}{C}}-Cl} \quad (nBuO)_2\overset{O}{\overset{\|}{P}}CF_2-\overset{O}{\overset{\|}{C}}-R$$

67-77%

I.A.7.a.3-25 V. B. Mochalin and T. V. Khenkina, J. Org. Chem. (USSR), 18, 583 (1982); M. Bellassoued, R. Arous-Chtara and M. Gaudemar, J. Organometal. Chem., 231, 185 (1982).

$$\underset{R^1}{\overset{Ar}{>}}C=N-CO_2R^2 \quad \xrightarrow{BrZnCH_2CO_2R^2} \quad \underset{R^1}{\overset{Ar}{>}}\underset{\underset{CH_2CO_2R^2}{|}}{C-NHCO_2R^2}$$

50-88%

I.A.7.a.3-26 M. Kumada et al., J. Amer. Chem. Soc., 104, 4962, 4963 (1982); D. Seyferth, J. Pornet and R. M. Weinstein, Organometallics, 1, 1651 (1982).

27-82%

(>85% ee)

I.A.7.a.3-27 A. Ricci et al., Tetrahedron Lett., 23, 5079 (1982); T. H. Yan and L. A. Paquette, ibid, 23, 3227 (1982).

$$\phi CH_2SiMe_3 \xrightarrow[\text{CsF or TBAF, SiO}_2]{E^+} \phi CH_2\text{-}E$$

35-90%

E^+ = ϕCHO, δ-valerolactone, cyclohexen-2-one.

I.A.7.a.3-28 A. J. Pratt and E. J. Thomas, Chem. Commun., 1115 (1982); M. Koreeda and Y. Tanaka, Chem. Lett., 1297, 1299 (1982); G. Tagliavini et al., J. Organometal. Chem., 226, 149, 307 (1982).

CHO

1) Bu$_3$SnLi

  THF, -78°C

2) MeOCH$_2$Cl

  iPr$_2$NEt

3) RCHO, ϕCH$_3$

  Δ

27-73%

I.A.7.a.3-29 M. T. Reetz et al., Tetrahedron Lett., 23, 5259 (1982); M. T. Reetz et al., Angew. Chem., Int. Ed. Engl., 21, 135 (1982).

RCHO (1 part)

+

$R^1\text{-}\overset{O}{\underset{\|}{C}}\text{-}R^2$ (1 part)

$\xrightarrow[\text{THF, -78°C}]{\text{Ti(NMe}_2)_4\text{Li}^+}$

98% Ketone

Selective

I.A.7.a.3-30   D. Seebach et al., Helv. Chim. Acta, 65, 1085, 1972, 2598 (1982);   E. Klei et al., J. Organometal. Chem., 224, 327 (1982).

$$CH_3CH=CH-CH_2-Ti(O\phi)_3 \xrightarrow{RCHO}_{THF, -100°C} \underset{R}{\overset{OH}{\text{product}}}$$

56-94%

(85-96% Diasteriosel.)

I.A.7.a.3-31   D. Hoppe et al., Angew. Chem., Int. Ed. Engl., 21, 372 (1982);   G. A. Tolstikov, F. K. Valitov and A. V. Kuchin, J. Gen. Chem. (USSR), 52, 1170 (1982).

$$\underset{OCN(iPr)_2}{\overset{AlR_2}{\text{compound}}} \xrightarrow{R^1CHO} R^1 \text{—product—} OCN(iPr)_2$$

88-95%

Also, homoaldol with (1-Oxyallyl) titanium Derivatives.

Major Diasteriomer (78-90%)

I.A.7.a.3-32   U. Hartkopf and A. de Meijere, Angew. Chem., Int. Ed. Engl., 21, 443 (1982).

$$R^1 \overset{O}{\underset{}{\text{—}}} R^2 \xrightarrow[THF, -100°C]{CF_3NO, NaN(SiMe_3)_2} R^1 \underset{}{\overset{HO\ \ CF_3}{\text{—}}} R^2$$

30-34%

I.A.7.b.1. Conjugate Additions of Enolate-type Carbanions

I.A.7.b.1-1 K. Takaki et al., <u>J. Org. Chem.</u>, 47, 1200 (1982); J. Bertrand et al., <u>Tetrahedron Lett.</u>, 23, 3267 (1982).

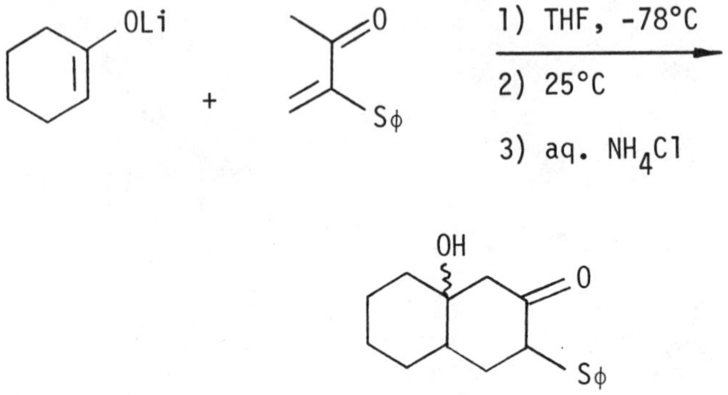

cyclohexenyl-OLi + CH$_2$=C(C(=O))–Sφ

1) THF, -78°C
2) 25°C
3) aq. NH$_4$Cl

→ decalin with OH, C=O, and Sφ substituents

80%

Products readily transformed into fused phenols.

I.A.7.b.1-2 G. Stork, C. S. Shiner and J. D. Winkler, <u>J. Amer. Chem. Soc.</u>, 104, 310, 3767 (1982); R. W. Thies and S. T. Yue, <u>Chem. Commun.</u>, 174 (1982); J. W. ApSimon, R. P. Sequin and C. P. Huber, <u>Can. J. Chem.</u>, 60, 509 (1982).

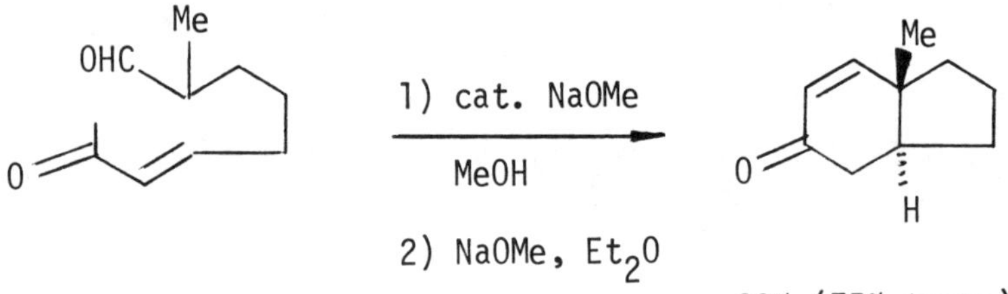

1) cat. NaOMe, MeOH
2) NaOMe, Et$_2$O

80% (75% trans)

I.A.7.b.1-3 S. J. Blarer, W. B. Schweizer and D. Seebach, Helv. Chim. Acta, 65, 1637 (1982); K. Yamamoto, M. Iijima and Y. Ogimura, Tetrahedron Lett., 23, 3711 (1982); E. Valentin et al., ibid, 23, 2683 (1982); Tetrahedron, 38, 1499 (1982); H. K. Hall, Jr., M. Abdelkader and M. E. Glogowski, J. Org. Chem., 47, 3691 (1982).

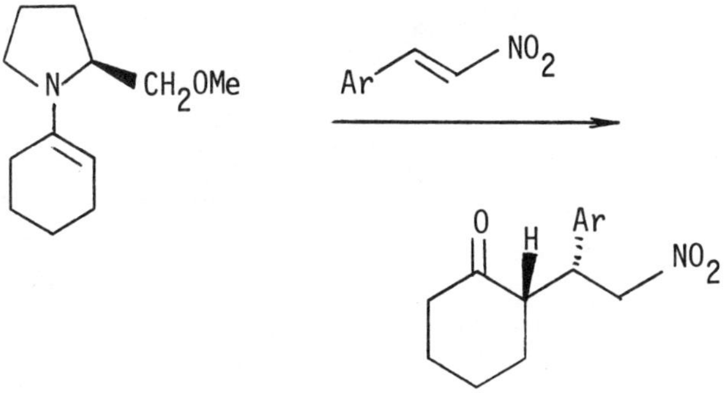

63-81%

(>90% ee)

I.A.7.b.1-4 J. W. Huffman, C. D. Rowe and F. J. Matthews, J. Org. Chem., 47, 1438 (1982).

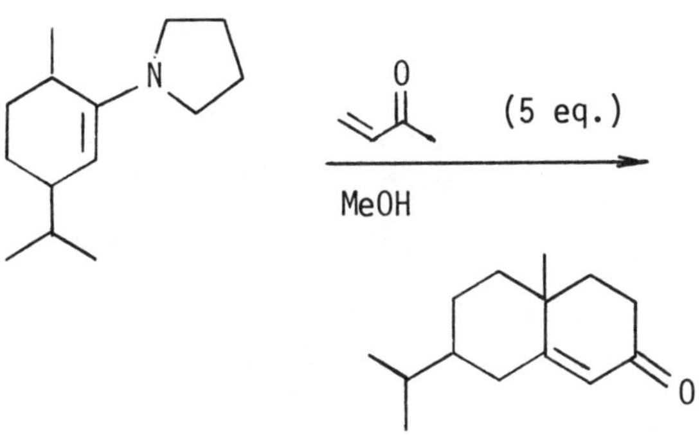

Abnormal Product

I.A.7.b.1-5 T. Fujisawa, M. Takeuchi and T. Sato, Chem. Lett., 1521, 1795 (1982).

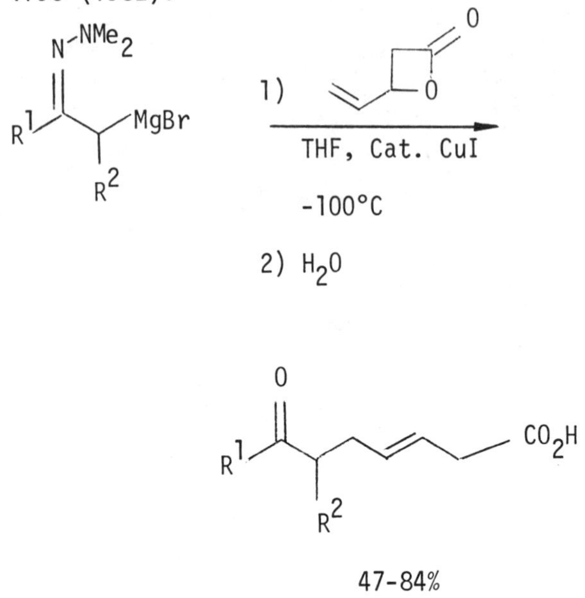

$$R^1\text{-C(=N-NMe}_2)\text{-CH(R}^2)\text{-MgBr} \xrightarrow[\text{2) H}_2\text{O}]{\text{1) vinyl-β-lactone, THF, Cat. CuI, -100°C}} R^1\text{-CO-CH(R}^2)\text{-CH}_2\text{-CH=CH-CH}_2\text{-CO}_2\text{H}$$

47-84%

I.A.7.b.1-6 P. Metzner, Chem. Commun., 335 (1982); M. Gaudemar et al., J. Organometal. Chem., 226, 209 (1982).

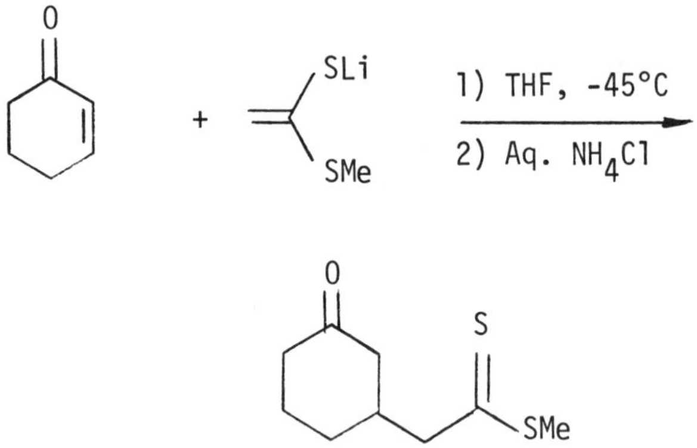

cyclohexenone + CH$_2$=C(SLi)(SMe) $\xrightarrow[\text{2) Aq. NH}_4\text{Cl}]{\text{1) THF, -45°C}}$ 3-(CH$_2$-C(=S)-SMe)-cyclohexanone

I.A.7.b.1-7 M. Miyashita, R. Yamaguchi and A. Yoshikoshi, Chem. Lett., 1505 (1982); Y. Tamura et al., J. Chem. Soc., Perkin I, 1099 (1982).

$$\underset{O_2N}{\overset{R^4}{\diagdown}}C=C\underset{H}{\overset{R^3}{\diagup}} \quad \xrightarrow[\substack{\text{THF, -100°C} \\ \text{2) } H_3O^+ \\ \text{3) } CH_2N_2}]{\text{1) } R^1R^2C(Li)(CO_2Li)} \quad R^4-C(=O)-CH(R^3)-C(R^2)(R^1)-CO_2Me$$

24-88%

I.A.7.b.1-8 D. W. Chasar, Synthesis, 841 (1982); N. Ono, A. Kaji et al., Tetrahedron Lett., 23, 2957 (1982); R. C. Cookson and P. S. Ray, ibid, 23, 3521 (1982); T. L. Ho, Synth. Commun., 12, 339 (1982).

$$\underset{R^2}{\overset{R^1}{\diagdown}}CH-NO_2 \quad \xrightarrow[\substack{\text{NaOH, } H_2O \\ CH_2Cl_2, \text{ 20°C}}]{CH_2=CH-CO_2Me} \quad R^1-\underset{\underset{NO_2}{|}}{\overset{\overset{R^2}{|}}{C}}-CH_2-CH_2-CO_2Me$$

45-65%

I.A.7.b.1-9 T. Miyakoshi, S. Saito and J. Kumanotani, Chem. Lett., 83 (1982).

$$CH_2=CH-C(=O)-R \quad \xrightarrow[\text{DMSO}]{\text{HOAc, NaNO}_2} \quad R-C(=O)-CH=CH-CH_2-C(=O)-R$$

58-86%

I.A.7.b.1-10 K. Rustemeier and E. Breitmaier, Chem. Ber., 115, 3898 (1982); L. Wartski and M. El Bouz, Tetrahedron, 38, 3285 (1982); S. R. Wilson and M. F. Price, Synth. Commun., 12, 657 (1982); G. Massiot, T. Mulamba and J. Levy, Bull. Soc. Chim. Fr. II, 241 (1982).

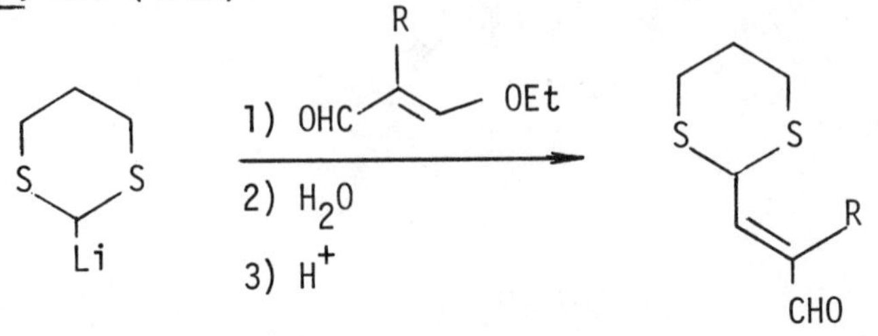

51-75%

I.A.7.b.1-11 F. E. Ziegler, et al., Tetrahedron Lett., 23, 3237 (1982); J. Amer. Chem. Soc., 104, 7174 (1982).

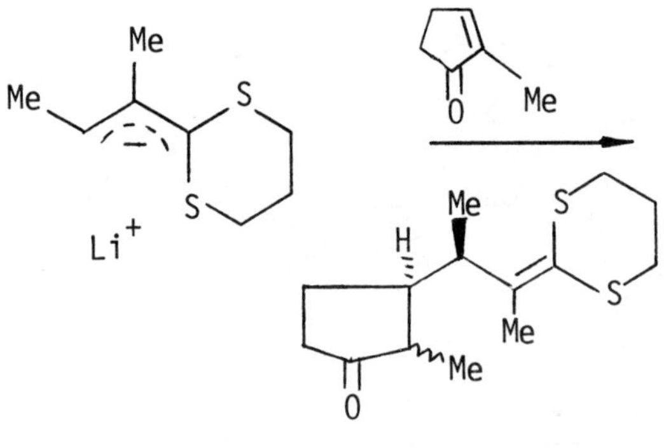

High Diasterioselectivity through an alkoxy-Cope rearrangement.

I.A.7.b.1-12 J. Nokami et al., Bull. Chem. Soc. Jpn., 55, 3043 (1982); J. Nokami et al., Chem. Lett., 607 (1982); T. Minami et al., J. Org. Chem., 47, 2360 (1982); I. M. Bazavova, V. M. Neplyuev and M. O. Lozinskii, J. Org. Chem. (USSR), 18, 750 (1982).

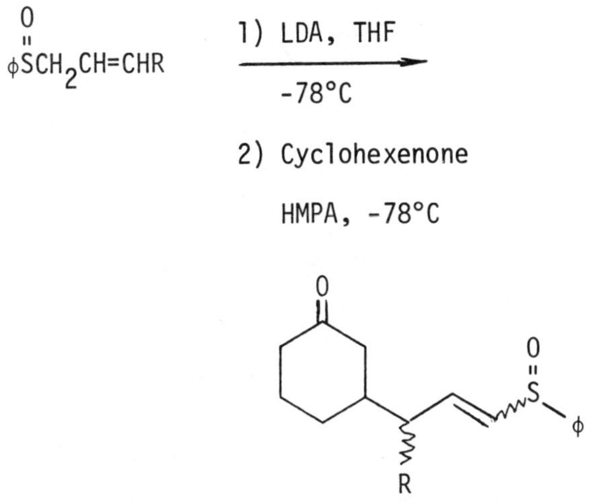

ϕSCH$_2$CH=CHR

1) LDA, THF, $-78°C$
2) Cyclohexenone, HMPA, $-78°C$

70%

I.A.7.b.1-13 T. Yoshida and S. Saito, Chem. Lett., 1587 (1982); J. Lucchetti and A. Krief, Chem. Commun., 127 (1982).

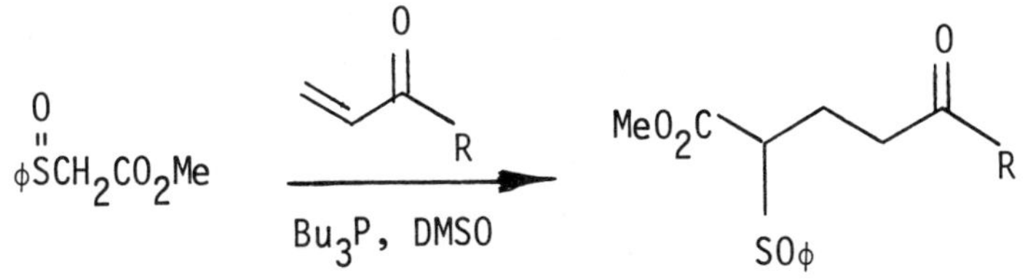

ϕSCH$_2$CO$_2$Me

Bu$_3$P, DMSO

86%

I.A.7.b.1-14 C. Chuit, R. J. P. Corriu and C. Reye, *Tetrahedron Lett.*, **23**, 5531 (1982); C. P. Fei and T. H. Chan, *Synthesis*, 467 (1982).

$$\text{CH}_3\text{CH=CHC(O)NR}_2 \xrightarrow[\text{CsF, (MeO)}_4\text{Si}]{\text{CH}_2(\text{CO}_2\text{Et})_2} \text{(EtO}_2\text{C)}_2\text{CHCH(iPr)CH}_2\text{C(O)NR}_2$$

88%

I.A.7.b.1-15 H. J. Liu and I. V. Oppong, *Can. J. Chem.*, **60**, 94 (1982); R. Cruz and R. M. Martinez, *Aust. J. Chem.*, **35**, 451 (1982); J. M. Fang, *J. Org. Chem.*, **47**, 3464 (1982).

cyclohex-2-enone $\xrightarrow[\text{2) H}_3\text{O}^+ \text{ 3) Ni(R)}]{\text{1) CH}_2(\text{CSEt})_2, \text{ DME, RT}}$ 3-(2-hydroxyethyl)cyclohexanone

74%

I.A.7.b.1-16 R. D. Little et al., *Tetrahedron Lett.*, **23**, 1339 (1982); *J. Org. Chem.*, **47**, 362 (1982).

$$\text{Br(CH}_2)_3\text{CH=C(CO}_2\text{Me})_2 \xrightarrow[\text{THF, 0°C}]{\text{Li(s-Bu)}_3\text{BH}_3} \text{1,1-bis(methoxycarbonyl)cyclopentane}$$

65%

$$\xrightarrow[\substack{\text{DMF, R}_4\text{NBr} \\ 25°\text{C}}]{-1.85 \text{ V (SCE)}}$$

[cyclobutyl]–CH(CO$_2$Et)$_2$

65-80%

I.A.7.b.1-17 A. Garcia-Raso et al., <u>Synthesis</u>, 1037 (1982); M. G. Ahmed et al., <u>Ind. J. Chem.</u>, <u>21B</u>, 470 (1982); J. L. Soto et al., <u>Org. Prep. Proc. Int.</u>, <u>14</u>, 319 (1982).

Ar^1–CH=C(Ar^2)–C(=O)– $\xrightarrow[\substack{\text{Ba(OH)}_2, \text{ EtOH} \\ \Delta}]{\text{CH}_2(\text{CO}_2\text{Et})_2}$

[cyclohexenone with Ar^1, Ar^2, EtO$_2$C substituents]

55-80%

I.A.7.b.1-18 S. Danishefsky and S. J. Etheredge, <u>J. Org. Chem.</u>, <u>47</u>, 4791 (1982); E. G. Gibbons, <u>J. Amer. Chem. Soc.</u>, <u>104</u>, 1767 (1982).

Me–C(Me)(CH(OMe)(OMe))–C(=O)–CH$_2$–CO$_2$Me

1) cyclohexenone, NaOMe, MeOH

2) pTsOH, PhCH$_3$, H$_2$O, Δ

38%

I.A.7.b.1-19 H. Irie et al., J. Chem. Soc., Perkin I, 25 (1982); M. Harre and E. Winterfeldt, Chem. Ber., 115, 1437 (1982).

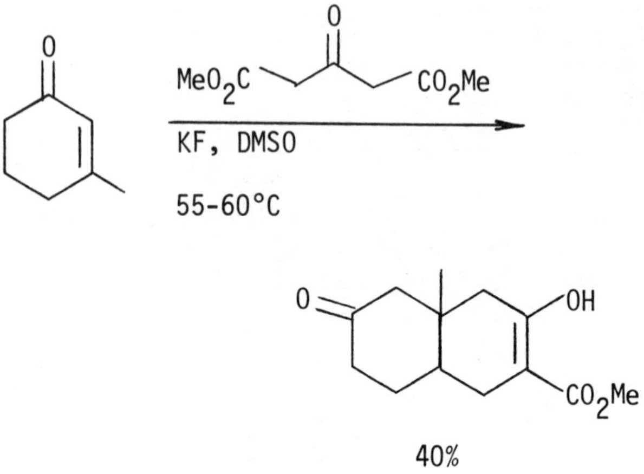

$$\text{cyclohexenone} + MeO_2C\text{-}CH_2\text{-}CO\text{-}CH_2\text{-}CO_2Me \xrightarrow[55-60°C]{KF, DMSO} \text{bicyclic product}$$

40%

I.A.7.b.2. Counjugate Additions of Organometallic Reagents

I.A.7.b.2-1 S. H. Bertz, G. Dabbagh et al., J. Amer. Chem. Soc., 104, 5824 (1982); Chem. Commun., 1030 (1982); C. R. Johnson and D. S. Dhanoa, Chem. Commun., 358 (1982).

$$RCu(P\phi_2)Li \qquad\qquad RCu(NCy_2)Li$$

Heterocuprates with Improved Thermal Stability (Cy = cyclohexyl).

I.A.7.b.2-2 J. L. Luche et al., J. Org. Chem., 47, 3805 (1982).

Formation of Organocopper Reagents with Ultrasound.

I.A.7.b.2-3 Y. Tamura, Z. Yoshida et al., <u>Tetrahedron Lett.</u>, <u>23</u>, 2383 (1982).

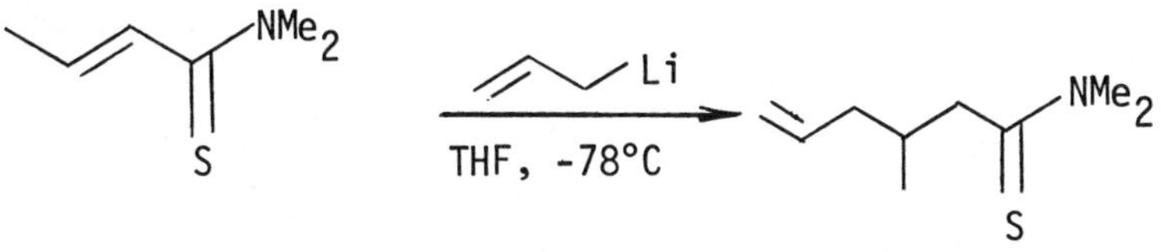

$$\underset{S}{\overset{NMe_2}{\diagdown}} \quad \xrightarrow[THF, -78°C]{\diagup\!\!\diagup Li} \quad \underset{S}{\overset{NMe_2}{\diagdown}}$$

47-89%

I.A.7.b.2-4 M. Semmelhack et al., <u>J. Org. Chem.</u>, <u>47</u>, 4382 (1982).

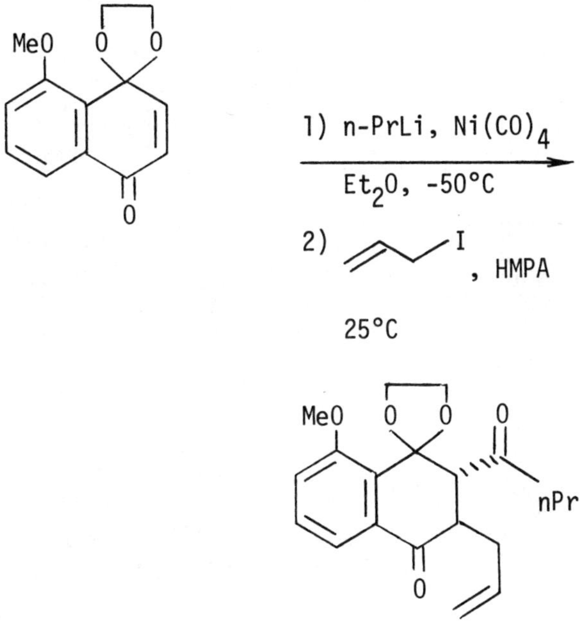

1) n-PrLi, Ni(CO)$_4$, Et$_2$O, -50°C

2) allyl–I, HMPA, 25°C

81%

I.A.7.b.2-5 Y. Yamamoto et al., J. Org. Chem., 47, 119 (1982).

$$\phi CH=CH-\underset{\underset{}{\|}}{\overset{O}{C}}-CH_3 \xrightarrow{nBuCu \cdot BF_3} \phi\underset{\underset{nBu}{|}}{CH}-CH_2-\overset{O}{\underset{\|}{C}}-CH_3$$

90%

Full Paper.

I.A.7.b.2-6 S. F. Martin and P. J. Garrison, Synthesis, 394 (1982); F. Naf, R. Decorzant and S. D. Escher, Tetrahedron Lett., 23, 5043 (1982).

1) Me$_2$CuLi
2) H$_2$O
3) nBuLi
4) ϕCHO

42%

I.A.7.b.2-7 M. Bourgain-Commercon, J. P. Foulon and J. F. Normant, J. Organometal. Chem., 228, 321 (1982); X. Huang, C. C. Chan and Q. L. Wu, Tetrahedron Lett., 23, 75 (1982); D. L. J. Clive, V. Farina and P. L. Beaulieu, J. Org. Chem., 47, 2572 (1982); D. Nasipuri, A. Sarkar and S. K. Konar, J. Org. Chem., 47, 2840 (1982).

$$\underset{R^2}{\overset{R^1}{\diagdown}}C=C\underset{CHO}{\overset{R^3}{\diagup}} \xrightarrow[THF, Me_3SiCl]{R^4CuMgCl \cdot Me_2S} R^2-\underset{R^4}{\overset{R^1}{\underset{|}{\overset{|}{C}}}}-\overset{R^3}{\underset{}{C}}=CHOSiMe_3$$

52-100%

I.A.7.b.2-8 Y. Gaoni, Tetrahedron Lett., 23, 5215, 5219
(1982); P. Yates and K. E. Stevens, Can. J. Chem., 60, 825
(1982); R. Jullien et al., Tetrahedron, 38, 2671 (1982).

$$ArSO_2-\triangleleft\!\triangleright \xrightarrow[\text{Hexane-Et}_2O]{n\text{-Bu}_2CuLi} ArSO_2-\square-n\text{-Bu}$$

87%

I.A.7.b.2-9 T. Fujisawa et al., Bull. Chem. Soc. Jpn., 55, 3555 (1982); Chem. Lett., 71, 219 (1982); Tetrahedron Lett., 23, 3583, 3587 (1982).

$$\xrightarrow[\text{Et}_2O, -78°C]{\text{RMgX, CoI}_2}$$

6-84%

I.A.7.b.2-10 M. Gill, A. J. Herlt and R. W. Rickards, Tetrahedron, 38, 3527 (1982); G. A. Kraus and M. E. Krolski, Synth. Commun., 12, 521 (1982); J. H. Dodd, R. S. Garigipati and S. M. Weinreb, J. Org. Chem., 47, 4045 (1982).

1) RLi, Et$_2$O, -78°C
2) Aq. NH$_4$Cl

40-99%

I.A.7.b.2-11 R. K. Dieter et al., Tetrahedron Lett., 23, 3747, 3751 (1982); E. Piers, K. F. Cheng and I. Nagakura, Can. J. Chem., 60, 1256 (1982).

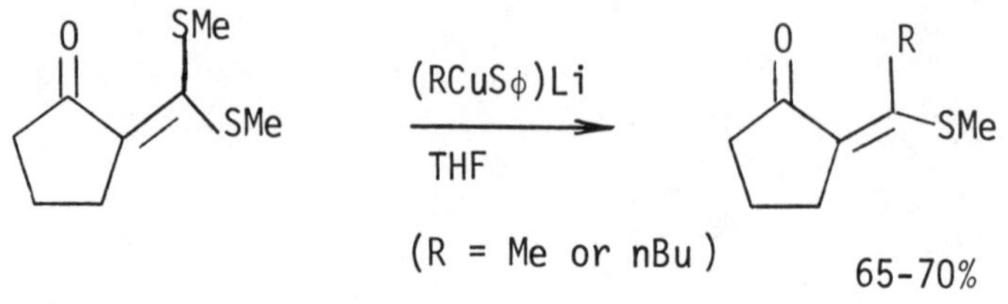

[cyclopentanone with =C(SMe)₂ ketene dithioacetal] + (RCuSφ)Li, THF → [cyclopentanone with =C(R)(SMe)] (R = Me or nBu) 65-70%

I.A.7.b.2-12 C. J. Kowalski, A. E. Weber and K. W. Fields, J. Org. Chem., 47, 5088 (1982).

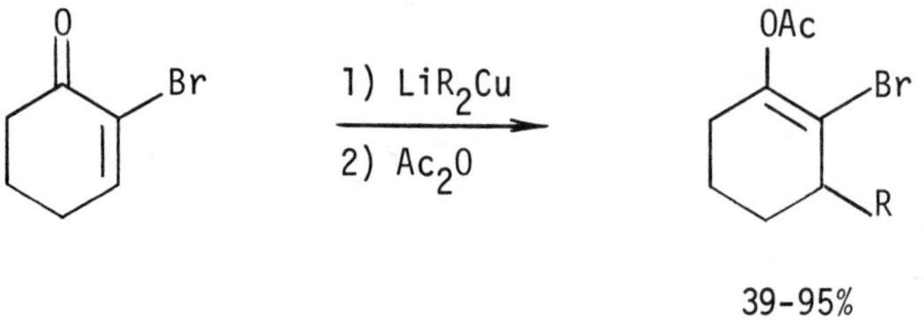

[2-bromocyclohex-2-enone] 1) LiR₂Cu 2) Ac₂O → [1-OAc-2-Br-6-R-cyclohexene] 39-95%

Extension to acyclic bromo enones largely unsuccessful.

I.A.7.b.2-13 W. C. Still and I. Galynker, J. Amer. Chem. Soc., 104, 1774 (1982).

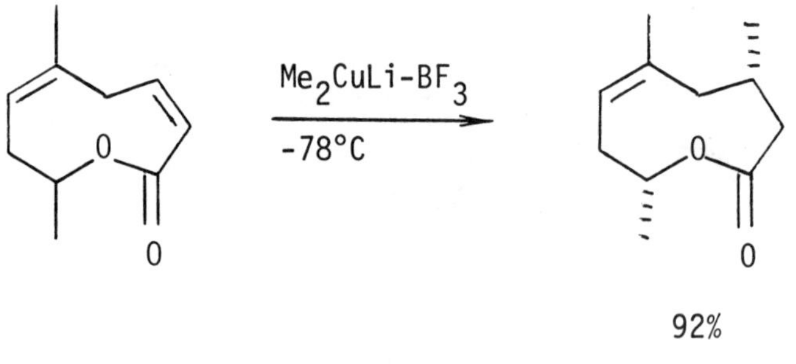

[macrocyclic unsaturated lactone] Me₂CuLi-BF₃, -78°C → [saturated lactone product] 92%

I.A.7.b.2-14 Y. Naruta, H. Uno and K. Maruyama, Chem. Lett., 609 (1982).

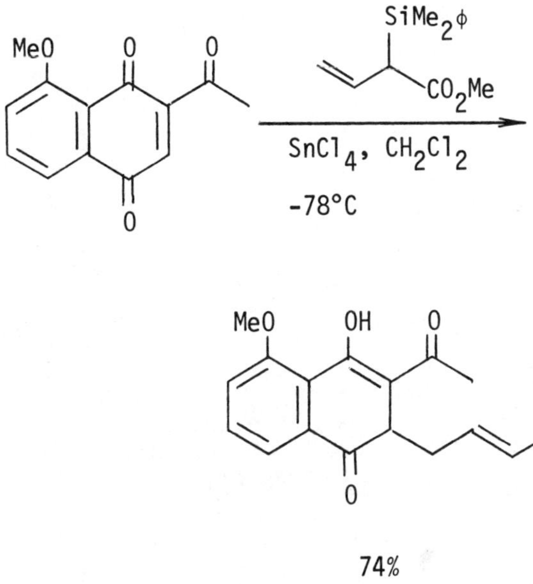

[Reaction scheme: methoxy-naphthoquinone with acetyl group + CH$_2$=CH-CH(SiMe$_2\phi$)-CO$_2$Me, SnCl$_4$, CH$_2$Cl$_2$, -78°C → product (74%)]

I.A.7.b.2-15 R. Noyori et al., Tetrahedron Lett., 23, 4057 (1982); K. Narasaka and T. Uchimaru, Chem. Lett., 57 (1982).

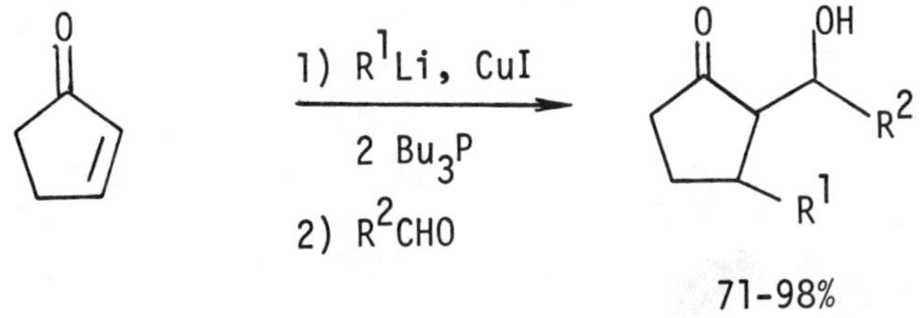

[Reaction scheme: cyclopentenone 1) R^{1}Li, CuI, 2 Bu$_3$P; 2) R^{2}CHO → 2,3-disubstituted cyclopentanone with R^1 and CH(OH)R^2 (71-98%)]

I.A.7.b.2-16 B. M. Trost and B. P. Coppola, *J. Amer. Chem. Soc.*, <u>104</u>, 6879 (1982); H. Stetter and K. Marten, <u>Liebigs Ann. Chem.</u>, 240, 250 (1982).

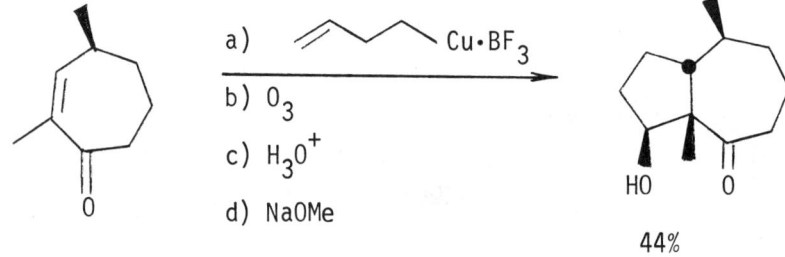

93%

I.A.7.b.2-17 C. H. Heathcock, C. M. Tice and T. C. Germroth, *J. Amer. Chem. Soc.*, <u>104</u>, 6081 (1982); S. A. Bal, A. Marfat and P. Helquist, *J. Org. Chem.*, <u>47</u>, 5045 (1982).

a) ∕=∕∕∕∕ Cu·BF$_3$
b) O$_3$
c) H$_3$O$^+$
d) NaOMe

44%

I.A.7.b.2-18 B. H. Lipshutz, R. S. Wilhelm and J. Kozlowski, *Tetrahedron Lett.*, <u>23</u>, 3755 (1982); P. J. De Clercq et al., *ibid*, 3283, 3287, 3291 (1982); H. Malmberg and M. Nilsson, *Tetrahedron*, <u>38</u>, 1509 (1982); A. Risaliti et al., *ibid*, <u>38</u>, 1459 (1982).

φ$_2$Cu(CN)Li$_2$ / Et$_2$O, -78°C

82%

I.A.7.b.2-19 G. Stork and D. H. Sherman, J. Amer. Chem. Soc., 104, 3758 (1982).

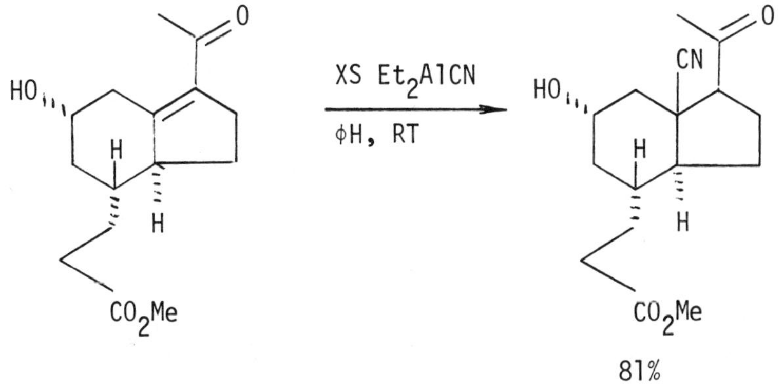

XS Et$_2$AlCN, φH, RT

81%

I.A.7.b.2-20 M. Nilsson and C. Ullenius, et al., Tetrahedron Lett., 23, 3823, (1982); Tetrahedron, 38, 389 (1982); G. H. Posner et al., J. Amer. Chem. Soc., 104, 4180 (1982).

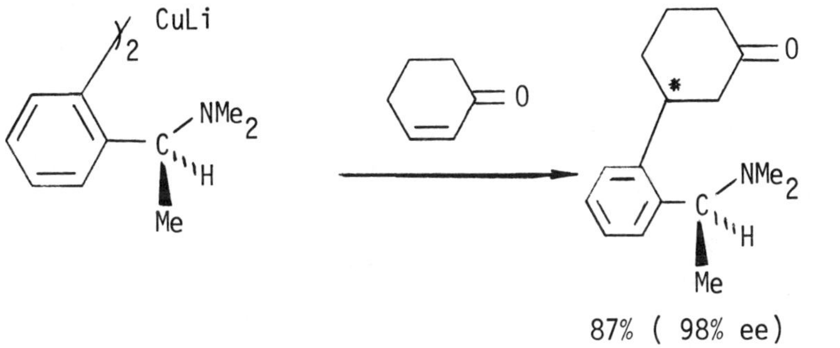

87% (98% ee)

I.A.7.b.3. Other Conjugate Additions

I.A.7.b.3-1 B. M. Trost, et al., Organometallics, 1, 1543 (1982); J. Amer. Chem. Soc., 104, 3733 (1982).

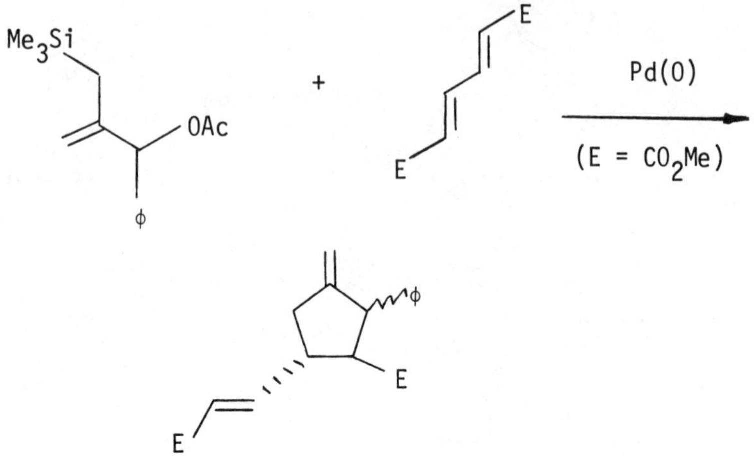

(E = CO_2Me)

70-75%

I.A.7.b.3-2 A. Bucheister, P. Klemarczyk and M. Rosenblum, Organometallics, 1, 1679 (1982).

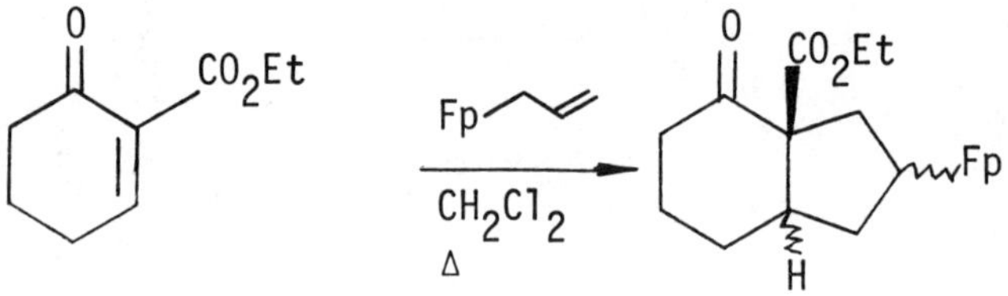

63%

I.A.7.b.3-3 S. Danishefsky, S. Chackalamannil and B. J. Uang, J. Org. Chem., 47, 2231 (1982).

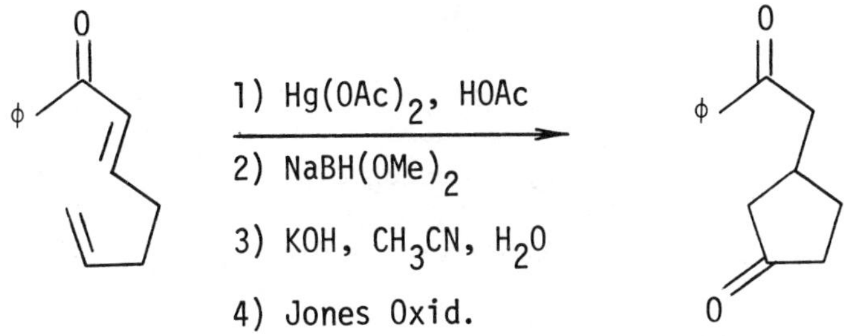

φ-CO-CH=CH-CH2-CH=CH2

1) Hg(OAc)$_2$, HOAc
2) NaBH(OMe)$_2$
3) KOH, CH$_3$CN, H$_2$O
4) Jones Oxid.

→ φ-CO-CH$_2$-(3-oxocyclopentyl)

56%

I.A.7.b.3-4 J. M. Pons and M. Santelli, Tetrahedron Lett., 23, 4937 (1982); A. Citterio, A. Arnoldi and A. Griffini, Tetrahedron, 38, 393 (1982).

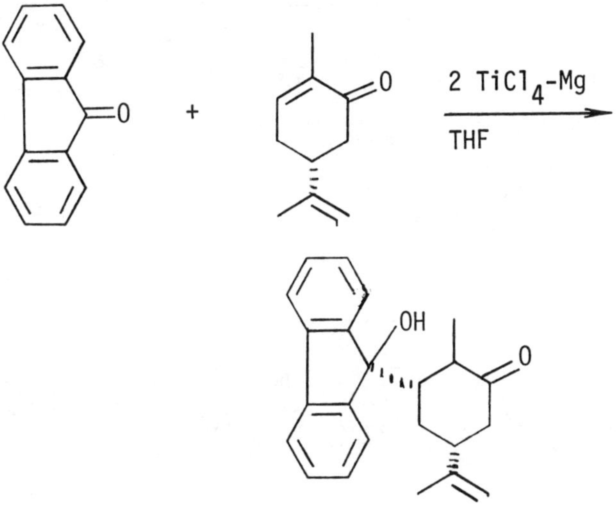

fluorenone + carvone →[2 TiCl$_4$-Mg, THF]

→ adduct (fluorenyl-OH attached to cyclohexanone with isopropenyl)

70%

I.A.7.b.3-5 F. Guibe, D. S. Grierson and H. P. Husson, Tetrahedron Lett., 23, 5055 (1982).

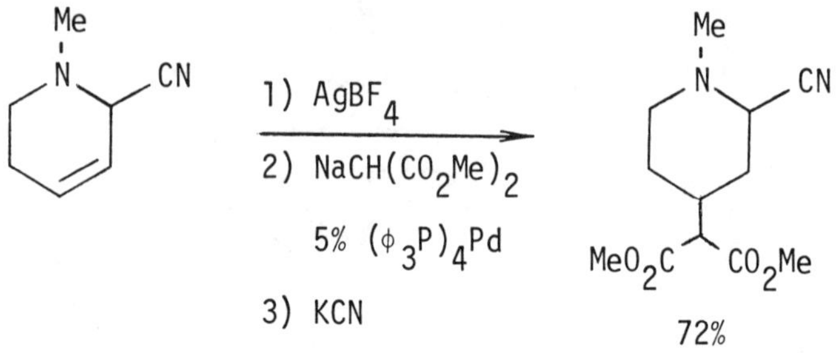
Me
N
CN
1) $AgBF_4$
2) $NaCH(CO_2Me)_2$
5% $(\phi_3P)_4Pd$
3) KCN
Me
N
CN
MeO_2C
CO_2Me
72%

I.A.8. Other Carbon-Carbon Single Bond Forming Reactions

I.A.8-1 E. W. Petrillo, Jr. et al., J. Med. Chem., 25, 250 (1982); T. Shono et al., J. Amer. Chem. Soc., 104, 6697 (1982).

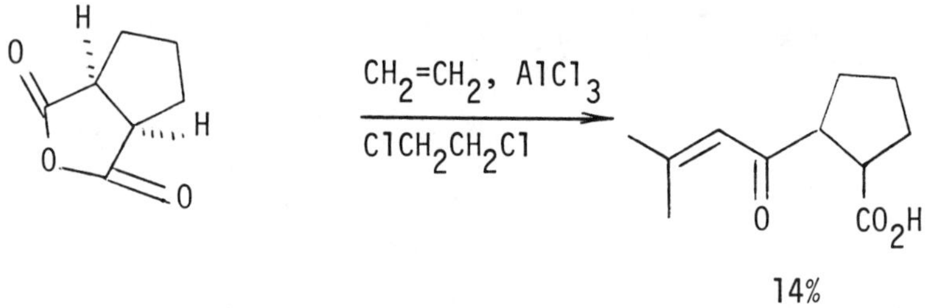
H
O
H
O
O
$CH_2=CH_2$, $AlCl_3$
$ClCH_2CH_2Cl$
O
CO_2H
14%

I.A.8-2 S. E. Denmark and T. K. Jones, J. Amer. Chem. Soc., 104, 2642 (1982); J. Org. Chem., 47, 4595 (1982); P. Magnus et al., Organometallics, 1, 1240, 1243 (1982).

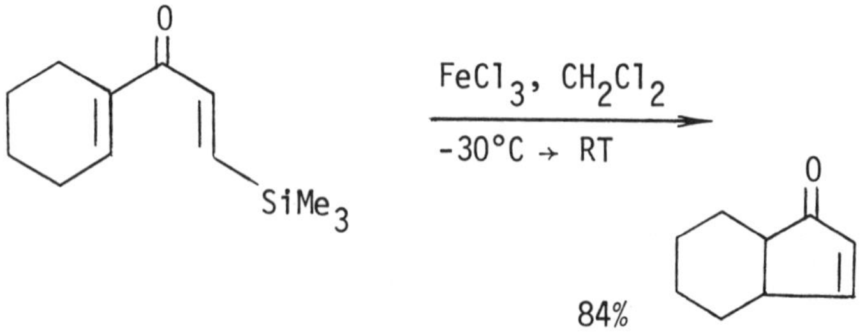
O
$SiMe_3$
$FeCl_3$, CH_2Cl_2
-30°C → RT
O
84%

I.A.8-3 B. B. Snider et al., J. Org. Chem., 47, 4538 (1982);
M. J. Smith and S. E. Wilson, Tetrahedron Lett., 23, 5013 (1982).

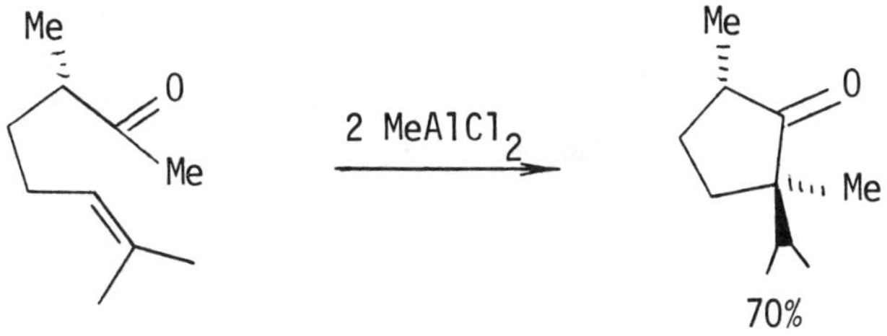

[Reaction: acyclic methyl ketone with pendant trisubstituted alkene + 2 MeAlCl$_2$ → cyclopentanone with Me substituent, 70%]

I.A.8-4 H. Suzuki, Y. Moro-Oka et al., Tetrahedron Lett., 23, 4031, 1079 (1982); G. Pattenden and S. Teague, ibid, 23, 1403 (1982).

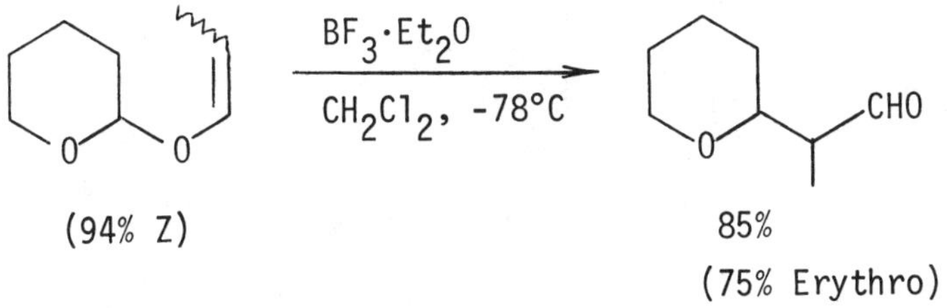

[Reaction: 2-(propenyl)tetrahydropyran (94% Z) + BF$_3$·Et$_2$O, CH$_2$Cl$_2$, -78°C → 2-(1-methyl-2-oxoethyl)tetrahydropyran, 85% (75% Erythro)]

I.A.8-5 N. Bluthe, M. Malacria and J. Gore, Tetrahedron Lett., 23, 4263 (1982); T. Matsumoto et al., ibid, 23, 2099 (1982).

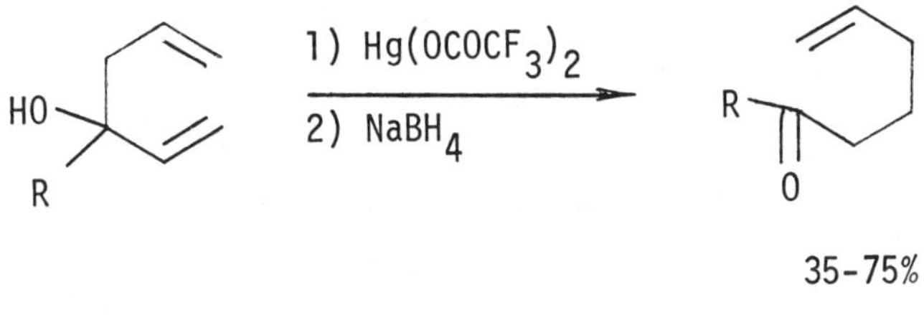

[Reaction: diallyl carbinol (HO, R) 1) Hg(OCOCF$_3$)$_2$ 2) NaBH$_4$ → cyclohexenone derivative, 35-75%]

I.A.8-6 C. Giordano et al., Tetrahedron Lett., 23, 1385 (1982); J. Chem. Soc., Perkin I, 2575 (1982); K. Itoh et al., Chem. Commun., 1232 (1982).

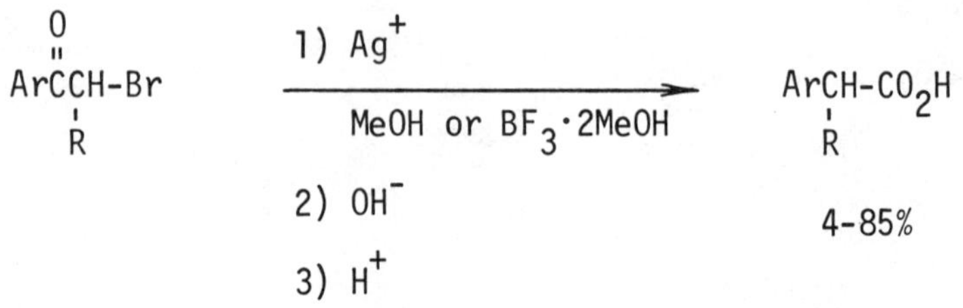

$$\underset{R}{ArC(O)CH-Br} \xrightarrow[\substack{\text{2) OH}^- \\ \text{3) H}^+}]{\substack{\text{1) Ag}^+ \\ \text{MeOH or BF}_3\cdot\text{2MeOH}}} \underset{R}{ArCH-CO_2H}$$

4-85%

I.A.8-7 C. Cambillau and M. Charpentier-Morize, Chem. Commun., 211 (1982).

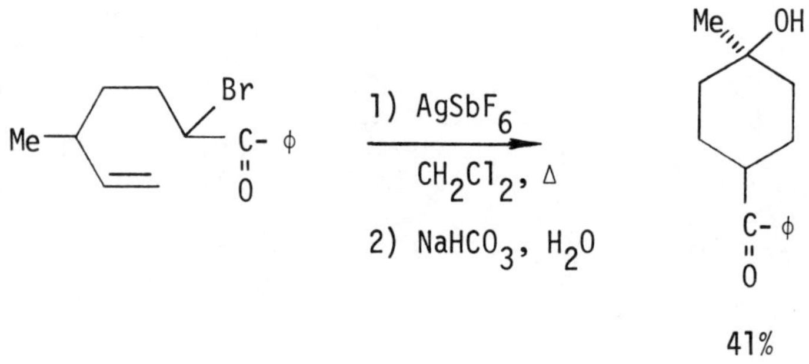

41%

I.A.8-8 Y. Masaki et al., Tetrahedron Lett., 23, 1481 (1982); R. J. Armstrong, F. L. Harris and L. Weiler, Can. J. Chem., 60, 673 (1982).

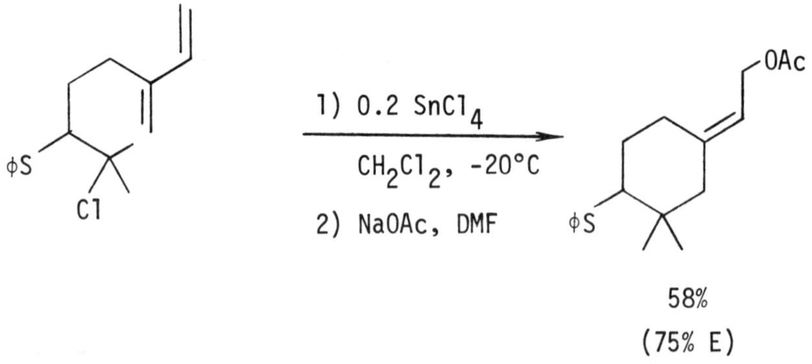

58%
(75% E)

I.A.8-9 S. V. Ley et al., Chem. Commun., 1251, 1252 (1982);
A. Toshimitsu, S. Uemura and M. Okano, ibid, 87 (1982).

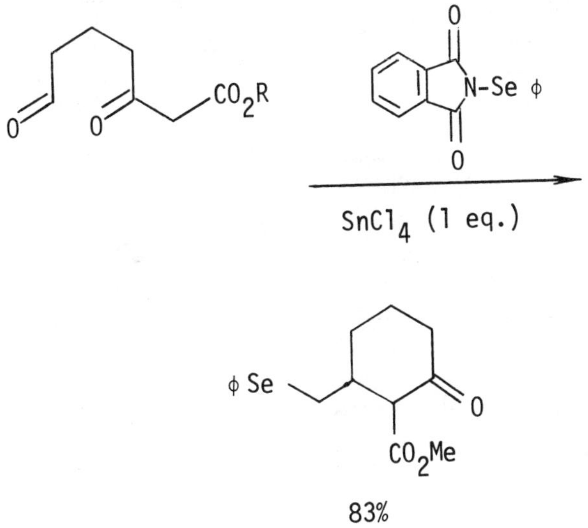

$$\xrightarrow{SnCl_4 \text{ (1 eq.)}}$$

83%

I.A.8-10 C. Schmidt, N. H. Chishti and T. Breining, Synthesis, 391 (1982); J. H. Rigby, Tetrahedron Lett., 23, 1863 (1982).

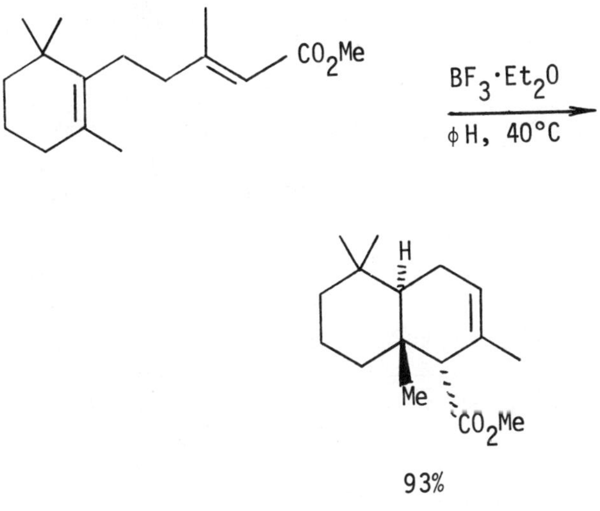

$$\xrightarrow[\phi H, 40°C]{BF_3 \cdot Et_2O}$$

93%

I.A.8-11 E. J. Brunke, F. J. Hammerschmidt and H. Struwe, Chem. Ber., 115, 3128 (1982); T. S. Sorensen et al., Can. J. Chem., 60, 2993 (1982); L. I. Zakharkin, et al., J. Org. Chem. (USSR), 18, 80, 83, 281 (1982).

[Structure] →(1) HCO$_2$H, 2) NaOH)→ [Structure] 61%

I.A.8-12 W. W. Epstein, J. R. Grua and D. Gregonis, J. Org. Chem., 47, 1128 (1982); J. Ackroyd, K. A. Pover and F. Scheinmann, Tetrahedron Lett., 23, 5583 (1982); R. Henning and H. M. R. Hoffmann, ibid, 23, 2305 (1982).

[Structure] →(CF$_3$CO$_2$H, 0°C)→ [Structure] 95%

I.A.8-13 M. S. Baird, et al., Chem. Commun., 224 (1982); J. Chem. Soc. (S), 290 (1982); M. G. Banwell, Chem. Commun., 847 (1982); R. Menicagli, C. Malanga and L. Lardicci, J. Org. Chem., 47, 2288 (1982).

[Structure] →(AgClO$_4$, MeOH, RT)→ [Structure] 75%

I.A.8-14 A. M. Birch and G. Pattenden, <u>Tetrahedron Lett.</u>, <u>23</u>, 991 (1982); J. A. Miller and G. M. Ullah, <u>Chem. Commun.</u>, 874 (1982).

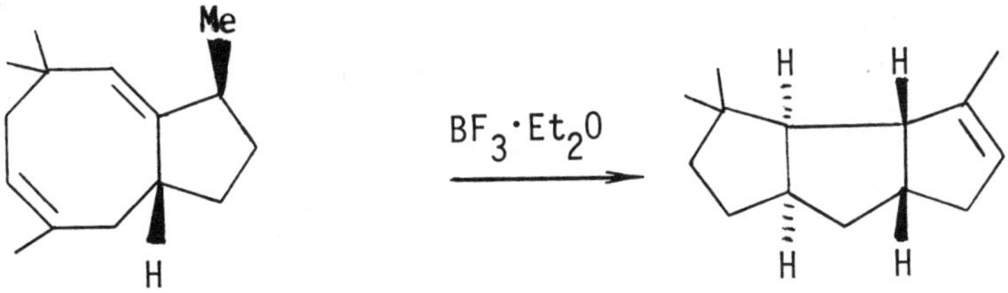

I.A.8-15 T. Masamune et al., <u>Chem. Commun.</u>, 511, 513, 32 (1982); N. Lamb et al., <u>Can. J. Chem.</u>, <u>60</u>, 1055 (1982).

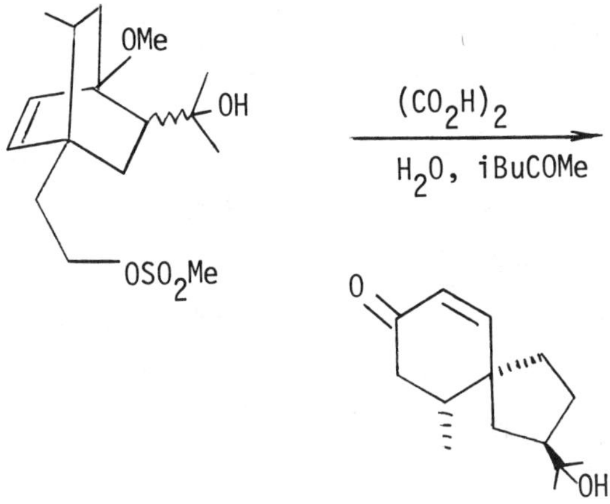

35%

I.A.8-16 H. Shirahama et al., Bull. Chem. Soc. Jpn., 55, 2691 (1982); Chem. Lett., 1417 (1982).

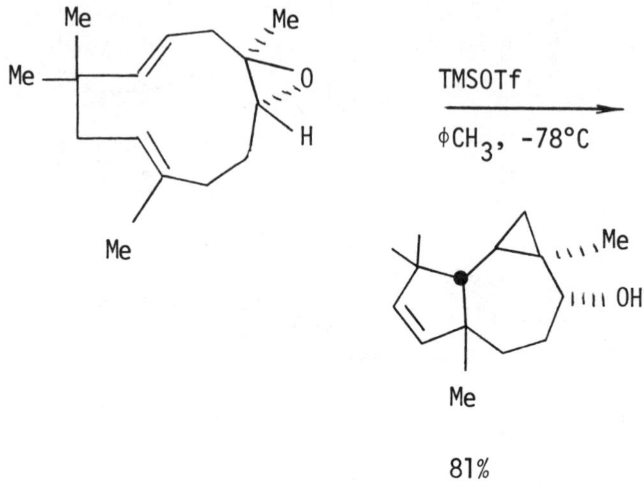

81%

I.A.8-17 W. S. Johnson et al., J. Amer. Chem. Soc., 104, 3508, 3510 (1982); Tetrahedron, 38, 1397 (1982); J. Org. Chem., 47, 161 (1982); M. B. Groen et al., Tetrahedron Lett., 23, 3611 (1982); Rec. Trav. Chim., 101, 148 (1982).

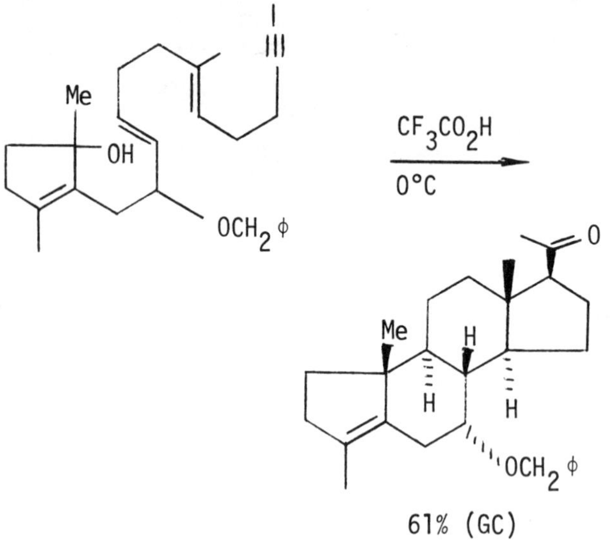

61% (GC)

I.A.8-18 E. E. van Tamelen et al., J. Amer. Chem. Soc., 104, 1785, 2061, 6479, 6480 (1982); W. Herz and J. S. Prasad, J. Org. Chem., 47, 4171 (1982); T. A. Bryson and L. T. McElligott, Synth. Commun., 12, 307 (1982).

$$\xrightarrow{SnCl_4, CH_2Cl_2, 0°C}$$

> 51%

I.A.8-19 J. C. Mullis and W. P. Weber, J. Org. Chem., 47, 2873 (1982); P. G. Gassman and T. L. Guggenheim, J. Amer. Chem. Soc., 104, 5849 (1982); F. G. de las Heras and P. Fernandez-Resa, J. Chem. Soc., Perkin I, 903 (1982); J. L. Belletire, H. Howard and K. Donahue, Synth. Commun., 12, 763 (1982); F. Duboudin et al., Synthesis, 212 (1982); M. T. Reetz and I. Chatziiosifidis, ibid, 330 (1982).

$$\xrightarrow{Me_3SiCN, Et_2AlCl} NC-CH_2\overset{CH_3}{\underset{}{CH}}-OSiMe_3$$

83%

I.A.8-20 S. Tomoda, Y. Takeuchi and Y. Nomura, Chem. Commun., 871 (1982); Tetrahedron Lett., 23, 1361 (1982).

$$\xrightarrow{\phi SeCN, SnCl_4 \text{ (1 eq.)}, CH_2Cl_2, 15°C}$$

96%

I.A.8-21 J. F. King et al., J. Amer. Chem. Soc., 104, 7108 (1982); O. Meth-Cohn, A. J. Reason and S. M. Roberts, Chem. Commun., 90 (1982).

$$ROSO_2\text{-}CH_2CH_2\text{-}\overset{+}{N}Me_3 \quad FSO_3^- \xrightarrow[20°C]{KCN, H_2O} ROSO_2\text{-}CH_2CH_2\text{-}CN \quad 90\%$$

I.A.8-22 A. Nudelman and E. Keinan, Synthesis, 687 (1982).

$$RCH=CH\text{-}CHO \xrightarrow{\begin{array}{l}1)\ KCN,\ Ac_2O\\ 2)\ Pd,\ THF\\ 3)\ NaOMe,\ MeOH\\ 4)\ Cl\text{-}\overset{O}{\underset{\|}{C}}\text{-}\overset{O}{\underset{\|}{C}}\text{-}Cl,\ DMSO\end{array}} R\overset{O}{\underset{\|}{C}}CH=CHCN$$

I.A.8-23 W. R. Jackson et al., Tetrahedron Lett., 23, 1621 (1982); Aust. J. Chem., 35, 2041 (1982); H. Bock, J. Wittmann and H. J. Arpe, Chem. Ber., 115, 2326 (1982).

[Reaction: cyclohexene with tBu substituent + DCN, Pd(DIOP)$_2$ → two cyclohexane products with CN and D substituents and tBu group]

No axial cyanides.

I.A.8-24 W. Kantlehner and E. Haug, Synthesis, 146 (1982).

$$R^2N\text{-}CH\begin{array}{l}OMe\\ CN\end{array} \xrightarrow{HCN} \begin{array}{c}NC\\ R^2N\end{array}C=C\begin{array}{c}N=C\\ CN\end{array}\begin{array}{c}NR_2\\ H\end{array} \quad 62\text{-}85\%$$

I.A.8-25 M. Lounasmaa and A. Koskinen, Tetrahedron Lett., 23, 349 (1982).

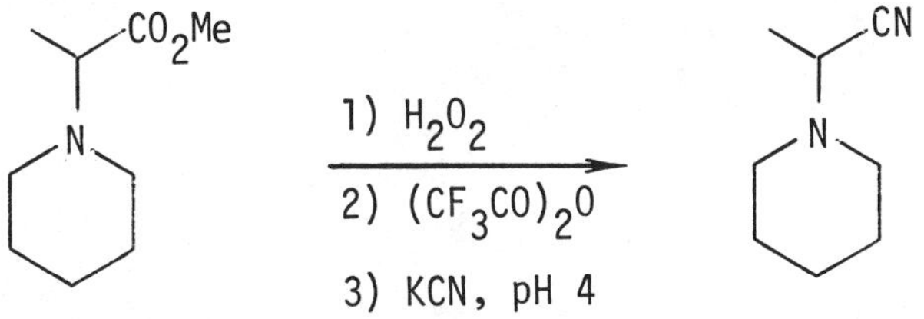

piperidine-CH(CO$_2$Me)Me →
1) H$_2$O$_2$
2) (CF$_3$CO)$_2$O
3) KCN, pH 4
→ piperidine-CH(CN)Me

25%

I.A.8-26 T. Saegusa et al., J. Amer. Chem. Soc., 104, 6449 (1982).

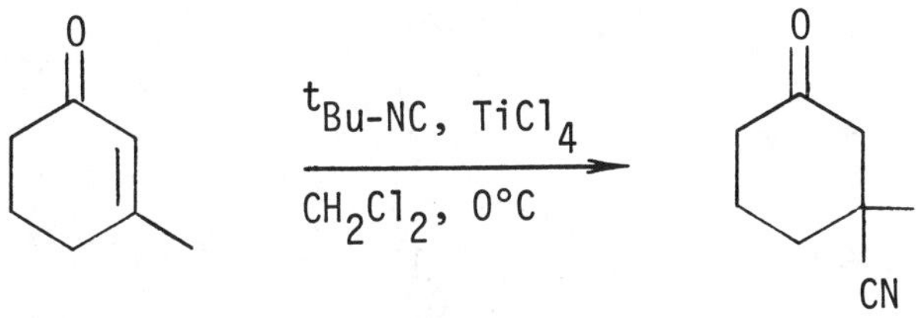

3-methylcyclohex-2-enone
^{t}Bu-NC, TiCl$_4$
CH$_2$Cl$_2$, 0°C
→ 3-methyl-3-cyanocyclohexanone

84%

I.A.8-27 B. M. Trost et al., J. Amer. Chem. Soc., 104, 3225, 3228 (1982).

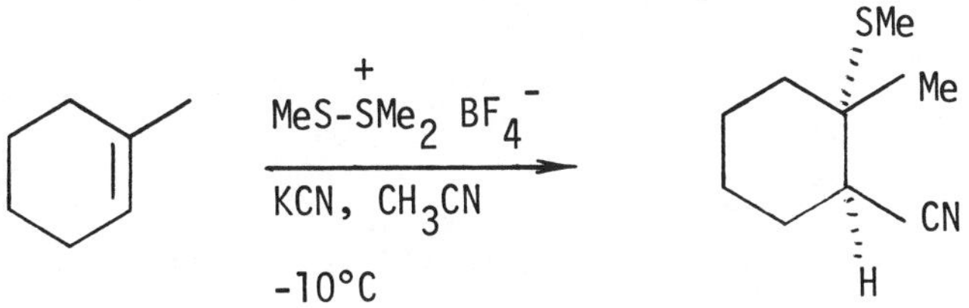

1-methylcyclohexene + MeS-SMe$_2^+$ BF$_4^-$
KCN, CH$_3$CN
−10°C
→ 1-methyl-1-(SMe)-2-(CN)cyclohexane

99%
(92% E)

I.A.8-28 M. F. Lappert and R. K. Maskell, Chem. Commun., 580 (1982); C. S. Sell and L. A. Dorman, ibid, 629 (1982); J. Castells et al., Tetrahedron, 38, 337 (1982); M. Yokoyama, K. Hoshi and T. Imamoto, Chem. Lett., 1615 (1982).

$$\phi CHO \xrightarrow[\text{(Benzoin Catalyst)}]{\begin{bmatrix} N & N \\ \diagdown \\ N & N \end{bmatrix}} \phi\text{-CH-C-}\phi \quad \begin{array}{c} OH\ O \\ |\ \ \| \end{array}$$

60%   84%

I.A.8-29 S. Hunig and R. Schaller, Angew. Chem., Int. Ed. Engl., 21, 36 (1982).

Review: "The Chemistry of Acyl Cyanides."

I.A.8-30 H. M. R. Hoffmann, et al., Angew. Chem., Int. Ed. Engl., 21, 83 (1982); Chem. Ber., 115, 3880 (1982).

$$\underset{}{\text{R-C-I}} \xrightarrow[\underset{\Delta}{CH_2Cl_2 \text{ or } CH_3CN}]{CuCN} \underset{27-78\%}{\text{R-C-CN}}$$
(with O double bonds on each carbonyl)

I.A.8-31 G. B. Schuster, Tetrahedron, 38, 1027-1122 (1982).

Review: "Electron-Transfer Initiated Reactions" (Symposium - In-Print, 10 Papers).

I.A.8-32 M. Chanon and M. L. Tobe, Angew. Chem., Int. Ed. Engl., 21, 1 (1982).

Review: "ETC (Electron-Transfer Catalysis): A Mechanistic Concept for Inorganic and Organic Chemistry."

I.A.8-33 J. M. Tedder, Angew. Chem., Int. Ed. Engl., 21, 401 (1982).

Review: "Which Factors Determine the Reactivity and Regioselectivity of Free Radical Substitution and Addition Reactions?"

I.A.8-34 H. Wendt, Angew. Chem., Int. Ed. Engl., 21, 256 (1982).

Review: "The Reactivity of Primary Free Radicals and Radical Ions, Mass Transfer, and Electrosorption - The Fundamental Factors for Selectivity in Electrochemical Syntheses of Organic Compounds."

I.A.8-35 M. Chanon, Bull. Soc. Chim. Fr. II, 197 (1982).

Review: "Electron Transfer Catalysis Applied to Organometallics. Part I. Application to the Activation of $C_{sp}3$ X Bonds and Other σ Bonded Species."

I.A.8-36   M. Dagonneau, Bull. Soc. Chim. Fr. II, 269 (1982).

Review: "Radical Reactions of Grignard Reagents."

I.A.8-37   G. Stork and N. H. Baine, J. Amer. Chem. Soc., 104, 2321 (1982); M. D. Johnson et al., ibid, 104, 5230 (1982); R. N. Renaud, C. J. Stephens and D. Beruba, Can. J. Chem., 60, 1687 (1982).

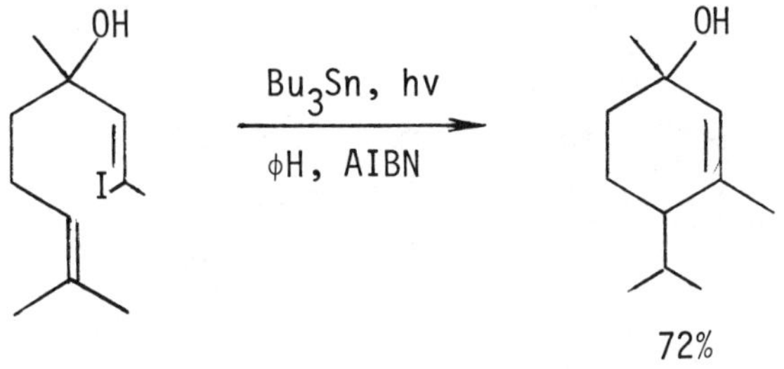

$$\text{substrate} \xrightarrow[\phi H, \text{AIBN}]{Bu_3Sn, h\nu} \text{product} \quad 72\%$$

I.A.8-38   B. Giese, et al., Tetrahedron Lett., 23, 931, 2765 (1982); Angew. Chem., Int. Ed. Engl., 21, 130 (1982); Chem. Ber., 115, 2526 (1982); Synthesis, 735 (1982).

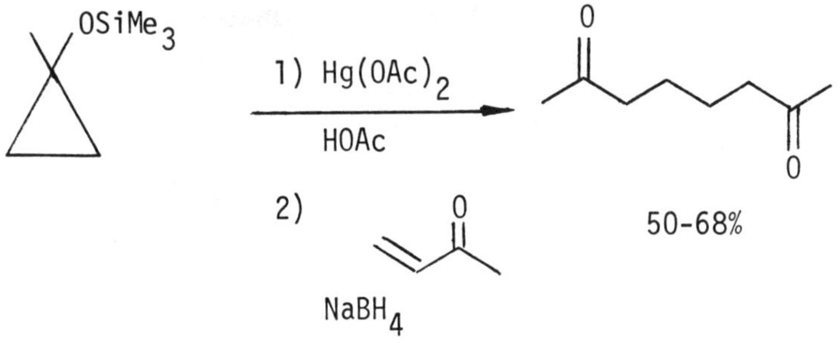

$$\text{cyclopropane-OSiMe}_3 \xrightarrow[\substack{2) \text{ methyl vinyl ketone} \\ NaBH_4}]{1) Hg(OAc)_2, HOAc} \text{diketone} \quad 50\text{-}68\%$$

I.A.8-39 J. J. Villenave et al., Tetrahedron Lett., 23, 3487 (1982); C. Filliatre et al., Bull. Soc. Chim. Fr. II, 352 (1982).

$$CH_3CH_2COMe \;+\; \text{CH}_2=\text{CHO-CO-O-O}^t\text{Bu} \xrightarrow{140°C} CH_3CH(CO_2Me)CH_2CHO \quad 43\%$$

I.A.8-40 W. C. Agosta and S. Wolff, Pure Appl. Chem., 54, 1579 (1982).

Review: "Photochemistry of Carbonyl-Substituted Hexadienes."

I.A.8-41 M. Demuth and K. Schaffner, Angew. Chem., Int. Ed. Engl., 21, 820 (1982).

Review: "Tricyclo[3.3.0.0^{2,8}]octan-3-ones: Photochemically Prepared Building Blocks for Enantiospecific Total Syntheses of Cyclopentanoid Natural Products."

I.A.8-42 P. A. Wender and J. J. Howbert, Tetrahedron Lett., 23, 3983 (1982); J. P. Morizur and J. Tortajada, ibid, 23, 5275 (1982); S. Katsumura and S. Isoe, Helv. Chim. Acta, 65, 1927 (1982).

Reagents: 1) hv 2) LAH 3) 10-Camphorsulfonic acid   13%

I.A.8-43   D. Pletcher, Chem. Ind., 358 (1982).

Review: "Organic Electrosynthesis in the Fine Chemicals Industry."

I.A.8-44   T. Shono et al., Tetrahedron Lett., 23, 1609 (1982); C. Degrand, P. L. Compagnon and F. Gasquez, J. Org. Chem., 47, 4586 (1982); P. Margaretha and P. Tissot, Helv. Chim. Acta, 65, 1949 (1982).

$$\text{RCHO} \xrightarrow[\substack{CCl_4,\ CHCl_3 \\ \text{2) NaH, MeI, THF} \\ \text{3) } + e^-,\ MeOH,\ H_2O \\ \text{4) KOH, EtOH} \\ \text{5) } H_3O^+}]{\text{1) } + e^-} \underset{31-56\%}{R-\overset{O}{\overset{\|}{C}}CH_2Cl}$$

I.A.8-45   M. Steiniger and H. J. Schafer, Angew. Chem., Int. Ed. Engl., 21, 79 (1982); Y. Rollin, J. F. Fauvarque et al., Tetrahedron Lett., 23, 3573 (1982).

$$\phi CCl_3 \xrightarrow[\substack{R^1\overset{O}{\overset{\|}{C}}CH_2R^2 \\ \text{THF, 0°C}}]{+\ 2e^-,\ NaH} \underset{58-65\%}{\phi\overset{O}{\overset{\|}{C}}\underset{R^1}{C}{=}CHR^2}$$

I.A.8-46   U. Hess and R. Thiele, J. Prakt. Chem., 324, 385 (1982).

$$Ar^1-CH{=}N-Ar^2 \xrightarrow[CO_2\ \text{Saturated DMF}]{\text{Electroredn.}} \underset{10-60\%}{Ar^1-\underset{CO_2H}{CH}-NHAr^2}$$

I.A.8-47 S. Torii et al., Bull. Chem. Soc. Jpn., 55, 3947 (1982); D. D. M. Wayner and D. R. Arnold, Chem. Commun., 1087 (1982).

$$\text{cyclopentene-R,CO}_2\text{Me} \xrightarrow[\text{t}_{BuOH}]{-e^-,\ Et_3N,\ AcOH,\ EtOAc} \text{AcO-cyclopentene-R} \quad 98\%$$

I.A.8-48 S. Torii, T. Inokuchi and R. Oi, J. Org. Chem., 47, 47 (1982); T. Iwasaki et al., ibid, 47, 3799 (1982).

$$\underset{R^2}{\text{cyclopentanone-}R^1,OX} \xrightarrow[\text{LiClO}_4,\ (Pt)]{-2e^-} \underset{R^2}{R^1\text{-CO-CH}_2\text{-CH}_2\text{-CH(CO}_2\text{Me})}$$

(X = H or Ac)

82-97%

Also electrooxidative cleavage of enol acetates.

I.A.8-49 T. G. Back and R. G. Kerr, Tetrahedron Lett., 23, 3241 (1982); T. Shioiri et al., Chem. Pharm. Bull., 30, 119, 526, 899, 3380 (1982); D. Krois and H. Lehner, J. Chem. Soc., Perkin I, 477 (1982); P. Eisenbarth and M. Regitz, Chem. Ber., 115, 3796 (1982).

$$R^1\text{-}\underset{\|}{\overset{O}{C}}\text{-SeR}^2 \xrightarrow[\text{Cu or CuI}]{CH_2N_2} R^1\text{-}\underset{\|}{\overset{O}{C}}\text{-CH}_2\text{-SeR}^2$$

42-65%

I.A.8-50   H. J. Callot and F. Metz, Tetrahedron Lett., 23, 4321 (1982).

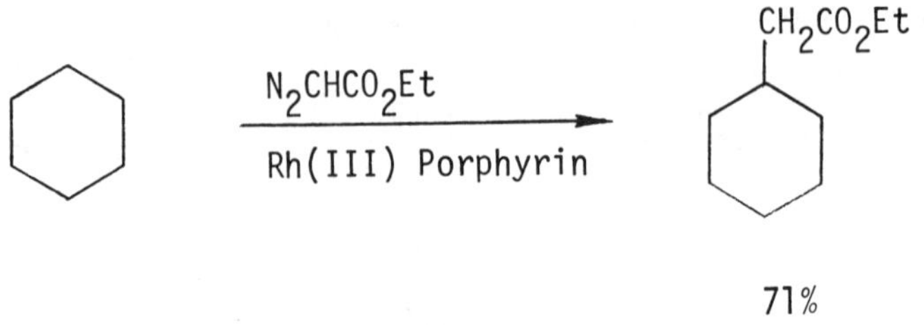

cyclohexane + N_2CHCO_2Et →[Rh(III) Porphyrin] cyclohexyl-CH_2CO_2Et

71%

I.A.8-51   D. F. Taber and E. H. Petty, J. Org. Chem., 47, 4808 (1982);   S. K. Maity, S. Bhattacharyya and D. Mukherjee, Ind. J. Chem., 21B, 269 (1982); T. Takahashi et al., Chem. Lett., 863 (1982).

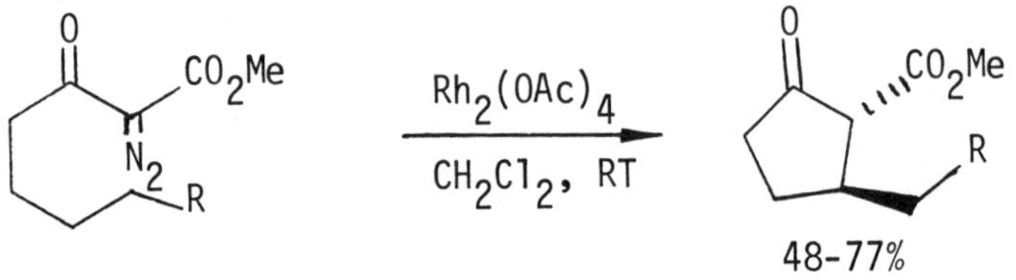

cyclohexanone with CO_2Me and N_2-R →[Rh$_2$(OAc)$_4$; CH_2Cl_2, RT] cyclopentanone with CO_2Me and R

48-77%

I.A.8-52   N. Slougui and G. Rousseau, Synth. Commun., 12, 401 (1982).

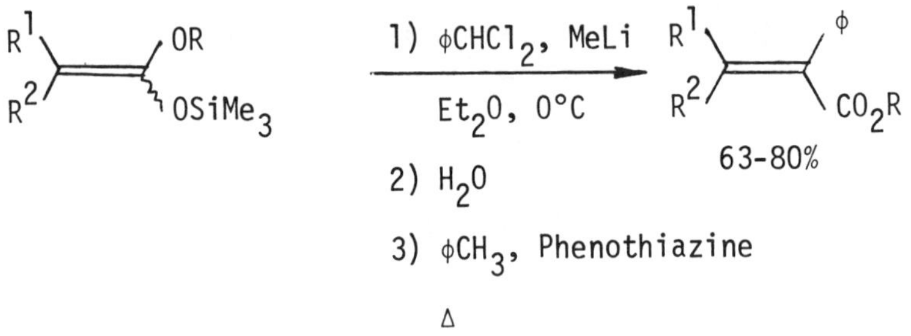

R^1R^2C=C(OR)(OSiMe$_3$) →[1) φCHCl$_2$, MeLi, Et$_2$O, 0°C; 2) H$_2$O; 3) φCH$_3$, Phenothiazine, Δ] R^1R^2C=C(φ)(CO$_2$R)

63-80%

I.A.8-53 L. A. Yanovskaya et al., Tetrahedron Lett., 23, 3607 (1982).

$$RCH(OAc)_2 \xrightarrow[\text{50\% aq. NaOH} \atop \text{QX}]{CHCl_3} RCH(OAc)(CCl_3)$$

50-72%

I.A.8-54 A. Clerica and O. Porta, J. Org. Chem., 47, 2852 (1982); Tetrahedron Lett., 23, 3517 (1982); T. Imamoto et al., ibid, 23, 1353 (1982); B. P. Mundy, R. J. Warnet et al., J. Org. Chem., 47, 1657 (1982).

$$R^1-\underset{O}{C}-X \xrightarrow[\text{H}_2\text{O/HOAc}]{R^2COR^3 \atop 2\ TiCl_3} R^1-\underset{OH}{\underset{|}{C}}(X)-\underset{OH}{\underset{|}{C}}(R^2)-R^3$$

28-95%

X = CN, CO$_2$H, CO$_2$Me, 2-Pyridyl

I.A.8-55 J. E. Pauw and A. C. Weedon, Tetrahedron Lett., 23, 5485 (1982); M. Oda et al., ibid, 23, 2117 (1982).

$$\xrightarrow[\text{THF}]{TiCl_3,\ K}$$

I.A.8-56 E. von Angerer, H. Schonenberger et al., J. Med. Chem., 25, 832, 1374 (1982); L. Brandsma et al., Chem. Commun. 1214 (1982).

$$ArCH=NR \xrightarrow[\text{EtOH}]{\text{Act. Al.}} Ar-\underset{NHR}{\underset{|}{CH}}-\underset{NHR}{\underset{|}{CH}}-Ar$$

8-42%

I.A.8-57 G. W. Griffin et al., J. Org. Chem., 47, 2342 (1982).

$$Ar\text{-}\underset{\underset{O}{\|}}{C}\text{-}CO_2Me \xrightarrow[\phi H,\ Reflux]{(Me_2N)_3P} \underset{Ar}{MeO_2C}\!\!\!\diagdown\!\!\!\overset{O}{\triangle}\!\!\!\diagup\!\!\!\underset{Ar}{CO_2Me}$$

50-94%

I.A.8-58 D. J. Pasto and D. K. Mitra, J. Org. Chem., 47, 1381 (1982); D. L. J. Clive et al., ibid, 47, 1641 (1982); J. J. Doney, C. H. Chen and H. R. Luss, Tetrahedron Lett., 23, 1747 (1982).

$$\underset{Cl}{\overset{Me}{Me\text{-}C\text{-}C\!\equiv\!C\text{-}R}} \xrightarrow[THF,\ 0°C]{(\phi_3P)_4Ni(0)}$$

(R = H or Me)

65-75%

I.A.8-59 M. Sato and K. Oshima, Chem. Lett., 157 (1982).

$$\bigcirc\!\!\text{-}OH \xrightarrow{NbCl_5,\ NaAlH_4} \bigcirc\!\!\text{-}\!\!\bigcirc$$

75%

I.A.8-60 K. Mach, F. Turecek et al., Tetrahedron Lett., 23, 1105 (1982).

$$\xrightarrow[190°C]{FHT}$$

cis:trans = 42:45 (GC)

FHT = μ(n^5:n^5-fulvalene)-di-μ-hydrido-bis(cyclopentadienyltitanium).

I.A.8-61 A. S. Kende et al., J. Amer. Chem. Soc., 104, 1784 (1982); J. Amer. Chem. Soc., 104, 5808 (1982).

$$\text{[vinyl cyclohexadiene-OSiMe}_3\text{]} \xrightarrow[\substack{CH_3CN,\ CH_2Cl_2 \\ 25°C}]{Pd(OAc)_2} \text{[bicyclic methylene ketone]} \quad 68\%$$

I.A.8-62 L. S. Hegedus and M. A. McGuire, Organometallics, 1, 1175 (1982); A. Solladie-Cavallo, J. E. Backvall et al., Tetrahedron Lett., 23, 939, 943 (1982); M. Hidai et al., J. Organometal. Chem., 232, 89 (1982).

$$R^1CH=CH_2 \xrightarrow[\substack{HMPA,\ RT \\ 2)\ 2\ Et_3N,\ -78°C \\ 3)\ \phi Li \\ 4)\ H_2}]{1)\ PdCl_2(R^2CH_2CN)_2} R^1CH_2CH_2-CH\!\!\begin{array}{c}R^2\\CN\end{array} \quad 50\text{-}71\%$$

I.A.8-63 I. Shimizu and J. Tsuji, J. Amer. Chem. Soc., 104, 5844 (1982); M. P. Cooke, Jr. and D. L. Burman, J. Org. Chem., 47, 4955, 4963 (1982); P. v. R. Schleyer et al., Chem. Ber., 115, 808 (1982).

$$\text{[2-(allyloxycarbonyl)-2-(CH}_2\text{CH}_2\text{CO}_2\text{Me)-cyclohexanone]} \xrightarrow[\substack{\phi_2PCH_2CH_2P\phi_2 \\ CH_3CN,\ \Delta}]{Pd(OAc)_2\ (cat.)} \text{[2-(CH}_2\text{CH}_2\text{CO}_2\text{Me)-cyclohexenone]}$$

I.A.8-64 M. Nanasawa and H. Kamogawa, Bull. Chem. Soc. Jpn., 55, 3655 (1982); C. R. Engel, Y. Merand and J. Cote, J. Org. Chem., 47, 4485 (1982); P. Ceccherelli, R. Pellicciari, E. Wenkert et al., ibid, 47, 3172, 3242 (1982); R. C. Cambie et al., Austr. J. Chem., 35, 183 (1982).

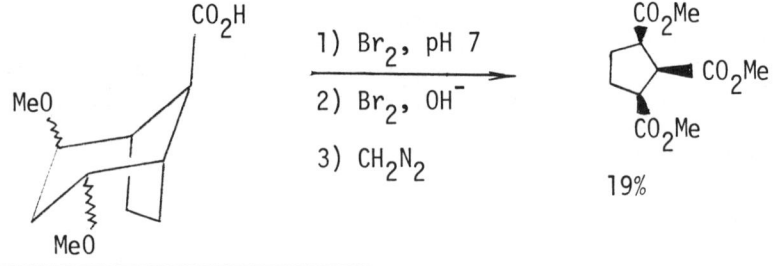

81%

(Favorskii-type Rearrangement)

I.A.8-65 P. Camps and C. Jaime, Can. J. Chem., 60, 2358 (1982).

I.A.8-66 C. H. Heathcock, E. G. Del Mar and S. L. Graham, J. Amer. Chem. Soc., 104, 1907 (1982); B. M. Trost and H. Hiemstra, ibid, 104, 886 (1982); M. E. Garst, V. A. Roberts and C. Prussin, J. Org. Chem., 47, 3969 (1982).

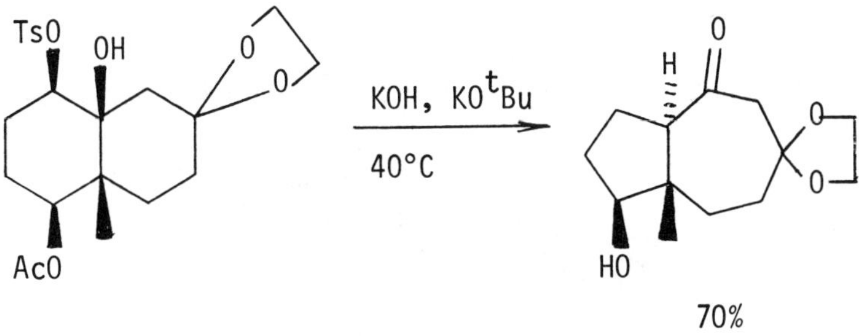

I.A.8-67 H. Yamamoto et al, Tetrahedron Lett., 23, 1933 (1982).

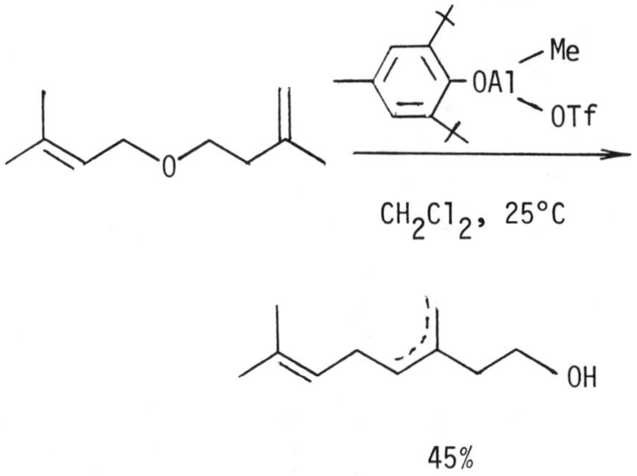

I.A.8-68 S. Halazy and A. Krief, Chem. Commun., 1200 (1982).

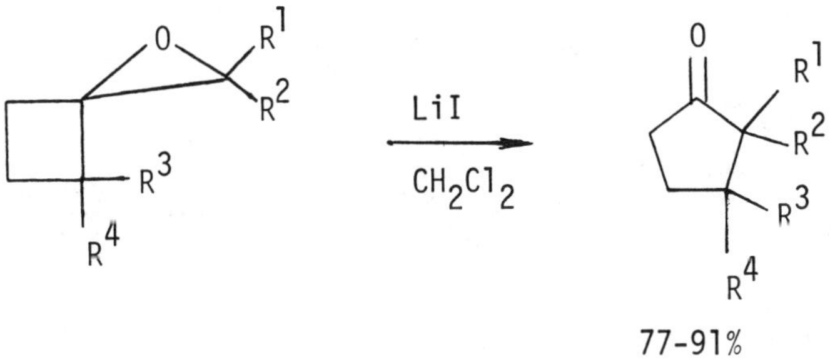

I.A.8-69 H. G. Henning, Zeit. Chem., 22, 77 (1982).

   Review: "Nucleophilic and Radicalic Aminoalkylations."

I.A.8-70 G. Piancatelli, Heterocycles, 19, 1735 (1982).

   Review: "Advances in Cyclopentenone Synthesis from Furans."

I.A.8-71 B. M. Trost, Chem. Soc. Rev., 11, 141 (1982).

   Review: "Cyclopentanoids: A Challenge for New Methodology."

I.A.8-72 F. Montanari, D. Landini and F. Rolla, Topics Curr. Chem., 101, 149 (1982).

   Review: "Phase-Transfer Catalyzed Reactions."

I.A.8-73 H. Wynberg, CHEMTECH, 116 (1982).

   Review: "Chance, Necessity and Asymmetric Catalysis."

I.A.8-74 E. Winterfeldt et al., Angew. Chem., Int. Ed. Engl., 21, 480 (1982).

   Review: "4-Oxo-2-Cyclopentenyl Acetate - A Synthetic Intermediate."

I.A.8-75 I. Ugi, Angew. Chem., Int. Ed. Engl., 21, 810 (1982).

Review: "From Isocyanides via Four-Component Condensations to Antibiotic Synthesis."

I.A.8-76 H. Paulsen, Angew. Chem., Int. Ed. Engl., 21, 155 (1982).

Review: "Advances in Selective Chemical Syntheses of Complex Oligosaccharides."

I.A.8-77 W. Bartmann and G. Beck, Angew. Chem., Int. Ed. Engl., 21, 751 (1982).

Review: "Prostacyclin and Synthetic Analogues."

I.A.8-78 T. A. Hase and J. K. Koskimies, Aldrichimica Acta, 15, 35 (1982).

Review: "A Compilation of References on R-Functional Acyl Anion Synthons, RCO^-."

I.A.8-79 K. Smith, Chem. Brit., 18, 29 (1982).

Review: "Lithiation and Organic Synthesis."

I.A.8-80 K. Drauz, A. Kleeman and J. Martens, Angew. Chem., Int. Ed. Engl., 21, 584 (1982).

Review: "Induction of Asymmetry by Amino Acids."

I.A.8-81 F. A. Carey and M. E. Kuehne, J. Org. Chem., 47, 3811 (1982).

"Beyond Erythro and Threo. A Proposal for Specifying Relative Configuration in Molecules with Multiple Chiral Centers."

I.A.8-82 D. Seebach and V. Prelog, Angew. Chem., Int. Ed. Engl., 21, 654 (1982).

Review: "The Unambiguous Specification of the Steric Course of Asymmetric Synthesis."

I.A.8-83 V. Prelog and G. Helmchen, Angew. Chem., Int. Ed. Engl., 21, 567 (1982).

Review: "Basic Principles of the CIP-System (Cahn-Ingold-Prelog) and Proposals for a Revision."

I.B. Carbon-Carbon Double Bonds
(see also: I.E.1, III.G, VI.A.16).

I.B.1. Wittig Type Olefination Reactions

I.B.1-1 M. Schlosser and B. Schaub, *Chimia*, 36, 396 (1982); J. Amer. Chem. Soc., 104, 5821 (1982).

$$\begin{array}{c} R^1 \\ R^2 \end{array}\!\!\!\!CH\text{-}P\phi_3 \;\; Br^-$$

\+

$NaNH_2$ (Powder)

Mixtures stored indefinately. Ylid generated on mixing with ether: "Instant Ylid."

I.B.1-2 J. L. Belletire, D. R. Walley and M. J. Bast, *Synth. Commun.*, 12, 469 (1982); M. A. Fox, C. A. Triebel and R. Rogers, *ibid*, 12, 1055 (1982); M. Orfanopoulos, *J. Chem. Res. (S)*, 188 (1982); K. J. McCullough, *Tetrahedron Lett.*, 23, 2223 (1982); L. Lombardo, *ibid*, 23, 4293 (1982).

$$Me_2C{<}^{CO_2Me}_{\overset{+}{P}\phi_3\;I^-} \quad \xrightarrow[125°C\;(Melt)]{ArCHO\;\;(LiCl)_x} \quad ArCH{=}C{<}^{Me}_{Me}$$

50-90%

I.B.1-3 H. J. Bestmann and A. Bomhard, *Angew. Chem., Int. Ed. Engl.*, 21, 545 (1982); G. L. Larson and D. Hernandez, *Tetrahedron Lett.*, 23, 1035 (1982).

$$2\;R^1CH{=}P\phi_3 \quad \xrightarrow[\substack{1)\;Me_3SiCl\\2)\;R^2X\\3)\;CsF\\4)\;R^3CHO}]{} \quad \begin{array}{c}R^1\\R^2\end{array}\!\!\!\!C{=}CH\text{-}R^3$$

39-78%

I.B.1-4 R. R. Mehta, V. L. Pardini and J. H. P. Utley, J. Chem. Soc., Perkin I, 2921 (1982); M. A. Christie, R. L. Webb and A. M. Tickner, J. Org. Chem., 47, 2802 (1982); D. Nagarathnam and P. C. Srinivasan, Synthesis, 926 (1982).

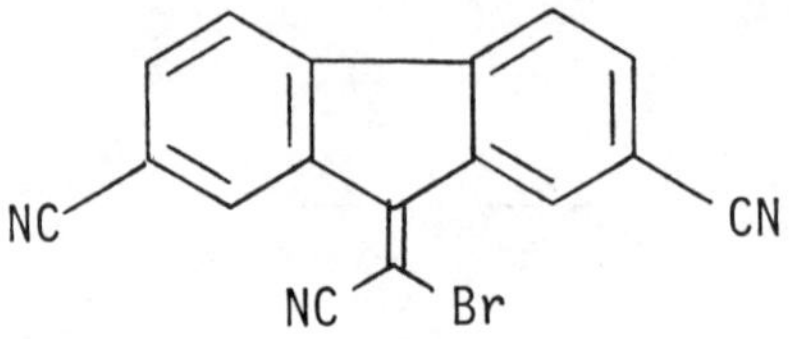

1) Cathode Redn. to Dianion
2) $R^1CH_2P\phi_3^+ \ X^-$
3) R^2CHO

$$R^1CH=CHR^2$$

Electrogenerated Base for Ylide Formation.

I.B.1-5 Y. LeBigot, M. Delmas and A. Gaset, Synth. Commun., 12, 107 (1982); O. I. Paynter, D. J. Simmonds and M. C. Whiting, Chem. Commun., 1165 (1982).

$$CH_3(CH_2)_8CHO \xrightarrow[\substack{K_2CO_3,\ \text{Dioxane} \\ H_2O,\ \Delta}]{\phi_3\overset{+}{P}-CH_2CH_2CH_2CH_3 \ Br^-}$$

$$CH_3(CH_2)_8CH=CHCH_2CH_2CH_3$$
72%

Solid-Liquid transfer using K_2CO_3 in Wittig reaction.

I.B.1-6 F. Watjen, O. Dahl and O. Buchardt, Tetrahedron Lett., 23, 4741 (1982); E. G. Baggiolini et al., J. Amer. Chem. Soc., 104, 2945 (1982).

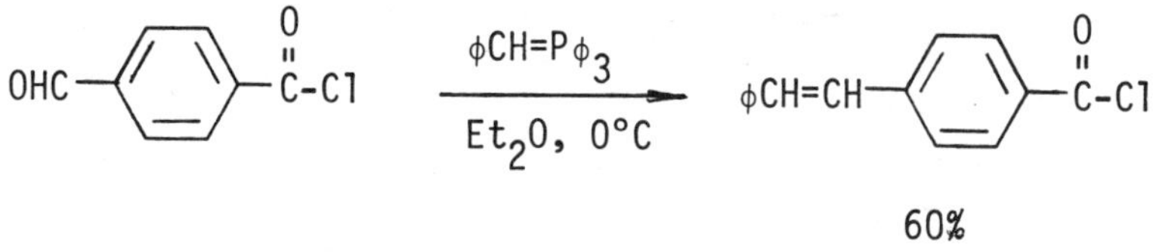

OHC—⌬—C(=O)—Cl $\xrightarrow[\text{Et}_2\text{O, 0°C}]{\phi\text{CH=P}\phi_3}$ φCH=CH—⌬—C(=O)—Cl

60%

I.B.1-7 W. R. Roush et al., Tetrahedron Lett., 23, 2331, 4879 (1982); A. H. Al-Hakim and A. H. Haines, ibid, 23, 5295 (1982).

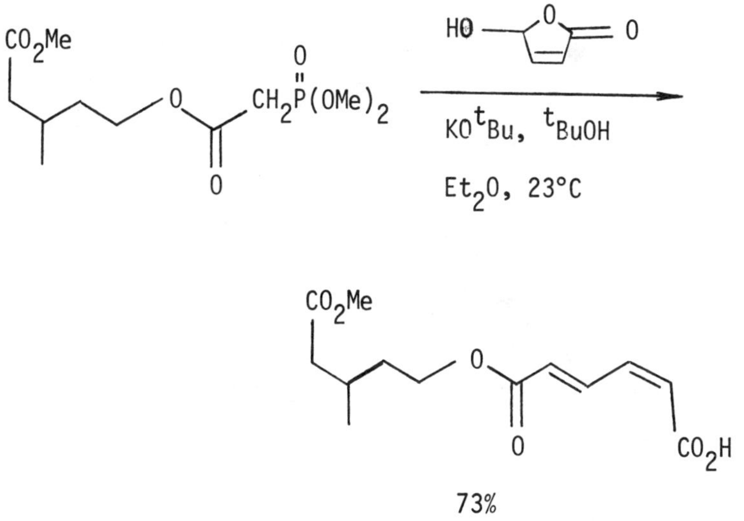

$\xrightarrow[\text{Et}_2\text{O, 23°C}]{\text{KO}^t\text{Bu, }^t\text{BuOH}}$

73%

I.B.1-8 K. M. Sun and B. Fraser-Reid, Synthesis, 28 (1982); P. M. Collins, W. G. Overend and T. S. Shing, Chem. Commun., 297 (1982); K. Olejniczak and R. W. Franck, J. Org. Chem., 47, 380 (1982).

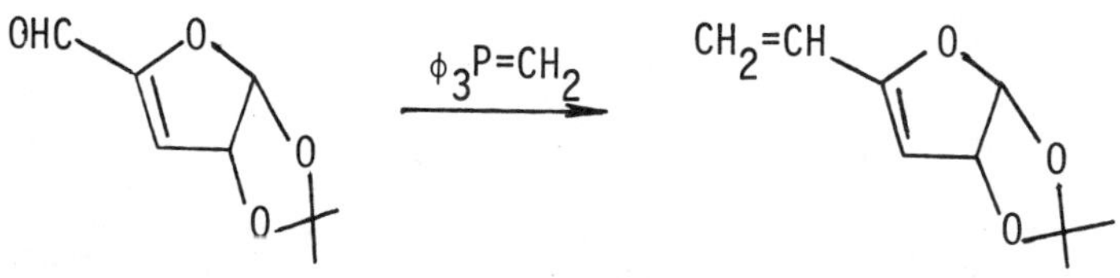

$\xrightarrow{\phi_3\text{P=CH}_2}$

I.B.1-9 E. J. Corey and J. Kang, J. Amer. Chem. Soc., 104, 4724 (1982).

$\phi_3P=CH_2$ → 1) ^tBuLi, Et_2O, $-78°C$ 2) 2 RCHO → R-CH(OH)-CH=CH-R 54-60%

I.B.1-10 A. Donetti et al., Tetrahedron Lett., 23, 2219 (1982).

AcO-CH$_2$-C(=O)-CH$_3$ → 1) $\phi_3\overset{+}{P}CH_2CH_2NR_2$ Br$^-$ (R = nBu), $KN(SiMe_3)_2$, THF, HMPA 2) $ClCO_2Et$, ϕH → AcO-CH$_2$-C(CH$_3$)=CH-CH=CH-Cl 38%

I.B.1-11 H. J. Bestmann, K. Roth and M. Ettlinger, Chem. Ber., 115, 161 (1982); J. M. Conia et al., J. Chem. Res. (S), 246, 248 (1982).

$\phi_3P=CH-CH(OEt)_2$ → 1) RCHO 2) pTsOH → (R)(H)C=C(H)(CHO) 49-77%

I.B.1-12 M. Suda, Tetrahedron Lett., 23, 427 (1982).

[methylenecyclohexene with =Pϕ_3] + [cyclopentene with CH$_2$OCHO and CH$_3$] → 1) THF 2) Xylene, Δ → [spiro product with OHC] 50%

Wittig then Claissen.

I.B.1-13 I. Ernest, A. J. Main and R. Menasse, Tetrahedron Lett., 23, 167 (1982); J. C. Buck, F. Ellis and P. C. North, ibid, 23, 4161 (1982).

OHC—[epoxide with H, CH(O)]—CO$_2$Me $\xrightarrow[\text{CH}_2\text{Cl}_2,\ 25°\text{C}]{\text{OHC}-\text{CH}=\text{CH}-\text{P}\phi_3}$

OHC—CH=CH—CH=CH—[epoxide]—CO$_2$Me

73%

I.B.1-14 J. Villieras and M. Rambaud, Synthesis, 924 (1982); A. Takeda et al., J. Org. Chem., 47, 1101 (1982); A. J. H. Labuschagne and D. F. Schneider, Tetrahedron Lett., 23, 4135 (1982); C. H. Eugster et al., Helv. Chim. Acta, 65, 353, 896 (1982); E. Widmer et al., ibid, 944, 958 (1982); H. J. Bestmann et al., Liebigs Ann. Chem., 363, 536, 1478 (1982).

(EtO)$_2$P(=O)-CH$_2$-CO$_2$Et $\xrightarrow[\text{2) aq. NH}_4\text{Cl}]{\text{1) 4 eq. CH}_2\text{O (30\% aq.)}, \text{K}_2\text{CO}_3\ (2\ \text{eq.}), \text{H}_2\text{O}}$

H$_2$C=C(CO$_2$Et)-CH$_2$OH

77%

I.B.1-15 H. Schubert and M. Regitz, Synthesis, 149 (1982); T. Koizumi et al., ibid, 917 (1982).

$$\text{pyrazole-CH=C(CN)}_2 \xrightarrow{\phi_3P=CH-\overset{O}{\underset{\|}{C}}-R} \phi_3P=C\begin{Bmatrix}CH=C(CN)_2 \\ C-R \\ \| \\ O\end{Bmatrix}$$

30-87%

I.B.1-16 U. Schmidt et al., Angew. Chem., Int. Ed. Engl., 21, 776 (1982); A. M. van Leusen and J. Wildeman, Rec. Trav. Chim., 101, 202 (1982).

$$R^1NH-\underset{PO(OEt)_2}{CH}-CO_2Et \xrightarrow[R^2CHO]{NaH, THF} R^1NH-\underset{CHR^2}{\overset{\|}{C}}-CO_2Et$$

73-85%

I.B.1-17 D. H. R. Barton, W. B. Motherwell and S. Z. Zaid, Nouv. J. Chim., 6, 295 (1982); Chem. Commun., 551 (1982); W. Reuther and A. Ruland, Liebigs Ann. Chem., 372 (1982); M. Faulques, L. Rene and R. Royer, Synthesis, 260 (1982).

1) CH$_3$CH(N=C)-PO(OEt)$_2$, KH, DME
2) HCO$_2$H, EtOAc

90%

(Full Paper)

I.B.1-18 L. Capuano and A. Willmes, Liebigs Ann. Chem., 80 (1982).

$\phi\text{CH=CH-}\underset{\underset{\text{Me}}{|}}{\text{C}}\text{=P}\phi_3$ →
1) nPrN=C=O
2) $MeO_2C-C≡C-CO_2Me$

→ [product, Me, H, φ, H, •, N-nPr] 95%

I.B.1-19 E. J. Corey and C. Rucker, Tetrahedron Lett., 23, 719 (1982); T. H. Chan and J. S. Li, Chem. Commun., 969 (1982).

$(iPr)_3Si-C≡C-CH_2-Si(iPr)_3$

1) nBuLi, THF, -20°C
2) RCHO, -78°C

→ H, R, C=C, H, C≡C-Si(iPr)$_3$

57-79%

Reaction in THF, HMPA gives trans enyne.

I.B.1-20 S. Warren and A. T. Zaslona, Tetrahedron Lett., 23, 4167 (1982); S. Kano et al., Heterocycles, 19, 1079 (1982); T. Agawa et al., Bull. Chem. Soc. Jpn., 55, 1205 (1982); J. V. Comasseto and C. A. Brandt, J. Chem. Res. (S), 56 (1982).

$\phi_2\overset{O}{\overset{\|}{P}}$-S$\phi$ (=CH$_2$)

1) R^1Li
2) R^2CHO

→ R^2, Sφ, R^1

25-93%

I.B.1-21 Y. Thebtaranonth et al., Synthesis, 579 (1982); M. Ishida, H. Sato and S. Kato, ibid, 927 (1982).

$$\text{[dithiane-CH-Li]} \xrightarrow[\substack{\text{THF, 0°C} \\ \text{2) Me}_3\text{SiCl, -78°C} \\ \text{3) nBuLi} \\ \text{4) Aq. NH}_4\text{Cl}}]{1)\ R^1R^2CO} \text{[ketene dithioacetal } R^1, R^2\text{]} \quad 57\text{-}97\%$$

I.B.1-22 C. N. Hsiao and H. Shechter, Tetrahedron Lett., 23, 3455 (1982).

$$\text{Me}_3\text{Si-CH}_2\text{-CH(Cl)-SO}_2\phi \xrightarrow[\substack{\text{2) E}^+ \\ \text{3) Bu}_4\text{NF}}]{\text{1) nBuLi}} \text{CH}_2=\text{C}(E)(\text{SO}_2\phi) \quad 90\text{-}97\%$$

E^+ = RX or RCHO

I.B.1-23 K. Thangaraj, P. C. Srinivasan and S. Swaminathan, Synthesis, 855 (1982); J. J. Salley, Jr. and R. A. Glennon, J. Het. Chem., 19, 545 (1982); H. J. Altenbach and R. Korff, Angew. Chem., Int. Ed. Engl., 21, 371 (1982); J. C. Canevet and F. Sharrard, Tetrahedron Lett., 23, 181 (1982).

$$\text{[2-formyl-2-methylcyclohexanone]} \xrightarrow[\substack{\text{NaH, DME} \\ \text{2) KOH, H}_2\text{O, MeOH}}]{1)\ \text{CH}_3\text{CCH}_2\text{PO(OEt)}_2} \text{[octahydronaphthalenone]} \quad 40\%$$

I.B.1-24 H. J. Bestmann and G. Schade, Tetrahedron Lett., 23, 3543 (1982); K. C. Nicolaou, M. R. Pavia and S. P. Seitz, J. Amer. Chem. Soc., 104, 2027, 2030 (1982).

$$CH_2\overset{O}{\overset{\|}{C}}-CH=P\phi_3 \longrightarrow$$

51%

I.B.1-25 C. R. Johnson et al., J. Amer. Chem. Soc., 104, 7041 (1982); Tetrahedron Lett., 23, 5005 (1982); M. Rosenberger et al., J. Org. Chem., 47, 1698, 1779, 1782, 2130 (1982); Y. Huang, Y. Xu and Z. Li, Org. Prep. Proc. Int., 14, 373 (1982).

1) $\phi-\overset{\overset{S}{\|}}{\underset{NMe_2}{P}}-CH_2Li$

2) H^+

3) MeI, Pyridine

99%

Alternative to Wittig for sluggish ketones.

I.B.1-26 M. Jawdosiuk and M. Uminski, Chem. Commun., 979 (1982); N. Ono et al., J. Org. Chem., 47, 5017 (1982); K. Hafner et al., Tetrahedron Lett., 23, 5131, 5135 (1982).

$\phi_2\ddot{C}H-\ddot{N}=\ddot{C}$ $\xrightarrow[\phi H]{Cl-CH_2-C_6H_4-NO_2, \; QX}{50\% \; aq. \; NaOH}$ $\phi_2C=CH-C_6H_4-NO_2$

85%

I.B.1-27 V. V. Tyuleneva, E. M. Rokhlin and I. L. Knunyants, Russ. Chem. Rev., 51, 1 (1982); G. M. Blackburn and M. J. Parratt, Chem. Commun., 1270 (1982); A. J. Lovey and B. A. Pawson, J. Med. Chem., 25, 71 (1982); J. Leroy and C. Wakselman, Synthesis, 496 (1982).

Review: "Fluorine-Containing Phosphorous Ylids."

I.B.1-28 H. Gross and I. Keitel, Zeit. Chem., 22, 117 (1982).

Review: "Heterosubstituted Olefins by Reaction of Horner with α-Substituted Phosphonates."

I.B.2.a. Eliminations of Alcohols and Derivatives to Form Double Bonds

I.B.2.a-1 E. J. Corey and P. B. Hopkins, Tetrahedron Lett., 23, 1979 (1982); N. C. Barua et al., Chem. Ind., 956 (1982).

1) $Cl_2C=S$, 4-DMAP
2) Me-N-P(φ)-N-Me (1,3-dimethyl-2-phenyl-1,3,2-diazaphospholidine)

75-86%

I.B.2.a-2 H. J. Reich et al., J. Amer. Chem. Soc., 104, 7051 (1982); J. Org. Chem., 47, 1618 (1982); G. Cardillo et al., Gazz. Chim. Ital., 112, 231 (1982); D. Berner, D. P. Cox and H. Dahn, Helv. Chim. Acta, 65, 2061 (1982).

ArSeCl, Et_3N ([2,3]Sigmatropic then Syn. Elim.)

17-100%

I.B.2.a-3   D. Cavalla and S. Warren, Tetrahedron Lett., 23, 4505 (1982).

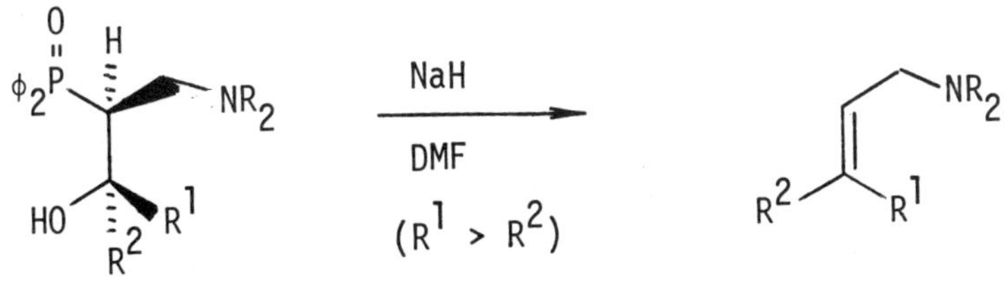

$\phi_2P(O)CH(\cdots)CH(OH)\cdots$ Erythro $\xrightarrow[DMF]{NaH}$ (R^1 > R^2) → alkene, 71-90% (Z)

I.B.2.a-4   J. Mulzer et al., Chem. Ber., 115, 3453 (1982).

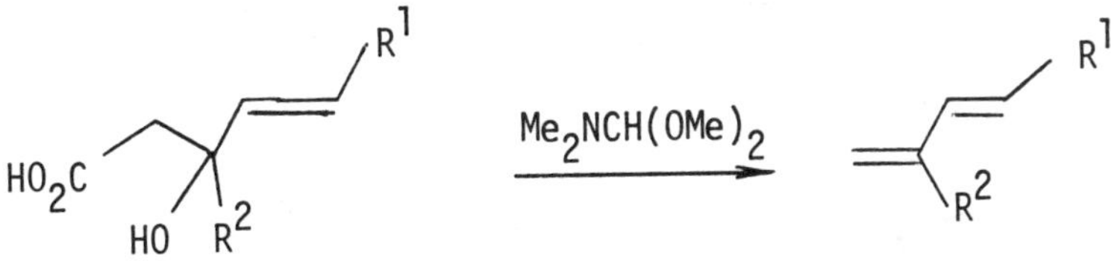

$\xrightarrow{Me_2NCH(OMe)_2}$ 59-86%

I.B.2.a-5   A. J. Bridges and J. W. Fischer, Chem. Commun., 665 (1982); H. M. Walborsky and H. H. Wust, J. Amer. Chem. Soc., 104, 5807 (1982); H. Matsushita and E. Negishi, J. Org. Chem., 47, 4161 (1982).

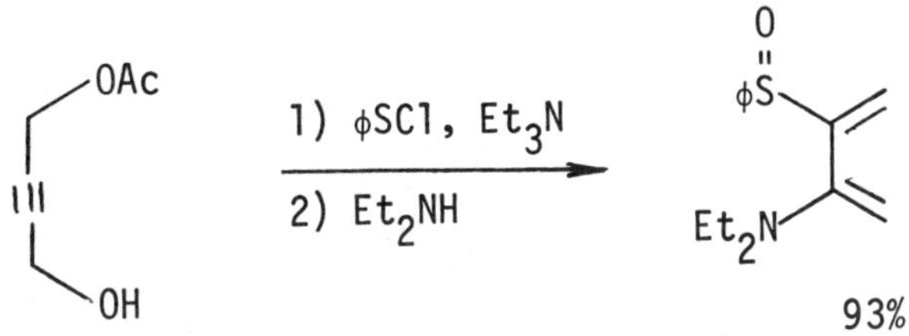

1) φSCl, Et$_3$N
2) Et$_2$NH

93%

I.B.2.b. Eliminations of Halides to Form Double Bonds

I.B.2.b-1 P. Wolkoff, J. Org. Chem., 47, 1944 (1982); J. Villieras and M. Rambaud, Compt. Rend. II, 294, 37 (1982); C. W. Spangler and D. A. Little, J. Chem. Soc., Perkin I, 2379 (1982).

$$\underset{R^2}{\overset{R^1}{\diagdown}} CH-\underset{Br}{CH}-CH_3 \xrightarrow[85°C]{DBU} \underset{R^2}{\overset{R^1}{\diagdown}} C=CHCH_3$$

Study of Dehydrobromination of 2° and 3° Alkyl and Cycloalkyl Bromides.

I.B.2.b-2 W. Chin-Hsien, Synthesis, 494 (1982); A. G. Martinez and J. L. M. Contelles, ibid, 742 (1982).

$$Br\diagdown\underset{\underset{Br}{|}}{CH}\diagup Br \xrightarrow[\underset{\Delta}{NaOH, H_2O}]{n-C_{16}H_{33}-N^+\diagdown\diagup Br^-} \diagdown=\diagup\diagdown Br \quad \underset{Br}{}$$

88-90%

I.B.2.b-3 G. D. Hartman and R. D. Hartman, Synthesis, 504 (1982); L. Avar, Org. Prep. Proc. Int., 14, 197 (1982).

$$\underset{R^2}{\overset{R^1}{\diagdown}} CH-SO_2-\underset{X}{CH}-R^3 \xrightarrow[CH_2Cl_2]{aq. \ NaOH, \ QX} \underset{R^2}{\overset{R^1}{\diagdown}} C=CHR^3$$

79-94%

I.B.2.b-4 F. Sato et al., Synthesis, 1025 (1982); L. Engman, Tetrahedron Lett., 23, 3601 (1982).

$$R^1-\underset{Br}{CH}-\underset{Br}{CH}-R^2 \xrightarrow[THF, \ 0°C]{Zn, \ TiCl_4 \ (cat)} R^1CH=CHR^2$$

82-91%

I.B.2.c. Other Eliminations to Form Double Bonds

I.B.2.c-1 B. Issari and C. J. M. Stirling, Chem. Commun., 684 (1982).

Nucleofugalities in 1,2 and 1,3 Eliminations.

I.B.2.c-2 A. R. Katritzky and A. M. El-Mowafy, J. Org. Chem., 47, 3506 (1982).

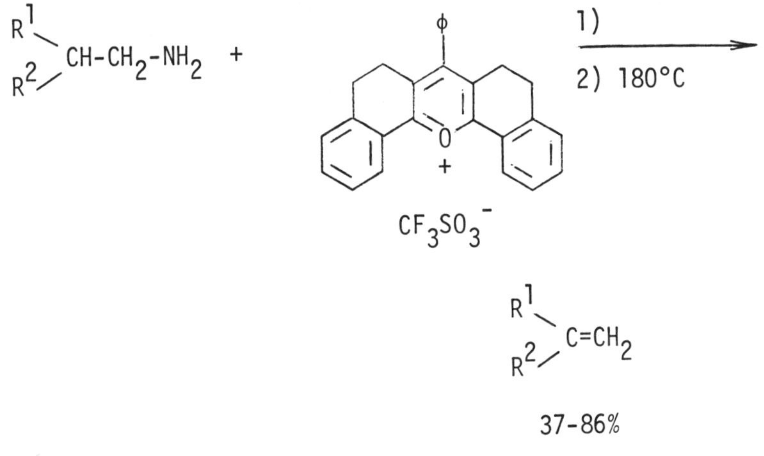

37-86%

I.B.2.c-3 I. Fleming, J. Goldhill and D. A. Perry, J. Chem. Soc., Perkin I, 1563 (1982); E. Fujita et al., Chem. Commun., 281 (1982); B. Psaume, M. Montury and J. Gore, Synth. Commun., 12, 409 (1982).

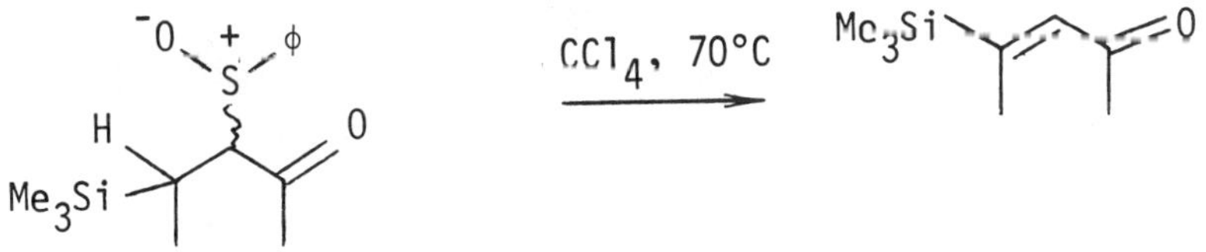

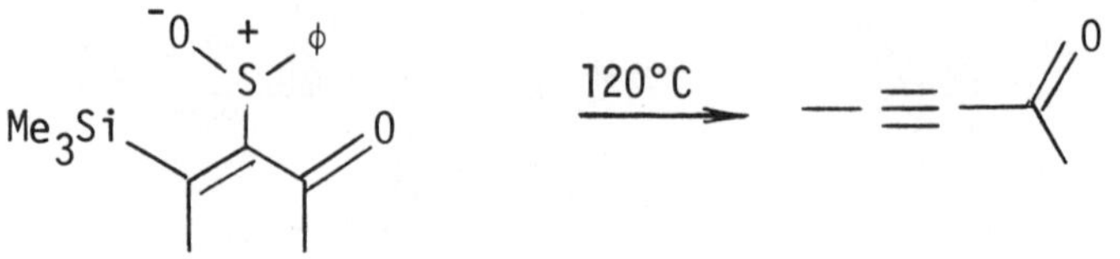

I.B.2.c-4 N. V. Bac and Y. Langlois, _J. Amer. Chem. Soc._, **104**, 7666 (1982).

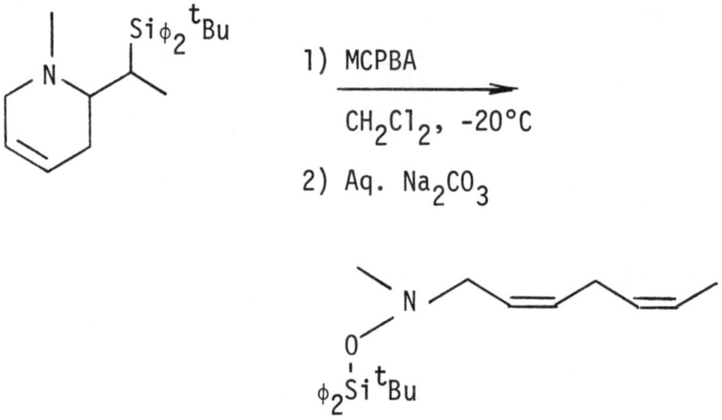

"Sila-Cope Elimination"

I.B.2.c-5 T. Yoshida and S. Saito, _Chem. Lett._, 165 (1982); J. H. Babler and R. A. Haack, _J. Org. Chem._, **47**, 4801 (1982); E. Fujita et al., _Tetrahedron Lett._, **23**, 2205 (1982).

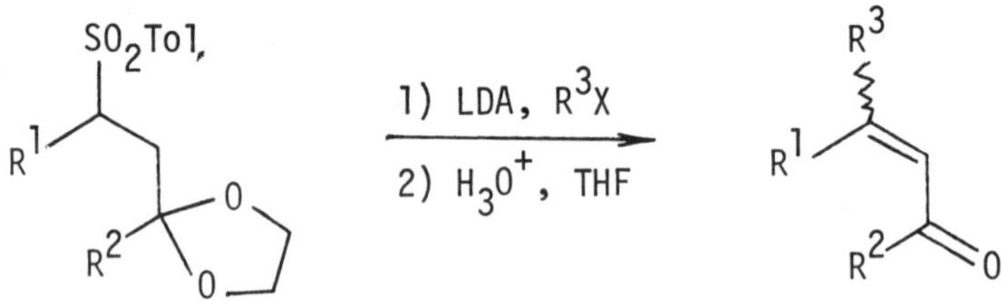

50-90%

I.B.2.c-6 D. Liotta, M. Saindane and D. Brothers, J. Org. Chem., 47, 1598 (1982).

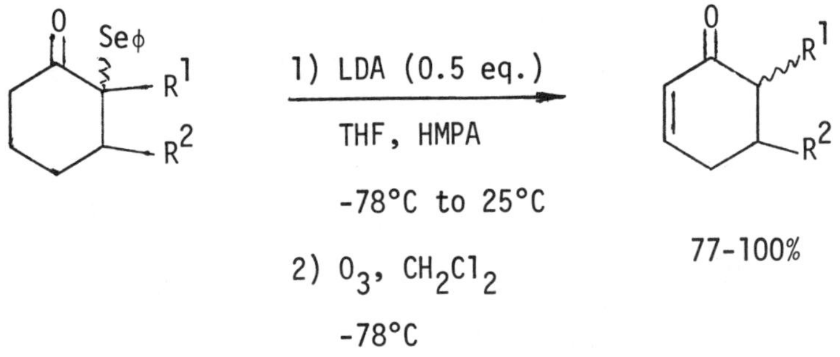

O
Seϕ
R^1
R^2
1) LDA (0.5 eq.)
THF, HMPA
-78°C to 25°C
2) O_3, CH_2Cl_2
-78°C
O
R^1
R^2
77-100%

I.B.2.c-7 C. J. M. Stirling et al., Chem. Commun., 236, 237 (1982); M. S. Baird and P. D. Slowey, Tetrahedron Lett., 23, 3795 (1982).

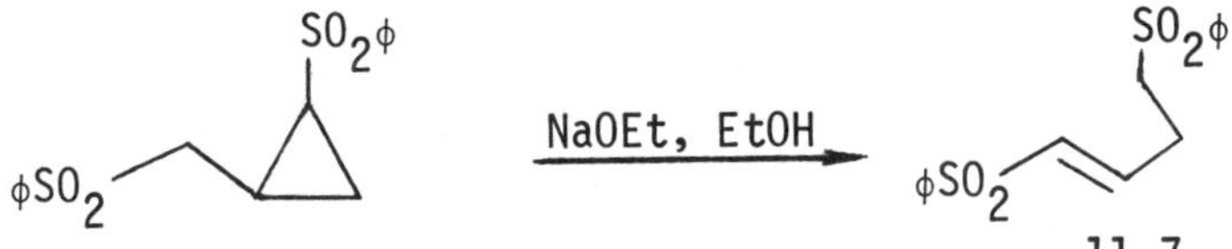

$SO_2ϕ$
$ϕSO_2$
NaOEt, EtOH
$SO_2ϕ$
$ϕSO_2$

Eliminative ring fission in cyclopropane ($10^{11.7}$) vs. acyclic analog (1) (Relative Rates).

I.B.2.c-8 O. G. Kulinkovich, I. G. Tishchenko and N. A. Roslik, Synthesis, 931 (1982); M. Ochiai, K. Sumi and E. Fujita, Chem. Lett., 79 (1982); I. Bohm, R. Schulz and H. U. Reissig, Tetrahedron Lett., 23, 2013 (1982); R. W. Lang and C. Djerassi, ibid, 23, 2063 (1982); Helv. Chim. Acta, 65, 407 (1982).

O
R^1
Sϕ
Sϕ
R^2
pTsOH, CH_2Cl_2
RT
O
R^2
R^1
Sϕ
Sϕ
74-95%

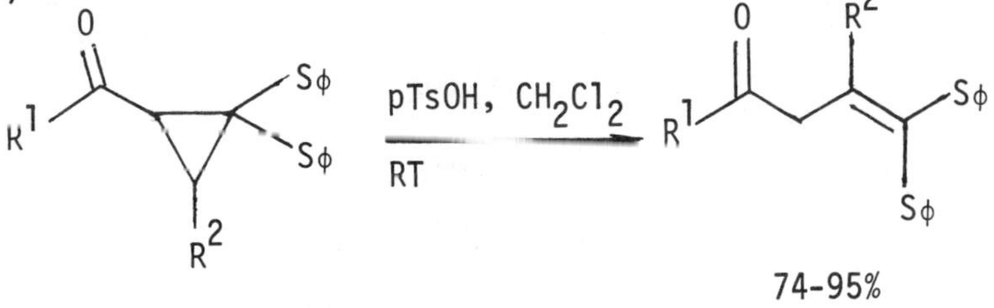

I.B.2.c-9 T. Hirao, Y. Ohshiro et al., <u>Chem. Lett.</u>, 1997 (1982); C. J. M. Stirling et al., <u>Chem. Commun.</u>, 658, 660 (1982).

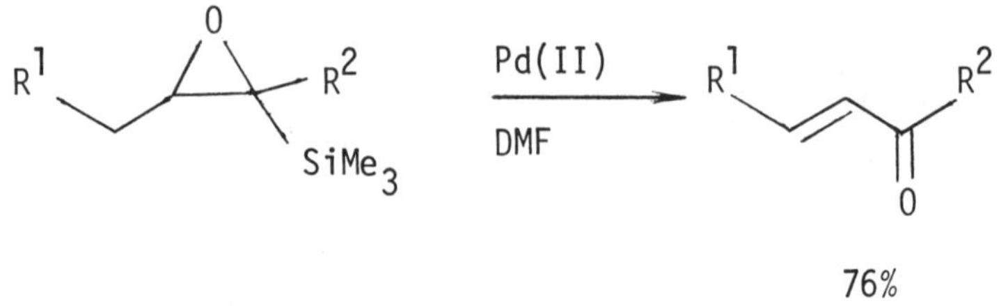

76%

I.B.2.c-10 J. Taoufik, J. Couquelet and J. Paris, <u>Synthesis</u>, 660 (1982); B. M. Trost and P. L. Ornstein, <u>J. Org. Chem.</u>, $\underline{47}$, 748 (1982); Y. Guindon et al., <u>Tetrahedron Lett.</u>, $\underline{23}$, 739 (1982); S. Fernandez and E. Hernandez, <u>Synth. Commun.</u>, $\underline{12}$, 915 (1982).

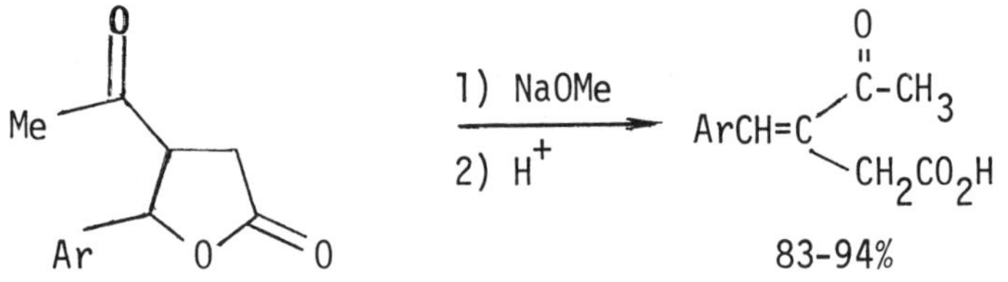

83-94%

I.B.3. Other Carbon-Carbon Double Bond Forming Reactions

I.B.3-1 P. A. Brown and P. R. Jenkins, <u>Tetrahedron Lett.</u>, $\underline{23}$, 3733 (1982).

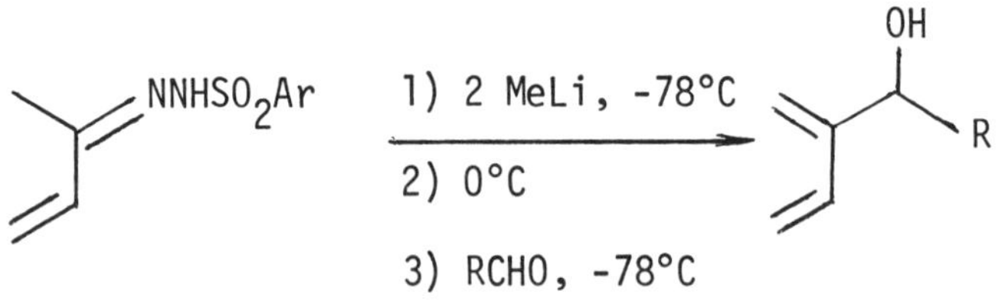

Ar = 2,4,6-^{i}Pr$_3$C$_6$H$_2$-

32-55%

I.B.3-2 O. Miyata and R. R. Schmidt, *Angew. Chem., Int. Ed. Engl.*, 21, 637 (1982); *Tetrahedron Lett.*, 23, 1793 (1982); N. G. Clemo and G. Pattenden, *ibid*, 23, 581, 585 (1982).

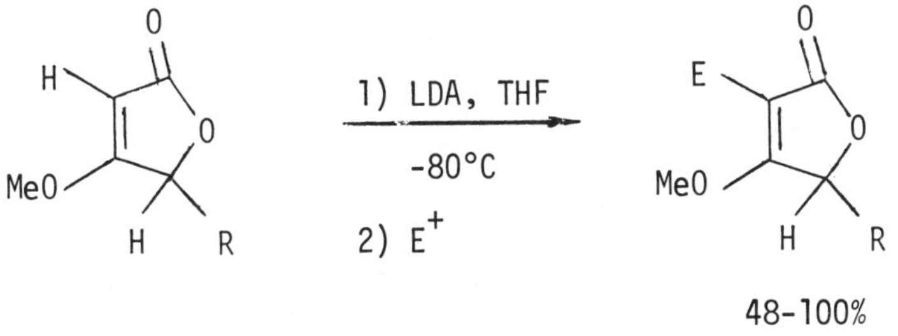

1) LDA, THF, $-80°C$
2) E^+

48-100%

E^+ = MeI, CH_3CH_2CHO, D_2O

I.B.3-3 L. Duhamel, J. Chauvin and A. Messier, *J. Chem. Res. (S)*, 48 (1982); R. W. Saylor and J. F. Sebastian, *Synth. Commun.*, 12, 579 (1982).

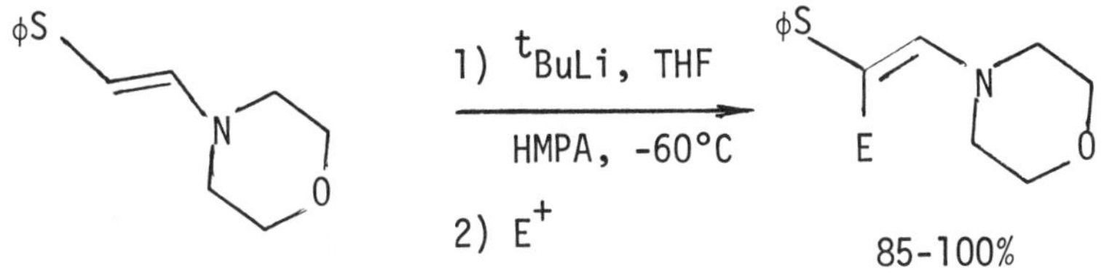

1) ^tBuLi, THF, HMPA, $-60°C$
2) E^+

85-100%

E^+ = RX, RCHO, D_2O.

I.B.3-4 J. P. Gillet, R. Sanvetre and J. F. Normant, *Synthesis*, 297 (1982); N. Ishikawa et al., *Bull. Chem. Soc. Jpn.*, 55, 2956 (1982).

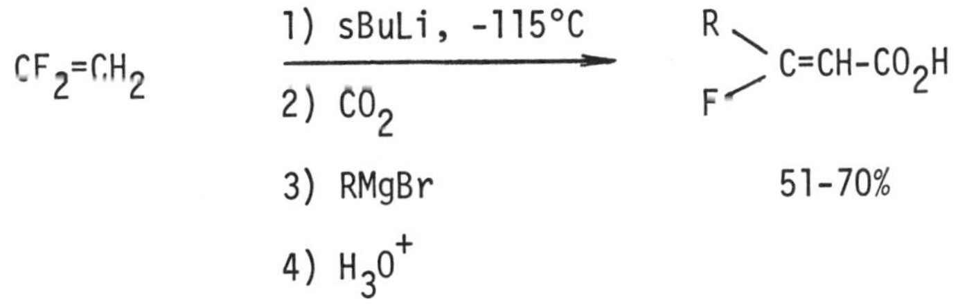

$CF_2=CH_2$

1) sBuLi, $-115°C$
2) CO_2
3) RMgBr
4) H_3O^+

$\underset{F}{\overset{R}{>}}C=CH-CO_2H$

51-70%

I.B.3-5 M. J. Marks and H. M. Walborsky, *J. Org. Chem.*, **47**, 52 (1982); J. Heinicke and A. Tzschach, *Tetrahedron Lett.*, **23**, 3643 (1982).

$$\text{R}_2\text{C}(\text{N=C})\text{CR}_2\text{Li} \xrightarrow[2)\ H_3O^+]{1)\ E^+} \text{product (ketone-E)} \quad 26\text{-}90\%$$

E^+ = ArX, RCH=CHI, ϕC≡CBr

I.B.3-6 Y. Takahashi, H. Kosugi and H. Uda, *Chem. Lett.*, 815 (1982); *Chem. Commun.*, 496 (1982).

$$\phi S\text{-C(Me)=C(CO}_2\text{Me)Li} + \text{CH}_2=\text{CH-CH(CO}_2\text{Me)-CH}_2\text{OSi}^t\text{BuMe}_2 \xrightarrow[\text{(Inverse addn.)}]{-50°C}$$

cyclopentenone product with ϕS, Me, CO_2Me, CH_2OSiR_3 substituents

---

I.B.3-7 C. Shih and J. S. Swenton, *J. Org. Chem.*, **47**, 2825 (1982); A. B. Smith, III et al., *ibid*, **47**, 1855 (1982); L. Duhamel and J. M. Poirier, *Bull. Soc. Chim. Fr. II*, 297 (1982).

$$\text{dithiolane-cyclohexene(R)(Br)} \xrightarrow[2)\ E^+]{1)\ nBuLi} \text{dithiolane-cyclohexene(R)(E)} \quad 75\text{-}92\%$$

I.B.3-8 J. N. Denis and A. Krief, Tetrahedron Lett., 23, 3407, 3411 (1982).

$$RCH=C\overset{SeMe}{\underset{SeMe}{}} \quad \xrightarrow[\text{2) E}^+]{\text{1) nBuLi, THF}} \quad RCH=C\overset{H}{\underset{E}{}}$$

3) Bu_3SnH, AIBN   40-66%

I.B.3-9 M. Kumada et al., J. Amer. Chem. Soc., 104, 180 (1982); E. Negishi, F. T. Luo and C. L. Rand, Tetrahedron Lett., 23, 27 (1982); F. Naso et al., Chem. Commun., 647 (1982).

$$\phi\text{-CH-MgCl} \atop Me \quad + \quad Br\diagup\!\!\!\diagdown\phi \quad \xrightarrow[\text{cat.}]{\text{(S)-(R)-PPFA/NiCl}_2} \quad \phi\text{-}\overset{*}{C}H\diagup\!\!\!\diagdown\phi \atop Me$$

62% (52% ee)

Nickel- and Palladium-Catalyzed Asymmetric Grignard Cross-Coupling (PPFA = Diphenylphosphino-ferrocenyl ethyl amine).

I.B.3-10 T. Kitazume and N. Ishikawa, Chem. Lett., 137, 1453 (1982); R. Yamaguchi, H. Kawasaki and M. Kawanisi, Synth. Commun., 12, 1027 (1982); N. K. Kapoor, R. B. Gupta and R. N. Khanna, Ind. J. Chem., 21B, 189 (1982).

$$R\diagup\!\!\!\diagdown Br \quad \xrightarrow[\text{Ultrasound}]{R_fI,\ Zn \atop THF,\ (\phi_3P)_4Pd\ (cat.)} \quad R\diagup\!\!\!\diagdown R_f$$

59-87%

Also Allylic and Aryl Halides.
R_f = Perfluoroalkyl.

I.B.3-11 E. Wenkert and T. W. Ferreira, Chem. Commun., 840 (1982); M. Julia et al., Tetrahedron Lett., 2465, 2469 (1982).

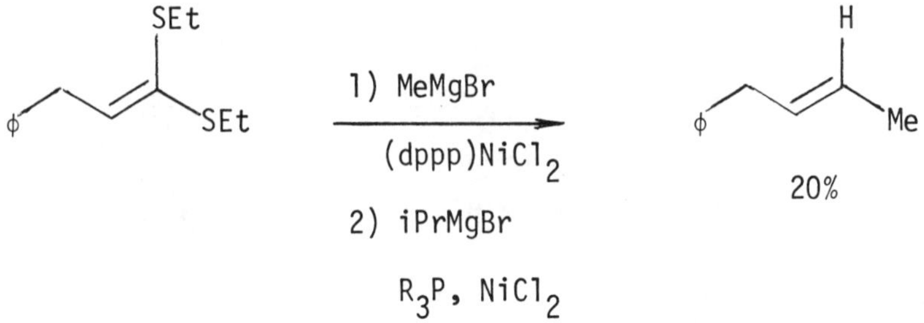

φ-CH₂-CH=C(SEt)₂

1) MeMgBr
   (dppp)NiCl$_2$
2) iPrMgBr
   R$_3$P, NiCl$_2$

→ φ-CH₂-CH=C(H)(Me)   20%

I.B.3-12 S. Araki, T. Sato and Y. Butsugan, Chem. Commun., 285 (1982).

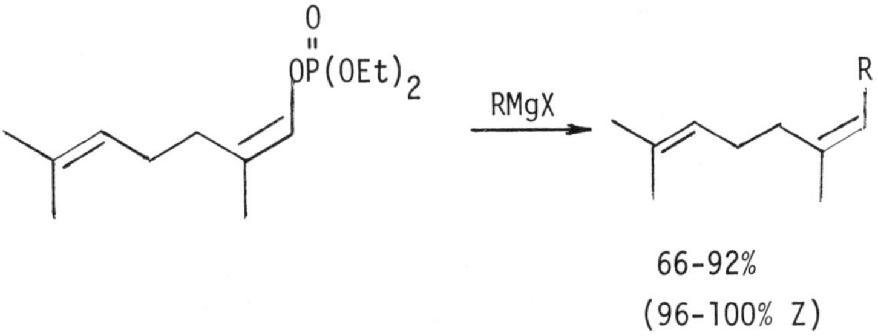

[diene-OP(O)(OEt)$_2$] —RMgX→ [diene-R]

66-92%
(96-100% Z)

I.B.3-13 R. C. Larock and S. S. Hershberger, J. Organometal. Chem., 225, 31 (1982); S. Uemura and S. I. Fukuzawa, Tetrahedron Lett., 23, 1181 (1982).

RCH=CHHgCl $\xrightarrow[\text{10 LiCl, HMPA}]{\text{MeRhI}_2(\text{P}\phi_3)_2}$ RCH=CHCH$_3$
                          70°C   90-99% (GC)

Also methylation of arylmercurials.

I.B.3-14 K. Fujita, E. Moret and M. Schlosser, Chem. Lett., 1819 (1982); B. B. Snider, R. Cordova and R. T. Price, J. Org. Chem., 47, 3643 (1982).

$$\text{HO}\diagup\diagdown\diagup\!\!\!\diagdown \xrightarrow[\text{TiCl}_4,\ \text{THF}]{\text{Me}_2\text{TiCl}_2\ \text{or}\ \text{Me}_3\text{Al}} \text{HO}\diagup\diagdown\diagup\!\!=\!\!\diagdown$$

57%

Δ

I.B.3-15 R. J. K. Taylor, R. F. Newton et al., Tetrahedron Lett., 23, 327 (1982); A. G. Cameron and A. T. Hewson, ibid, 23, 561 (1982); T. Fujisawa et al., Chem. Lett., 1641 (1982).

1) R–CH=CH–Cu(C≡CPr)Li, Et$_2$O, -78°C

2) CH$_2$=C(OMe)CH$_2$Br, NH$_3$

16%

I.B.3-16 N. Jabri, A. Alexakis and J. F. Normant, Tetrahedron Lett., 23, 1589 (1982); D. Michelot, A. Guerrero and V. Ratovelomanana, J. Chem. Res. (S), 93 (1982); R. F. Heck et al., J. Org. Chem., 47, 1267, 1278 (1982); M. Kumada et al., Organometallics, 1, 542 (1982).

$$R^1R^2C=CH\text{–Cu, MgX}_2\ +\ \text{I–C}(R^3)=CHR^4 \xrightarrow[\text{THF}]{(\phi_3P)_4Pd\ (5\%)}$$

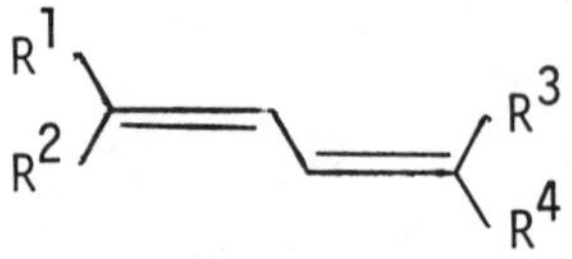

R¹R²C=CH-CH=CR³R⁴

53-78%

(98.2-99.8 Isomeric Purity)

I.B.3-17   J. S. Temple, M. Riediker and J. Schwartz, *J. Amer. Chem. Soc.*, 104, 1310 (1982); P. Vincent, J. P. Beaucourt and L. Pichat, *Tetrahedron Lett.*, 23, 63 (1982).

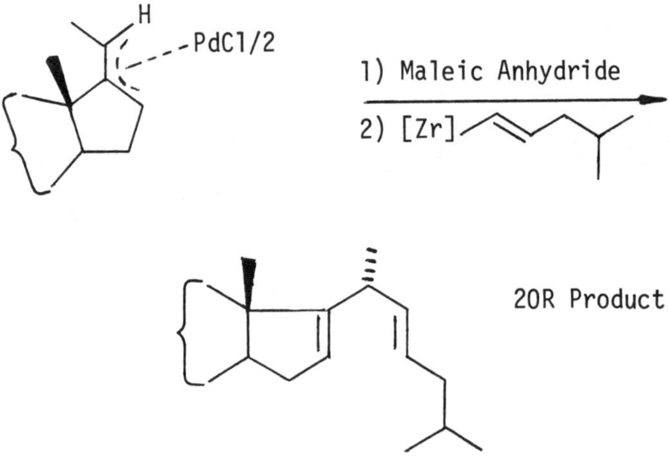

1) Maleic Anhydride
2) [Zr]

20R Product

78%

I.B.3-18 G. R. Stephenson, *J. Chem. Soc., Perkin I*, 2449 (1982).

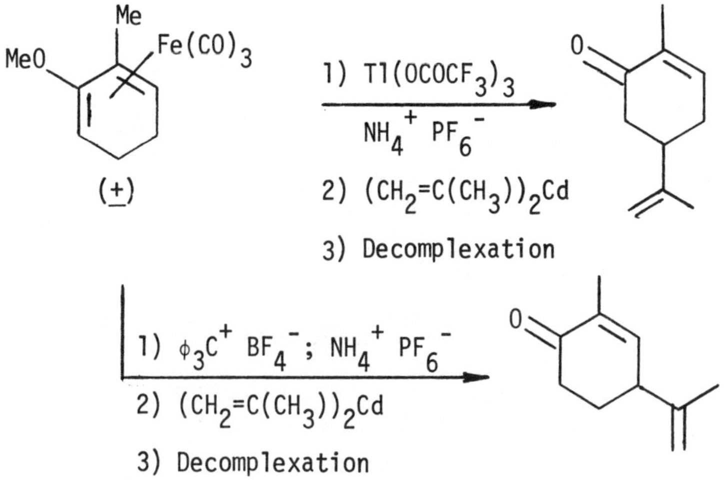

1) $Tl(OCOCF_3)_3$ / $NH_4^+ PF_6^-$
2) $(CH_2=C(CH_3))_2Cd$
3) Decomplexation

1) $\phi_3C^+ BF_4^-$; $NH_4^+ PF_6^-$
2) $(CH_2=C(CH_3))_2Cd$
3) Decomplexation

I.B.3-19 N. Miyaura, K. Suzuki et al., *J. Organometal. Chem.*, **233**, C13 (1982); H. Suginome et al., *J. Org. Chem.*, **47**, 2117 (1982); N. Miyaura, H. Suginome and A. Suzuki, *Bull. Chem. Soc. Jpn.*, **55**, 2221 (1982).

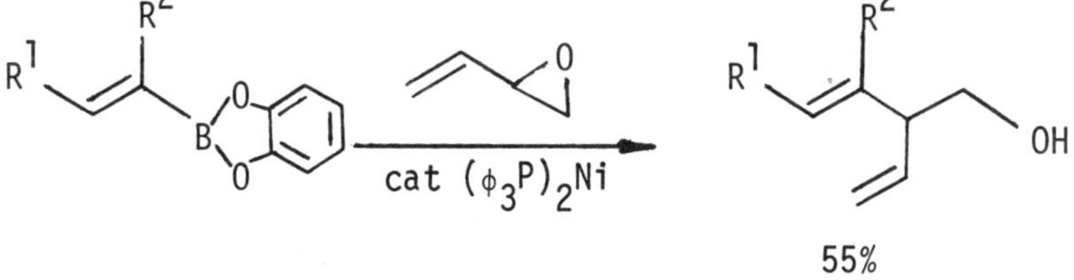

cat $(\phi_3P)_2Ni$

55%

Regioselectivity controlled by nature of catalyst.

I.B.3-20 Y. Ban et al., J. Org. Chem., 47, 4713 (1982); H. Ehrhardt and H. Mildenberger, Liebigs Ann. Chem., 989 (1982).

$$\text{Et-C(CO}_2\text{Et)}_2^- \text{Na}^+ \xrightarrow[\text{THF, }-80°\text{C}]{\begin{array}{l}1)\ \phi\text{SO}_2\text{C}\equiv\text{C-SiMe}_3\\ 2)\ \text{HOAc}\\ 3)\ \text{Al(Hg), CH}_3\text{CN}\end{array}} \text{Et-C(CO}_2\text{Et)}_2\text{-CH=CH}_2 \quad 65\%$$

I.B.3-21 P. Vermeer et al., Tetrahedron Lett., 23, 2797 (1982); J. F. Normant et al., ibid, 23, 5151, 5155 (1982); E. Piers and J. M. Chong, J. Org. Chem., 47, 1602 (1982); A. Carpita, M. Benetti and R. Rossi, Gazz, Chim. Ital., 112, 415 (1982).

$$\text{H-C}\equiv\text{C-H} \xrightarrow[\text{2) RX}]{\text{1) }\phi_3\text{SnCu}} \begin{array}{c}\text{H}\\ \phi_3\text{Sn}\end{array}\!\!\!\!\!\!\!\!\!\!\!\!\!\!\!\!\text{C=C}\!\!\!\!\!\!\!\!\!\!\!\!\!\!\!\!\begin{array}{c}\text{H}\\ \text{R}\end{array}$$

~ 80%

I.B.3-22 B. Giese and S. Lachhein, Angew. Chem., Int. Ed. Engl., 21, 768 (1982).

$$\text{RHgX} \xrightarrow[\text{X-C}\equiv\text{C-Y}]{\text{NaBH}_4} \begin{array}{c}\text{R}\\ \text{X}\end{array}\!\!\!\!\text{C=CHY}$$

I.B.3-23 E. Negishi et al., Chem. Commun., 160 (1982); Tetrahedron Lett., 23, 2085 (1982); A. P. Kozikowski and Y. Kitigawa, ibid, 23, 2087 (1982); T. Yoshida, Chem. Lett., 293, 429 (1982).

$$\underset{Me}{\overset{nBu}{>}}=\underset{AlMe_2}{\overset{H}{<}} \quad + \quad \text{AcO, MeO}_2\text{C-cyclohexenyl} \quad \xrightarrow{\text{cat } (\phi_3P)_4Pd}$$

$$\underset{Me}{\overset{nBu}{>}}=\underset{\text{(cyclohexenyl-MeO}_2\text{C)}}{\overset{H}{<}}$$

86% (90-98% Inversion)

I.B.3-24 F. Sato et al., Chem. Commun., 1126 (1982); R. Yamaguchi et al., Chem. Lett., 1485 (1982); K. J. H. Kruithof and G. W. Klumpp, Tetrahedron Lett., 23, 3101 (1982).

$$Me_3Si-\equiv-CH_2OH \quad \xrightarrow[\text{2) } H_3O^+]{\text{1) 2 }^tBuMgCl, \text{ } Cp_2TiCl_2} \quad \underset{H}{\overset{^tBu}{>}}=\underset{H}{\overset{CH_2OH}{<}}$$

60%

(> 93% Z)

I.B.3-25 H. C. Brown et al., J. Org. Chem., 47, 3806, 3808, 171, 1792 (1982); J. Organometal. Chem., 225, C1 (1982).

$$R^2C\equiv CH \quad \xrightarrow[\substack{\text{2) NaOMe} \\ \text{3) NaOMe, } I_2}]{\text{1) } R^1BHBr \cdot SMe_2} \quad \underset{H}{\overset{R^2}{>}}=\underset{H}{\overset{R^1}{<}}$$

59-74%

Also, stereospecific synthesis of trans alkenes.

I.B.3-26 H. C. Brown and D. Basavaiah, J. Org. Chem., 47, 754 (1982); A. Lattes et al., Tetrahedron Lett., 23, 2785 (1982); Tetrahedron, 38, 2355 (1982).

$$R_2BH \xrightarrow[\substack{\text{2) NaOMe} \\ \text{3) NaOMe}/I_2}]{\text{1) BrC≡CR}^1} \begin{array}{c} R \\ R \end{array}\!\!\!>\!\!=\!\!<\!\!\!\begin{array}{c} H \\ R^1 \end{array}$$

69%

I.B.3-27 J. Leimner and P. Weyerstahl, Chem. Ber., 115, 3697 (1982); J. Janssen and W. Luttke, ibid, 115, 1234 (1982).

$$\underset{\text{Ar-C-R}}{\overset{O}{\|}} \xrightarrow[\text{Pyridine}]{TiCl_4, \text{ Zinc}} \begin{array}{c} Ar \\ R \end{array}\!\!\!>\!\!=\!\!<\!\!\!\begin{array}{c} Ar \\ R \end{array}$$

Z-Product Predominates

I.B.3-28 T. H. Chan et al., Tetrahedron Lett., 23, 837 (1982); J. E. McMurry et al., ibid, 23, 1777, 2723 (1982); R. Dams, M. Malinowski and H. J. Geise, Rec. Trav. Chim., 101, 112 (1982); C. Broquet and H. Riviere, J. Organometal. Chem., 226, 1 (1982).

$$R^1\underset{|}{\overset{OSiMe_3}{CH}}\!-\!S\!-\!\underset{|}{\overset{OSiMe_3}{CHR^2}} \xrightarrow[\text{THF}]{4:1\ TiCl_3 \cdot LAH} R^1CH\!=\!CHR^2$$

18-98% (GC)

I.B.3-29 B. K. R. Shanker and H. Shechter, Tetrahedron Lett., 23, 2277 (1982); T. Nakano et al., Chem. Lett., 613 (1982).

$$ArCH=N_2 \xrightarrow[\text{tetraphenylporphyrin}]{\text{Rh(II) Acetate or Iodorhodium(III)}} \begin{array}{c} Ar \\ H \end{array}\!\!\!>\!\!=\!\!<\!\!\!\begin{array}{c} Ar \\ H \end{array}$$

38-99%

I.B.3-30 F. Barba et al., J. Org. Chem., 47, 142 (1982); H. M. Walborsky et al., Organometallics, 1, 667 (1982); M. Julia et al., Tetrahedron Lett., 23, 2453, 2457 (1982).

$$\phi\text{-}\overset{O}{\underset{\|}{C}}\text{-Cl} \quad \xrightarrow[\text{Acetone, LiClO}_4]{+\ 4e^-} \quad \phi\overset{O}{\underset{\|}{C}}\text{-}\underset{\underset{\phi}{|}}{C}\text{=}\underset{\underset{\phi}{|}}{C}\text{-}\overset{O}{\underset{\|}{C}}\phi$$

95% (68% trans)

I.B.3-31 Y. Sakakibara et al., Chem. Lett., 1565 (1982); H. Yamamoto et al., ibid, 1093 (1982); Y. Sato and Y. Niinomi, Chem. Commun., 56 (1982); W. R. Jackson and C. G. Lovel, ibid, 1231 (1982); T. Funabiki et al., J. Amer. Chem. Soc., 104, 1560 (1982); N. B. H. Henis and L. L. Miller, ibid, 104, 2526 (1982).

$$\underset{H}{\overset{R^1}{>}}\!\!=\!\!\underset{X}{\overset{R^2}{<}} \quad \xrightarrow[\substack{\text{NiBr}_2(P\phi_3)_2 \\ \text{Zn, } \phi_3 P}]{\text{KCN}} \quad \underset{H}{\overset{R^1}{>}}\!\!=\!\!\underset{CN}{\overset{R^2}{<}}$$

(X = Cl or Br) 64-100% (20-96% Stereosel.)

I.B.3-32 S. Hunig et al., Chem. Ber., 115, 261 (1982).

$$\underset{R^2}{\overset{R^1}{>}}\!\!\text{CH-}\overset{O}{\underset{\|}{C}}\text{-Cl} \quad \xrightarrow[\text{2) Me}_3\text{SiCN}]{\text{1) Et}_3\text{N}} \quad \underset{R^2}{\overset{R^1}{>}}C\!\!=\!\!C\!\!\underset{CN}{\overset{OSiMe_3}{<}}$$

Replacement of Me$_3$Si in Product with
$\overset{O}{\underset{\|}{R C}}\text{-}$ and MeSO$_2$-.

I.B.3-33 S. De Lombaert, B. Lesur and L. Ghosez, Tetrahedron Lett., 23, 4251 (1982); N. Slougui, G. Rousseau and J. M. Conia, Synthesis, 58 (1982).

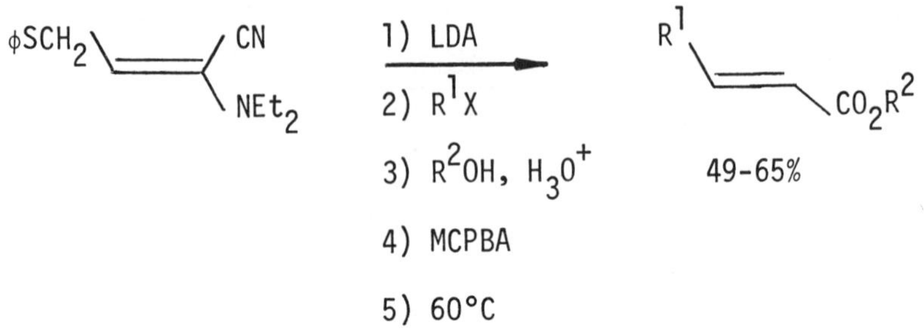

φSCH$_2$-C(=)-C(CN)(NEt$_2$)

1) LDA
2) R^{1}X
3) R^{2}OH, H$_3$O$^+$
4) MCPBA
5) 60°C

→ R^1-CH=CH-CO$_2$R^2 49-65%

I.B.3-34 D. J. Ager, Tetrahedron Lett., 23, 1945 (1982).

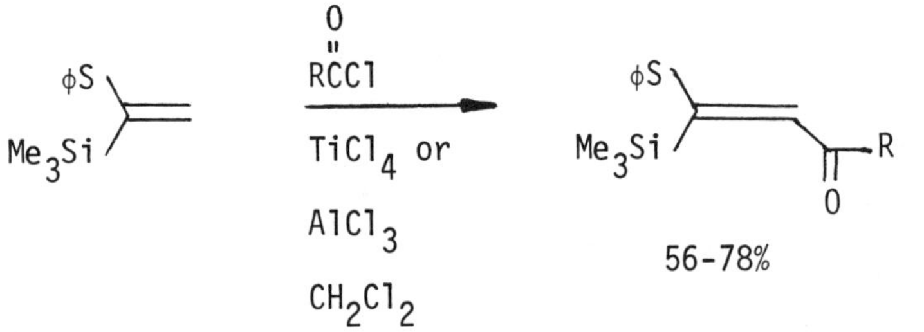

φS, Me$_3$Si substituted alkene

RCCl (O)
TiCl$_4$ or AlCl$_3$
CH$_2$Cl$_2$

→ φS, Me$_3$Si substituted enone with R-C(=O)   56-78%

I.B.3-35 E. I. Negishi, Acct. Chem. Res., 15, 340 (1982).

Review: "Palladium or Nickel-Catalyzed Cross Coupling. A New Selective Method for Carbon-Carbon Bond Formation."

I.B.4. Allene Forming Reactions

I.B.4-1 G. Linstrumelle, et al., <u>Synthesis</u>, 738 (1982); Synth. Commun., <u>12</u>, 739 (1982); B. Psaume and J. Gore, <u>Compt. Rend. II</u>, <u>294</u>, 177 (1982); P. Vermeer et al., <u>J. Organometal. Chem.</u>, <u>224</u>, 399 (1982).

$$R^1R^2C=C=CH_2 \xrightarrow[\substack{2)\ ArI \\ (\phi_3P)_4Pd}]{1)\ nBuLi,\ THF,\ -70°C} R^1R^2C=C=CHAr \quad 78\text{-}90\%$$

Also, vinylation.

I.B.4-2 B. Myrboh, H. Ila and H. Junjappa, <u>Synthesis</u>, 1100 (1982).

$$\underset{H}{\underset{|}{N}}\text{-pyrazolinone}(R^1, R^2) \xrightarrow[(R^2 = H)]{Pb(OAc)_4,\ MeOH} R^1\text{-}C{\equiv}C\text{-}CO_2Me \quad 35\text{-}50\%$$

$$\downarrow \begin{array}{c} Pb(OAc)_4,\ MeOH \\ \hline BF_3\cdot Et_2O \\ (R^1 = CH_2R^3,\ R^2 = \text{Alkyl}) \end{array} \quad R^3HC=C=CR^2(CO_2Me) \quad 60\text{-}76\%$$

I.B.4-3 J. Jullien et al., Tetrahedron Lett., 23, 4943 (1982).

$$\underset{Me_3SiO}{\overset{R^2}{>}}C=C\underset{CH-SiMe_3}{\overset{CO_2Me}{<}} \quad \xrightarrow[\text{2) } H_2O]{\text{1) } 680°C} \quad R^1CH=C=C\underset{R^2}{\overset{CO_2H}{<}}$$
$$\qquad\qquad\qquad R^1 \qquad\qquad\qquad\qquad 43\text{-}60\%$$

I.B.4-4 R. Ruzziconi and M. Schlosser, Angew. Chem., Int. Ed. Engl., 21, 855 (1982); A. Roedig and W. Ritschel, Chem. Ber., 115, 3324 (1982).

55%

I.B.4-5 N. R. Pearson, G. Hahn and G. Zweifel, J. Org. Chem., 47, 3364 (1982).

$$R-C\equiv C-CH_3 \quad \xrightarrow[\text{2) } R_3Al]{\text{1) } ^tBuLi, \text{ TMEDA}, \text{ Et}_2O, -78°C} \quad \underset{E}{\overset{R}{>}}=\bullet= $$
$$\qquad\qquad\qquad\qquad\qquad\qquad 71\text{-}84\%$$
$$\qquad\qquad\qquad \text{3) } E^+$$

E^+ = Allylic Halides, $R_2C=O$, CO_2.

I.B.4-6 A. Claesson et al., *Acta Chem. Scand.*, **36B**, 179 (1982); *Tetrahedron*, **38**, 363 (1982); L. Brandsma et al., *J. Organometal. Chem.*, **232** C1, **233** C25 (1982); *Rec. Trav. Chim.*, **101**, 180 (1982); P. Vermeer et al., *ibid*, **101**, 97 (1982).

$$R^2-\underset{\underset{OMe}{|}}{\overset{\overset{R^1}{|}}{C}}-C\equiv C-CH_2-NR_2 \quad \xrightarrow[\text{2) } H_2O]{\text{1) } R^3MgX, \text{ Cat CuX, THF, Et}_2O} \quad \underset{R^2}{\overset{R^1}{\diagdown}}C=C=C\underset{CH_2NR_2}{\overset{R^3}{\diagup}} \quad 20\text{-}70\%$$

I.B.4-7 A. Haces, E. M. G. A. van Kruchten and W. H. Okamura, **23**, 2707 (1982); P. Vermeer, L. A. van Dijck et al., *Chem. Commun.*, 84 (1982).

[structure with C_8H_{17} substituent, GO group] $\xrightarrow[(G = Bz, Ac, SOMe)]{Me_2CuLi}$ [product ketone with C_8H_{17} and Me substituents]

64-67%

I.B.4-8 G. E. Keck and R. R. Webb, II, *Tetrahedron Lett.*, **23**, 3051 (1982); A. Doutheau, A. Saba and J. Gore, *Synth. Commun.*, **12**, 557 (1982).

$HOCH_2-\equiv$—OMe (propenyl) $\xrightarrow[\text{2) Solid } I_2]{\text{1) LAH, THF, NaOMe}}$ HO-allene-vinyl product

40-98%

I.B.4-9 J. Pornet, L. Miginiac et al., J. Organometal. Chem., **236**, 177 (1982); Tetrahedron Lett., **23**, 4083 (1982).

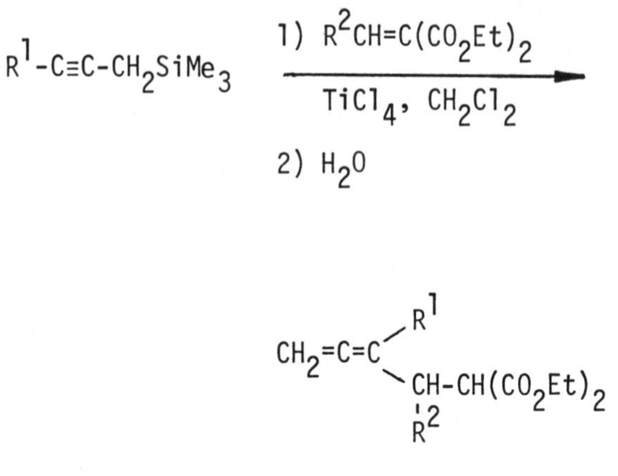

$$R^1-C\equiv C-CH_2SiMe_3 \xrightarrow[\text{2) } H_2O]{\text{1) } R^2CH=C(CO_2Et)_2, \text{ TiCl}_4, \text{ CH}_2\text{Cl}_2}$$

$$CH_2=C=C\begin{array}{l}R^1\\ \diagdown CH-CH(CO_2Et)_2\\ R^2\end{array}$$

5-84%

I.B.4-10 M. Ishiguro, N. Ikeda and H. Yamamoto, J. Org. Chem., **47**, 2225 (1982); B. Cazes, C. Verniere and J. Gore, Tetrahedron Lett., **23**, 3501 (1982).

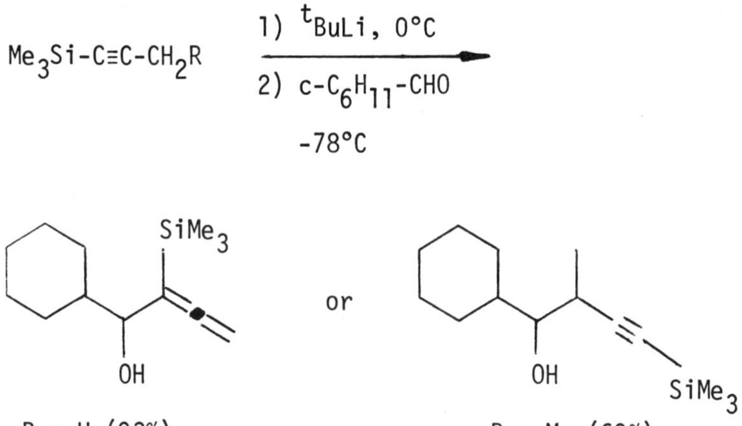

$$Me_3Si-C\equiv C-CH_2R \xrightarrow[\text{2) } c-C_6H_{11}-CHO]{\text{1) } ^tBuLi, 0°C}$$

−78°C

or

R = H (93%)   R = Me (69%)

I.B.4-11 P. Vermeer et al., J. Organometal. Chem., 234, 117 (1982); J. Org. Chem., 47, 2194 (1982).

$$\underset{R^1}{\overset{R^2}{\diagdown}}\!\!=\!\!=\!-X \quad \xrightarrow[\text{2) } H_3O^+]{\text{1) } R^2Ag \text{ or } R^2_2AgMgCl} \quad \underset{R^1}{\overset{R^2CH_2}{\diagdown}}\!\!=\!\!\bullet\!=\!\!\underset{H}{\overset{X}{\diagup}}$$

80-90%

X = SMe, SOMe or Pϕ_2.

I.B.4-12 P. Vermeer et al., J. Org. Chem., 47, 371 (1982); Rec. Trav. Chim., 101, 382, 405 (1982); J. Organometal. Chem., 240, 329 (1982).

$$HC\equiv C-C\equiv C-\underset{R^2}{\overset{R^1}{\underset{|}{C}}}-\overset{O}{\overset{\|}{C}}-OSCH_3 \quad \xrightarrow[\text{THF, HMPA}]{^tBuAg} \quad ^tBuCH=C=C=C\underset{R^2}{\overset{R^1}{\diagup}}$$

60-80%

I.C. Carbon-Carbon Triple Bonds

(See also: VI.A.16).

I.C-1 F. Marcuzzi, G. Modena and G. Melloni, J. Org. Chem., 47, 4577 (1982).

$$PhC\equiv CH \quad \xrightarrow[CH_2Cl_2]{Ph_2CH-OTf} \quad Ph-C\equiv C-CHPh_2$$

73%

I.C-2 A. S. Kende and P. Fludzinski, Tetrahedron Lett., 23, 2369, 2373 (1982).

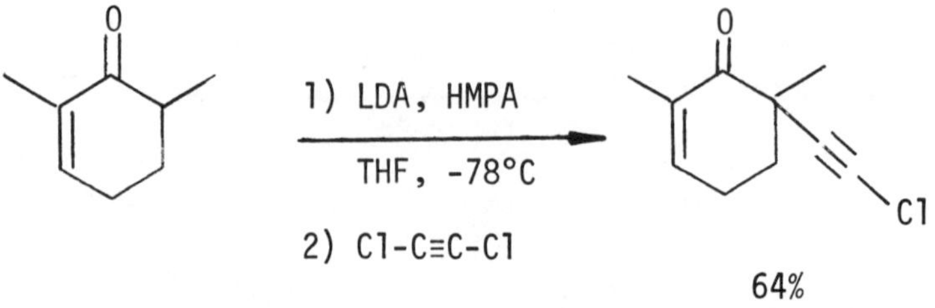

1) LDA, HMPA
   THF, -78°C
2) Cl-C≡C-Cl

64%

I.C-3 S. W. Russell and H. J. J. Pabon, J. Chem. Soc., Perkin I, 545 (1982); J. R. Schauder and A. Krief, Tetrahedron Lett., 23, 4389 (1982).

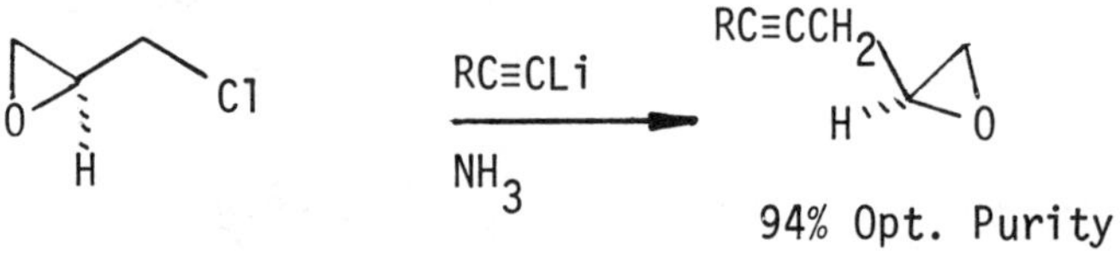

RC≡CLi
―――――→
NH_3

94% Opt. Purity

I.C-4 A. Fisch, J. M. Coisne and H. P. Figeys, Synthesis, 211 (1982); E. V. Dehmlow and A. R. Shamout, Liebigs Ann. Chem., 1750 (1982); C. Santelli-Rouvier and M. Santelli, Tetrahedron Lett., 23, 4945 (1982); K. F. West and H. W. Moore, J. Org. Chem., 47, 3591 (1982).

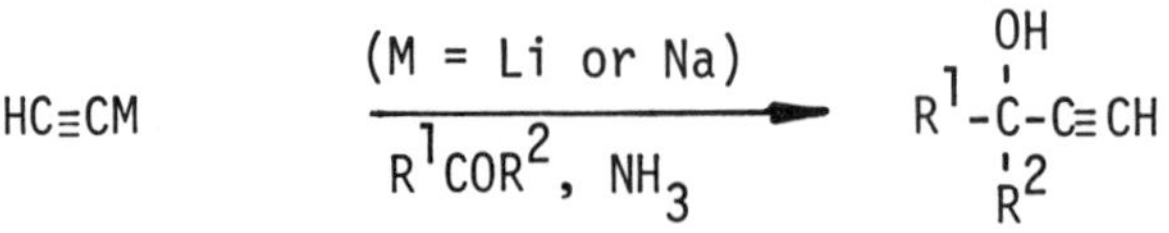

HC≡CM $\xrightarrow[R^1COR^2, NH_3]{(M = Li \text{ or } Na)}$ $R^1\text{-}\underset{R^2}{\overset{OH}{C}}\text{-}C≡CH$

Improved Procedure for Prep. and Use of Alkali Metal Acetylides.

I.C-5 R. Sauvetre, J. F. Normant et al., Tetrahedron Lett., **23**, 4325, 4329 (1982); K. Oshima et al., Bull. Chem. Soc. Jpn., **55**, 3941 (1982).

$$CF_2=CH_2 \quad \xrightarrow[\text{2) } CH_3CHO]{\text{1) }^tBuLi} \quad ^tBu-C\equiv C-\overset{\overset{OH}{|}}{C}HCH_3$$
$$63\%$$

I.C-6 M. Olomucki, J. Y. Le Gall and I. Barrand, Chem. Commun., 1290 (1982); R. M. Carlson et al., Synth. Commun., **12**, 977 (1982).

$$H-C\equiv C-CH_2Cl \quad \xrightarrow[\substack{\text{2) } ClCO_2R,\ -50°C \\ \text{3) } H_2O}]{\substack{\text{1) MeLi (1 eq.)} \\ Et_2O,\ -60°C}} \quad RO_2C-C\equiv C-CH_2Cl$$
$$60-73\%$$

I.C-7 H. J. Bestmann and K. Li, Chem. Ber., **115**, 828 (1982).

$$R^1CHO \quad \xrightarrow[\substack{\text{2) 2 BuLi} \\ \text{3) } B(CH_2CH_2R^2)_3 \\ \text{4) } I_2}]{\text{1) } CBr_4,\ \phi_3P} \quad R^1-C\equiv C-CH_2CH_2R^2$$
$$63-72\%$$

I.C-8 M. W. Logue and K. Teng, J. Org. Chem., 47, 2549 (1982); G. Himbert and L. Henn, Org. Prep. Proc. Int., 14, 189 (1982); M. Fenstel and G. Himbert, Liebigs Ann. Chem., 196 (1982); G. Capozzi, G. Romeo and F. Marcuzzi, Chem. Commun., 959 (1982); G. E. Jones and A. B. Homes, Tetrahedron Lett., 23, 3203 (1982); P. Babin, P. Lapouyade and J. Dunogues, Can. J. Chem., 60, 379 (1982).

$$R^1-C\equiv C-SnBu_3 \xrightarrow[\substack{(\phi_3P)_2PdCl_2 \text{ (cat)} \\ ClCH_2CH_2Cl, 84°C \\ 2) \text{ aq. KF}}]{1) R^2\overset{O}{\overset{\|}{C}}Cl}$$

$$R^1-C\equiv C-\overset{O}{\overset{\|}{C}}-R^2$$

31-71%

I.C-9 H. Yamamoto et al., J. Amer. Chem. Soc., 104, 7667 (1982).

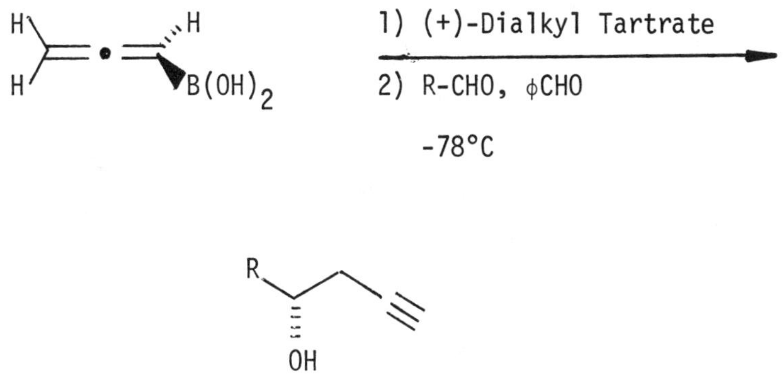

$$\text{H}_2\text{C}=\text{C}=\text{CH}-\text{B(OH)}_2 \quad \xrightarrow[\text{2) R-CHO, }\phi\text{CHO}]{\text{1) (+)-Dialkyl Tartrate}}$$

$$-78°\text{C}$$

$$\underset{\text{OH}}{\text{R}}\diagdown\text{CH}-\text{CH}_2-\text{C}\equiv\text{CH}$$

39-85%

(60->95% ee)

I.C-10 E. J. Corey and J. Kang, Tetrahedron Lett., 23, 1651 (1982).

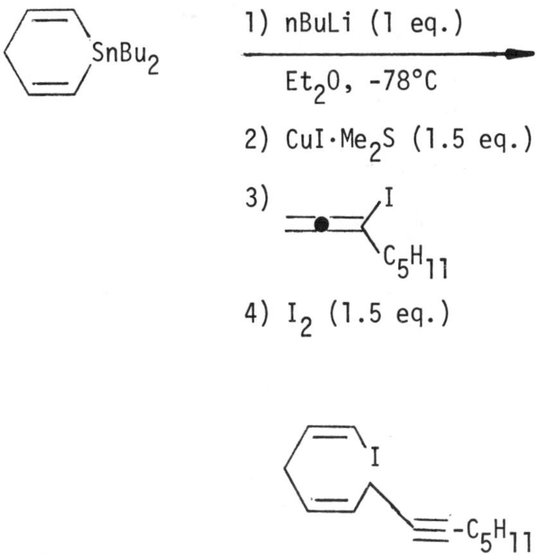

cyclohexadienyl-SnBu$_2$

1) nBuLi (1 eq.)

   Et$_2$O, -78°C

2) CuI·Me$_2$S (1.5 eq.)

3) $\text{CH}_2=\text{C}=\text{C}(\text{I})(\text{C}_5\text{H}_{11})$

4) I$_2$ (1.5 eq.)

cyclohexadienyl(I)—C≡C-C$_5$H$_{11}$

73%

I.C-11 A de Meijere et al., Tetrahedron Lett., 23, 3341 (1982); Angew. Chem., Int. Ed. Engl., 21, 65 (1982); G. Himbert and M. Feustel, ibid, 21, 282 (1982); P. Dureja, J. E. Casida and L. O. Ruzo, Tetrahedron Lett., 23, 5003 (1982); M. A. Pericas, A. Riera and F. Serratosa, Tetrahedron, 38, 1505 (1982).

$$\text{R}\overset{\triangle}{\underset{Cl}{\diagup}}\overset{Cl}{\underset{Cl}{\diagdown}}\!\!=\!\!\overset{Cl}{\underset{Cl}{\diagdown}} \quad \xrightarrow[\text{2) E}^+]{\text{1) 2 BuLi}} \quad \text{R}\overset{\triangle}{\diagup}\!\!-\!\!\text{C}\!\equiv\!\text{C}\!-\!\text{E}$$

59-95%

$E^+ = ClCO_2Me, CO_2, Me_3SiCl, H_2O$.

I.C-12 M. Shibasaki, Y. Torisawa and S. Ikegami, Tetrahedron Lett., 23, 4607 (1982); P. F. Schuda and M. R. Heimann, J. Org. Chem., 47, 2484 (1982).

$$RCH_2CH(SnBu_3)(Br) \quad \xrightarrow[\phi CH_3,\ 110°C]{3\ DBU} \quad RC\equiv CH$$

α-Bromostannane prepared from aldehyde.

I.C-13 T. Miura and M. Kobayashi, Chem. Commun., 438 (1982).

$$\underset{H}{\overset{ArSO_2}{\diagdown}}\!\!C\!\!=\!\!C\underset{Se\phi}{\overset{R}{\diagup}} \quad \xrightarrow[\text{THF, RT}]{30\%\ H_2O_2} \quad ArSO_2\text{-}C\!\equiv\!C\text{-}R$$

64-93%

I.C-14 J. C. Gilbert and U. Weerasooriya, J. Org. Chem., 47, 1837 (1982).

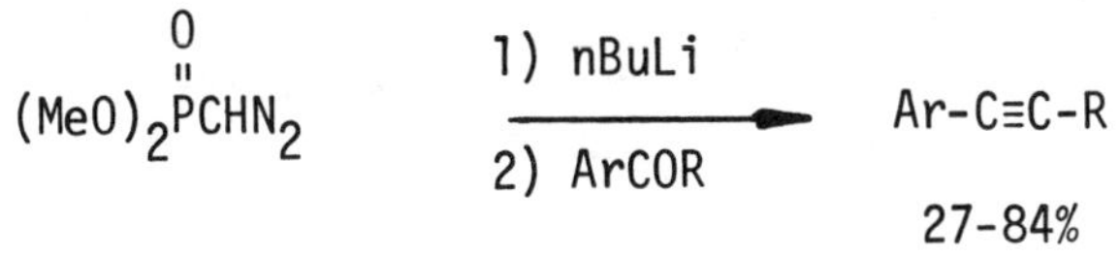

$$(MeO)_2\overset{O}{\overset{\|}{P}}CHN_2 \quad \xrightarrow[\text{2) ArCOR}]{\text{1) nBuLi}} \quad Ar-C\equiv C-R$$

27-84%

I.C-15 Y. Kobayashi et al., Tetrahedron Lett., 23, 343 (1982).

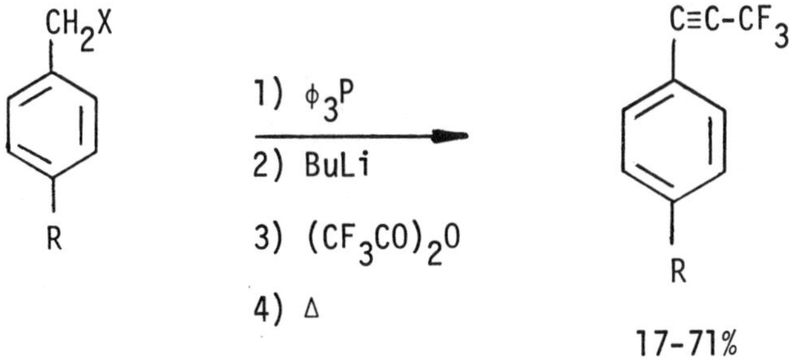

4-R-C$_6$H$_4$-CH$_2$X $\xrightarrow[\text{4) }\Delta]{\text{1) }\phi_3P \text{; 2) BuLi; 3) }(CF_3CO)_2O}$ 4-R-C$_6$H$_4$-C$\equiv$C-CF$_3$

17-71%

I.C-16 R. T. Logan, R. G. Roy and G. F. Woods, J. Chem. Soc., Perkin I, 1079 (1982).

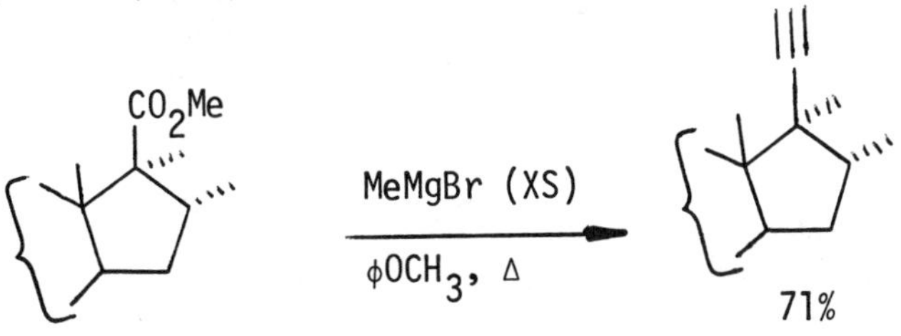

bicyclic-CO$_2$Me $\xrightarrow[\phi OCH_3, \Delta]{\text{MeMgBr (XS)}}$ bicyclic-C$\equiv$CH

71%

I.C-17 P. Calas, P. Moreau and A. Commeyras, Chem. Commun., 433 (1982); T. Umemoto, Y. Kuriu and O. Miyano, Tetrahedron Lett., 23, 3579 (1982).

$$HC\equiv C-\underset{Me}{\underset{|}{\overset{Me}{\overset{|}{C}}}}-OH \xrightarrow[\text{2) KOH, MeOH}]{\begin{array}{c}1) C_6F_{13}I, H_2O \\ \text{Electrolysis}\end{array}} C_6F_{13}-C\equiv CH$$
3) NaOH, Δ   78%

I.C-18 M. Catellani and G. P. Chiusoli, Tetrahedron Lett., 23, 4517 (1982); R. C. Larock, J. P. Burkhart and K. Oertle, ibid, 23, 1071 (1982).

$$\xrightarrow[\text{80°C}]{\phi Br,\ \phi C\equiv CH,\ Pd(0)\ Cat.}$$

42-86%

I.C-19 G. Struve and S. Seltzer, J. Org. Chem., 47, 2109 (1982); V. Thaller et al., J. Chem. Res. (S), 199 (1982); R. Rossi et al., Tetrahedron, 38, 631 (1982); H. Priebe and H. Hopf, Angew. Chem., Int. Ed. Engl., 21, 286 (1982).

$$MeO_2C-CH=CH-I \xrightarrow[\text{DMF}]{CuC\equiv C-R} MeO_2C-CH=CH-C\equiv C-R$$

< 57%

I.C-20 E. B. Merkushev and T. S. Skorokhodova, J. Org. Chem. (USSR), 18, 308 (1982).

$$Ar^1I \xrightarrow[\text{Et}_2\text{NH, CuI}]{\underset{PdCl_2,\ \phi_3P}{Ar^2C\equiv CH}} Ar^1-C\equiv C-Ar^2$$

43-80%

I.C-21 G. J. Leigh, M. T. Rahmen and D. R. M. Walton, Chem. Commun., 541 (1982).

Acetylene Metathesis

I.D. Cyclopropanations

I.D.1. Carbene or Carbenoic Additions to Multiple Bonds
(See also: VI.A.7.)

I.D.1-1 K. G. Taylor, Tetrahedron, 38, 2751 (1982).

Review: "Carbenes and Carbenoids with Neighboring Heteroatoms."

I.D.1-2 Z. I. Yoshida, Pure Appl. Chem., 54, 1059 (1982).

Review: "Novel Pi Systems Possessing Cyclopropenylidene Moiety."

I.D.1-3 P. J. Stang, Acct. Chem. Res., 15, 348 (1982).

Review: "Recent Developments in Unsaturated Carbenes and Related Chemistry."

I.D.1-4 E. V. Dehmlow and M. Prashad, J. Chem. Res. (S), 354 (1982); N. I. Kobesheva, Y. I. Kheruze and A. A. Petrov, J. Org. Chem. (USSR), 18, 828 (1982); R. Barlett, R. Le Goaller and C. Gey, Can. J. Chem., 60, 1933 (1982).

$$\text{limonene} \xrightarrow[\text{Me}_4\text{N}^+ \text{Cl}^-]{:\text{CCl}_2} \text{dichlorocarbene adduct} \quad 68\%$$

I.D.1-5 S. L. Regen and A. Singh, J. Org. Chem., 47, 1587 (1982); P. Muller and M. Rey, Helv. Chim. Acta, 65, 1191 (1982); B. H. Jennings et al., Steroids, 39, 371 (1982); A. A. Formanovskii, N. Y. Kozotsyna and I. G. Bolesov, J. Org. Chem (USSR), 18, 71 (1982).

$$\text{alkene} \xrightarrow[\substack{\text{NaOH/CHCl}_3 \\ 30\text{-}40°\text{C} \\ \text{No PT Catalyst}}]{\text{Ultrasound}} \text{dichlorocyclopropane} \quad 57\%$$

I.D.1-6 R. Fields, R. N. Haszeldine et al., J. Chem. Soc., Perkin I, 2203 (1982).

$$\text{(CF}_3\text{)}_2\text{C=C=CF}_2 \xrightarrow{:CF_2} \text{cyclopropane product}$$

52%

I.D.1-7 R. A. Moss et al., J. Org. Chem., 47, 4177 (1982); Chem. Commun., 432 (1982); W. Bruck and H. Durr, Angew. Chem., Int. Ed. Engl., 21, 916 (1982).

$$\text{Cl,}\phi\text{O-diazirine} + R^1R^2C=CR^3R^4 \xrightarrow{25°C} \text{cyclopropane}$$

10-40%

I.D.1-8 E. C. Friedrich and G. Biresaw, J. Org. Chem., 47, 1615, 2426 (1982); C. R. Johnson and M. R. Barbachyn, J. Amer. Chem. Soc., 104, 4290 (1982); O. Repic and S. Vogt, Tetrahedron Lett., 23, 2729 (1982); W. Hartmann and D. Wendisch, Tetrahedron Lett., 23, 2841 (1982).

$$\text{cyclopentenol} \xrightarrow[\text{Et}_2\text{O}]{\text{CH}_3\text{CHI}_2, \text{Zn-CuCl}} \text{bicyclic product}$$

71%

I.D.1-9 T. Hiyama and M. Kai, Tetrahedron Lett., 23, 2103 (1982); H. Abdallah, R. Gree and R. Carrie, ibid, 23, 503 (1982).

$$R^1\text{-CH=C}(CO_2R^2)\text{-N}_3 \xrightarrow[2) \Delta, CCl_4]{1) CH_2N_2} R^1\text{-cyclopropane-}(N_3)(CO_2R^2)$$

11-93%

I.D.1-10 M. S. Baird, S. R. Buxton and M. Mitra, Tetrahedron Lett., 23, 2701 (1982); T. Hudlicky and R. P. Short, J. Org. Chem., 47, 1522 (1982).

$$R^1_2C=C(R^2)\text{-CH}_2\text{-C(Br)}_2\text{SiMe}_3 \xrightarrow[20-35°C]{MeLi, Et_2O} \text{bicyclobutane}(R^1,R^1,R^2,SiMe_3)$$

47-53%

I.D.1-11 M. P. Doyle et al., Tetrahedron Lett., 23, 2261 (1982); J. Org. Chem., 47, 4059 (1982); H. J. Callot, F. Metz and C. Piechocki, Tetrahedron, 38, 2365 (1982); O. Pelletier and K. Jankowski, Can. J. Chem., 60, 2383 (1982); T. Aratani, Y. Yoneyoshi and T. Nagase, Tetrahedron Lett., 23, 685 (1982); A. R. Daniewski and T. Kowalczyk-Przewloka, ibid, 23, 2411 (1982).

$$\text{diene}(R^2,R^1) \xrightarrow[ML_n]{N_2CHCO_2Et} \text{cyclopropane}(CO_2Et, R^2, \text{vinyl-}R^1) \quad +/\text{or}$$

ML_n = $Rh_2(OAc)_4$, $Rh_6(CO)_{16}$, $CuCl \cdot P(OiPr)_3$, $PdCl_2 \cdot 2PhCN$

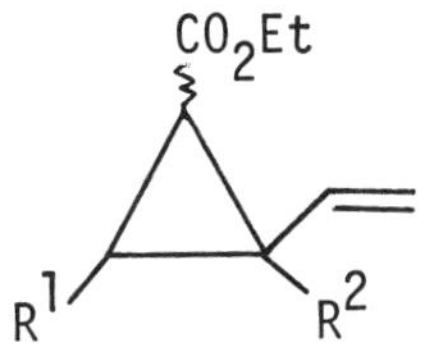

"Metal Carbene Regioselectivity Index."

I.D.2. Other Cyclopropanations

I.D.2-1 N. Kawabata, S. Yanao and J. I. Yoshida, <u>Bull. Chem. Soc. Jpn.</u>, <u>55</u>, 2687 (1982).

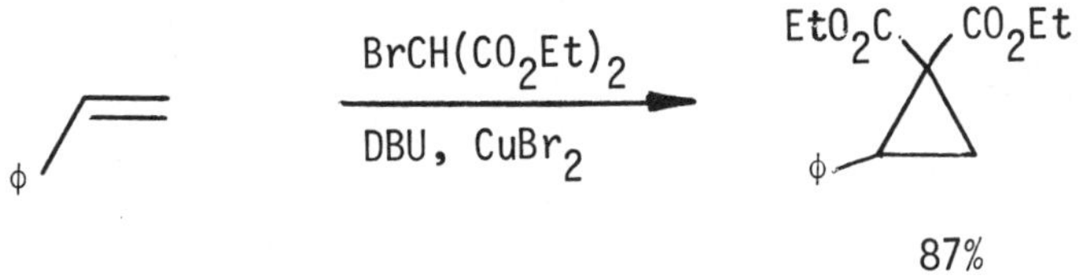

I.D.2-2 C. P. Casey et al., <u>J. Amer. Chem. Soc.</u>, <u>104</u>, 3761 (1982).

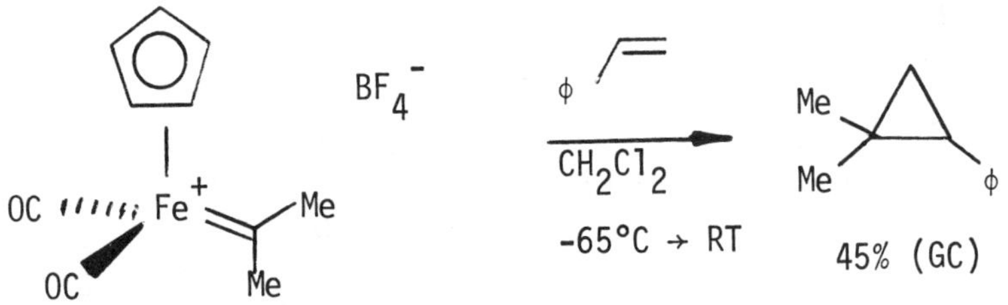

I.D.2-3 R. K. Freidlina, A. A. Kamyshova and E. T. Chukovskaya, <u>Russ. Chem. Rev.</u>, <u>51</u>, 368 (1982).

Review: "The Synthesis of Substituted Cyclopropanes and Cyclopropenes by the Reductive Cyclization of Polychloroalkanes."

I.D.2-4 S. S. Bhattacharjee, H. Ila and H. Junjappa, Synthesis, 301 (1982); R. Lantzsch, ibid, 955 (1982); T. Shono et al., J. Org. Chem., 47, 3090 (1982).

$$Me_3\overset{+}{N}-CH_2-CN \quad I^- \quad \xrightarrow[\text{2) } R^1CH=CH-COR^2]{\text{1) NaH, THF}} \quad \text{cyclopropane with } R^1, H, H, COR^2, CN, H$$

21-86%

I.D.2-5 J. P. Genet, M. Balabane and F. Charbonnier, Tetrahedron Lett., 23, 5027 (1982); T. L. Ho and S. H. Liu, Synth. Commun., 12, 995 (1982).

$$AcO-CH(Me)-CH=CH-CH_2-CH(CO_2Me)_2 \quad \xrightarrow[\text{2) Pd(DIPHOS)}_2]{\text{1) NaH, DME}}$$

Me-CH=CH-cyclopropane-(CO$_2$Me)$_2$

(+13% Z)

I.D.2-6 M. Joucla, L. Toupet et al., Chem. Commun., 858 (1982); T. Ikeda, S. Kobayashi and H. Taniguchi, Synthesis, 393 (1982).

$$R^1R^2C=N-OLi \quad + \quad 2 \; CH_2=C(Br)(CO_2Me) \quad \longrightarrow \quad R^1R^2C=N-O-\text{cyclopropane}(CO_2Me)_2(Br)$$

40-60%

I.D.2-7 J. D. Fourneron, L. M. Harwood and M. Julia, Tetrahedron, 38, 693 (1982); K. Tanaka et al., Bull. Chem. Soc. Jpn., 55, 2965 (1982).

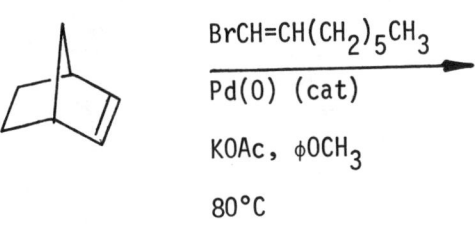

I.D.2-8 M. Majewski and V. Snieckus, Tetrahedron Lett., 23, 1343 (1982); Y. Gaoni, J. Org. Chem., 47, 2564 (1982); L. A. Last, E. R. Fretz and R. M. Coates, ibid, 47, 3211 (1982); E. R. Koft and A. B. Smith, III, J. Amer. Chem. Soc., 104, 2659 (1982).

I.D.2-9 G. P. Chiusoli et al., J. Organometal. Chem., 233, C21; 239, C35; 240, 311 (1982).

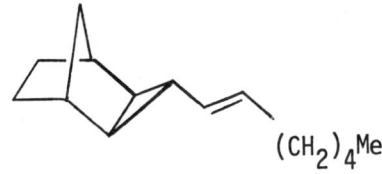

I.D.2-10 B. B. Snider and M. Karras, J. Org. Chem., 47, 4588 (1982).

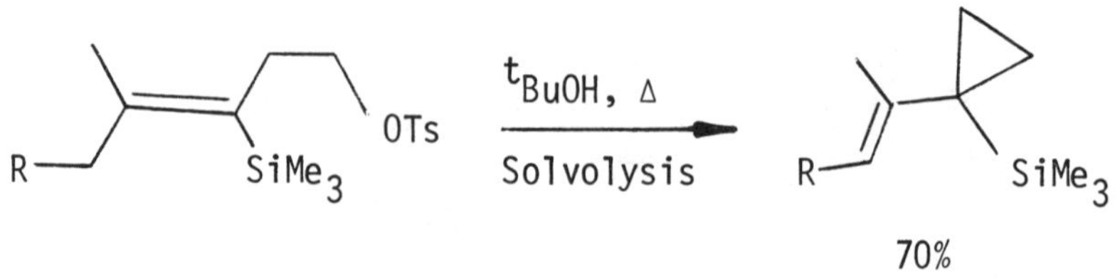

[Scheme: R-CH2-C(Me)=C(SiMe3)-CH2CH2-OTs → (tBuOH, Δ, Solvolysis) → R-CH=C(cyclopropyl with SiMe3), 70%]

I.D.2-11 T. H. Chan and I. H. M. Wallace, Tetrahedron Lett., 23, 799 (1982).

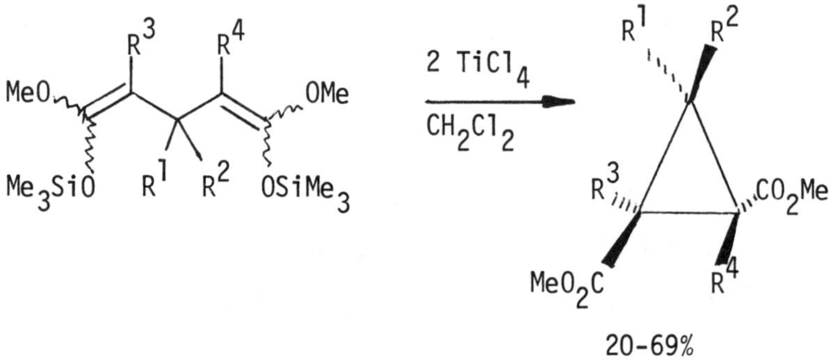

[Scheme: MeO-C(R^3)=...-C(R^4)-OMe with Me$_3$SiO, R^1, R^2, OSiMe$_3$ substituents → (2 TiCl$_4$, CH$_2$Cl$_2$) → cyclopropane with R^1, R^2, R^3, R^4, CO$_2$Me, MeO$_2$C substituents, 20-69%]

I.D.2-12 Y. Ueno, M. Ohta and M. Okawara, Tetrahedron Lett., 23, 2577 (1982); L. Birkofer and J. Kittler, Chem. Ber., 115, 3737 (1982).

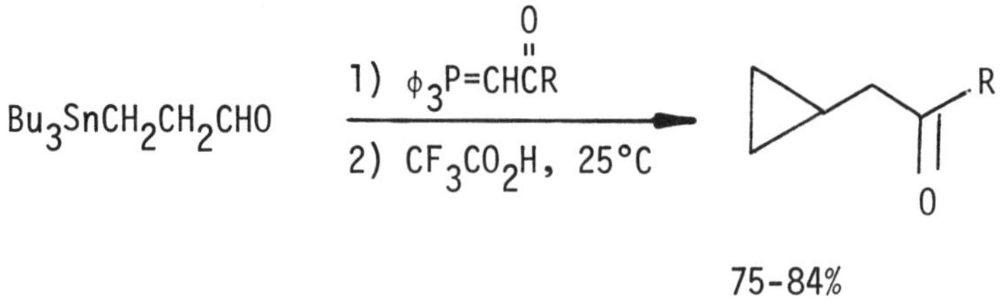

[Scheme: Bu$_3$SnCH$_2$CH$_2$CHO → 1) ϕ_3P=CHCR(=O) 2) CF$_3$CO$_2$H, 25°C → cyclopropyl-CH$_2$-C(=O)-R, 75-84%]

I.D.2-13 M. Franck-Neumann and M. Miesch, Tetrahedron Lett., 23, 1409 (1982); R. J. Bushby et al., J. Chem. Soc., Perkin I, 2647, 2655 (1982); R. F. Childs, G. S. Shaw and A. Varadarajan, Synthesis, 198 (1982); M. G. Steinmetz, R. T. Mayes and J. C. Yang, J. Amer. Chem. Soc., 104, 3518 (1982); A. Hassner, D. Middlemas et al., Tetrahedron, 38, 2539 (1982).

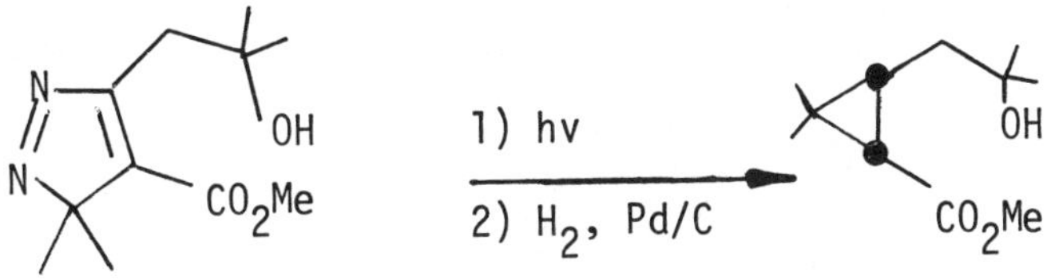

I.D.2-14 A. Bury, S. T. Corker and M. D. Johnson, J. Chem. Soc., Perkin I, 645 (1982).

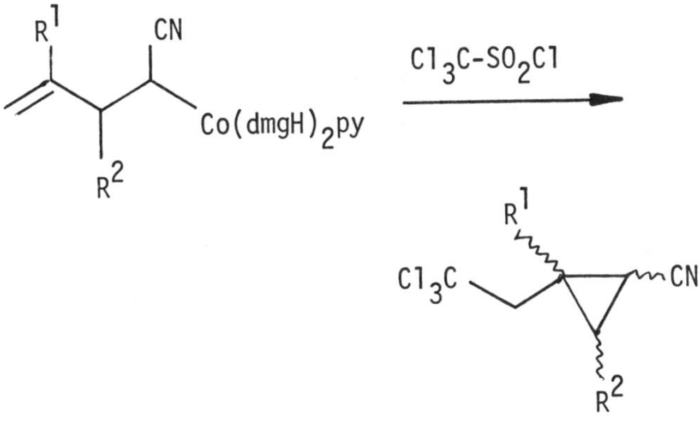

dmg = dimethylglyoximato, py = pyridine

I.D.2-15 H. H. Wasserman and R. P. Dion, Tetrahedron Lett., 23, 785, 1413 (1982); E. Vilsmaier et al., Chem. Ber., 115, 1209, 2795 (1982).

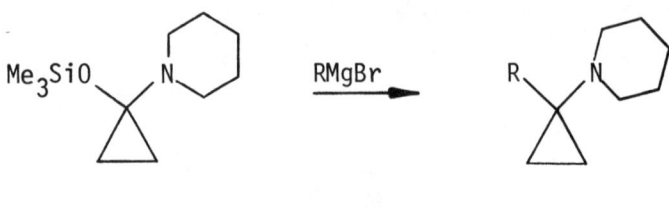

67-95%

Also, 1-hydroxy derivative of starting material reacts with nucleophiles in the presence of Lewis acids.

I.D.2-16 L. A. Paquette et al., Tetrahedron Lett., 23, 259, 263 (1982); C. L. Bumgardner, J. R. Lever and S. T. Purrinton, ibid, 23, 2379 (1982); P. M. Warner and D. Le, J. Org. Chem., 47, 893 (1982); H. U. Reissig and I. Bohm, J. Amer. Chem. Soc., 104, 1735 (1982).

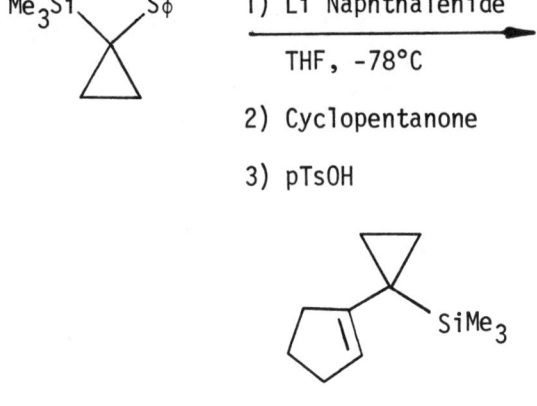

52-75%

Thermal rearr. of product to annulated derivatives.

I.D.2-17 T. Hiyama et al., Tetrahedron Lett., 23, 1279 (1982);
R. Hassig, H. Siegel and D. Seebach, Chem. Ber., 115, 1990
(1982); L. Skattebol et al., Acta Chem. Scand., 36B, 587, 593
(1982).

I.D.2-18 D. Seebach et al., Helv. Chim. Acta, 65, 137 (1982);
L. Fitjer, Chem. Ber., 115, 1035, 1047, 1061 (1982).

up to 60%

(Nitro-nitroso cmpd up to 45%)

I.D.2-19 O. A. Nesmeyanova et al., Synthesis, 296 (1982); H.
Lehmkuhl and K. Mehler, Liebigs Ann. Chem., 2244 (1982); R. B.
Mitra, Z. Muljiani and A. R. A. S. Deshmukh, Synth. Commun.,
12, 1063 (1982); A. M. Moiseenkov, B. A. Czeskis and A. V.
Semenovsky, Chem. Commun., 109 (1982).

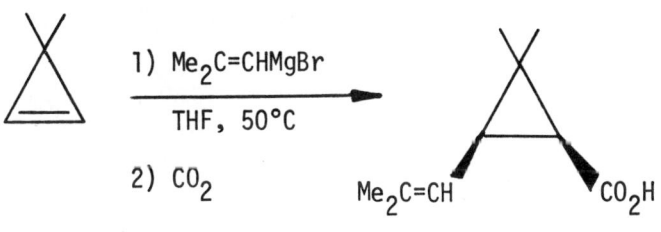

72%

I.D.2-20   M. Regitz et al., Chem. Ber., 115, 2965 (1982).

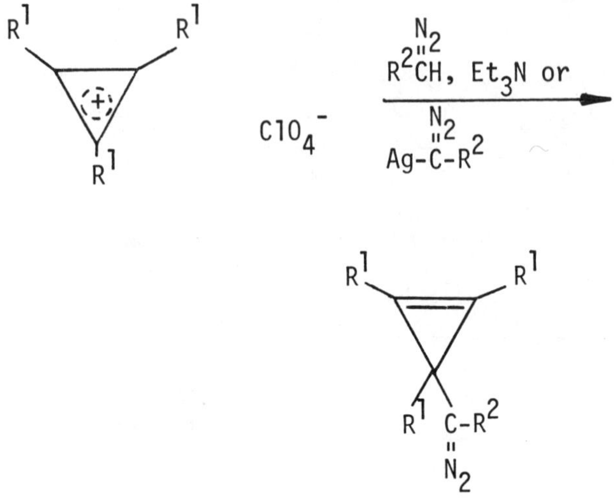

[cyclopropenyl cation with R^1 substituents] ClO_4^- $\xrightarrow{\substack{R^2CH=N_2,\ Et_3N\ or \\ Ag-C(=N_2)-R^2}}$

[cyclopropene product with R^1, R^1, R^1, and C(=N$_2$)-R^2 substituents]

18-96%

I.D.2-21   O. G. Kulinkovich, I. G. Tishchenko and N. V. Masalov, J. Org. Chem. (USSR), 18, 859 (1982); T. Ibuka and E. Tabushi, Chem. Commun., 703 (1982).

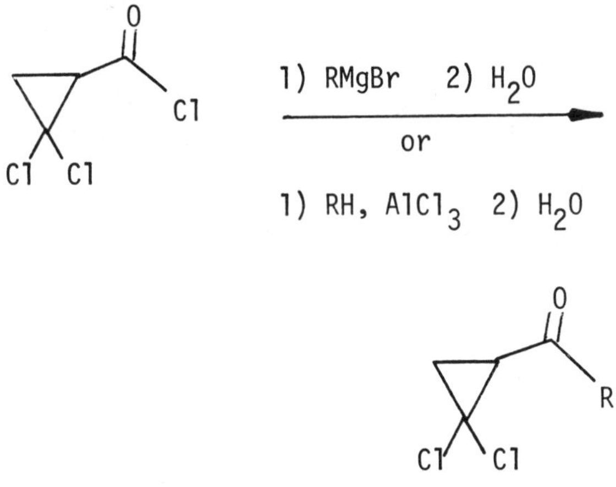

[2,2-dichlorocyclopropyl ketone with COCl group] $\xrightarrow[\text{or}]{\substack{1)\ RMgBr\quad 2)\ H_2O \\ \\ 1)\ RH,\ AlCl_3\quad 2)\ H_2O}}$

[2,2-dichlorocyclopropyl ketone C(=O)R]

40-86%

I.D.2-22 T. V. Akhachinskaya et al., J. Org. Chem. (USSR), 18, 403 (1982); T. Liese, G. Splettstosser and A. de Meijere, Angew. Chem., Int. Ed. Engl., 21, 790 (1982); D. Spitzner, A. de Meijere et al., ibid, 791; H. M. R. Hoffmann et al., ibid, 21, 83 (1982); H. Dahn, L. H. Dao and R. Hunma, Helv. Chim. Acta, 65, 2458 (1982).

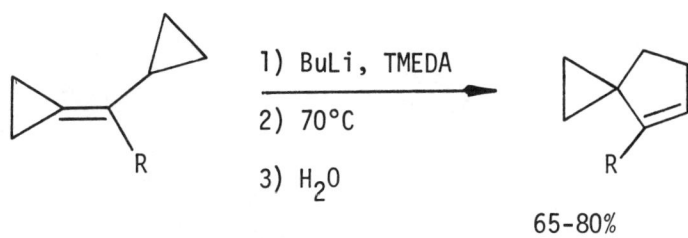

65-80%

I.D.2-23 M. L. Deem, Synthesis, 701 (1982).

Review: "Expanded Ring Systems from Cyclopropenes: 1,3-Dipolar and [2+2]-Additions Across the Cyclopropenyl π-Bond."

I.E. Thermal Reactions

I.E.1. Cycloadditions

I.E.1-1 K. Fukui, Angew. Chem., Int. Ed. Engl., 21, 801 (1982); Science, 218, 747 (1982).

Review: "The Role of Frontier Orbitals in Chemical Reactions (Nobel Lecture)."

I.E.1-2 U. E. Wiersum, Rec. Trav. Chim., 101, 317, 367 (1982).

Review: "Flash Vacuum Thermolysis, A Versatile Method in Organic Chemistry."

I.E.1-3 S. M. Weinrab and R. R. Staib, Tetrahedron, 38, 3087 (1982).

Review: "Synthetic Aspects of Diels-Alder Cycloadditions with Heterodienophiles."

I.E.1-4 W. Grundler, Zeit. Chem., 22, 235 (1982).

"Significant Electron Structures: Regioselectivity of Cycloaddition Reactions."

I.E.1-5 T. Cohen and Z. Kosarych, J. Org. Chem., 47, 4005 (1982); I. Ojima, M. Yatabe and T. Fuchikami, ibid, 47, 2051 (1982); A. Hosomi, H. Sakurai et al., Tetrahedron Lett., 23, 551 (1982); A. V. Rama Rao, V. H. Deshpande and N. L. Reddy, ibid, 23, 775 (1982); N. Ono, H. Miyake and A. Kaji, Chem. Commun., 33 (1982).

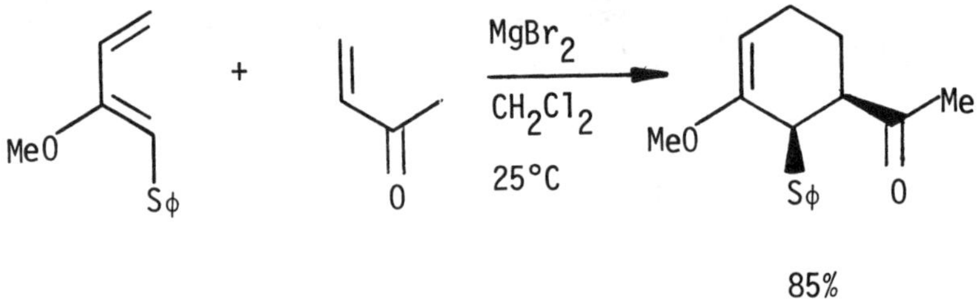

85%

I.E.1-6 F. Brion, <u>Tetrahedron Lett.</u>, <u>23</u>, 5299 (1982); P. F. Schuda and J. M. Bennett, <u>ibid</u>, <u>23</u>, 5525 (1982); C. Schmitz, J. M. Aubry and J. Rigaudy, <u>Tetrahedron</u>, <u>38</u>, 1425 (1982); D. P. G. Hamon and P. R. Spurr, <u>Chem. Commun.</u>, 372 (1982).

furan + CH$_2$=CH-CO$_2$Me

1) ZnI$_2$, 40°C
2) (Me$_3$Si)$_2$NLi
3) Aq. NH$_4$Cl

→ cyclohexadiene with CO$_2$Me and OH substituents

47%

I.E.1-7 S. Danishefsky, et al., <u>J. Org. Chem.</u>, <u>47</u>, 1981, 3183 (1982); K. Jankowski et al., <u>ibid</u>, <u>47</u>, 3649 (1982); H. A. A. Rasoul and H. K. Hall, Jr., <u>ibid</u>, <u>47</u>, 2080 (1982); O. Achmatowicz, Jr. and J. Szymoniak, <u>Tetrahedron</u>, <u>38</u>, 1299 (1982).

Me$_3$SiO-diene with OMe + aldehyde with NH^{t}BOC and CH$_2$CHMe$_2$

1) ZnCl$_2$, φH
2) O$_3$
3) H$_2$O$_2$

→ HO$_2$C–C(OH)(H)–CH(NH^{t}BOC)(CH$_2$CHMe$_2$)   S,S

I.E.1-8 Y. Ito, M. Nakatsuka and T. Saegusa, J. Amer. Chem. Soc., 104, 7609 (1982); R. W. Franck et al., ibid, 104, 1106 (1982); F. M. Hauser and S. Prasanna, J. Org. Chem., 47, 383 (1982); J. Mann and S. E. Piper, Chem. Commun., 430 (1982).

$$\text{o-}C_6H_4(CH_2SiMe_3)(CH_2\overset{+}{N}Me_3\ Cl^-) \xrightarrow[EtO_2C-C\equiv C-CO_2Et]{Bu_4N^+F^-,\ CH_2Cl_2}$$

[bicyclic product: 3,4-dihydronaphthalene-2,3-dicarboxylate diethyl ester]

76%

I.E.1-9 W. G. Dauben et al., Tetrahedron Lett., 23, 4875, 2611 (1982); J. Jurczak, C. H. Eugster et al., Helv. Chim. Acta, 65, 1021 (1982); M. Papadopoulos and G. Jenner, Bull. Soc. Chim. Fr. II, 313 (1982).

[p-benzoquinone] + [CH$_2$=CH-CH=CH-C(O)-R*] $\xrightarrow[20°C]{15\ \text{Kbar}}$ [cis-fused decalin-dione with C(O)-R* substituent]

60-98%

(up to 50% ee)

COR* = Chiral Ester or Amide.

I.E.1-10 Y. Ohfune and M. Tomita, J. Amer. Chem. Soc., 104, 3511 (1982); A. P. Kozikowski, E. Huie and J. P. Springer, ibid, 104, 2059 (1982); B. M. Trost and M. Shimizu, ibid, 104, 4299 (1982); T. J. Brocksom and M. G. Constantino, J. Org. Chem., 47, 3450 (1982).

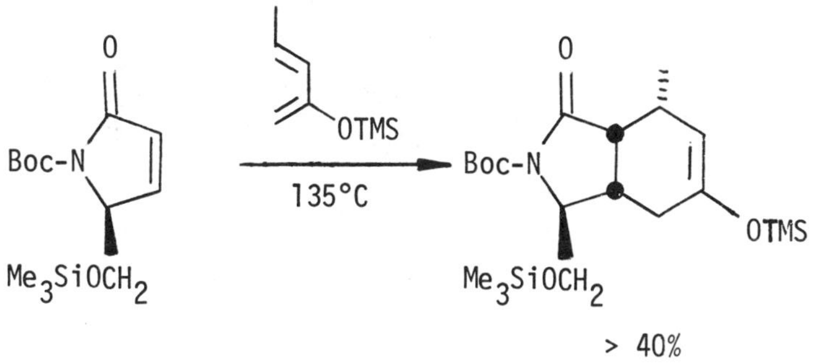

O
Boc-N
Me_3SiOCH_2
OTMS
135°C
O
Boc-N
OTMS
Me_3SiOCH_2
> 40%

I.E.1-11 J. H. Rigby, J. M. Sage and J. Raggon, J. Org. Chem., 47, 4815 (1982).

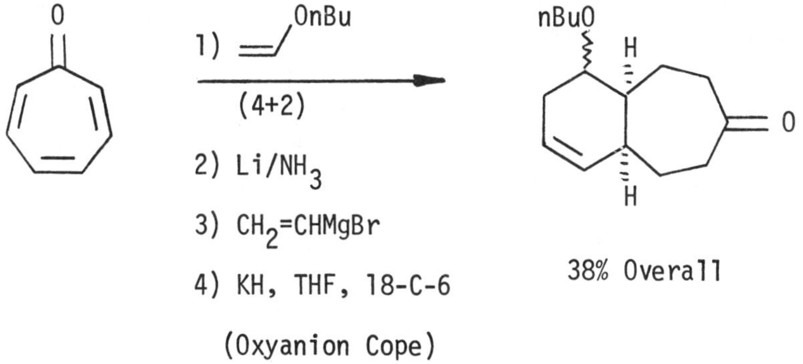

O
1) OnBu
(4+2)
2) Li/NH_3
3) CH_2=CHMgBr
4) KH, THF, 18-C-6
(Oxyanion Cope)
nBuO
H
H
O
38% Overall

I.E.1-12 C. H. Hassall et al., J. Chem. Soc., Perkin I, 2227, 2239, 2249 (1982); Chem. Commun., 158 (1982); R. C. Gupta, D. A. Jackson and R. J. Stoodley, ibid, 929 (1982); Y. Tamura et al., J. Org. Chem., 47, 4376 (1982).

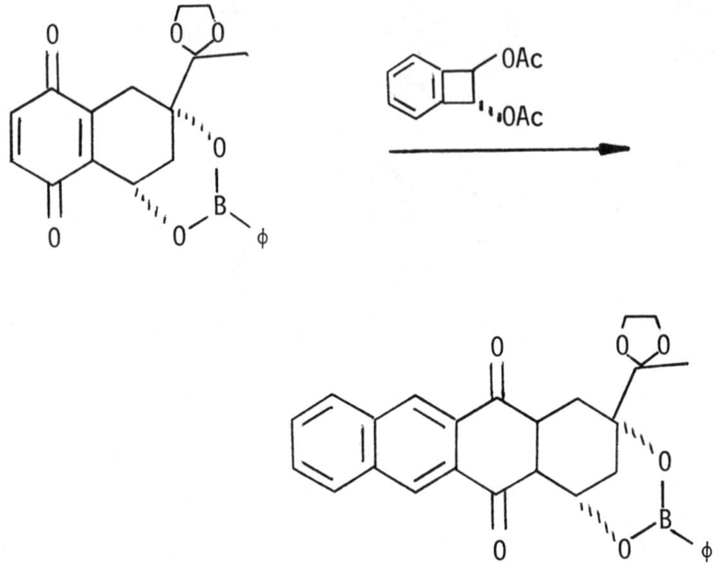

I.E.1-13 J. P. Gesson and M. Mondon, Chem. Commun., 421 (1982); T. R. Kelly, N. D. Parekh and E. N. Trachtenberg, J. Org. Chem., 47, 5009 (1982); N. L. Agarwal and H. W. Scheeren, Chem. Lett., 1057 (1982); A. V. Rama Rao, Tetrahedron Lett., 23, 1115 (1982).

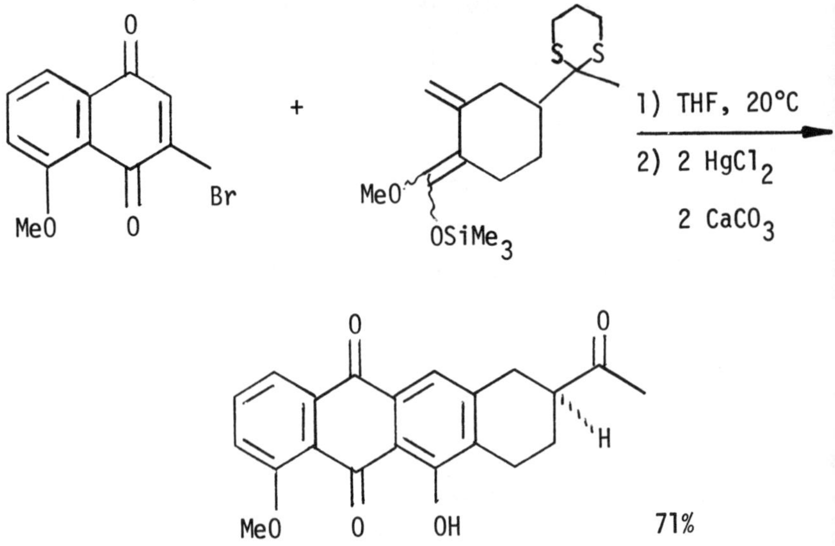

71%

I.E.1-14 A. P. Kozikowski and E. M. Huie, J. Amer. Chem. Soc., 104, 2923 (1982); P. D. Bartlett, W. H. Watson et al., ibid, 104, 3131 (1982); R. N. Warrener, R. A. Russell et al., Chem. Commun., 1134, 1136 (1982).

Diels-Alder then Aldol.

I.E.1-15 E. J. Corey and J. E. Munroe, J. Amer. Chem. Soc., 104, 6129 (1982); L. Stella and J. L. Boucher, Tetrahedron Lett., 23, 953 (1982); W. Oppolzer et al., ibid, 23, 4781 (1982); I. Gupta and P. Yates, Chem. Commun., 1227 (1982); A. Gonzalez and S. L. Holt, J. Org. Chem., 47, 3186 (1982).

I.E.1-16 D. J. Bellville and N. L. Bauld, J. Amer. Chem. Soc., 104, 2665 (1982); D. Spitzner, Angew. Chem., Int. Ed. Engl., 21, 636 (1982); K. Pramod and G. S. R. Subba Rao, Chem. Commun., 762 (1982).

Selectivity Profile of Cation Radical Diels-Alder

I.E.1-17 P. Dowd and W. Weber, <u>Tetrahedron Lett.</u>, 23, 2155 (1982); <u>J. Org. Chem.</u>, 47, 4774 (1982); H. Hiranuma and S. I. Miller, <u>ibid</u>, 47, 5083 (1982).

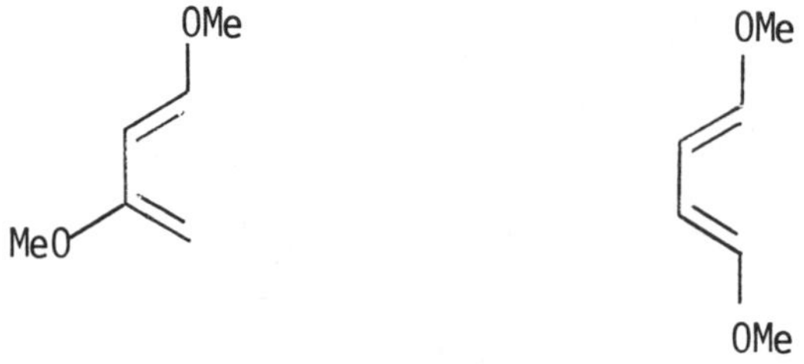

Diels-Alder Dienes.

I.E.1-18 M. Koreeda and M. A. Ciufolini, <u>J. Amer. Chem. Soc.</u>, 104, 2308 (1982); R. R. Schmidt and A. Wagner, <u>Synthesis,</u> 958 (1982); F. Fringuelli, E. Wenkert et al., <u>J. Org. Chem.</u>, 47, 5056 (1982).

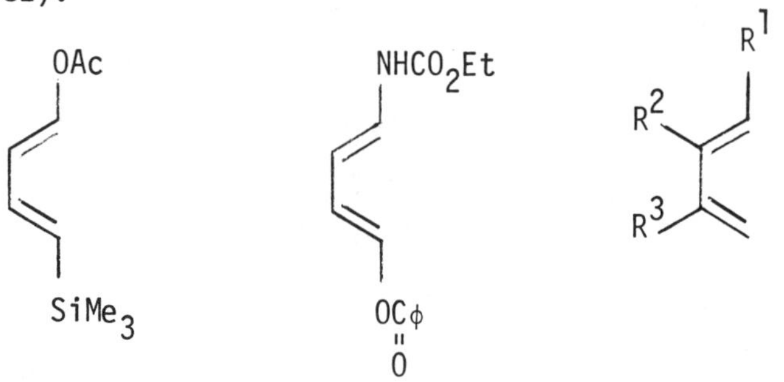

Diels-Alder Dienes.

I.E.1-19 Y. Lepage et al., <u>Bull. Soc. Chim. Fr. II</u>, 321 (1982); J. Dunogues et al., <u>Organometallics</u>, 1, 1525 (1982).

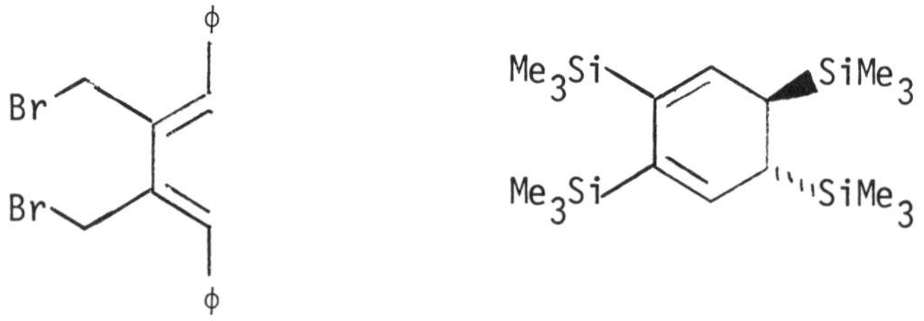

Diels-Alder Dienes.

I.E.1-20 P.D. Bartlett, W. H. Watson et al., J. Org. Chem., 47, 4491 (1982); M. E. Jung et al., ibid, 47, 1150 (1982); M. E. Jung and L. A. Light, ibid, 47, 1084 (1982).

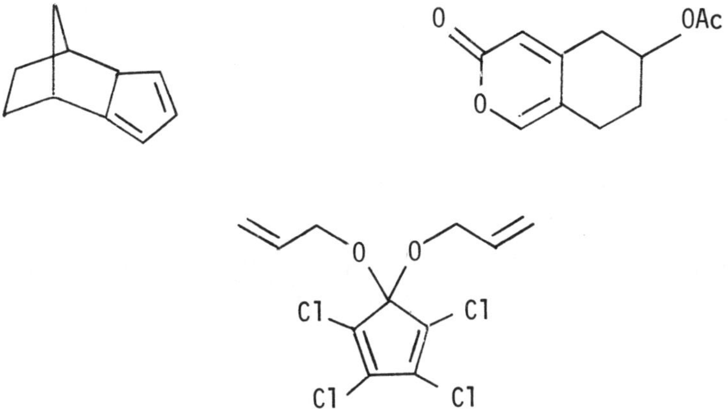

Diels-Alder Dienes.

I.E.1-21 P. Vogel et al., Helv. Chim. Acta, 65, 178, 188, 204, 866, 887 (1982); J. Org. Chem., 47, 3796 (1982); Angew. Chem., Int. Ed. Engl., 21, 430 (1982).

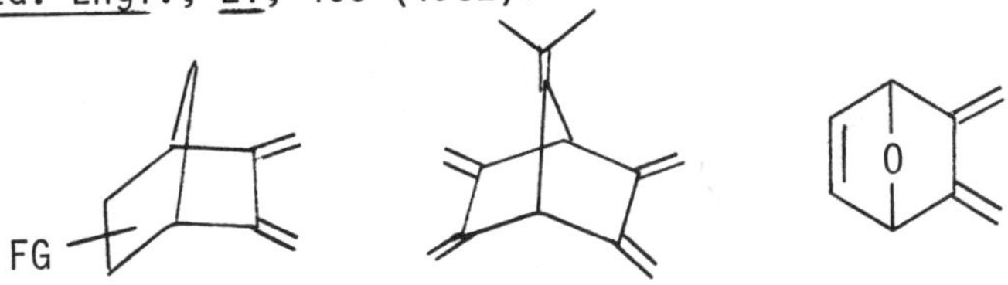

Diels-Alder Dienes (FG = Functional Groups).

I.E.1-22 T. R. Hoye, A. J. Caruso and A. S. Magee, J. Org. Chem., 47, 4152 (1982); R. J. Ardecky, D. Dominguez and M. P. Cava, ibid, 47, 409 (1982); B. M. Trost and P. G. McDougal, J. Amer. Chem. Soc., 104, 6110 (1982).

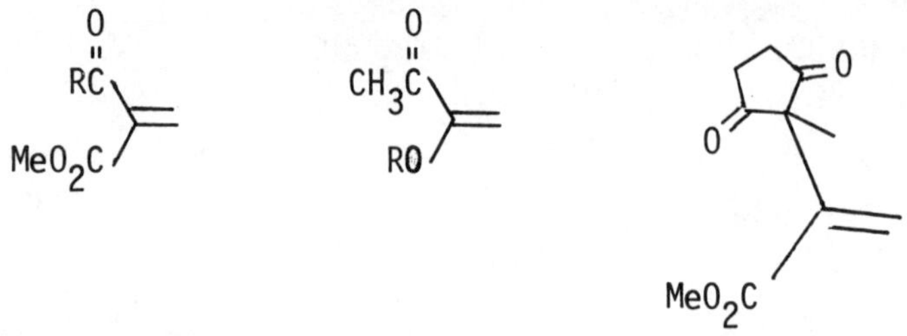

Diels-Alder Dienophiles.

I.E.1-23 P. Yates and S. P. Douglas, <u>Can. J. Chem.</u>, **60**, 2760 (1982); L. A. Paquette and W. A. Kinney, <u>Tetrahedron Lett.</u>, **23**, 5127 (1982).

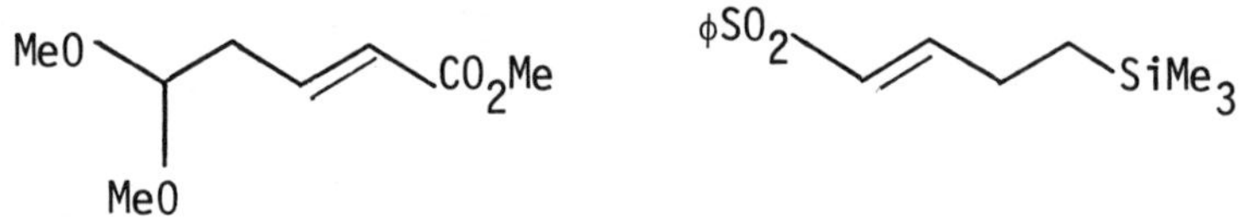

Diels-Alder Dienophiles.

I.E.1-24 H.D. Martin et al., <u>Tetrahedron Lett.</u>, **23**, 841 (1982); M.S. South and L. S. Liebeskind, <u>J. Org. Chem.</u>, **47**, 3815 (1982); V. V. Plemenkov et al., <u>J. Org. Chem. (USSR)</u>, **18**, 1442 (1982).

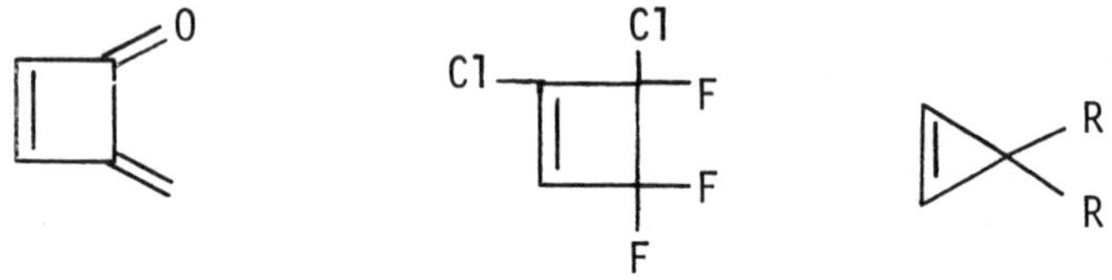

Diels-Alder Dienophiles.

I.E.1-25 P. Dowd and W. Weber, J. Org. Chem., 47, 4777 (1982); H. Takeshita et al., Bull. Chem. Soc. Jpn., 55, 2291 (1982).

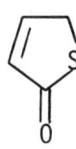
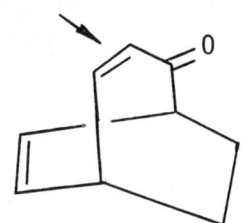

Diels-Alder Dienophiles.

I.E.1-26 H. K. Hall, Jr. et al., J. Org. Chem., 47, 1451, 3647 (1982); H. J. Liu, E. N. C. Browne and P. R. Pednekar, Can. J. Chem., 60, 921 (1982); H. S. Liu and T. K. Ngooi, Synth. Commun., 12, 715 (1982).

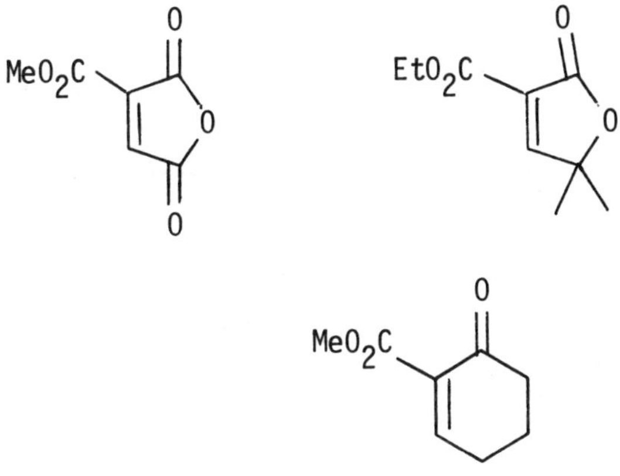

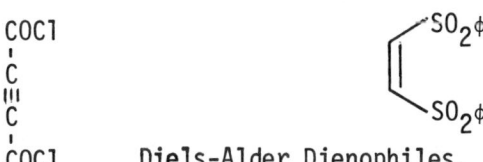

Diels-Alder Dienophiles.

I.E.1-27 G. Maier and W. A. Jung, Chem. Ber., 115, 804 (1982); O. De Lucchi and G. Modena, Chem. Commun., 914 (1982).

```
COCl
 |
 C
 |||
 C
 |
COCl
```

SO$_2\phi$ / SO$_2\phi$ (disubstituted alkene)

Diels-Alder Dienophiles.

I.E.1-28   J. M. J. Verlaak, A. J. H. Klunder and B. Zwanenburg, Tetrahedron Lett., 23, 5463 (1982);   J. V. N. V. Prasad, P. Iyer and C. N. Pillai, J. Org. Chem., 47, 1380 (1982);   T. Siwapinyoyos and Y. Thebtaranonth, ibid, 47, 598 (1982);   T. L. Ho and S. H. Liu, Chem. Ind., 371 (1982).

I.E.1-29   K. A. Parker and T. Iqbal, J. Org. Chem., 47, 337 (1982);   W. R. Roush, H. R. Gillis and A. I. Ko, J. Amer. Chem. Soc., 104, 2269 (1982);   P. L. Fuchs et al., ibid, 104, 5719, 5728 (1982).

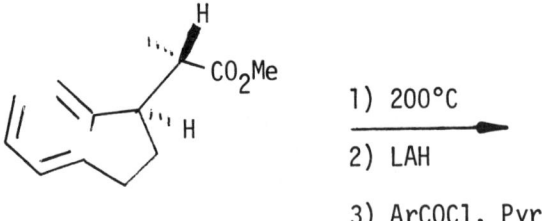

(cis:trans ~ 50:50)

I.E.1-30 D. F. Taber and S. A. Saleh, Tetrahedron Lett., 23, 2361 (1982); E. Yoshii et al., Chem. Pharm. Bull., 30, 4000 (1982); W. R. Roush et al., J. Org. Chem., 47, 4611, 4825 (1982); R. L. Funk and W. E. Zeller, ibid, 47, 180 (1982); B. J. Willis, F. W. Wehrli et al., ibid, 47, 4786 (1982); F. Naf, R. Decorzant and W. Thommen, Helv. Chim. Acta, 65, 2212 (1982); L. F. Tietze, G. von Kiedrowski and B. Berger, Angew. Chem., Int. Engl., 21, 221 (1982).

ϕCH_3, 195°C, Methylene Blue

69%

I.E.1-31 E. A. Deutsch and B. B. Snider, J. Org. Chem., 47, 2682 (1982); G. Himbert and L. Henn, Angew. Chem., Int. Ed. Engl., 21, 620 (1982); J. L. Gras, J. Chem. Res. (S), 300 (1982); M. Fink, H. Gaier and H. Gerlach, Helv. Chim. Acta, 65, 2563 (1982).

1) ϕH, 150°C, 0.5% BHT
2) L-Selectride

75%

I.E.1-32 K. J. Shea and E. Wada, <u>Tetrahedron Lett.</u>, <u>23</u>, 1523 (1982).

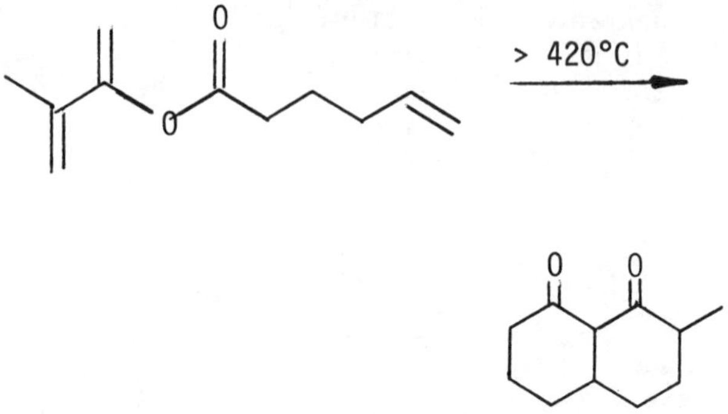

1,3-Acyl Shift then Intramol. Diels-Alder.

I.E.1-33 R. K. Boeckman, Jr. et al., <u>J. Org. Chem.</u>, <u>47</u>, 1789 (1982); <u>J. Amer. Chem. Soc.</u>, <u>104</u>, 1033, 3216 (1982).

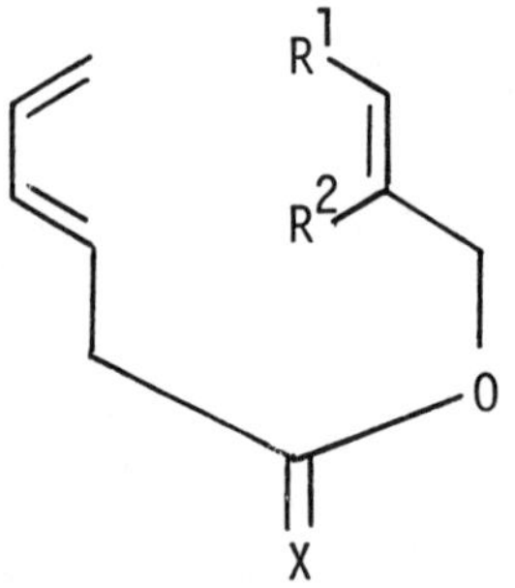

X = O   Sluggish Diels-Alder

X = H_2 Normal Diels-Alder

R^1, R^2 = H, CO_2Me or CO_2Me, H

I.E.1-34 K. J. Shea et al., <u>J. Amer. Chem. Soc.</u>, <u>104</u>, 5708, 5715 (1982); E. Piers and M. Winter, <u>Liebigs Ann. Chem.</u>, 973 (1982).

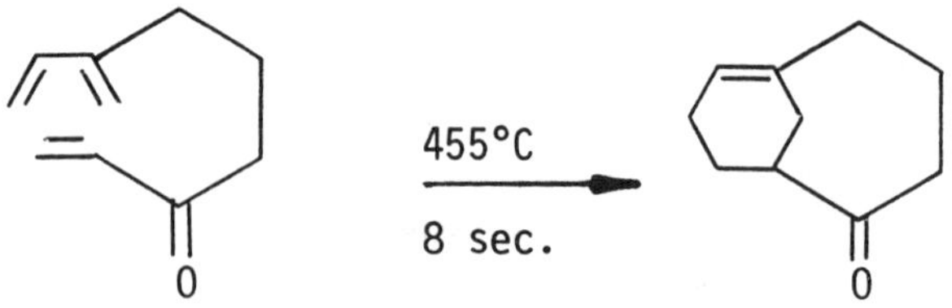

455°C
8 sec.

85%

I.E.1-35 L. F. Tietze et al., Angew. Chem., Int. Ed. Engl., 21, 863 (1982); B. A. Keay and R. Rodrigo, J. Amer. Chem. Soc., 104, 4725 (1982); G. A. Kraus and J. O. Pezzanite, J. Org. Chem., 47, 4337 (1982); G. M. Muschik, T. P. Kelly and W. B. Manning, J. Org. Chem., 47, 4709 (1982).

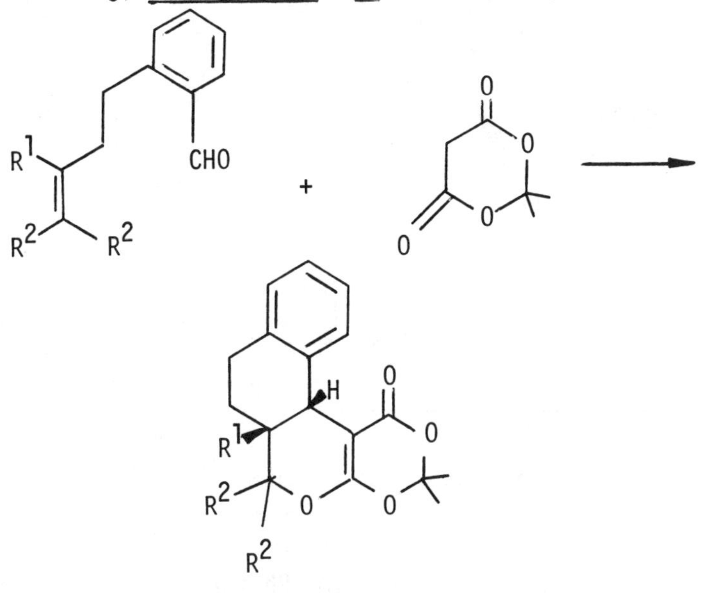

I.E.1-36 T. Gallagher, P. Magnus and J. C. Huffman, J. Amer. Chem. Soc., 104, 1140 (1982); L. Mandell, D. E. Lee and L. F. Courtney, J. Org. Chem., 47, 610 (1982).

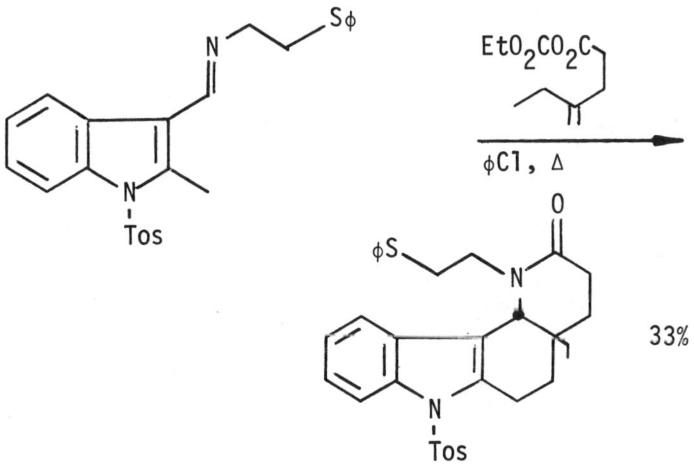

I.E.1-37 G. Quinkert et al., Liebigs Ann. Chem., 1999 (1982); T. Kametani et al., Chem. Commun., 699 (1982); J. Org. Chem., 47, 2331 (1982); Tetrahedron Lett., 23, 2973 (1982).

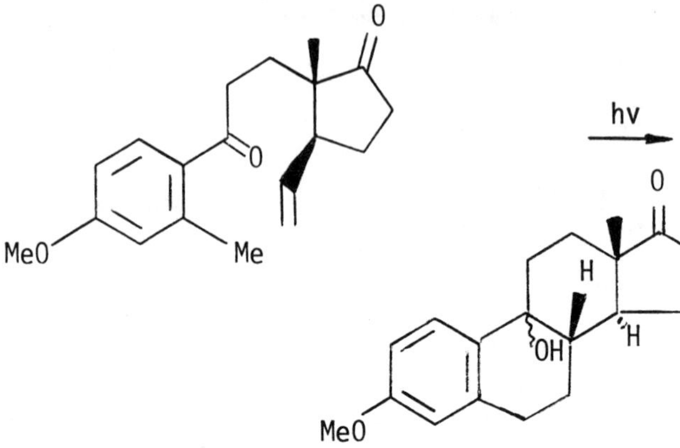

I.E.1-38 W. Oppolzer, Acct. Chem. Res., 15, 135 (1982).

Review: "Intramolecular [2+2] Photoaddition/Cyclobutane-Fragmentation Sequence in Organic Synthesis."

I.E.1-39 S. L. Mattes and S. Farid, Acct. Chem. Res., 15, 80 (1982).

Review: "Photochemical Cycloadditions via Exciplexes, Excited Complexes and Radical Ions."

I.E.1-40 E. Schaumann and R. Ketcham, Angew. Chem., Int. Ed. Engl., 21, 225 (1982).

Review: "[2+2] Cycloreversions."

I.E.1-46 M. Rosenblum and D. Scheck, Organometallics, 1, 397 (1982); K. Griesbaum, H. Mach and R. Hittich, Chem. Ber., 115, 1911 (1982); A. Bou, M. A. Pericas and F. Serratosa, Tetrahedron Lett., 23, 361 (1982); Y. Hanzawa and L. Paquette, Synthesis, 661 (1982).

$$Me-C\equiv C-CO_2Me \quad Fp^+ \quad BF_4^- \quad + \quad \bigcirc \quad \longrightarrow \quad \text{[bicyclic product]}-CO_2Me$$

53%

I.E.1-47 J. Ficini et al., Tetrahedron Lett., 23, 1821 (1982); J. J. Eisch, J. E. Galle and L. E. Hallenbeck, J. Org. Chem., 47, 1608 (1982).

cyclopentenone + $CH_2CH_2O^tBu$–C≡C–NEt_2

1) THF, CH_3CN
   Reflux
2) 5% HCO_2H
   20°C

50%

I.E.1-48 R. Huston, M. Rey and A. S. Dreiding, Helv. Chim. Acta, 65, 451 (1982); J. A. Duncan et al., J. Amer. Chem. Soc., 104, 2837 (1982); D. J. Pasto et al., ibid, 104, 3670, 3676 (1982); D. Becker et al., J. Org. Chem., 47, 3297 (1982); Z. Komiya and S. Nishida, Chem. Commun., 429 (1982).

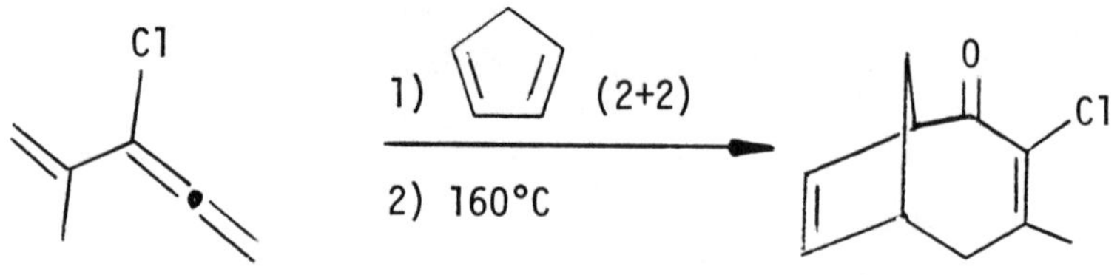

I.E.1-49 L. Ghosez et al., J. Amer. Chem. Soc., 104, 2920 (1982); H. Wynberg and E. G. J. Staring, ibid, 104, 166 (1982).

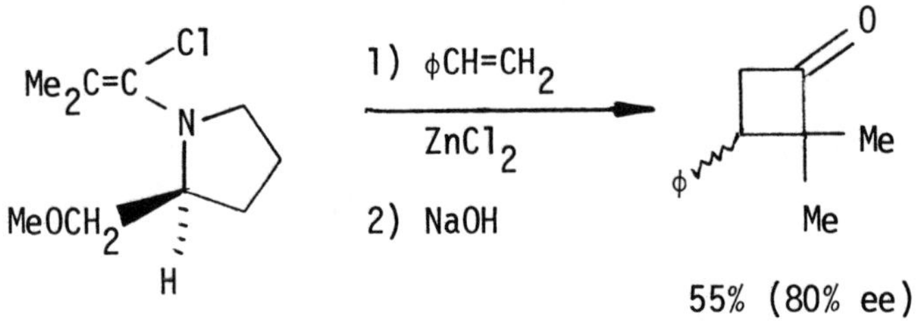

I.E.1-50 A. S. Dreiding et al., Helv. Chim. Acta, 65, 2230, 1563 (1982); A. S. Dreiding, L. Ghosez et al., Helv. Chim. Acta, 65, 703 (1982); R. L. Danheiser, S. K. Gee and H. Sard, J. Amer. Chem. Soc., 104, 7670 (1982).

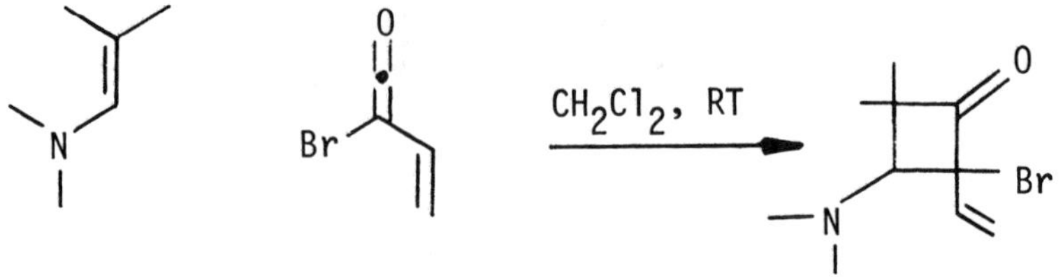

I.E.1-51   E. Lindner, M. Steinwand and S. Hoehne, Angew. Chem., Int. Ed. Engl., 21, 355 (1982); Chem. Ber., 115, 2181 (1982); L. Weiler et al., Can. J. Chem., 60, 872 (1982); P. W. Jeffs et al., J. Org. Chem., 47, 3871, 3876, 3881 (1982); Y. Ohshiro et al., Chem. Lett., 587 (1982).

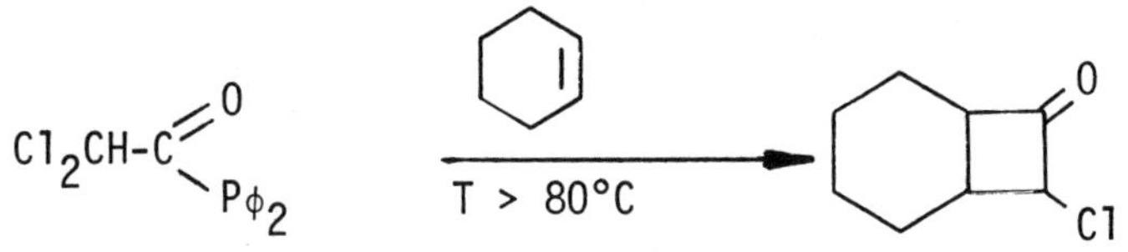

I.E.1-52   N. K. Hamer, Tetrahedron Lett., 23, 473 (1982).

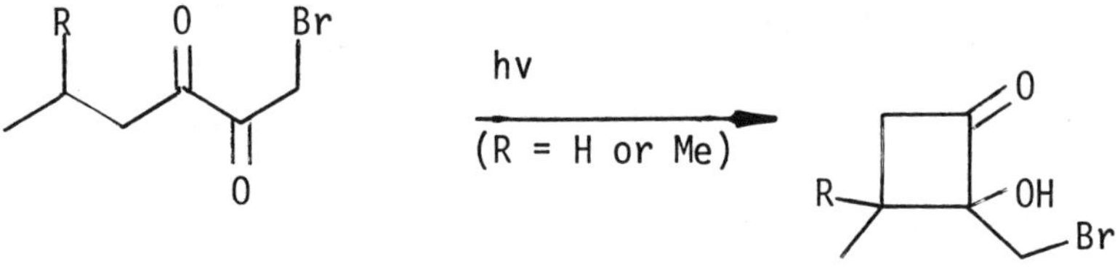

~ 100%

I.E.1-53   W. G. Dauben and D. M. Walker, Tetrahedron Lett., 23, 711 (1982); K. B. Becker et al., Helv. Chim. Acta, 65, 229, 235 (1982); S. R. Raychaudhuri, S. Ghosh and R. G. Salomon, J. Amer. Chem. Soc., 104, 6841 (1982); R. G. Salomon et al., J. Org. Chem., 47, 829 (1982); T. R. Hoye, S. J. Martin and D. R. Peck, ibid, 47, 331 (1982).

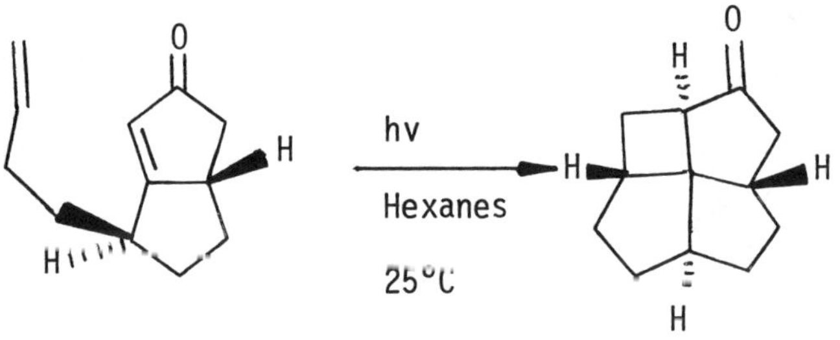

95%

I.E.1-54 A. Padwa and M. Pulwer, Chem. Commun., 783 (1982);
O. Tsuge et al., Chem. Lett., 993 (1982).

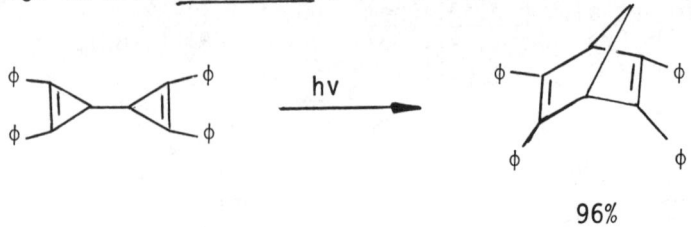

96%

I.E.1-55 A. Padwa, S. Goldstein and M. Pulwer, J. Org. Chem.,
47, 3893 (1982); R. M. Coates, P. D. Senter and W. R. Baker,
ibid, 47, 3597 (1982); P. A. Wender and G. B. Dreyer, J. Amer.
Chem. Soc., 104, 5805 (1982); S. F. Martin and J. B. White,
Tetrahedron Lett., 23, 23 (1982); P. Margaretha and K.
Grohmann, Helv. Chim. Acta, 65, 556 (1982); T. Kumagai, M.
Ichikawa and T. Mukai, Chem. Lett., 257 (1982).

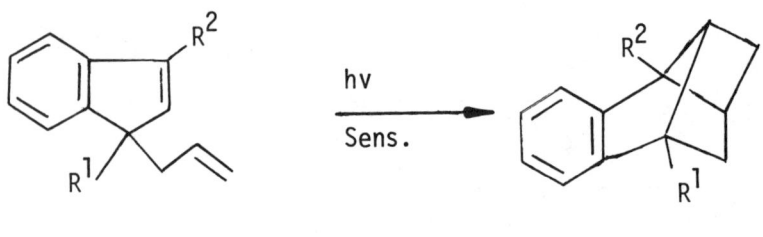

44-83%

I.E.1-56 N. Hanold, T. Molz and H. Meier, Angew. Chem., Int.
Ed. Engl., 21, 917 (1982); K. Hafner and M. Goltz, ibid, 21,
695 (1982); J. McRae, V. A. Moss and R. A. Raphael, Tetrahedron, 38, 2097 (1982); L. Fitjer et al., Tetrahedron Lett.,
23, 1661 (1982).

450-640°C
0.3 Torr

I.E.1-57 J. F. W. Keana, H. R. Taneja and M. Erion, Synth. Commun., 12, 167 (1982); Y. Nomura et al., Bull. Chem. Soc. Jpn., 55, 3343 (1982); M. Horner and S. Hunig, Liebigs Ann. Chem., 1409 (1982).

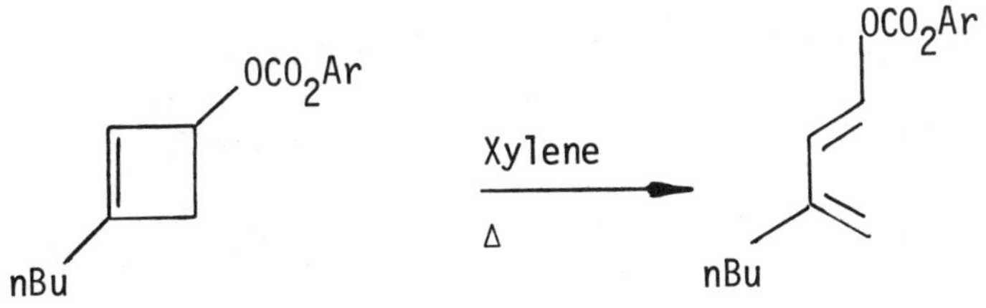

I.E.1-58 L. T. Scott et al., J. Amer. Chem. Soc., 104, 3530, 3659 (1982).

Competitive [6+2], [4+2] and [2+2] Cycloadditions.

I.E.1-59 I. Saito, K. Shimozono and T. Matsuura, J. Org. Chem., 47, 4356 (1982); H. Takeshita et al., Chem. Lett., 1153 (1982).

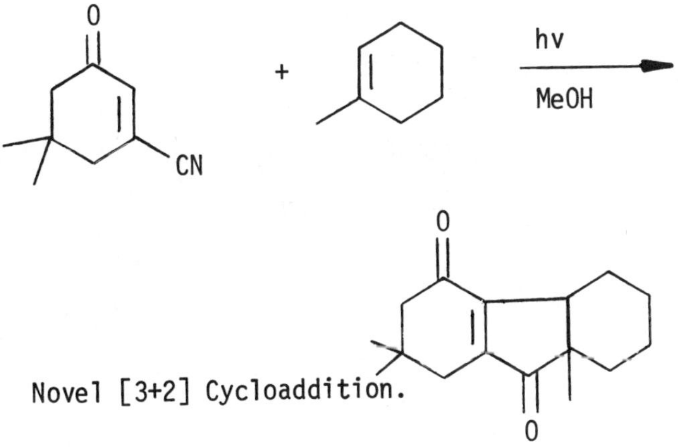

Novel [3+2] Cycloaddition.

35%

I.E.1-60 B. M. Trost and P. Renaut, J. Amer. Chem. Soc., 104, 6668 (1982); P. Binger and P. Bentz, Angew. Chem., Int. Ed. Engl., 21, 622 (1982).

[structure: norbornene with two CO_2Me groups] + [2-iodomethyl-3-(trimethylsilylmethyl)propene, with I and Me_3Si groups] $\xrightarrow{\text{Pd(OAc)}_2,\ (iPrO)_3P,\ THF,\ \Delta}$ [tricyclic product with exocyclic methylene, labeled E, E]

63%

I.E.1-61 D. C. Lathbury and P. J. Parsons, Chem. Commun., 291 (1982); K. B. G. Torssell et al., Acta Chem. Scand., 36B, 1 (1982); A. P. Kozikowski and P. D. Stein, J. Amer. Chem. Soc., 104, 4023 (1982); D. P. Curran, ibid, 4024 (1982).

φS—CH=CH—CH=CH$_2$

1) R-C≡N-O$^-$ (with + on N)
2) LAH
3) $(CF_3CO)_2O$, Na_2CO_3
4) $HgCl_2$, CH_3CN

[product: OHC-CH=CH-CH$_2$-CH(R)-NHC(O)CF$_3$]

25-33%

I.E.1-62 H. M. R. Hoffmann, R. Henning and O. R. Lalko, Angew. Chem., Int. Ed. Engl., 21, 442 (1982); R. Baker et al., J. Chem. Soc., Perkin I, 285, 295, 301 (1982).

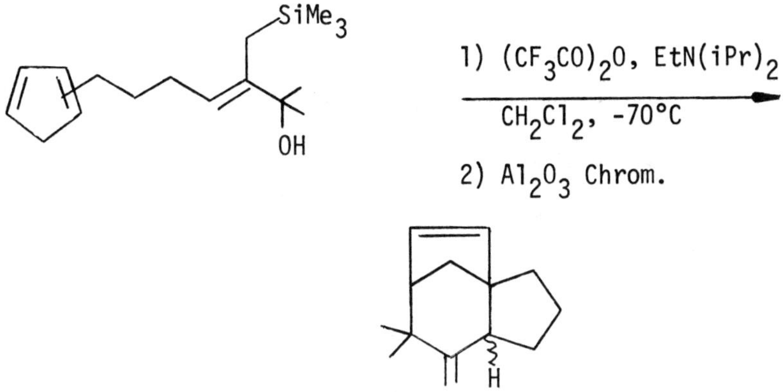
SiMe3
OH
1) (CF3CO)2O, EtN(iPr)2
CH2Cl2, -70°C
2) Al2O3 Chrom.
H

16%

I.E.1-63 T. Sasaki, Y. Ishibashi and M. Ohno, Tetrahedron Lett., 23, 1693 (1982).

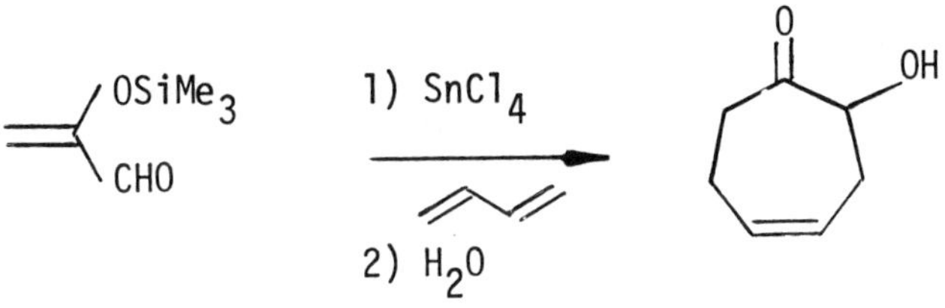
OSiMe3
CHO
1) SnCl4
2) H2O
O
OH

32%

I.E.1-64 B. Fohlisch et al., Chem. Ber., 115, 355, 381 (1982); Synthesis, 976 (1982); Angew. Chem., Int. Ed. Engl., 21, 137 (1982); H. Mayr et al., Chem. Ber., 115, 3479, 3516, 3528 (1982); N. Shimizu, M. Tanaka and Y. Tsuno, J. Amer. Chem. Soc., 104, 1330 (1982).

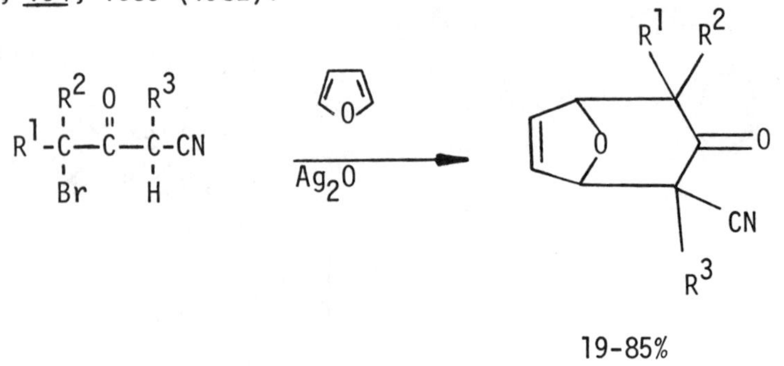

19-85%

I.E.1-65 K. N. Houk, et al., Tetrahedron Lett., 23, 495 (1982); J. Amer. Chem. Soc., 104, 7336 (1982); M. Neuenschwander et al. Helv. Chim. Acta, 65, 74, 89 (1982).

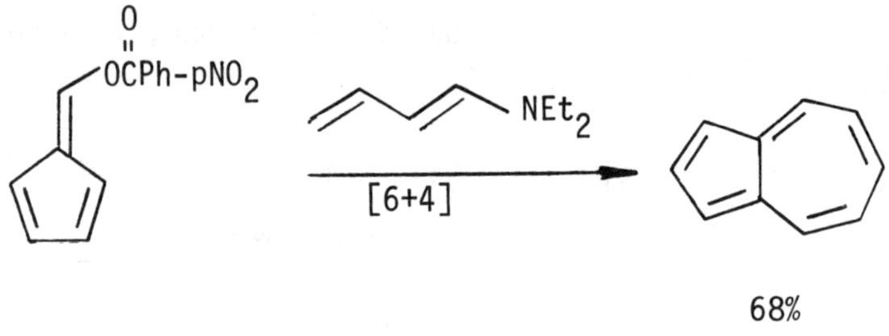

68%

I.E.2. Other Thermal Reactions

I.E.2-1 R. F. Childs, Tetrahedron, 38, 567 (1982).

Review: "Circumambulatory Rearrangements."

I.E.2-2   K. N. Houk, Pure Appl. Chem., 54, 1633 (1982).

Review: "Theory of Cycloadditions of Excited Aromatics to Alkenes."

I.E.2-3   B. B. Snider et al., J. Org. Chem., 47, 745 (1982); J. Amer. Chem. Soc., 104, 555, 1930 (1982).

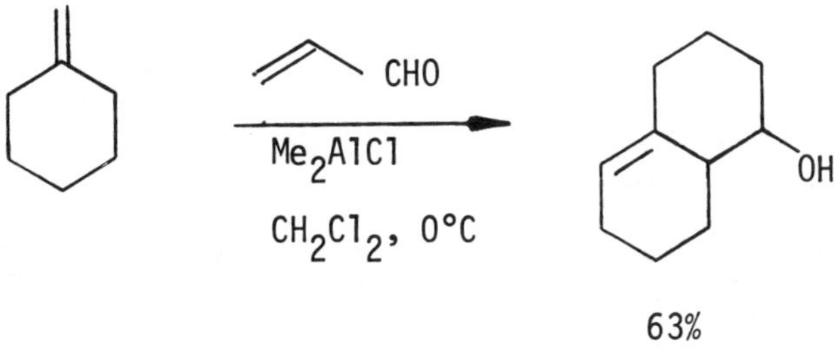

Two Sequencial Ene Reactions.

I.E.2-4   W. Oppolzer et al., Tetrahedron Lett., 23, 4669, 4673 (1982); J. Amer. Chem. Soc., 104, 6476, 6478 (1982).

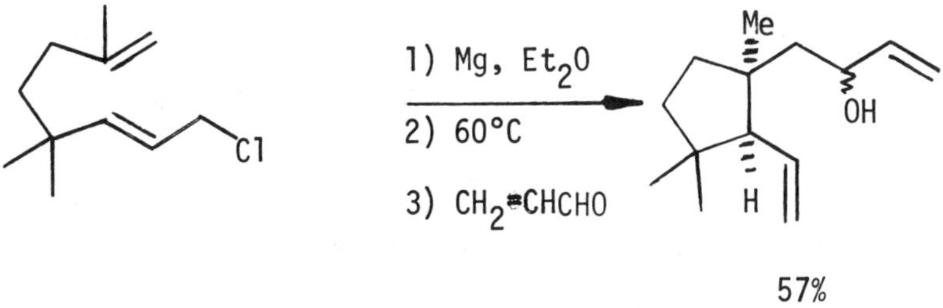

I.E.2-5 W. G. Dauben and T. Brookhart, J. Org. Chem., 47, 3921 (1982); G. Jenner and M. Papadopoulos, ibid, 47, 4201 (1982); J. K. Whitesell et al., Chem. Commun., 988, 989 (1982).

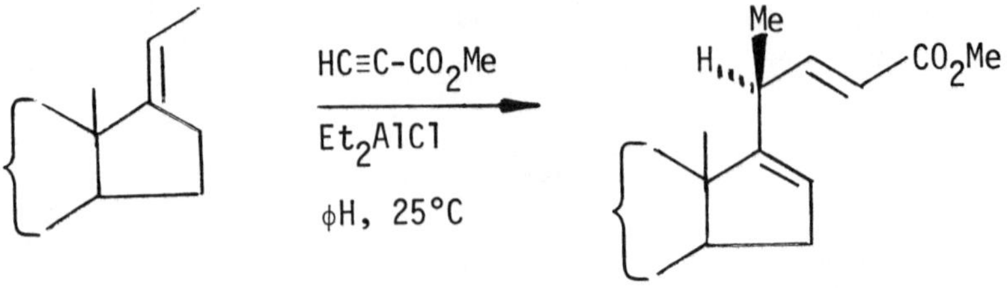

$HC \equiv C\text{-}CO_2Me$

Et_2AlCl

ϕH, 25°C

94%
(40% Conversion)

I.E.2-6 D. M. Tschaen and S. M. Weinreb, Tetrahedron Lett., 23, 3015 (1982); D. Armesto, A. Ramos and R. Perez-Ossorio, ibid, 23, 5195 (1982).

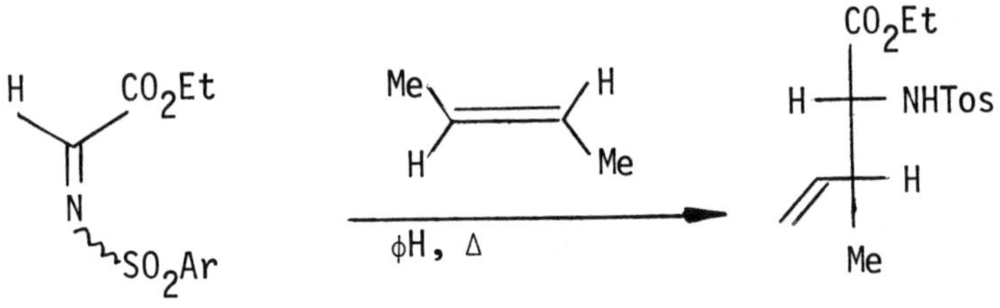

ϕH, Δ

77%
(90% Alloleucine Diast.)

I.E.2-7 G. B. Gill and K. S. Kirollos, Tetrahedron Lett., 23, 1399 (1982).

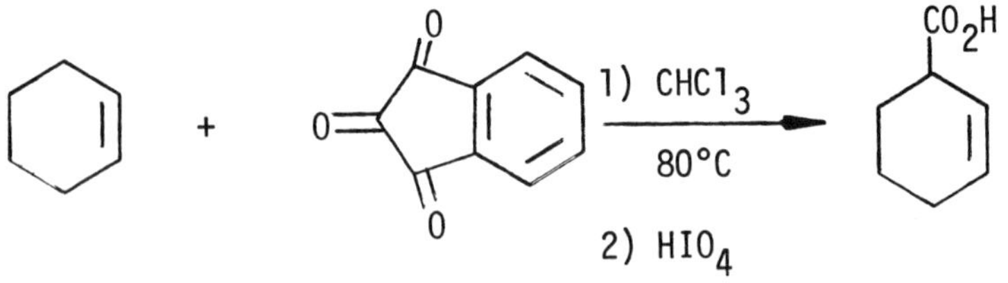

1) $CHCl_3$, 80°C
2) HIO_4

100%

I.E.2-8 Y. Tamura et al., Synthesis, 56 (1982).

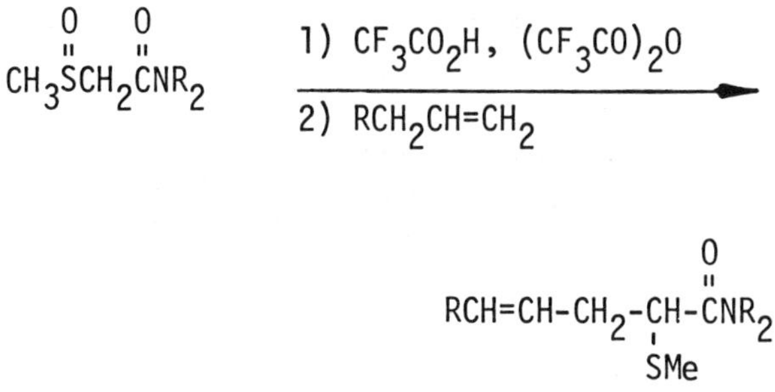

$CH_3\overset{O}{\overset{\|}{S}}CH_2\overset{O}{\overset{\|}{C}}NR_2$
1) CF_3CO_2H, $(CF_3CO)_2O$
2) $RCH_2CH{=}CH_2$
$RCH{=}CH{-}CH_2{-}CH(SMe){-}\overset{O}{\overset{\|}{C}}NR_2$

65-81%

(82-88% E)

I.E.2-9 D. L. Lindner, R. B. Woodward et al., Tetrahedron Lett., 23, 5111 (1982); J. R. Williams and T. P. Cleary, Chem. Commun., 626 (1982).

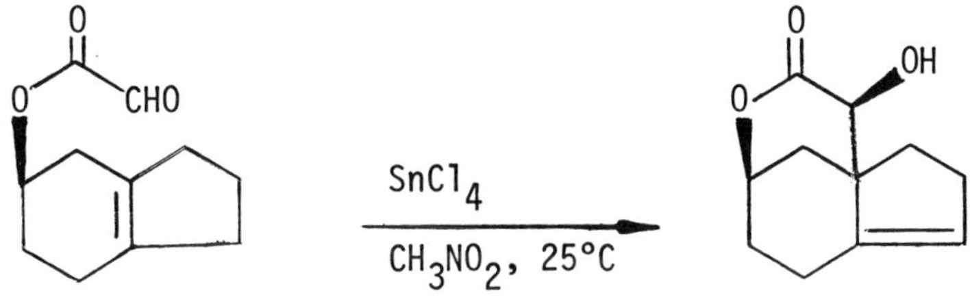

O
O
CHO
$SnCl_4$
CH_3NO_2, 25°C
O
OH
O

85%

I.E.2-10 L. E. Overman and E. J. Jacobsen, J. Amer. Chem. Soc., 104, 7225 (1982).

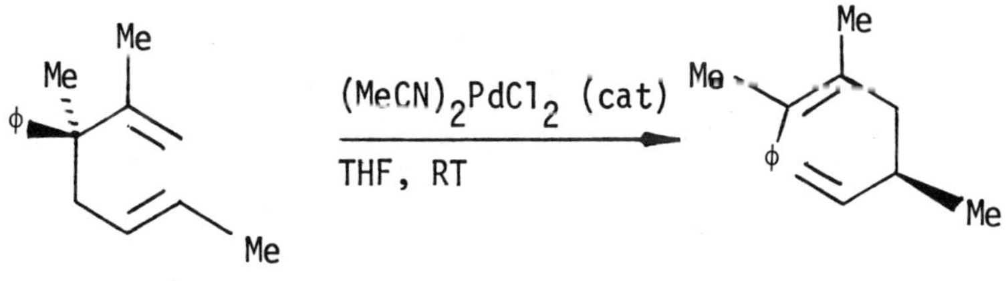

Me
Me
ϕ
Me
$(MeCN)_2PdCl_2$ (cat)
THF, RT
Me
Me
ϕ
Me

60%

I.E.2-11 M. Dollinger, W. Henning and W. Kirmse, Chem. Ber., 115, 2309 (1982); P. M. Cairns, L. Crombie and G. Pattenden, Tetrahedron Lett., 23, 1405 (1982); K. Gubernator and R. Gleiter, Angew. Chem., Int. Ed. Engl., 21, 686 (1982).

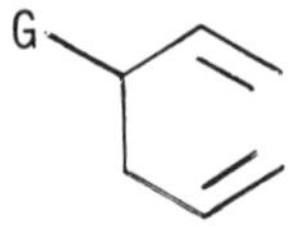

Donor Substituents Effects on Cope Rearr.

G = RO-, RS-, R_2N-

I.E.2-12 S. Swaminathan et al., Tetrahedron, 38, 2195, 569, 4983 (1982); S. F. Martin, J. B. White and R. Wagner, J. Org. Chem., 47, 3190 (1982); R. C. Gadwood and R. M. Lett, ibid, 47, 2268 (1982).

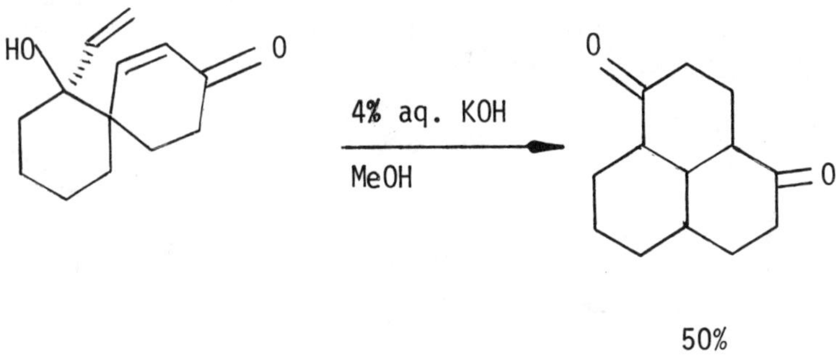

4% aq. KOH / MeOH

50%

I.E.2-13 L. E. Overman et al., Tetrahedron Lett., 23, 2733, 2737, 2741 (1982); A. Padwa and L. A. Cohen, ibid, 23, 915 (1982); I. B. Abdrakhmanov et al., J. Org. Chem. (USSR), 18, 1278 (1982).

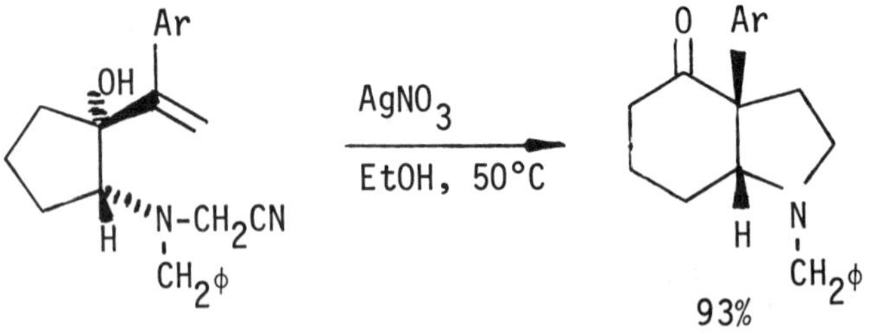

AgNO$_3$ / EtOH, 50°C

93%

I.E.2-14 R. Gompper and B. Kohl, Angew. Chem., Int. Ed. Engl., 21, 198, 199 (1982).

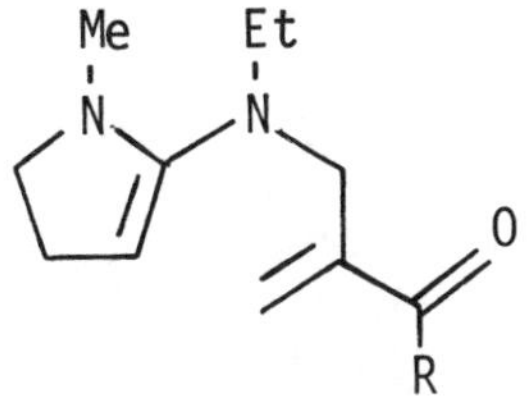

Aza-Cope vs. Aldol

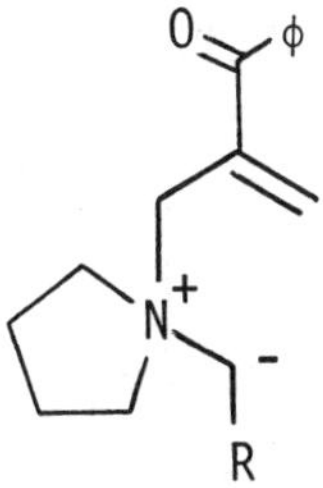

[2,3] Sigmatropic vs. Aldol

I.E.2-15 T. Yoshizawa et al., Chem. Lett., 1131 (1982); L. I. Bunina-Krivorukova et al., J. Org. Chem.(USSR), 18, 742, 745 (1982); L. M. Harwood, Chem. Commun., 1120 (1982); S. Terao et al., J. Chem. Soc., Perkin I, 2909 (1982).

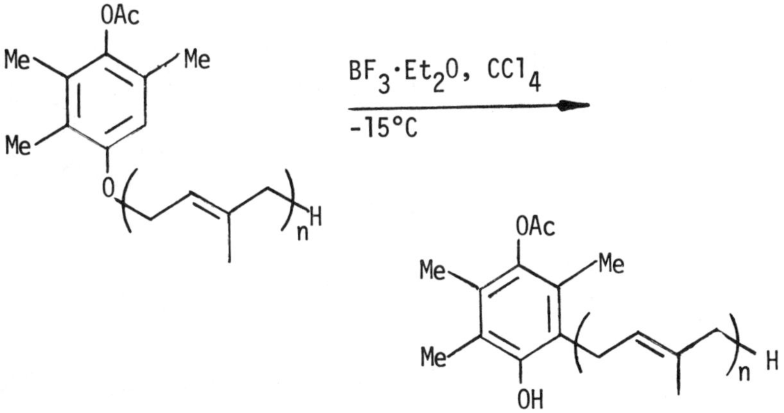

16-80%

I.E.2-16 P. S. Rutledge et al., Tetrahedron Lett., 23, 4407 (1982); J. E. Baldwin and A. J. Rajeckas, Tetrahedron, 38, 3079 (1982); I. Takahashi and S. Terashima, Chem. Pharm. Bull., 30, 4539 (1982).

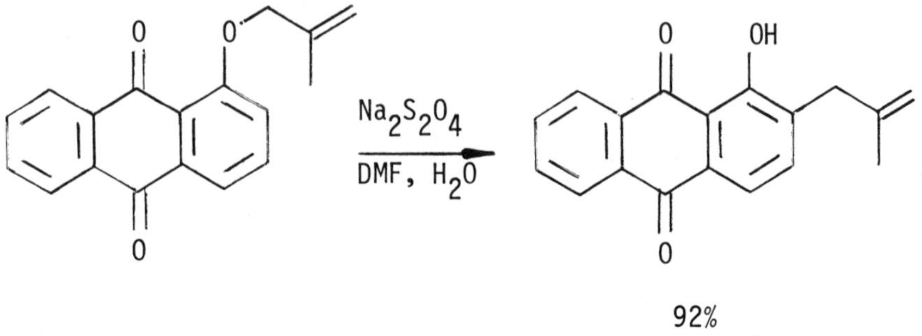

$$\xrightarrow{Na_2S_2O_4, DMF, H_2O}$$

92%

I.E.2-17 P. A. Bartlett et al., J. Org. Chem., 47, 3933, 3941 (1982); Tetrahedron Lett., 23, 619, 623 (1982); D. J. Ager, ibid, 23, 3419 (1982).

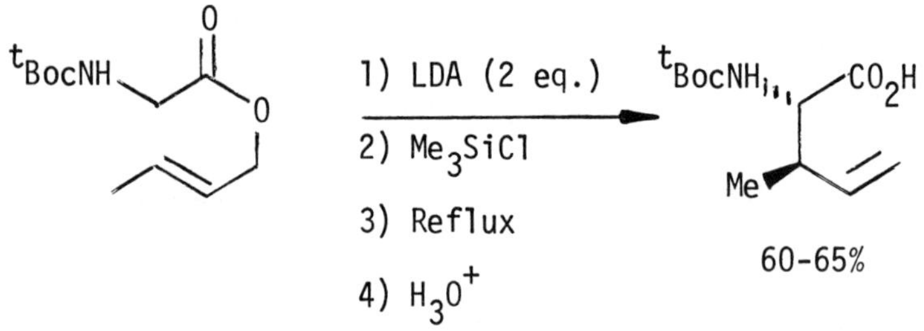

1) LDA (2 eq.)
2) Me$_3$SiCl
3) Reflux
4) H$_3$O$^+$

60-65%

I.E.2-18 G. Stork and K. S. Atwal, Tetrahedron Lett., 23, 2073 (1982).

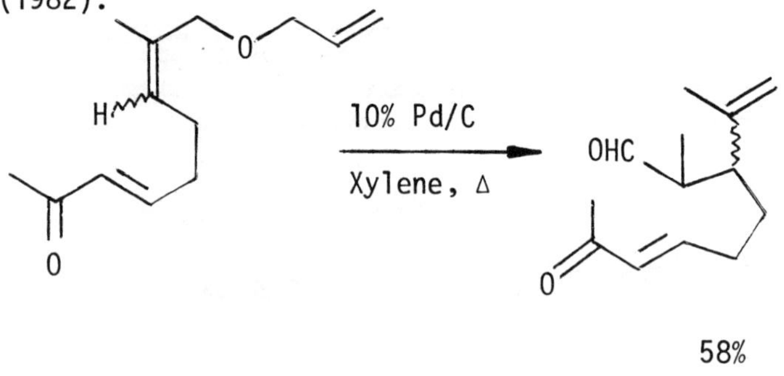

10% Pd/C, Xylene, Δ

58%

I.E.2-19 S. R. Wilson and M. F. Price, J. Amer. Chem. Soc., 104, 1124 (1982).

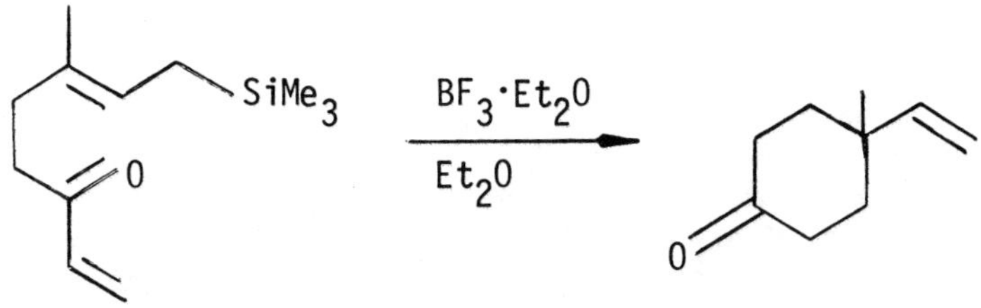

I.E.2-20 F. E. Ziegler et al., J. Amer. Chem. Soc., 104, 7181 (1982); J. Org. Chem., 47, 5229 (1982); R. Baker and D. L. Selwood, Tetrahedron Lett., 23, 3839 (1982).

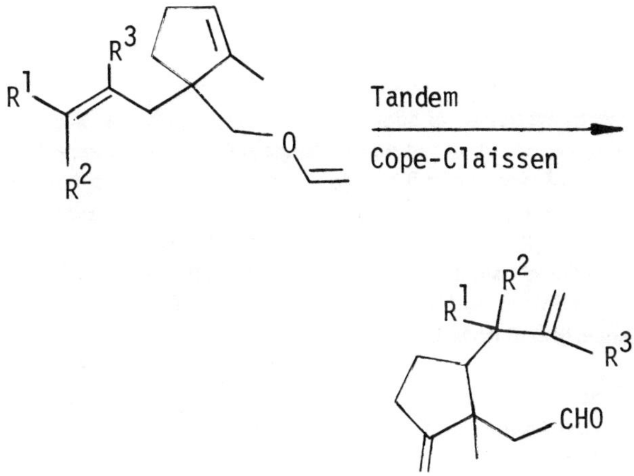

Full Paper

I.E.2-21 Y. Ishino et al., Synthesis, 740 (1982); H. J. Liu and P. R. Pednekar, Synth. Commun., 12, 395 (1982); T. Takeda and T. Fujiwara, Chem. Lett., 1113 (1982); G. W. Daub et al., J. Org. Chem., 47, 743 (1982); K. A. Parker et al., ibid, 47, 389 (1982).

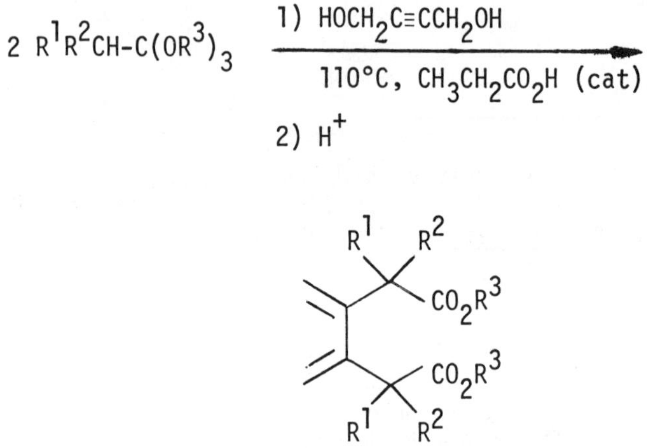

$$2\ R^1R^2CH\text{-}C(OR^3)_3 \xrightarrow[\substack{110°C,\ CH_3CH_2CO_2H\ (cat) \\ 2)\ H^+}]{1)\ HOCH_2C\equiv CCH_2OH}$$

[product structure with R^1, R^2, CO_2R^3 groups]

47-94%

I.E.2-22 C. H. Heathcock and E. T. Jarvi, Tetrahedron Lett., 23, 2825 (1982); S. E. Denmark and M. A. Harmata, J. Amer. Chem. Soc., 104, 4972 (1982).

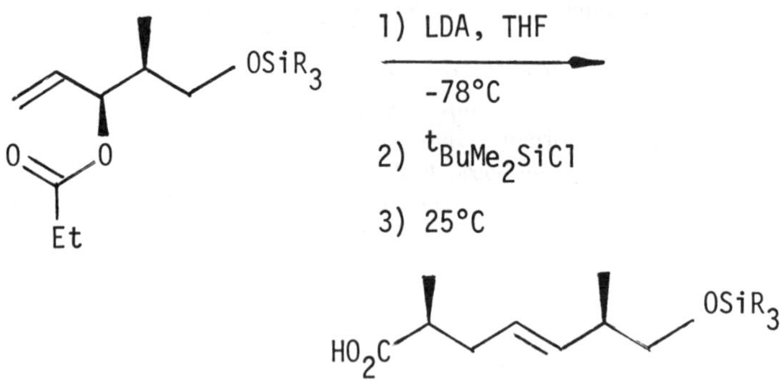

Reagents:
1) LDA, THF, -78°C
2) ^{t}BuMe$_2$SiCl
3) 25°C

58%

I.E.2-23 T. Kametani et al., Chem. Commun., 123 (1982); J. Zielinski, H. T. Li and C. Djerassi et al., J. Org. Chem., 47, 620, 2420 (1982).

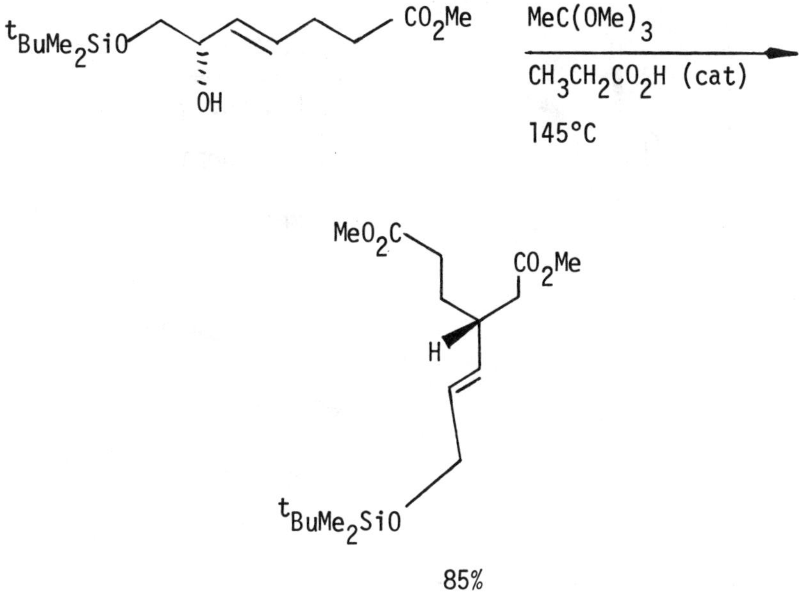

$^{t}BuMe_2SiO$–CH(OH)–CH=CH–CH_2CH_2–CO_2Me

$\xrightarrow[145°C]{MeC(OMe)_3 \atop CH_3CH_2CO_2H \text{ (cat)}}$

[product: branched compound with MeO_2C–CH_2CH_2–C(H)(CH_2–CO_2Me)–CH=CH–CH_2–$OSiMe_2^tBu$]

85%

I.E.2-24 M. M. Abelman, R. L. Funk and J. D. Munger, Jr., J. Amer. Chem. Soc., 104, 4030 (1982); A. G. Cameron and D. W. Knight, Tetrahedron Lett., 23, 5455 (1982).

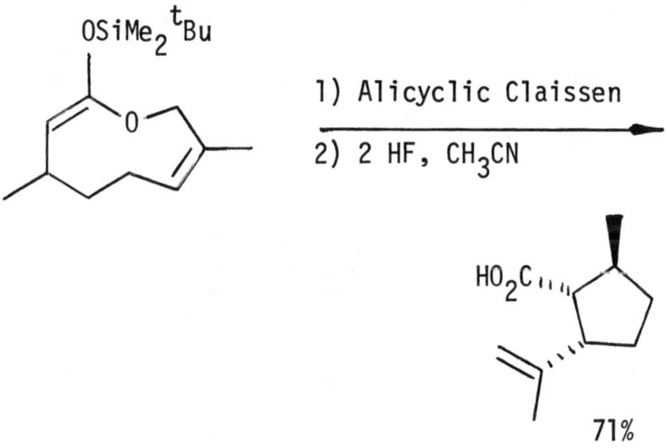

[starting material: oxacycle with $OSiMe_2^tBu$]

1) Alicyclic Claissen
2) 2 HF, CH_3CN

[product: cyclopentane with HO_2C and isopropenyl substituents]

71%

I.E.2-25 D. P. Curran, Tetrahedron Lett., 23, 4309 (1982);
F. E. Ziegler and J. K. Thottathil, ibid, 23, 3531 (1982).

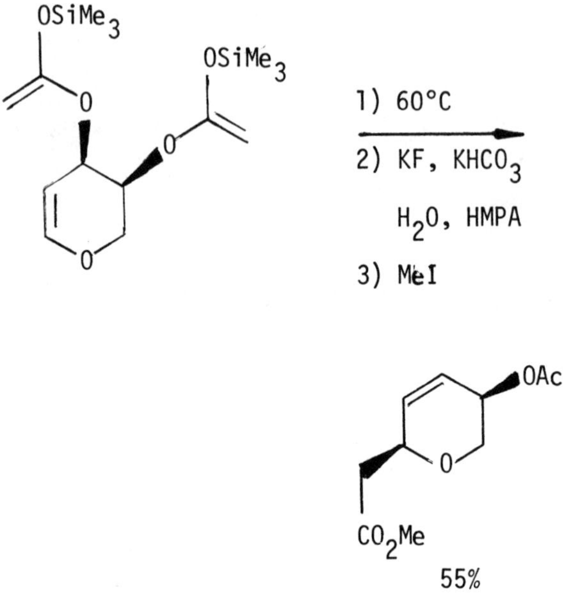

1) 60°C
2) KF, KHCO$_3$
   H$_2$O, HMPA
3) MeI

55%

I.E.2-26 J. W. S. Stevenson and T. A. Bryson, Tetrahedron Lett., 23, 3143 (1982); H. Monti, C. Corriol and M. Bertrand, ibid, 23, 947 (1982); T. Takahashi, H. Yamada and J. Tsuji, ibid, 23, 233 (1982).

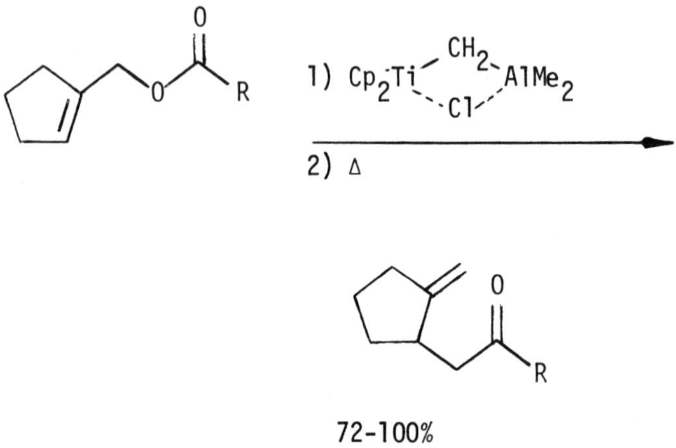

1) Cp$_2$Ti$\overset{CH_2}{\underset{Cl}{\cdots}}$AlMe$_2$
2) Δ

72-100%

I.E.2-27 Z. Yoshida et al., Tetrahedron Lett., 23, 5319
(1982); K. Hayakawa, Y. Kamikawaji and K. Kanematsu, ibid, 23,
2171 (1982); E. Nagashima, K. Suzuki and M. Sekiya, Chem.
Pharm. Bull., 30, 4384 (1982).

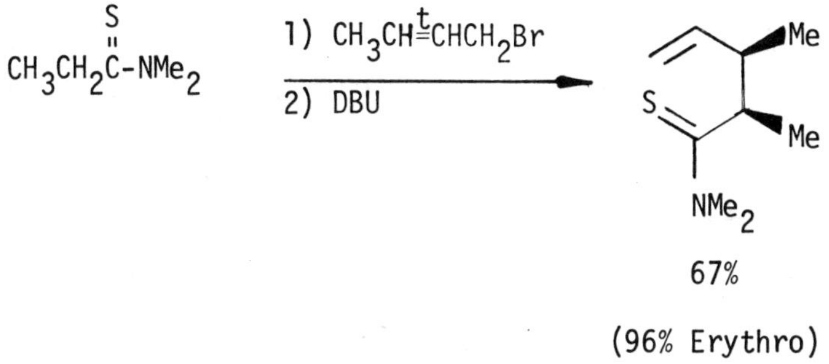

$$CH_3CH_2\overset{S}{\underset{\|}{C}}-NMe_2 \quad \xrightarrow[\text{2) DBU}]{\text{1) } CH_3CH\overset{t}{=}CHCH_2Br}$$

67%

(96% Erythro)

I.E.2-28 W. H. Okamura et al., J. Amer. Chem. Soc., 104, 6115
(1982); Tetrahedron Lett., 23, 1019 (1982); Z. Kosarych and
T. Cohen, ibid, 23, 3019 (1982); P. G. Gassman, T. Miura and
A. Mossman, J. Org. Chem., 47, 954 (1982); K. Hiroi and S.
Sato, Chem. Lett., 1871 (1982).

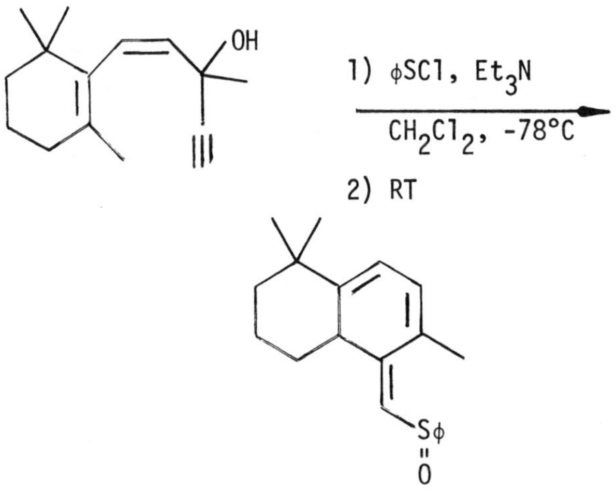

$$\xrightarrow[\text{2) RT}]{\text{1) } \phi SCl, Et_3N \atop CH_2Cl_2, -78°C}$$

I.E.2-29 W. D. Ollis et al., J. Chem. Soc., Perkin I, 893 (1982);   T. Nakai et al., Chem. Lett., 1349, 1643 (1982); Tetrahedron Lett., 23, 3931 (1982);   E. Vedejs et al., J. Org. Chem., 47, 4384 (1982).

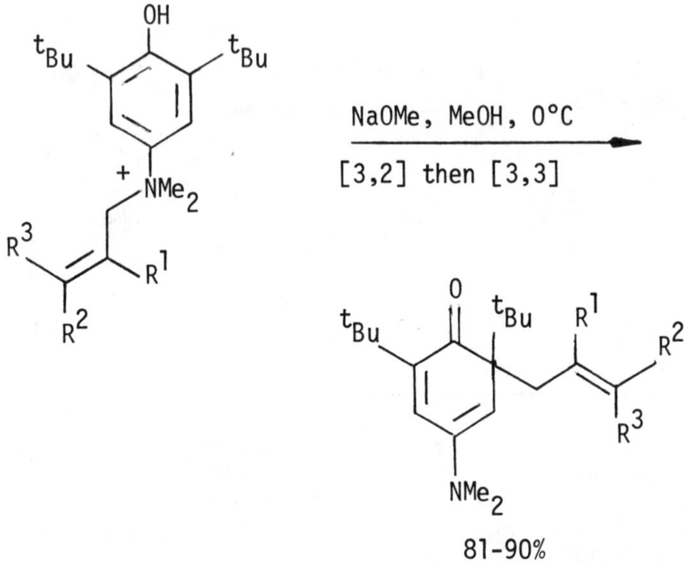

NaOMe, MeOH, 0°C
[3,2] then [3,3]

81-90%

I.E.2-30 W. D. Munslow and W. Reusch, J. Org. Chem., 47, 5096 (1982).

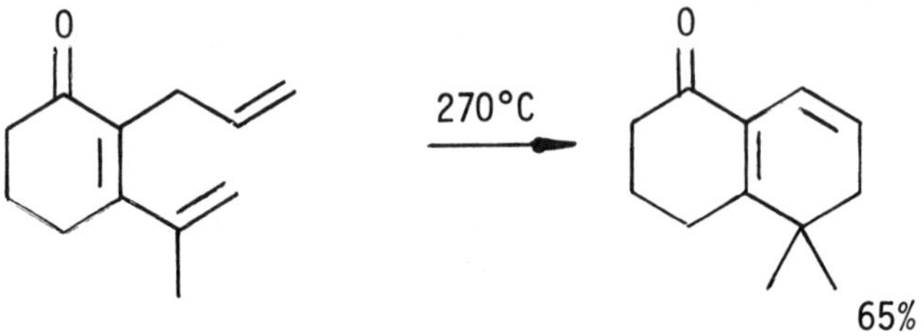

270°C

65%

I.E.2-31 J. I. G. Cadogan, I. Gosney et al., Chem. Commun., 325 (1982).

[Structure: bicyclic sulfone with two CO$_2$Me groups] $\xrightarrow{550°C,\ 10^{-3}\ mm\ Hg}$ [diene diester with two CO$_2$Me groups]

87%

I.E.2-32 A. S. Dreiding et al., Helv. Chim. Acta, 65, 13, 2413, 2517 (1982); E. Piers et al., Can. J. Chem., 60, 2965 (1982).

[ketone with alkyne] $\xrightarrow{620°C,\ 12\text{-}16\ Torr}$ [cyclopentenone]

68%

I.E.2-33 E. Vogel et al., Tetrahedron Lett., 23, 1797, 1801 (1982); J. Amer. Chem. Soc., 104, 3729 (1982); G. I. Fray, G. R. Geen and N. A. Whiteside, Synthesis, 956 (1982); G. Boche et al., Chem. Ber., 115, 3167, 3191 (1982).

[benzocyclobutene dibromide] + [bis(bromomethyl) cyclooctatetraene-benzo compound] $\xrightarrow[\text{2) NBS}\ \text{3) NaI}]{\text{1) Zn/DMF}}$

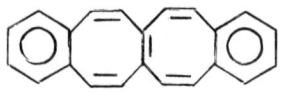

22-25%

I.E.2-34 G. V. Kalechits and N. G. Kozlov, J. Org. Chem. (USSR), 18, 585 (1982); W. Burgert, M. Grosse and D. Rewicki, Chem. Ber., 115, 309 (1982); A. G. Anderson, Jr. and L. G. Kao, J. Org. Chem., 47, 3589 (1982).

$$\xrightarrow[H_2 + Cat^*]{200-260°C}$$

78%

*Cat = 15% Cu + 6% LiOH on Al_2O_3.

I.E.2-35 R. Grigg, R. Scott and P. Stevenson, Tetrahedron Lett., 23, 2691 (1982); K. P. C. Vollhardt, et al., Tetrahedron, 38, 2911 (1982); J. Org. Chem., 47, 3447 (1982); Chem. Commun., 953 (1982); K. C. Nicolaou et al., J. Amer. Chem. Soc., 104, 5555, 5557, 5558, 5560 (1982).

$$\xrightarrow[EtOH, 25°C]{2\% \; RhCl(P\phi_3)_3}$$

75%

I.F. Aromatic Substitutions Forming a New Carbon-Carbon Bond

I.F.1. Friedel-Crafts Type Aromatic Substitution Reactions

I.F.1-1 D. Farcasiu, *Acct. Chem. Res.*, **15**, 46 (1982).

Review: "Protonation of Simple Aromatics in Superacids. A Reexamination."

I.F.1-2 L. I. Kruse and J. K. Cha, *Chem. Commun.*, 1333 (1982).

Explanation of Unexpected Regiochemistry in Electrophilic Aromatic Substitution - Stereoelectronic Control.

I.F.1-3 I. Fleming and J. Iqbal, *Synthesis*, 937 (1982); A. K. Sinhababu and R. T. Borchardt, *Synth. Commun.*, **12**, 983 (1982); J. E. Fitzpatrick, D. J. Milner and P. White, *ibid*, **12**, 489 (1982).

$$\underset{CH_3}{\underset{|}{\overset{OH}{\overset{|}{\bigcirc}}}} \quad \xrightarrow[\text{SnCl}_4,\ CH_2Cl_2]{1)\ \phi SCH_2Cl} \quad \underset{CH_3}{\underset{|}{\overset{OH}{\overset{|}{\bigcirc}}}}{-CH_3}$$

2) Ni(R), Acetone
EtOH

66%

I.F.1-4 A. Citterio, M. Serravalle and E. Vismara, Tetrahedron Lett., 23, 1831 (1982); J. K. Ruminski and K. D. Przewoska, Chem. Ber., 115, 3436 (1982); R. Bongue-Boma, J. Rinaudo and J. M. Bonnier, Bull. Soc. Chim. Fr. II, 52 (1982); C. W. Rees et al., Chem. Commun., 497, 499 (1982).

$$ArN_2^+ \; BF_4^- \xrightarrow[\text{DMSO}]{\substack{CH_3\overset{O}{\overset{\|}{C}}-\overset{O}{\overset{\|}{C}}CH_3 \\ h\nu \text{ or } FeSO_4 \cdot 7H_2O}} Ar-\overset{O}{\overset{\|}{C}}-CH_3$$

10-70%

I.F.1-5 G. Sartori et al., Synthesis, 879 (1982); A. Rahm, R. Guilhemat and M. Pereyre, Synth. Commun., 12, 485 (1982).

<chemical reaction: 2,3,4-substituted phenyl OLi with R^1 → treated with 1) AlCl$_3$, Xylene 2) φN=C=O → 2,3,4-substituted phenol with R^1 and CNHφ(=O) group>

15-36%

I.F.1-6 N. G. Kunda, J. Peck and D. W. Evangelatos, Org. Prep. Proc. Int., 14, 206 (1982); M. N. Magerramov, J. Org. Chem. (USSR), 18, 115 (1982).

<chemical reaction: m-methylbenzyl-NHAc → 1) BrCH$_2$O~~~OCH$_2$Br, AlCl$_3$, CH$_2$Cl$_2$, 0°C 2) Δ 3) H$_3$O$^+$>

[Structure: benzene ring with Me, CH2Br, CH2Br, CH2NHAc substituents]

72%

I.F.1-7 J. M. Briody and G. L. Marshall, Synthesis, 939 (1982); H. Suzuki, Y. Yoshida and A. Osuka, Chem. Lett., 135 (1982).

$$2 \text{ ArH} \xrightarrow[CF_3CO_2H]{B(OCOCF_3)_3} \text{Ar-}\underset{Ar}{\overset{CF_3}{C}}\text{-Ar}$$

63-90%

I.F.1-8 B. Miller et al., J. Org. Chem., 47, 5204, 710 (1982); E. Fujita et al., Chem. Pharm. Bull., 30, 3994 (1982); R. R. Schmidt and M. Hoffmann, Tetrahedron Lett., 23, 409 (1982).

[2,6-dimethylphenol/anisole] + $CH_2=CHCH_2X$ $\xrightarrow{ZnCl_2, CHCl_3}$ [4-allyl-2,6-dimethylphenol/anisole]

(R = H or Me)   (X = Cl or Br)

High Percentage of Meta-Allylation

I.F.1-9 A. Zanarotti, Tetrahedron Lett., 23, 3963 (1982); N. I. Ganushchak, N. D. Obushak and O. P. Polishchuk, J. Org. Chem. (USSR), 18, 633 (1982); L. M. Lubritskii, N. D. Romashchenkova and A. A. Petrov, ibid, 18, 578 (1982).

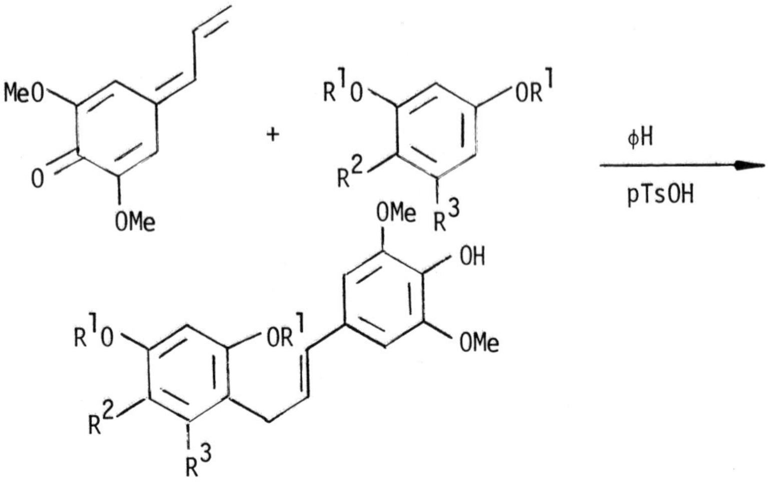

I.F.1-10 N. De Kimpe, M. Charpentier-Morize et al., Tetrahedron Lett., 23, 2853 (1982); T. Kato et al., Chem. Pharm. Bull., 30, 552 (1982); Y. Tamura et al., ibid, 30, 915, 3574 (1982).

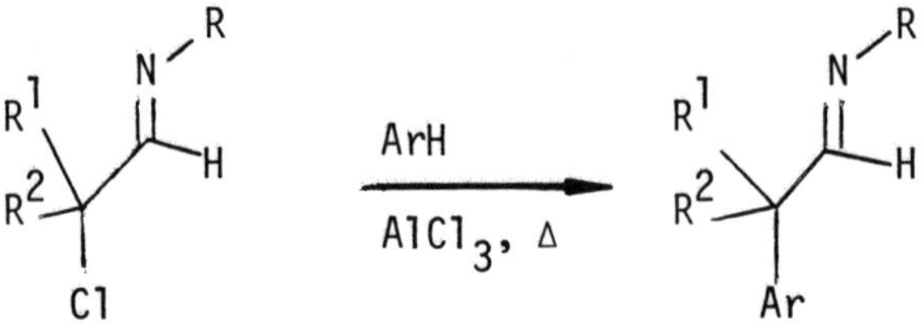

I.F.1-11 S. Ghosh, S. N. Pardo and R. G. Salomon, J. Org. Chem., 47, 4692 (1982).

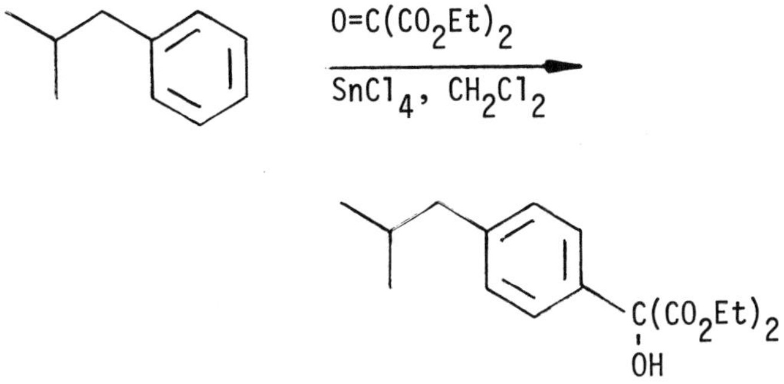

$$\text{iBuC}_6\text{H}_5 \xrightarrow[\text{SnCl}_4,\ \text{CH}_2\text{Cl}_2]{\text{O=C(CO}_2\text{Et})_2} \text{iBu-C}_6\text{H}_4\text{-C(OH)(CO}_2\text{Et})_2$$

54-100%

I.F.1-12 R. G. F. Giles et al., Tetrahedron Lett., 23, 3299 (1982); F. Effenberger and R. Gutmann, Chem. Ber., 115, 1089 (1982).

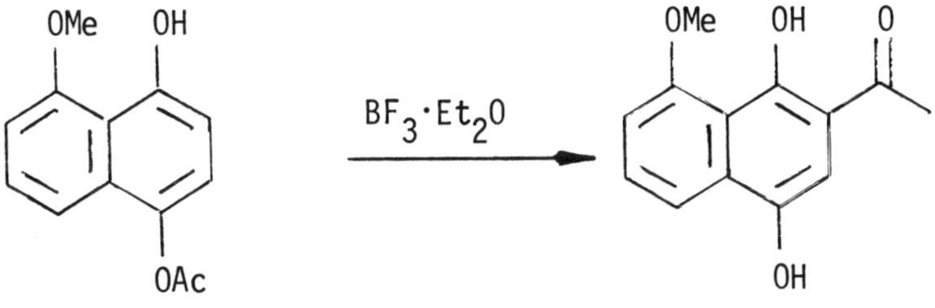

[Naphthalene with OMe, OH, OAc substituents] $\xrightarrow{\text{BF}_3\cdot\text{Et}_2\text{O}}$ [Naphthalene with OMe, OH, acetyl, OH substituents]

56%

Abnormal Fries Rearr.

I.F.1-13 G. I. Tsuchihashi, Tetrahedron Lett., 23, 5427 (1982); G. Frater, Chem. Commun., 521 (1982).

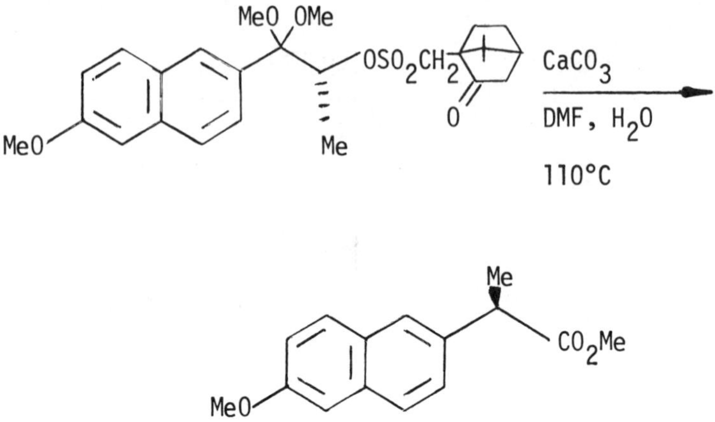

80%
(100% OP)

I.F.1-14 A. Marxer, Helv. Chim. Acta, 65, 392 (1982); G. Henbach, Liebigs Ann. Chem., 1017 (1982); L. Jalander and M. Broms, Acta Chem. Scand., 36B, 371 (1982); G. V. Pavel, M. N. Tilichenko and L. B. Smelik, J. Org. Chem. (USSR), 18, 581 (1982); A. Sen and R. R. Thomas, Organometallics, 1, 1251 (1982); K. Eichinger, H. Berbalk and R. Schuster, J. Chem. Res. (S), 226, 317 (1982).

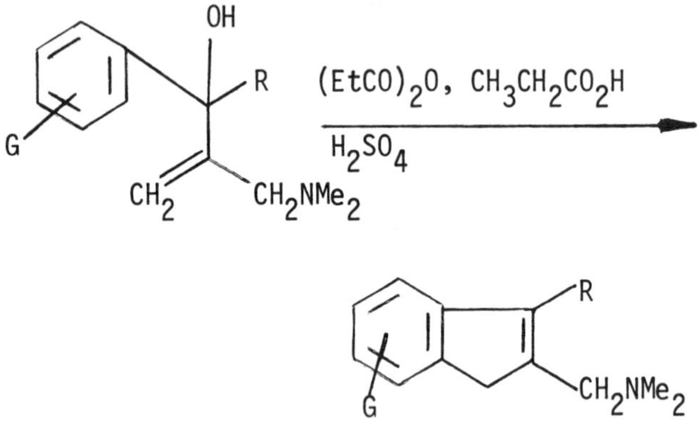

20-73%

I.F.1-15 J. D. P. Teresa, A. F. Mateos and R. R. Gonzalez, Tetrahedron Lett., 23, 3405 (1982); A. E. K. M. N. Gohar et al., Ind. J. Chem., 21B, 658 (1982); N. A. R. Hatam and D. A. Whiting, J. Chem. Soc., Perkin I, 461 (1982); W. S. Murphy and S. Wattanasin, ibid, 1029 (1982).

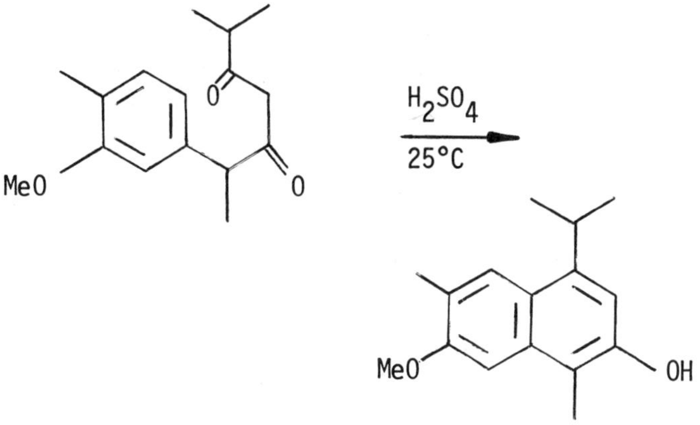

I.F.1-16 B. M. Trost and E. Murayama, Tetrahedron Lett., 23, 1047 (1982); R. A. Abramovitch et al., J. Org. Chem., 47, 4817, 4819 (1982); J. K. Ray and R. G. Harvey, ibid, 47, 3335 (1982); E. Lee-Ruff et al., Can. J. Chem., 60, 154 (1982).

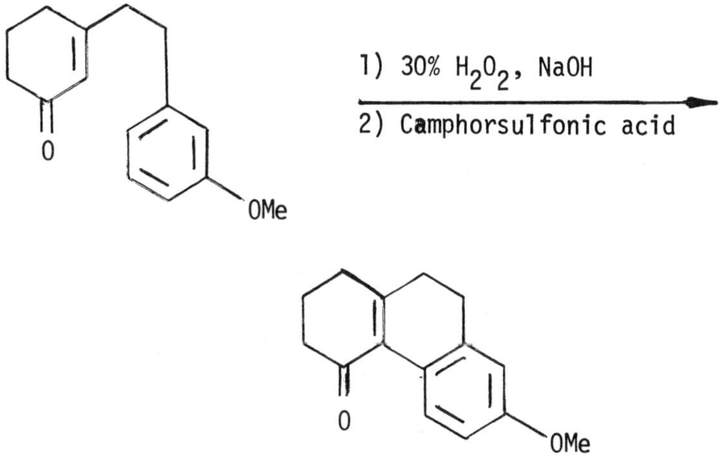

I.F.1-17 A. V. R. Rao, et al., Tetrahedron Lett., 23, 2415 (1982); Tetrahedron, 38, 3555 (1982); F. Johnson et al., Tetrahedron Lett., 23, 3871 (1982); L. Lepage and Y. Lepage, Synthesis, 882 (1982); M. Gates, J. Org. Chem., 47, 578 (1982).

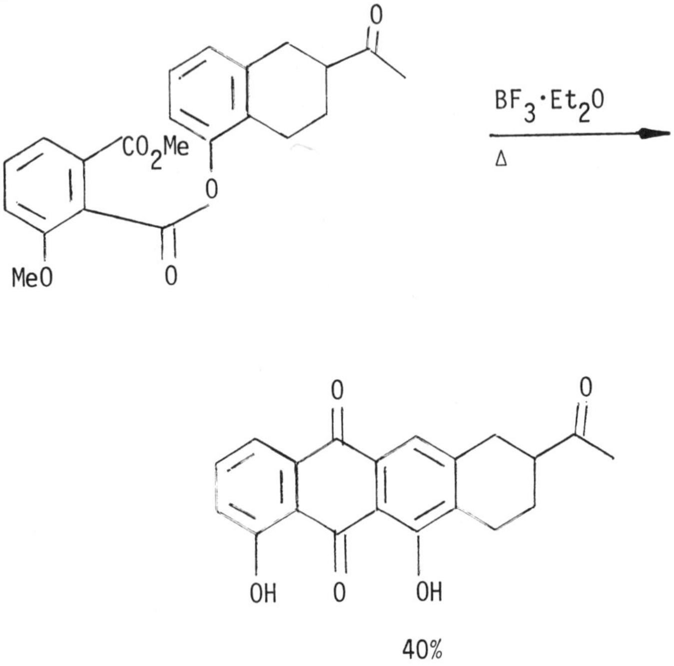

$$\xrightarrow{BF_3 \cdot Et_2O,\ \Delta}$$

40%

I.F.2. Coupling Reactions to Form an Aromatic Carbon-Carbon Bond.

I.F.2-1 R. S. Ward, Chem. Soc. Rev., 11, 75 (1982); A. Ronlan, B. Aalstad and V. D. Parker, Acta Chem. Scand., 36B, 317 (1982).

Review: "The Synthesis of Lignans and Neolignans."

I.F.2-2 S. I. Inaba, H. Matsumoto and R. D. Rieke, Tetrahedron Lett., 23, 4215 (1982); E. Balogh-Hergovich, G. Speier and Z. Tyeklar, Synthesis, 731 (1982).

$$ArX \xrightarrow[Glyme]{Act. Ni(0)} Ar-Ar$$
$$45-99\%$$

Also coupling of benzylic halides.

I.F.2-3 T. Yamagishi, K. Torizuka and T. Sato, Bull. Chem. Soc. Jpn., 55, 1140 (1982); M. Mehdi Nafissi-V, A. T. McPhail et al., J. Org. Chem., 47, 3345 (1982).

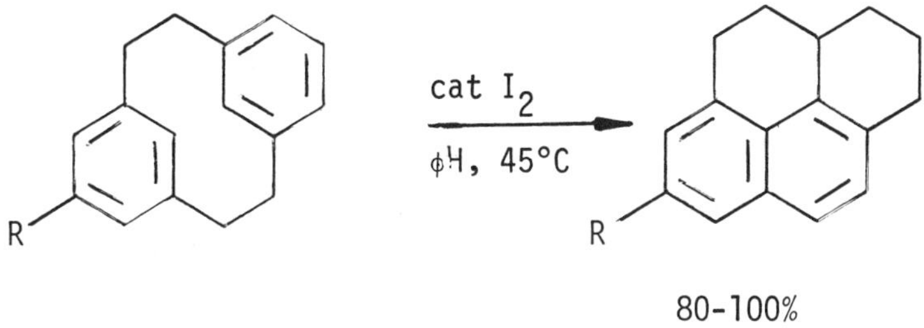

$$\xrightarrow[\phi H, 45°C]{cat\ I_2}$$

80-100%

I.F.2-4 M. Tiecco et al., Tetrahedron Lett., 23, 4629 (1982); S. Ozasa et al., Chem. Pharm. Bull., 30, 802, 2369 (1982); E. Ibuki et al., Bull. Chem. Soc. Jpn., 55, 845 (1982); M. Okubo and Y. Uematsu, ibid, 55, 1121 (1982).

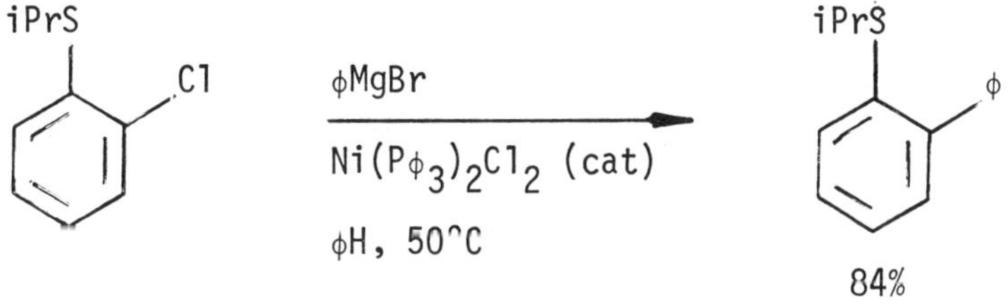

$$\xrightarrow[\phi H, 50°C]{\phi MgBr,\ Ni(P\phi_3)_2Cl_2\ (cat)}$$

84%

I.F.2-5 I. R. Girling and D. A. Widdowson, Tetrahedron Lett., 23, 1957 (1982); A. Hallberg and C. Westerlund, Chem. Lett., 1993 (1982); H. U. Blaser and A. Spencer, J. Organometal. Chem., 233, 267, 240, 209 (1982).

$$R\text{-}C_6H_4\text{-}CH=N\text{-}\text{\textit{t}Bu} \xrightarrow[\text{HOAc, 80°C}]{\substack{1)\ PdCl_2,\ NaOAc \\ 2)\ \phi CH=CH_2 \\ 3)\ H_3O^+}} R\text{-}C_6H_3(CHO)\text{-}CH=CH\text{-}\phi$$

73-86%

I.F.2-6 E. Negishi and L. D. Boardman, Tetrahedron Lett., 23, 3327 (1982); A. A. Moroz et al., J. Org. Chem. (USSR), 18, 1283 (1982).

$$\underset{Me}{\overset{R}{>}}\!\!=\!\!\underset{AlMe_2}{\overset{H}{<}} \xrightarrow[\substack{2)\ Cl_2ZrCp_2 \\ 3)\ \phi I,\ 5\%\ (\phi_3P)_4Pd}]{1)\ nBuLi} \underset{Me}{\overset{R}{>}}\!\!=\!\!\underset{\phi}{\overset{H}{<}} \quad 89\%$$

ZnCl$_2$
Trisubstituted olefins from Alkenylboranes also.

I.F.2-7 H. Taniguchi, Z. Rappoport et al., J. Org. Chem., 47, 5003 (1982).

$$\underset{R^3}{\overset{R^2}{>}}\!\!=\!\!\underset{Br}{\overset{R^1}{<}} \xrightarrow[\text{110°C, Lutidine}]{ArH,\ Aq.\ BF_4} \underset{R^3}{\overset{R^2}{>}}\!\!=\!\!\underset{Ar}{\overset{R^1}{<}}$$

57-89%

I.F.3. Other Aromatic Substitutions

I.F.3-1 D. H. R. Barton, W. B. Motherwell et al., Tetrahedron Lett., 23, 3365 (1982); Chem. Commun., 732 (1982); R. P. Kozyrod and J. T. Pinhey, Tetrahedron Lett., 23, 5365 (1982).

[cyclohexanone with CO_2Et at α-position] →
1) Guanidine Base
2) $\phi_4BiOCOCF_3$
→ [cyclohexanone with ϕ and CO_2Et at α-position] 91%

Regioselectivity of arylation controlled by pH.

I.F.3-2 I. Kuwajima and H. Urabe, J. Amer. Chem. Soc., 104, 6831 (1982); T. Migita et al., Chem. Lett., 939 (1982); Y. Fujiwara et al., J. Organometal. Chem., 226, C36 (1982).

R—C(OSiMe$_3$)=CH$_2$ $\xrightarrow[\phi H, \Delta]{ArBr,\ Bu_3SnF,\ PdCl_2(PAr_3)_2\ (cat)}$ R—CO—CH$_2$—Ar 15-86%

I.F.3-3 R. Beugelmans, M. Bois-Choussy and B. Boudet, Tetrahedron, 38, 3479 (1982); S. Sugai et al., Chem. Lett., 597 (1982); J. Setsune, K. Matsukawa and T. Kitao, Tetrahedron Lett., 23, 663 (1982).

[2-bromobenzonitrile] $\xrightarrow[\substack{hv,\ NH_3 \\ 2)\ H_3O^+}]{1)\ KCH(CO_2Et)_2}$ [2-cyanophenyl-CH(CO$_2$Et)$_2$] 78%

I.F.3-4　M. Stark and D. R. Arnold, Chem. Commun., 434 (1982).

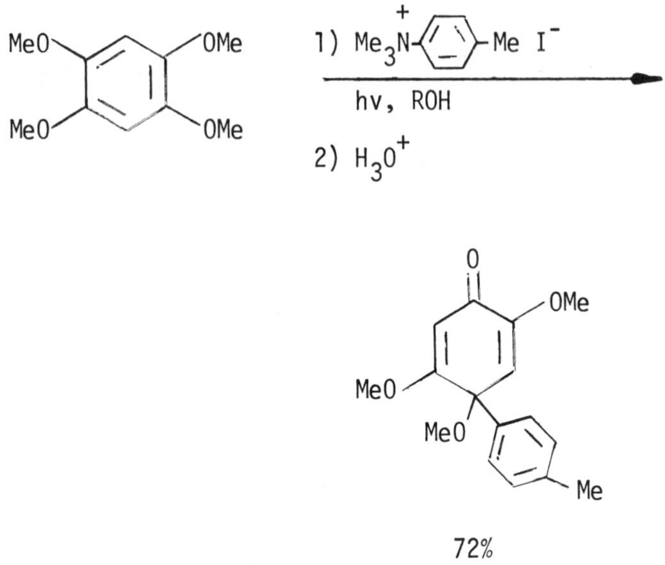

[Structure: 1,2,4,5-tetramethoxybenzene]

1) $Me_3\overset{+}{N}$-⟨C_6H_4⟩-Me I^-
   hv, ROH
2) H_3O^+

[Product structure, 72%]

I.F.3-5　W. R. Jackson, M. F. Semmelhack et al., Chem. Commun., 1359 (1982); Y. K. Chung, P. G. Williard and D. A. Sweigart, Organometallics, 1, 1053 (1982); A. J. Birch, A. J. Liepa and G. R. Stephenson, J. Chem. Soc., Perkin I, 713 (1982).

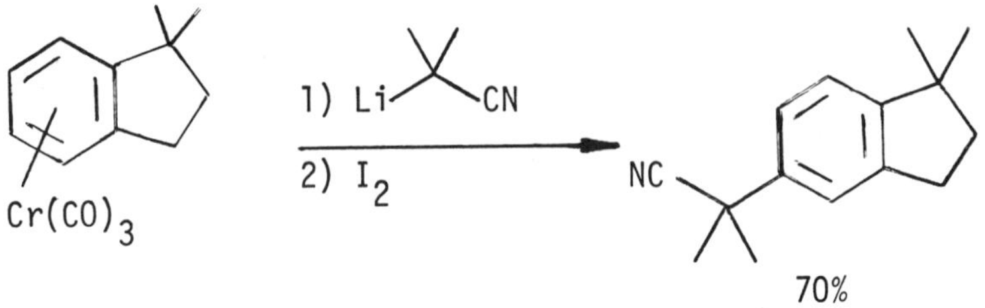

[Reactant: 1,1-dimethylindane-Cr(CO)₃]

1) Li-C(Me)₂-CN
2) I_2

[Product, 70%]

Stereoelectronic Control

I.F.3-6 K. M. Chen and M. M. Joullie, Tetrahedron Lett., 23, 4567 (1982); M. O. Fatope and J. I. Okogun, J. Chem. Soc., Perkin I, 1601 (1982); K. Krohn and W. Baltus, Liebigs Ann. Chem., 1579 (1982).

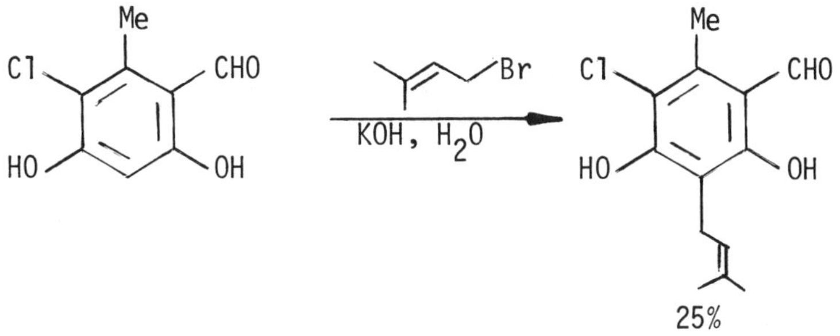

[Reaction scheme: 4-chloro-3-methyl-2,6-dihydroxybenzaldehyde + prenyl bromide, KOH, H_2O → prenylated product, 25%]

I.F.3-7 A. Pochini et al., Tetrahedron Lett., 23, 3803 (1982); J. Chem. Soc., Perkin I, 805 (1982); M. Soucek et al., Coll. Czech. Chem. Commun., 47, 59 (1982); K. Krohn and B. Behnke, Tetrahedron Lett., 23, 395 (1982).

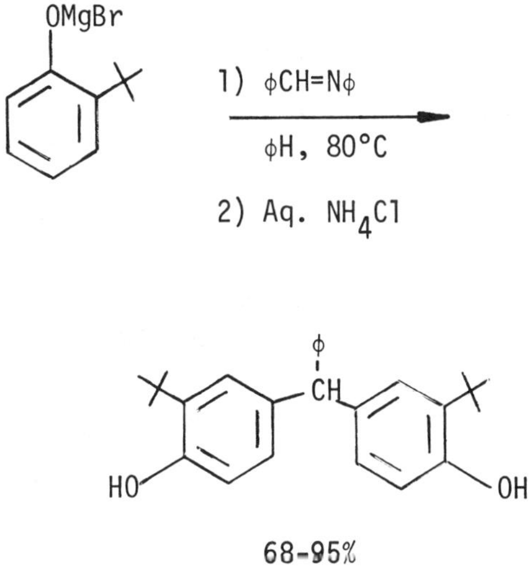

[Reaction scheme: ArOMgBr with 1) ϕCH=Nϕ, ϕH, 80°C; 2) Aq. NH_4Cl → diarylmethane product, 68-95%]

I.F.3-8 M. Makosza and J. Golinski, Angew. Chem., Int. Ed. Engl., 21, 451 (1982); G. Bartoli et al., Synthesis, 836 (1982); M. Zander, Chem. Ber., 115, 3449 (1982).

$$\text{Ar-NO}_2 + (MeO)_2\overset{O}{\underset{\|}{P}}CH(Cl)\phi \xrightarrow{NH_3(\ell),\ NaOH} p\text{-}O_2N\text{-}C_6H_4\text{-}CH(\phi)\text{-}\overset{O}{\underset{\|}{P}}(OMe)_2$$

I.F.3-9 M. A. Fox, A. C. Ranade and I. Madany, J. Organometal. Chem., 239, 269 (1982); G. Kaupp, H. W. Grüter and E. Teufel, Chem. Ber., 115, 3208 (1982); J. P. Tane and K. P. C. Vollhardt, Angew. Chem., Int. Ed. Engl., 21, 617 (1982); R. S. Kapil et al., Synthesis, 405, (1982).

$$\text{anthracene} \xrightarrow[\text{2) hv, -80°C}]{\text{1) }\phi CH_2Li,\ THF,\ -78°C} \text{9-benzylanthracene (47\%)}$$

I.F.3-10 K. Hirakawa, Y. Minami and S. Hayashi, J. Chem. Soc., Perkin I, 577 (1982); R. V. Stevens and G. S. Bisacchi, J. Org. Chem., 47, 2393, 2396 (1982); R. W. Thies and S. T. Yue, ibid, 47, 2685 (1982).

$$\text{10-diazoanthracen-9(10H)-one} \xrightarrow[\text{2) }\Delta,\ Ac_2O]{\text{1) } p\text{-tolyl}} \quad (R^1, R^2 = H,\ Me\ or\ Me,\ H)$$

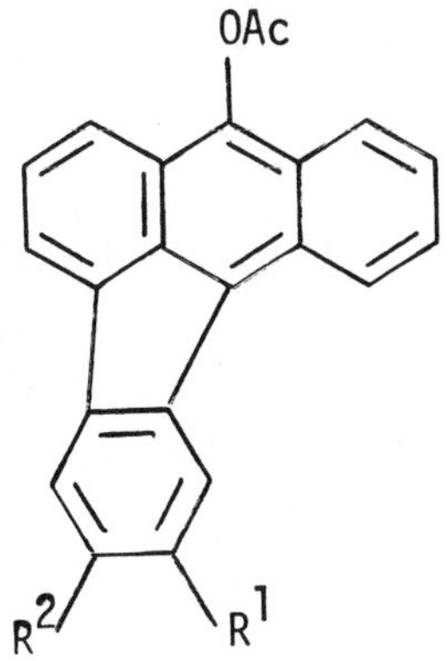

I.F.3-11 W. E. Parham and C. K. Bradsher, Acct. Chem. Res., 15, 300 (1982).

Review: "Aromatic Organolithium Reagents Bearing Electrophilic Groups. Preparation by Halogen-Lithium Exchange."

I.F.3-12 P. Beak and V. Snieckus, Acct. Chem. Res., 15, 306 (1982).

Review: "Directed Lithiation of Aromatic Tertiary Amides: An Evolving Synthetic Methodology for Polysubstituted Aromatics."

I.F.3-13 D. L. Comins, J. D. Brown and N. B. Mantlo, Tetrahedron Lett., 23, 3979 (1982).

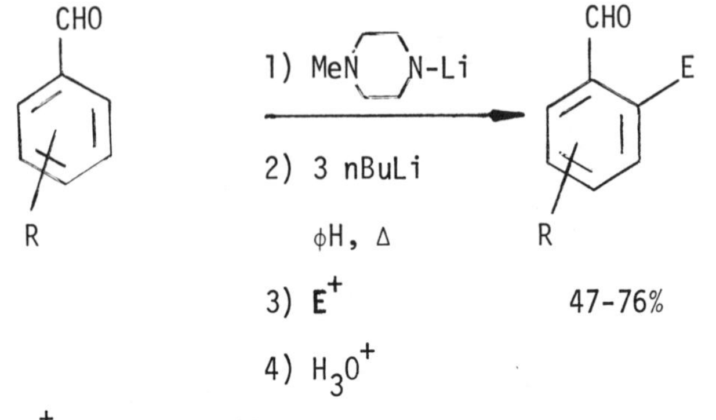
CHO
R
1) MeN N-Li
2) 3 nBuLi
ϕH, Δ
3) E+
4) H3O+
CHO
E
R
47-76%

E^+ = RX, Me_3SiCl.

I.F.3-14 A. I. Meyers et al., Tetrahedron Lett., 23, 2091 (1982); J. Amer. Chem. Soc., 104, 879 (1982); J. M. Wilson and D. J. Cram, ibid, 881 (1982); K. J. Edgar and C. K. Bradsher, J. Org. Chem., 47, 1585 (1982).

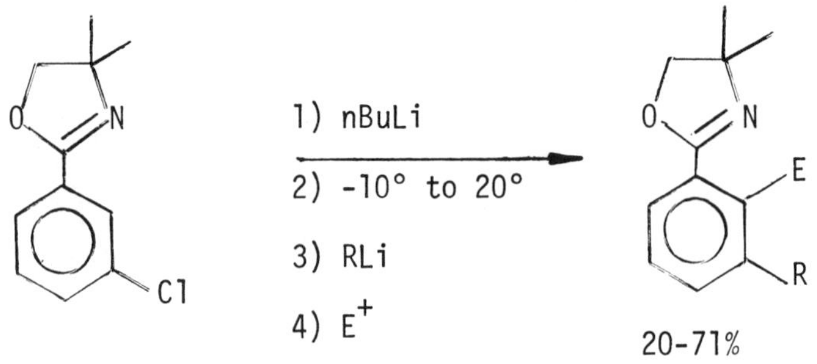
O
N
Cl
1) nBuLi
2) -10° to 20°
3) RLi
4) E+
O
N
E
R
20-71%

I.F.3-15 L. S. Hegedus et al., J. Org. Chem., 47, 2607 (1982); R. D. Clark and J. M. Caroon, ibid, 47, 2804 (1982).

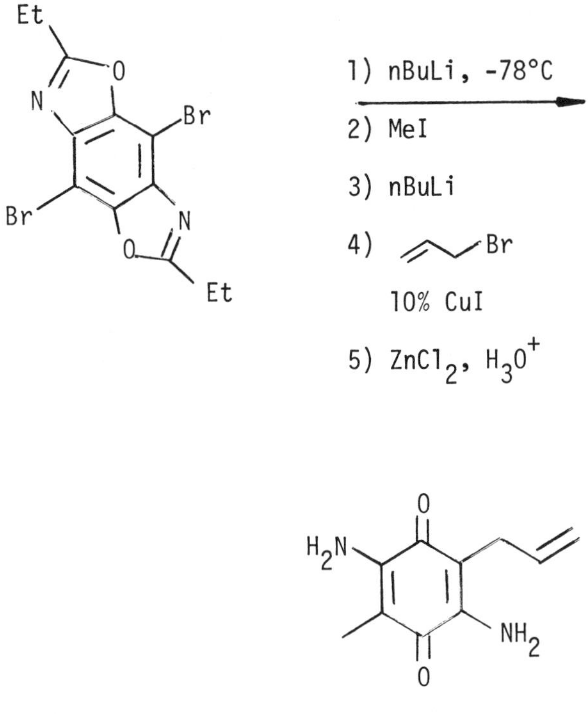
Et
O
N
Br
Br
N
O
Et
1) nBuLi, -78°C
2) MeI
3) nBuLi
4) Br
10% CuI
5) ZnCl2, H3O+
O
H2N
NH2
O

84%

I.F.3-16 P. Beak and R. A. Brown, J. Org. Chem., 47, 34 (1982); R. G. Harvey, C. Cortez and S. A. Jacobs, ibid, 47, 2120 (1982); M. Watanabe, V. Snieckus et al., Tetrahedron Lett., 23, 1647 (1982).

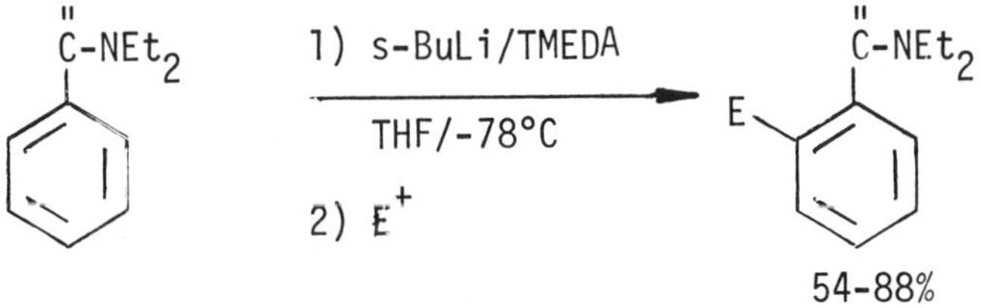
O
C-NEt2
1) s-BuLi/TMEDA
THF/-78°C
2) E+
O
C-NEt2
E

54-88%

Tertiary amido group more effective in directing metalation than chloro, methoxyl, sulfonamido, (dimethylamino) methyl, or oxazolino functions.

I.F.3-17 T. Gungor, F. Marsais and G. Queguiner, Synthesis, 499 (1982).

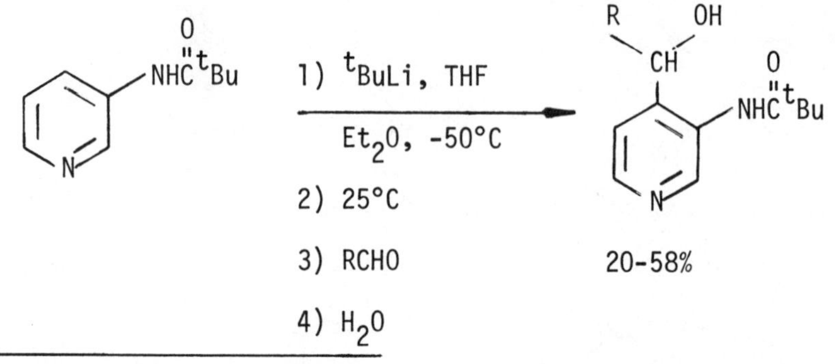

[pyridine-3-NHC(O)^{t}Bu]
1) ^{t}BuLi, THF, Et$_2$O, -50°C
2) 25°C
3) RCHO
4) H$_2$O
→ [4-CH(R)(OH)-3-NHC(O)^{t}Bu-pyridine] 20-58%

I.F.3-18 T. D. Krizan and J. C. Martin, J. Org. Chem., 47, 2681 (1982).

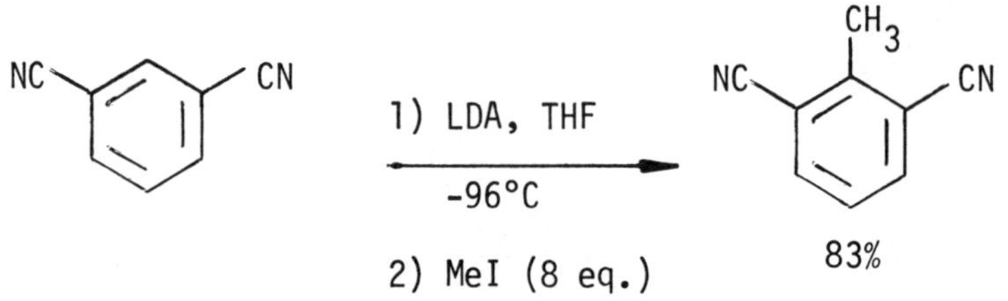

[1,3-dicyanobenzene]
1) LDA, THF, -96°C
2) MeI (8 eq.)
→ [2-methyl-1,3-dicyanobenzene] 83%

I.F.3-19 F. Marsais, G. Le Nard and G. Queguiner, Synthesis, 235 (1982); M. R. Winkle and R. C. Ronald, J. Org. Chem., 47, 2101 (1982).

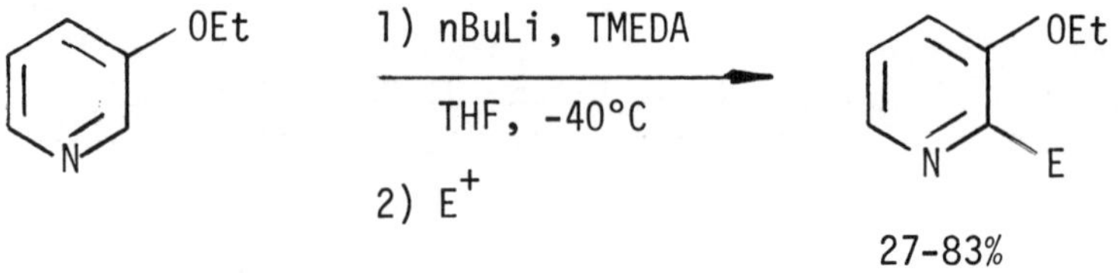

[3-ethoxypyridine]
1) nBuLi, TMEDA, THF, -40°C
2) E$^+$
→ [3-ethoxy-2-E-pyridine] 27-83%

E$^+$ = RCHO, R$_2$CO, Me$_3$SiCl, Me$_2$AsI.

I.F.3-20 M. Fukui, T. Ikeda and T. Oishi, Tetrahedron Lett., 23, 1605 (1982); T. R. Hoye and P. A. Kaese, Synth. Commun., 12, 49 (1982).

```
    Me   SiMe₂ᵗBu                                    Me   Ac
      \ N /                1) nBuLi, THF               \ N /
        |              ─────────────────────→            |
        ⌬                 2) E⁺                          ⌬
        |                                                |  E
   (CO)₃Cr               3) I₂, CSA, THF
                            10% HCl                61-73%
                                                (85-98% meta
                         4) Ac₂O, Pyr.              isomer)
```

E⁺ = MeI, φCHO, Me₂NCHO, φCN, MeSSMe

I.F.3-21 R. Stradi et al., Synthesis, 787, 789 (1982); H. Molines, M. Tordeux and C. Wakselman, Bull. Soc. Chim. Fr. II, 367 (1982).

```
       Ar
       |
       CH-Br           R₂N                              Ar
      /                    \                             |
  ⎡O  N⁺=CH⎤    Br⁻          ═                           ⌬
  ⎣        ⎦                 ⟋        NR₂            /      \
                                  ────────────→    NR₂
                             2 Et₃N, -50°C         NR₂
                                                  15-47%
```

I.F.3-22 D. H. R. Barton et al, J. Chem. Soc., Perkin I, 665 (1982); C. Ivanov and T. Tcholakova, Synthesis, 730 (1982).

```
                         CHO
    O⁻    O⁻         1) φ⌇                            CO₂Et
     \   /              ⎹  NMe₂                        |  OH
      ═══                                              ⌬
     ⟋   \OEt        2) SOCl₂                          |
                                                       φ
  Li⁺ and Na⁺        3) Pyrrolidine, Δ
                                                      43%
```

I.F.3-23 R. F. C. Brown et al., Aust. J. Chem., 35, 1373, 1385 (1982).

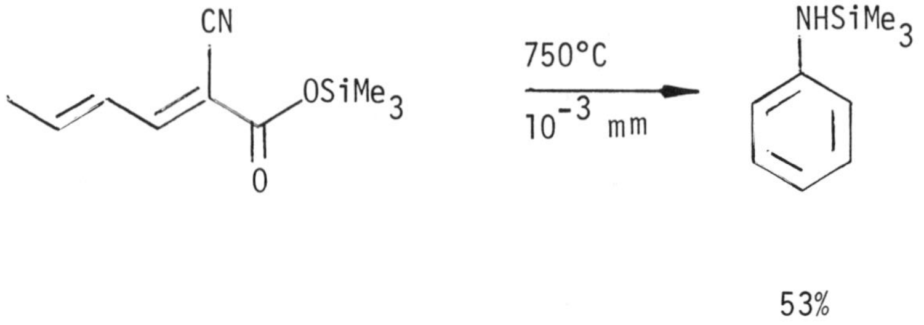

53%

I.F.3-24 Y. Kikuchi, Y. Hasegawa and M. Matsumoto, Tetrahedron Lett., 23, 2199 (1982); J. M. Bruce et al., Chem. Commun., 686 (1982); K. Mori and K. Sato, Tetrahedron, 38, 1221 (1982).

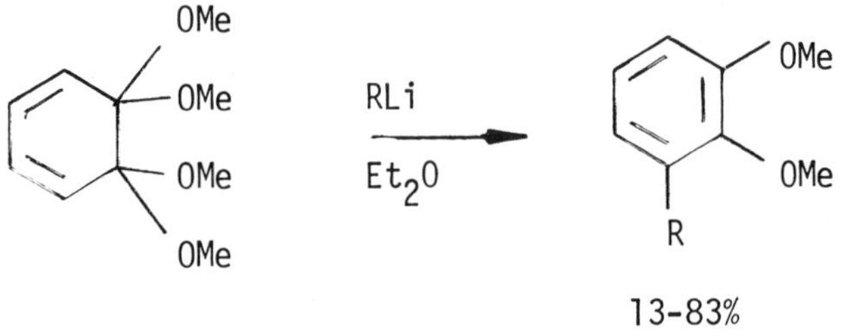

13-83%

I.F.3-25 G. Bringmann, Angew. Chem., Int. Ed. Engl., 21, 200 (1982); N. Katagiri, T. Kato and J. Nakano, Chem. Pharm. Bull., 30, 2440, 2590 (1982).

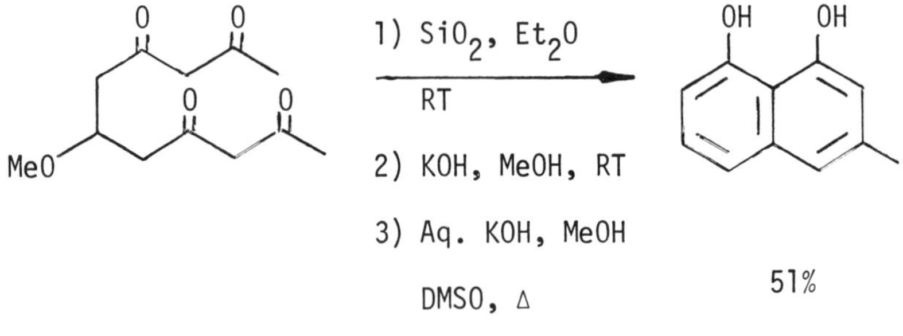

1) SiO_2, Et_2O
   RT

2) KOH, MeOH, RT

3) Aq. KOH, MeOH
   DMSO, Δ

51%

I.F.3-26 M. F. Semmelhack et al., Tetrahedron Lett., 23, 2931 (1982); J. Amer. Chem. Soc., 104, 5850 (1982).

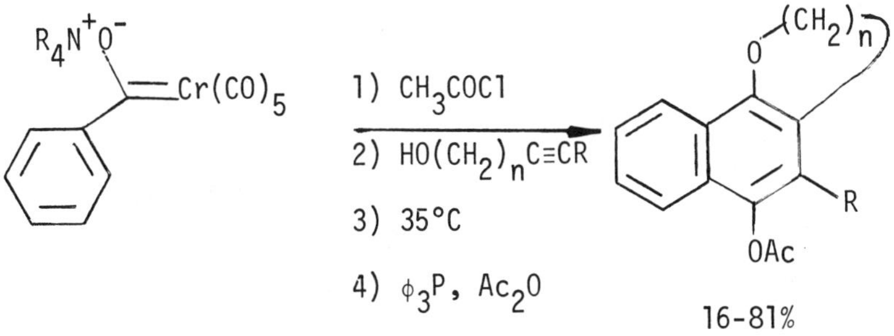

$$R_4N^+O^- \text{—Ph—}=Cr(CO)_5 \xrightarrow[\substack{1)\ CH_3COCl \\ 2)\ HO(CH_2)_nC\equiv CR \\ 3)\ 35°C \\ 4)\ \phi_3P,\ Ac_2O}]{} \text{naphthalene-}O(CH_2)_n,\ R,\ OAc$$

16-81%

Starting Material Available in Two Steps from PhLi.

I.F.3-27 A. M. Mehta and D. N. Patil, J. Chem. Res. (S), 4 (1982); G. Bringmann, Tetrahedron Lett., 23, 2009 (1982); M. V. Sargent et al., J. Chem. Soc., Perkin I, 3007 (1982).

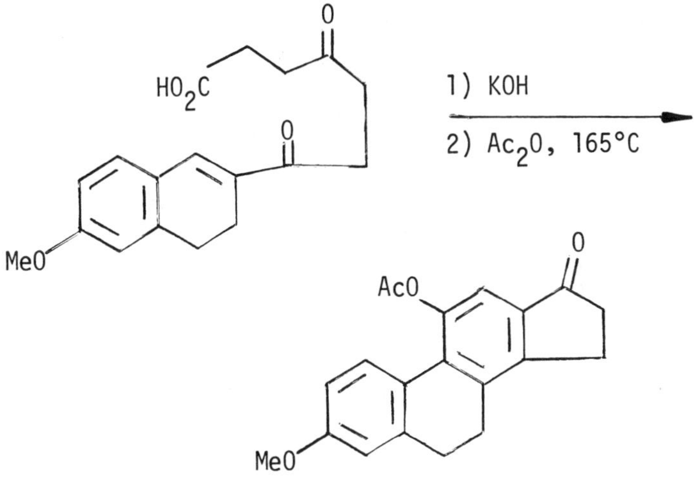

$$\xrightarrow[\substack{1)\ KOH \\ 2)\ Ac_2O,\ 165°C}]{}$$

I.F.3-28 G. P. Gisby, S. E. Royall and P. G. Sammes, J. Chem. Soc., 169 (1982); S. Manna, J. R. Falck and C. Mioskowski, J. Org. Chem., 47, 5021 (1982); M. E. Garst and J. D. Frazier, ibid, 47, 3553 (1982).

R^3, R^4, R^2, R^5, R^1 pyridinone + $MeO_2C-C\equiv C-CO_2Me$, 145°C → substituted benzene with R^2, R^3, R^4, R^5, CO_2Me, CO_2Me

21-96%

I.F.3-29 M. A. Tius et al., J. Org. Chem., 47, 3163 (1982); Tetrahedron Lett., 23, 2819, 2823 (1982); T. H. Chan and T. Chaly, ibid, 23, 2935 (1982).

cyclopentanone with =CHOH
1) Me_3SiCl, Et_3N
2) isobutenyl-MgCl
3) H_3O^+
4) pTsOH
→ methylindane

58-87%

I.F.3-30 D. L. Boger et al., Tetrahedron Lett., 23, 4551, 4555, 4559 (1982); D. W. Cameron et al., Aust. J. Chem., 35, 1501 (1982).

α-tetralone
1) LDA
2) CO_2Me, CO_2Me, MeO-substituted alkene
3) $(MeO)_2C=CH_2$, 95°C
→ phenanthrene derivative with OMe, CO_2Me

70%

I.F.3-31 M. N. Paddon-Row, H. K. Patney and L. N. Pasupuleti, Aust. J. Chem., 35, 307 (1982); P. A. Harland and P. Hodge, Synthesis, 223 (1982).

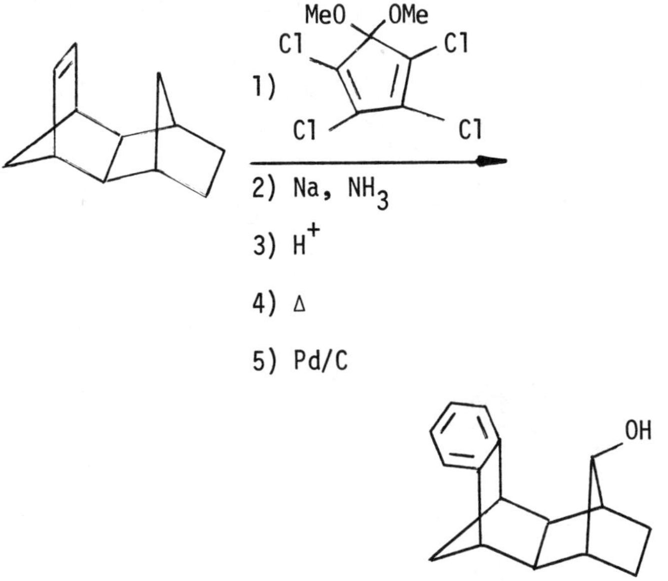

1) [tetrachloro-dimethoxy cyclopentadiene]
2) Na, NH$_3$
3) H$^+$
4) Δ
5) Pd/C

Benzene Annelation

I.F.3-32 H. Meier et al., Liebigs Ann. Chem., 914, 1366 (1982).

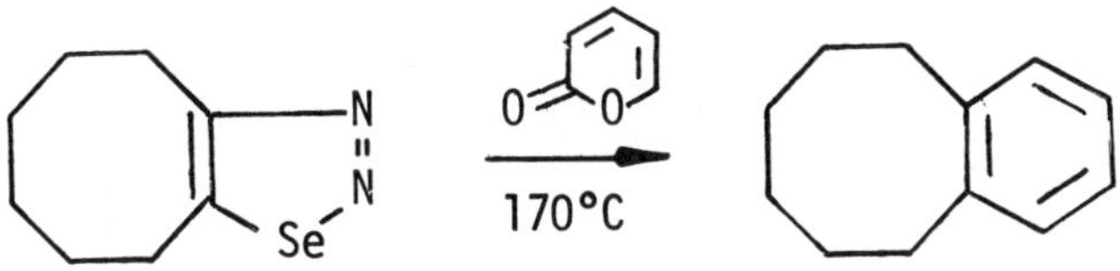

170°C

74%

I.F.3-33 T. Umemoto and O. Miyano, Tetrahedron Lett., 23, 3929 (1982); R. Lapouyade, N. Hanafi and J. P. Morand, Angew. Chem., Int. Ed. Engl., 21, 766 (1982); N. Suzuki, Y. Ayaguchi and Y. Izawa, Bull. Chem. Soc. Jpn., 55, 3349 (1982).

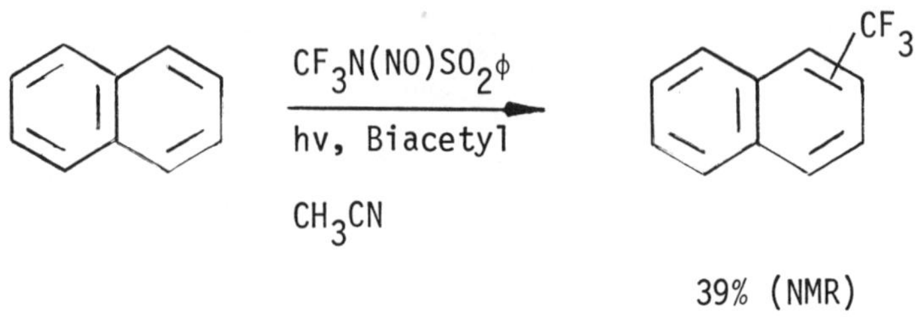

naphthalene + CF$_3$N(NO)SO$_2\phi$ / hv, Biacetyl / CH$_3$CN → CF$_3$-substituted naphthalene

39% (NMR)

I.F.3-34 R. Lapouyade, A. Couture et al., J. Org. Chem., 47, 1361 (1982); P. M. op den Brouw and W. H. Laarhoven, J. Chem. Soc., Perkin II, 795 (1982).

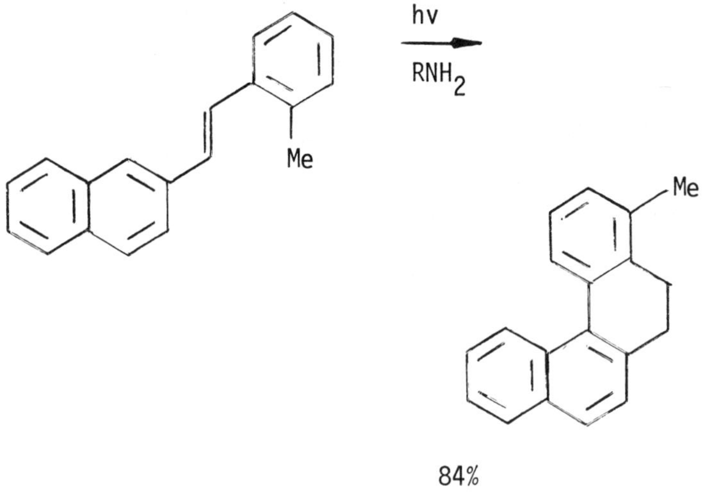

hv, RNH$_2$

84%

I.F.3-35 L. Capuano, C. Wamprecht and A. Willmes, *Chem. Ber.*, **115**, 3904 (1982).

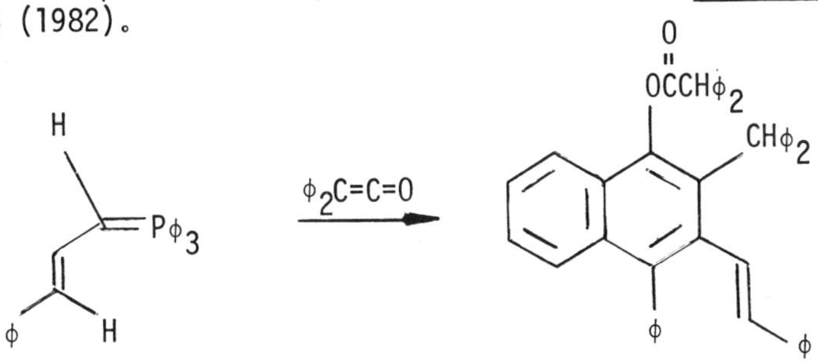

$\phi_2C=C=O$

29%

I.F.3-36 K. Tintel, J. Lugtenburg and J. Cornelisse, *Chem. Commun.*, 185 (1982).

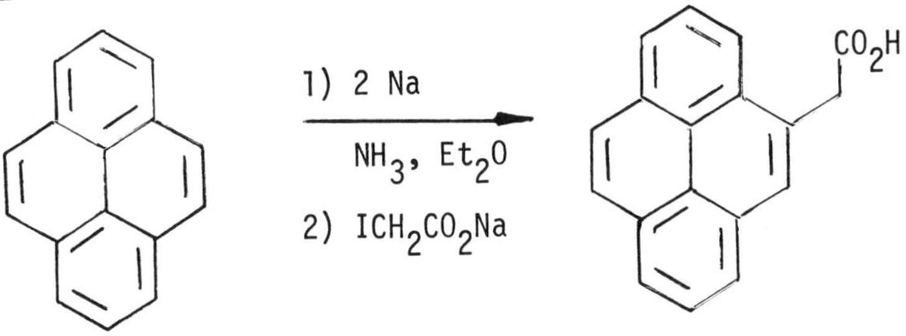

1) 2 Na, NH_3, Et_2O
2) ICH_2CO_2Na

95%

I.F.3-37 J. J. Eisch et al., *J. Org. Chem.*, **47**, 5051 (1982).

ArOH
1) Me_3SiCH_2Cl, Base
2) RLi
3) H_2O
4) KOH, EtOH
→ $ArCH_2OH$

I.F.3-38 A. Citterio, A. Gentile and F. Minisci, Tetrahedron Lett., 23, 5587 (1982).

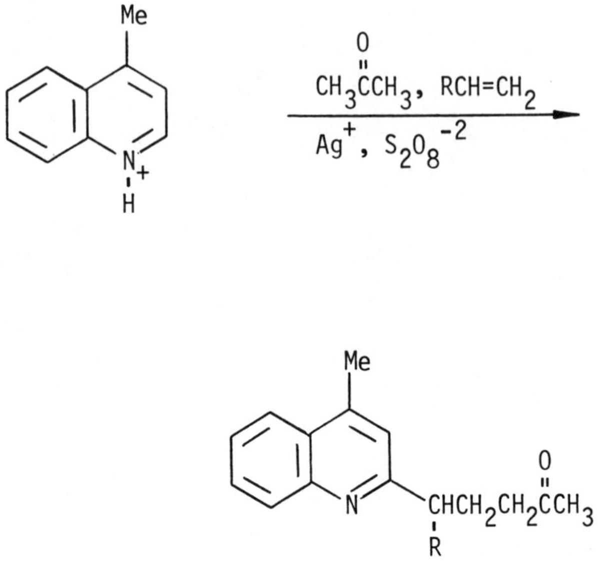

$$\underset{\substack{\text{4-methylquinolinium}}}{\text{Me-quinoline-N}^+\text{H}} \xrightarrow[\text{Ag}^+,\ S_2O_8^{-2}]{CH_3\overset{O}{\overset{\|}{C}}CH_3,\ RCH=CH_2} \underset{\substack{\text{Me-quinoline-N-CHR-CH}_2\text{CH}_2\text{C(O)CH}_3}}{}$$

42%

I.F.3-39 N. Pourahmady, E. H. Vickery and E. J. Eisenbraun, J. Org. Chem., 47, 2590 (1982).

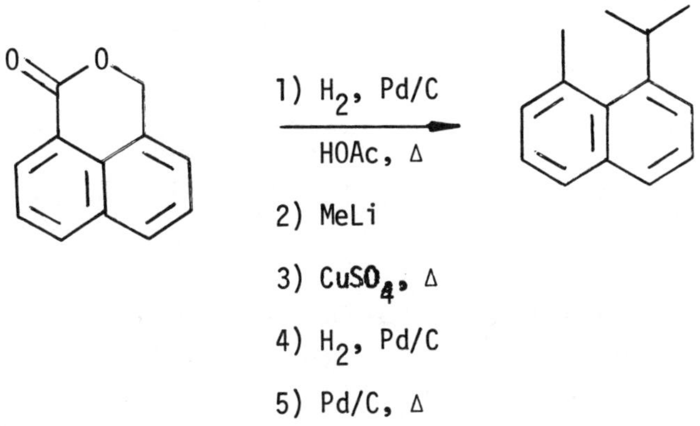

1) H_2, Pd/C, HOAc, Δ
2) MeLi
3) $CuSO_4$, Δ
4) H_2, Pd/C
5) Pd/C, Δ

I.F.3-40 L. T. Scott, Acct. Chem. Res., 15, 52 (1982).

Review: "Thermal Rearrangements of Aromatic Compounds."

I.F.3-41 R. A. Rossi, Acct. Chem. Res., 15, 164 (1982).

Review: "Phenomenon of Radical Anion Fragmentation in the Course of Aromatic $S_{RN}1$ Reactions."

I.F.3-42 E. Vogel, Pure Appl. Chem., 54, 1015 (1982).

Review: "Recent Advances in the Chemistry of Bridged Annulenes."

I.F.3-43 S. Ito, Pure Appl. Chem., 54, 957 (1982).

Review: "Nonbenzenoid Phanes."

I.F.3-44 K. Hafner, Pure Appl. Chem., 54, 939 (1982).

Review: "New Aspects of the Chemistry of Nonbenzenoid Polycyclic Conjugated π-Electron Systems."

I.G. Synthesis via Organometallics

I.G.1 Synthesis via Organoboranes

I.G.1-1 A. Pelter, Chem. Soc. Rev., 11, 191 (1982).

Review: "Carbon-Carbon Bond Formation Involving Boron Reagents."

I.G.1-2 H. C. Brown and S. U. Kulkarni, J. Organometal. Chem., 239, 23 (1982).

Review: "Haloboranes and their Alkyl Derivatives."

I.G.1-3   A. Suzuki, Acct. Chem. Res., 15, 178 (1982).

Review: "Organoborates in New Synthetic Reactions."

I.G.1-4   H. C. Brown, et al., J. Amer. Chem. Soc., 104, 6844 (1982); Synthesis, 193, 195 (1982).

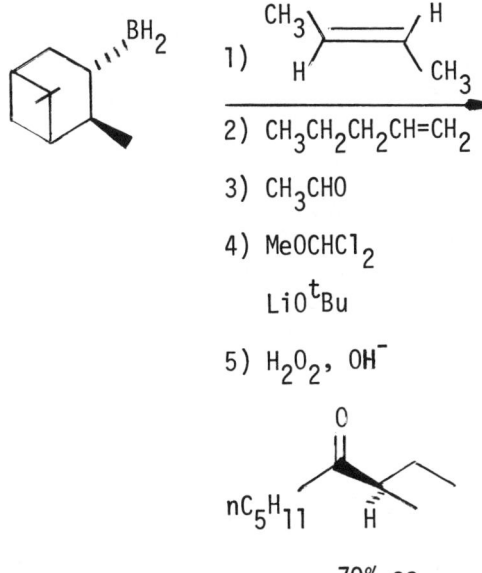

70% ee

I.G.1-5   D. S. Matteson et al., Organometallics, 1, 20, 280 (1982).

$CH_2(B\langle{}^O_O\rangle)_2$ $\xrightarrow[\text{3) NaBO}_3]{\text{1) LiTMP} \atop \text{2) RX}}$ R-CHO

49-71%

I.G.1-6 H. C. Brown et al., <u>Organometallics</u>, 1, 212 (1982); J. Org. Chem., 47, 863, 872 (1982).

$R^AR^BBX \cdot SMe_2$ $\xrightarrow{\begin{array}{l}\text{1) NaOMe, MeOH}\\ \text{2) Alkene C}\\ \text{1/3 LAH}\\ \text{3) Cl}_2\text{CHOMe}\\ \text{Et}_3\text{COLi}\\ \text{4) [O]}\end{array}}$ $R^AR^BR^CC\text{-OH}$

via Mixed Trialkylboranes

I.G.1-7 G. W. Kabalka et al., <u>Chem. Commun.</u>, 1273 (1982).

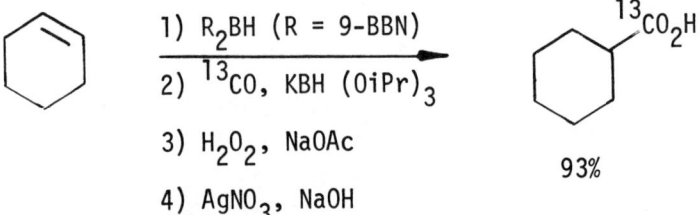

1) R_2BH (R = 9-BBN)
2) ^{13}CO, KBH $(OiPr)_3$
3) H_2O_2, NaOAc
4) $AgNO_3$, NaOH

93%

I.G.1-8 M. M. Midland and Y. C. Kwon, <u>Tetrahedron Lett.</u>, 23, 2077 (1982); A. Suzuki et al., <u>Synth. Commun.</u>, 12, 813 (1982).

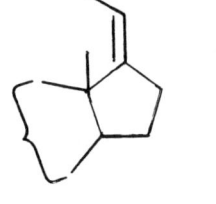

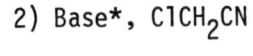
1) 9-BBN (2 eq.)
2) Base*, ClCH$_2$CN

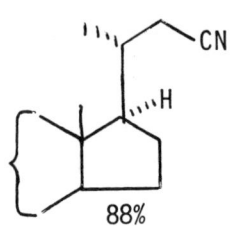

88%

* Base = Potassium 2,6-Di-t-butyl-4-methylphenoxide.

I.G.1-9 S. Hara, Y. Satoh and A. Suzuki, Chem. Lett., 1289 (1982).

$$R^1C\equiv C-CH_2BR^1_2 \xrightarrow[\substack{\text{LiOMe, CuI} \\ -78°C}]{\substack{BrCH_2 \diagup C(R^2) \diagdown\!\!=\!\!CH_2}} R^1C\equiv C-CH_2CH_2C(R^2)=CH_2$$

65-85% (GC)

I.G.1-10 A. Lattes et al., J. Organometal. Chem., 238, 281 (1982).

$$Me_2N-CH_2-C\equiv C-Br \xrightarrow[\substack{25°C \\ 2)\ R^1C\equiv CR^2 \\ 3)\ OH^-}]{1)\ \vdash\!\!\!\vdash\!\!-BH_2,\ THF} Me_2NCH_2C(R^1)\!=\!C(CHBr)\!-\!CHR^2$$

30-100%

I.G.1-11 A. Pelter, L. Hughes and J. M. Rao, J. Chem. Soc., Perkin I, 719 (1982).

$$\underset{R^4}{\overset{R^3}{\diagdown}}\!\!=\!\!\underset{Z^2}{\overset{Z^1}{\diagup}} \xrightarrow[\substack{2)\ [O]}]{1)\ R^1_3BC\equiv CR^2\ Li^+} R^1\!-\!\underset{R^2}{\overset{O}{C}}\!-\!\underset{Z^2}{\overset{R^3\ R^4}{C}}\!-\!Z^1$$

Z^1, Z^2 = NO_2, H; CO_2Et, CO_2Et; COMe, CO_2Et; SOφ, H; COR, H; CO_2Et, H.

I.G.1-12 M. Schlosser and K. Fujita, Angew. Chem., Int. Ed. Engl., 21, 309 (1982); Helv. Chim. Acta, 65, 1258 (1982); M. M. Midland and S. B. Preston, J. Amer. Chem. Soc., 104, 2330 (1982); R. W. Hoffmann et al., Chem. Ber., 115, 2357 (1982).

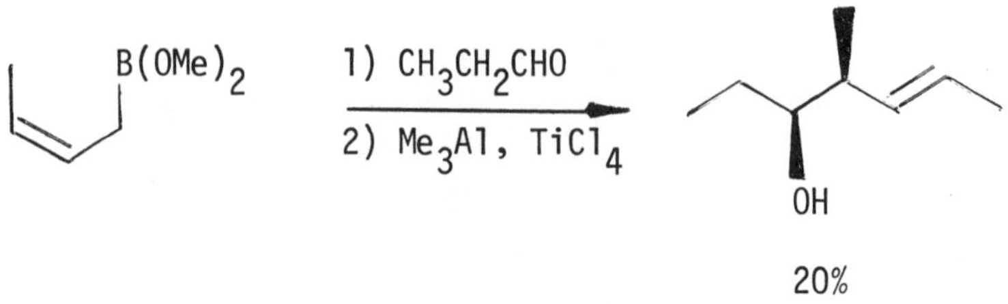

I.G.1-13 R. W. Hoffmann and B. Kemper, Tetrahedron Lett., 23, 845 (1982); P. G. M. Wuts and S. S. Bigelow, J. Org. Chem., 47, 2498 (1982); Synth. Commun., 12, 779 (1982); M. Koreeda and Y. Tanaka, Chem. Commun., 845 (1982); Y. Yamamoto, Y. Saito and K. Maruyama, ibid, 1326 (1982).

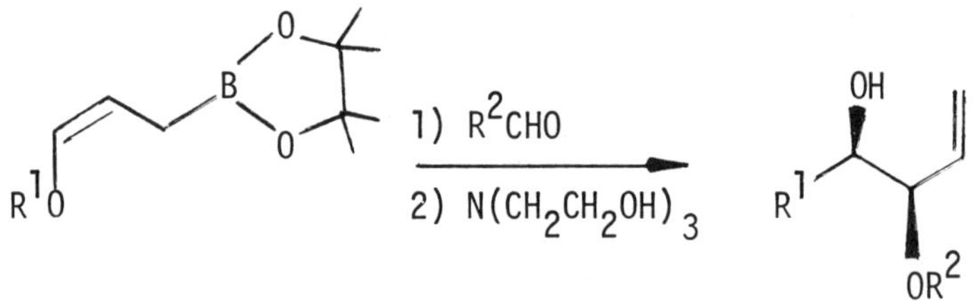

Increased steric bulk both on aldehyde or allylboronate causes decreased diasterioselectivity.

I.G.2. Carbonylation Reactions

I.G.2-1 H. M. Colquhoun, Chem. Ind., 747 (1982).

Review: "Cobalt-Catalyzed Carbonylation and Cyclisation of Organic Compounds."

I.G.2-2 K. Kikukawa et al., Chem. Lett., 35 (1982); Y. Fujiwara et al., Chem. Commun., 132 (1982); D. Farcasiu and R. H. Schlosberg, J. Org. Chem., 47, 151 (1982); N. S. Nudelman and P. Outumuro, ibid, 47, 4347 (1982).

$$\text{Ar-N}_2^+ \text{ BF}_4^- \xrightarrow[\text{CH}_3\text{CN}]{\substack{R_4Sn, CO \\ Pd(OAc)_2 \text{ (cat)}}} \text{Ar-}\underset{\underset{40\text{-}90\%}{}}{\overset{\overset{O}{\|}}{C}}\text{-R}$$

I.G.2-3 R. C. Larock and C. A. Fellows, J. Amer. Chem. Soc., 104, 1900 (1982).

$$\text{Ar-H} \xrightarrow[\substack{CF_3CO_2H \\ 2) CO, PdCl_2, CH_3OH}]{1) Tl(O_2CCF_3)_3} \text{Ar-CO}_2\text{CH}_3 \quad 42\text{-}80\%$$

I.G.2-4 T. Kobayashi and M. Tanaka, J. Organometal. Chem., 231, C12; 233, C64, (1982); H. Hoberg and H. J. Riegel, ibid, 236, C53 (1982); A. Yamamoto et al., Tetrahedron Lett., 23, 3383 (1982); Chem. Lett., 865 (1982).

$$\phi I \xrightarrow[\substack{(\phi_3P)_2PhPdI \text{ (cat)} \\ 120°C}]{Et_3N, CO} \phi\text{-}\overset{\overset{O}{\|}}{C}\text{-NEt}_2 \quad 74\%$$

Also, double carbonylation procedure.

I.G.2-5 H. Alper and J. L. Fabre, Organometallics, 1, 1037 (1982); M. Yamashita et al., Bull. Chem. Soc. Jpn., 55, 1663 (1982).

$$R^1SCH\text{-}Li \atop R^2 \quad \xrightarrow[\text{THF, -78°C}]{\text{1) Fe(CO)}_5} \quad \begin{array}{c} O \\ \| \\ R^1SCH\text{-}CCH_3 \\ R^2 \end{array}$$

2) RT

3) MeI

5-100%

I.G.2-6 F. Serratosa et al., Chem. Commun., 1305 (1982).

$$^tBuO\text{-}C\equiv C\text{-}O^tBu \quad \xrightarrow[\text{Pentane, -78°C}]{\text{1) (C}_5\text{H}_5\text{)Co(CO)}_2}$$

2) Electrochem. Oxid.

CH_3CN, $Q^+ ClO_4^-$

[cyclopentadienone with four O^tBu groups]

40%

I.G.2-7 L. S. Hegedus and Y. Inoue, J. Amer. Chem. Soc., 104, 4917 (1982); T. Imamoto, T. Kusumoto and M. Yokoyama, Bull. Chem. Soc. Jpn., 55, 643 (1982).

RX

1) NaCo(CO)$_4$

2) CO (1 atm)

3) ⌇⌇

4) MeC(CO$_2$Et)$_2^-$

[product: R-C(O)-CH$_2$-CH=CH-CH$_2$-C(Me)(CO$_2$Et)$_2$]

49%

I.G.2-8 L. S. Hegedus and R. Tamura, Organometallics, 1, 1188 (1982); D. Milstein, ibid, 1, 888 (1982); T. Y. Luh and C. L. Lung, Chem. Commun., 57 (1982).

$$\text{\Large{$\langle$}}\!\!-\text{PdP}\phi_3{}^+\ \text{BF}_4{}^- \xrightarrow[\text{-78°C to RT}]{\substack{\text{CH}_3\overset{\text{O}}{\text{C}}\text{Ni(CO)}_x\text{Li} \\ \text{THF}}} \phi\!\diagup\!\!\diagdown\!\!\diagup\!\!\text{C(O)CH}_3$$

61%

I.G.2-9 F. Francalanci and M. Foa, J. Organometal. Chem., 232, 59 (1982); H. Alper, K. Hashem and J. Heveling, Organometallics, 1, 775 (1982).

$$\underset{\text{ArCH-Br}}{\overset{\text{CH}_3}{|}} \xrightarrow[\substack{50\%\ \text{KOH, nBuOH} \\ Q^+ X^-,\ 35°C}]{\text{CO, Co}_2(\text{CO})_8\ (\text{cat})} \underset{\text{ArCH-CO}_2\text{H}}{\overset{\text{CH}_3}{|}}$$

35-54%

I.G.2-10 G. Cometti and G. P. Chiusoli, J. Organometal. Chem., 236, C31 (1982); J. Tsuji, K. Sato and H. Nagashima, Tetrahedron Lett., 23, 893 (1982); F. Jachimowicz and J. W. Raksis, J. Org. Chem., 47, 445 (1982); P. Hong, T. Mise and H. Yamazaki Chem. Lett., 361, 401 (1982).

$$\phi\text{CH=CH}_2 \xrightarrow[\substack{\text{Pd(0) Complex*} \\ \text{CF}_3\text{CO}_2\text{H}}]{\text{CO, MeOH}} \underset{*}{\overset{\text{CH}_3}{\phi\text{CH-CO}_2\text{Me}}}$$

94% (54% ee)

*Neomenthyldiphenylphosphine Ligand.

I.G.2-11 J. Tsuji, K. Sato and H. Okumoto, Tetrahedron Lett., 23, 5189 (1982).

R–CH=CH–CH$_2$–OC(O)R^1 $\xrightarrow[\text{50°C}]{\text{CO, Pd(OAc)}_2\text{-Ph}_3\text{P (cat)}}$ R–CH=CH–CH$_2$–CO$_2$R^1

67-94%

I.G.2-12 N. Sonoda et al., Chem. Commun., 1283 (1982).

2'-hydroxyacetophenone $\xrightarrow[\text{DBU, THF}]{\text{CO, Se}}$ 4-hydroxycoumarin

100%

I.G.2-13 K. Hirai, Y. Takahashi and I. Ojima, Tetrahedron Lett., 23, 2491 (1982).

$\underset{R^3}{\underset{|}{R^1\text{–C}=\text{C}(R^2)\text{–CH}_2\text{OH}}}$ $\xrightarrow[\substack{\text{Co}_2(\text{CO})_8 \\ \text{Co-catalyst} \\ \text{H}_2, \text{Dioxane}}]{\text{H}_2\text{NCOR}^4, \text{CO}}$ $R^1\text{–CH}(R^2)\text{–CH}(\text{NHCOR}^4)\text{–CH}(R^3)\text{–CO}_2\text{H}$

34-77%

Co-catalyst = Transition metal catalyst.

I.G.2-14 D. Seyferth and R. M. Weinstein, *J. Amer. Chem. Soc.*, **104**, 5534 (1982).

$$RLi \xrightarrow[\substack{THF, Et_2O \\ -110°C}]{CO, Me_3SiCl} R\underset{}{\overset{O}{\|}}C-SiMe_3 \quad 50-71\%$$

I.G.2-15 A. A. Schegolev, R. Caple et al., *Tetrahedron Lett.*, **23**, 4419 (1982).

$$\underset{Co_2(CO)_6}{HC\equiv C-\underset{CH_3}{\overset{|}{C}}=CH_2} \xrightarrow[\substack{1) \ ^tBuC^+\overset{O}{\|}\ BF_4^- \\ 2) \ MeOH \\ 3) \ Fe(III)}]{} HC\equiv C-\underset{MeO}{\overset{CH_3}{\underset{|}{C}}}-CH_2-\overset{O}{\overset{\|}{C}}-{^t}Bu \quad 64\%$$

I.G.2-16 A. Yamashita and T. A. Scahill, *Tetrahedron Lett.*, **23**, 3765 (1982).

$$\underset{Ar-\overset{\|}{C}-OCH_3}{Cr(CO)_5} \xrightarrow[\substack{EtOH, THF \\ 60°C}]{HC\equiv C-CO_2Et} \underset{Ar-\overset{\|}{C}-OCH_3}{CHCH(CO_2Et)_2} \quad 80-87\%$$

I.G.3. Other Syntheses via Organometallics

I.G.3-1 H. Hoberg and D. Schaefer, *J. Organometal. Chem.*, **236**, C28 (1982).

1) CO_2, Ni(0), 2,2'-Bipyridine
2) H_3O^+

88%

I.G.3-2 T. Kauffmann et al., Tetrahedron Lett., 23, 2301
(1982); J. Souppe, J. L. Namy and H. B. Kagan, ibid, 23, 3497
(1982); T. Imamoto, T. Kusumoto and M. Yokoyama, Chem. Commun.,
1042 (1982); T. Hiyama et al., Bull. Chem. Soc. Jpn., 55,
561 (1982).

$Me_2Nb(OiPr)_3$, $Me_2Ta(OiPr)_3$, $MeNbCl_4$, $MeTaCl_4$ and $nBuNbCl_4$ selective reactions with aldehydes to add alkyl group.

I.G.3-3 M. D. Lewis and Y. Kishi, Tetrahedron Lett., 23, 2343
(1982); T. Okano, J. Kiji et al., ibid, 23, 4967 (1982); J.
Thivolle-Cazat and I. Tkatchenko, Chem. Commun., 1128 (1982).

φ-C(Me)=CH-CHO + $CH_3CH=CHCH_2Br$ →[$CrCl_2$] product with Me, Me, OH substituents

---

I.G.3-4 G. P. Chiusoli, L. Pallini and G. Salerno, J. Organometal. Chem., 238, C85 (1982); S. Miyano et al., Chem. Lett.,
1379 (1982); L. I. Zakharkin and E. A. Petrushkina, J. Org.
Chem. (USSR), 18, 1419 (1982).

isoprene + $CH_2=CHCH_2CO_2H$ →[Rh Cat.] diene carboxylic acid

---

I.G.3-5 S. Padmanabhan and K. M. Nicholas, Tetrahedron Lett.,
23, 2555 (1982).

alkynyl-$Co_2(CO)_6$ carbinol + allyl-$SiMe_3$ →[$BF_3 \cdot Et_2O$, CH_2Cl_2, -78°C] product-$Co_2(CO)_6$, 81%

I.G.3-6   Y. Morizawa, K. Oshima and H. Nozaki, Tetrahedron Lett., 23, 2871 (1982).

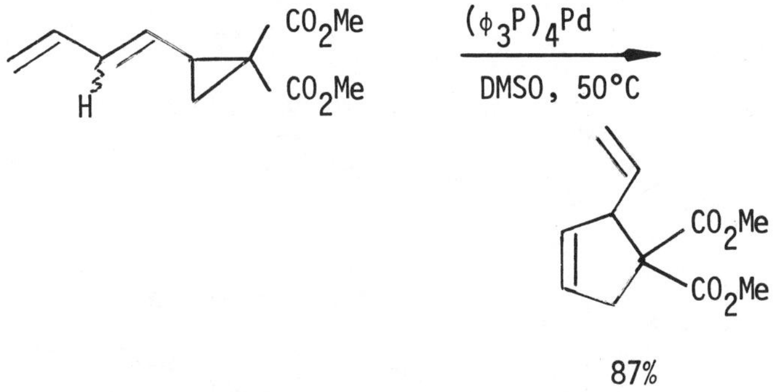

Vinylcyclopropene-cyclopentene rearrangement at mild temperature.

I.G.3-7   S. L. Baysdon and L. S. Liebeskind, Organometallics, 1, 771 (1982).

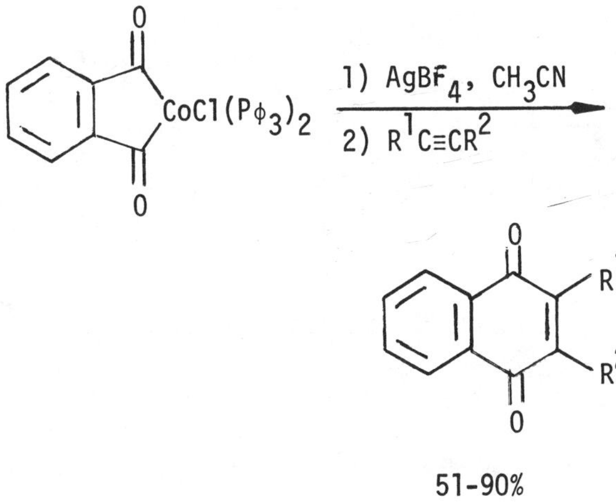

I.G.3-8 S. Warwel, H. Ridder and W. Winkelmuller, Angew. Chem., Int. Ed. Engl., 21, 700 (1982); D. G. Daly and M. A. McKervey, Tetrahedron Lett., 23, 2997 (1982).

cyclohexenyl-CH=CH$_2$

+

RCH=CHR

$\xrightarrow{\substack{\text{1) Selective Metathesis} \\ \text{2) Dehydrogenation}}}$

phenyl-CH$_2$CH$_2$R

I.G.3-9 D. Villemin and P. Cadiot, Tetrahedron Lett., 23, 5139 (1982); M. Petit, A. Mortreux and F. Petit, Chem. Commun., 1385 (1982).

ϕ-C≡C-CH$_2$CH$_2$-OAc $\xrightarrow[\substack{4\text{-ClC}_6\text{H}_4\text{OH} \\ \text{Octane}}]{\text{Mo(CO)}_6}$ AcO-CH$_2$CH$_2$-C≡C-CH$_2$CH$_2$-OAc

Acetylene Metathesis

I.G.4. Organometallic Reviews

I.G.4-1 R. Hoffmann, Angew. Chem., Int. Ed. Engl., 21, 711 (1982).

Review: "Building Bridges Between Inorganic and Organic Chemistry (Nobel Lecture)."

I.G.4-2 C. Floriani, Pure Appl. Chem., 54, 59 (1982).

Review: "Metal-Carbon and Carbon-Carbon Bond Formation from Small Molecules and One Carbon Functional Groups."

I.G.4-3 T. Kauffmann, Angew. Chem., Int. Ed. Engl., 21, 410 (1982).

Review: "New Possible Applications of Heavy Main-Group Elements in Organic Synthesis."

I.G.4-4 T. H. Black, Aldrichimica Acta, 15, 13 (1982).

Review: "Recent Applications of Homogeneous Catalysis to Organic Synthesis."

I.G.4-5 L. D. Freedman and G. O. Doak, Chem. Rev., 82, 15 (1982).

Review: "Preparation Reactions and Physical Properties of Organobismuth Compounds."

I.G.4-6 T. A. Ahlbright, Tetrahedron, 38, 1339 (1982).

Review: "Structure and Reactivity in Organometallic Chemistry. An Applied Molecular Orbital Approach."

I.G.4-7   R. C. Larock, Tetrahedron, 38, 1713 (1982).

Review: "Organomercurials in Organic Synthesis."

I.G.4-8   L. Miginiac, J. Organometal. Chem., 238, 235 (1982).

Review: "The Synthetic Possibilities of Addition Reactions Between Common Organometallic Compounds and Conjugated Dienes."

I.G.4-9   T. Hayashi and M. Kumada, Acct. Chem. Res., 15, 395 (1982).

Review: "Asymmetric Synthesis Catalyzed by Transition-Metal Complexes with Functionalized Chiral Ferrocenylphosphine Ligands."

II
OXIDATIONS

II.A. C—O Oxidations

1. Alcohol ⟶ Ketone, Aldehyde

II.A.1-1   S. O. Nwaukwa and P. M. Keehn, <u>Tetrahedron Lett.</u>, <u>23</u>, 35 (1982).

$$R-\underset{\underset{H}{|}}{\overset{\overset{OH}{|}}{C}}-R' \quad \xrightarrow[CH_3CN]{Ca(OCl)_2} \quad R-\overset{O}{\underset{\|}{C}}-R'$$

>90%

R, R' = alkyl, Ph

II.A.1-2   R. V. Stevens et al., <u>Tetrahedron Lett.</u>, <u>23</u>, 4647 (1982).

$$\underset{R \quad R'}{\overset{\overset{OH}{|}}{\underset{}{CH}}} \quad \xrightarrow{NaOCl, HOAc} \quad \underset{R \quad R'}{\overset{O}{\underset{\|}{C}}}$$

R, R' = alkyl, cyclic   70-90%

Secondary alcohols may be selectively oxidized in the presence of primary alcohols.

$$R-CHO \quad \xrightarrow[CH_3OH]{NaOCl, HOAc} \quad R-\overset{O}{\underset{\|}{C}}-OCH_3$$

58-90%

R = alkyl, subst. Ph

II.A.1-3 H. Tomioka, K. Oshima, and H. Nozaki, Tetrahedron Lett., 23, 539 (1982).

$$\underset{R-CH-R'}{\overset{OH}{|}} \xrightarrow[NaBrO_3]{Ce^{4+}} \underset{R-C-R'}{\overset{O}{\|}}$$

R, R' = alkyl, Ph   ~80-100%

Allows oxidation of secondary alcohols in the presence of primary alcohols.

II.A.1-4 K. Antonakis, J.C.S. Perkin I, 1967 (1982).

$$\underset{R \quad R'}{\overset{OH}{\underset{|}{CH}}} \xrightarrow[\text{4A molecular seives}]{PCC^* \text{ or } PDC} \underset{R \quad R'}{\overset{O}{\|}{C}}$$

R, R' = H, alkyl, aryl   50-100%

*PCC = pyridinium chlorochromate
PDC = pyridinium dichromate

II.A.1-5 F. S. Guziec, Jr. and F. A. Luzzio, J. Org. Chem., 47, 1787 (1982).

$$R\text{-}C_6H_4\text{-}CH_2OH \xrightarrow[H^{\oplus}]{\underset{}{4\text{-}NMe_2\text{-}pyridine}, CrO_3Cl^{\ominus}} R\text{-}C_6H_4\text{-}CHO$$

Also works with allylic alcohols.   43-98%

R = alkyl, alkoxy, nitro

II.A.1-6   M. K. Chaudhuri et al., Synthesis, 588 (1982).

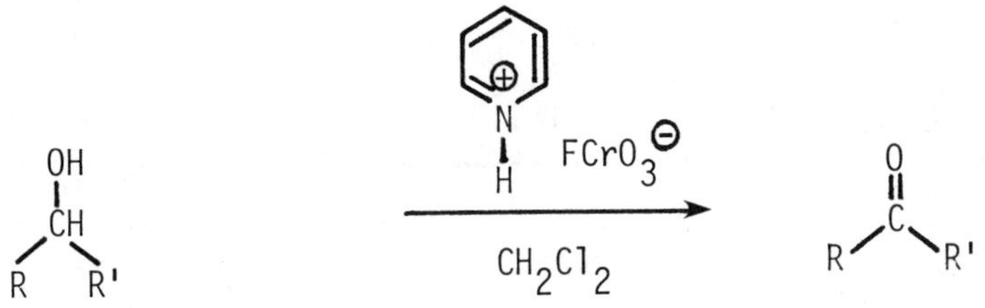

$$\underset{RR'}{\overset{OH}{\underset{|}{CH}}} \xrightarrow[CH_2Cl_2]{PyH^+ \ FCrO_3^-} \underset{RR'}{\overset{O}{\underset{\|}{C}}}$$

R, R' = H, alkyl, aryl   84-98%

II.A.1-7   X. Huang and C. -C. Chan, Synthesis, 1091 (1982).

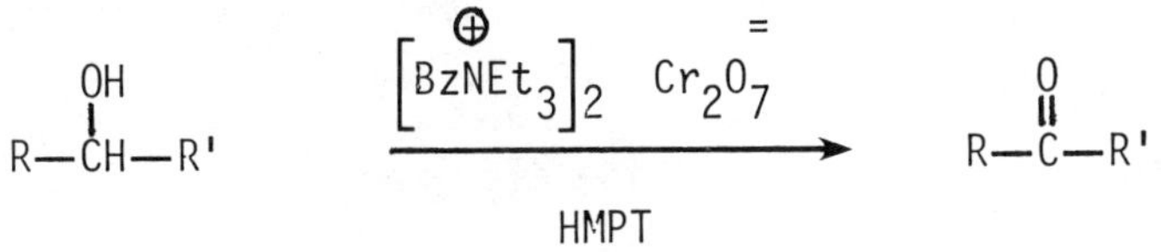

$$R-\overset{OH}{\underset{|}{CH}}-R' \xrightarrow[HMPT]{[BzNEt_3]_2^+ \ Cr_2O_7^=} R-\overset{O}{\underset{\|}{C}}-R'$$

30-99%

R, R' = H, Ph, styryl, alkyl

II.A.1-8   I. Kuwajima, M. Shimizu, and H. Urabe, J. Org. Chem., 47, 837 (1982).

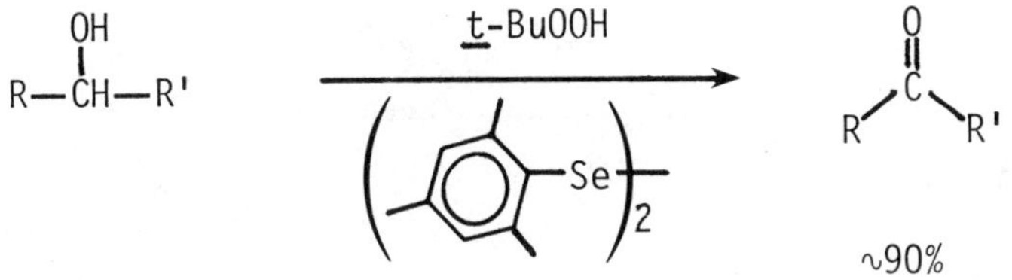

$$R-\overset{OH}{\underset{|}{CH}}-R' \xrightarrow[(Mes-Se)_2]{\underline{t}-BuOOH} \underset{RR'}{\overset{O}{\underset{\|}{C}}}$$

∼90%

R, R' = H, alkyl, Ph

II.A.1-9 J. Tsuji, H. Nagashima, and K. Sato, Tetrahedron Lett., 23, 3085 (1982).

$$R\underset{X}{\overset{OH}{-CH-CH}}R' \xrightarrow[K_2CO_3]{\underset{P(\underline{o}\text{-Tol})_3}{Pd(OAc)_2}} R\text{-CH}_2\text{-C(=O)-}R'$$

∼40-90%

X = Cl, Br, I
R, R' = H, alkyl, aryl

II.A.1-10/II.A.2-1 J. Kaulen and H. -J. Schafer, Tetrahedron, 38, 3299 (1982).

$$R\text{-CH}_2\text{OH} \xrightarrow[\text{NaOH, H}_2\text{O}]{\text{nickel hydroxide electrode}} R\text{-COO}^{\ominus}$$

∼60-90%

$$R\text{-CH(OH)-}R' \xrightarrow{\text{similar conditions}} R\text{-C(=O)-}R'$$

∼60-90%

II.A.1-11/II.A.2-2 N. A. Noureldin and D. G. Lee, J. Org. Chem., 47, 2790 (1982).

$$\underset{R\ \ \ R'}{\overset{H\ \ \ OH}{C}} \xrightarrow[CH_2Cl_2]{Cu(MnO_4)_2 \cdot 8H_2O} \underset{R\ \ \ R'}{\overset{O}{\underset{\|}{C}}}$$

R, R' = alkyl, aryl, cyclic,
        vinyl, acetylenic, etc.

51-100%

$$R\text{-CH}_2\text{OH} \xrightarrow{\text{similar conditions}} R\text{-COOH}$$

R = alkyl, aryl

81-99%

II.A.2. Alcohol, Aldehyde ⟶ Acid, Acid Derivative

II.A.2-3   J. B. Jones et al., J. Am. Chem. Soc., **104**, 4659 (1982).

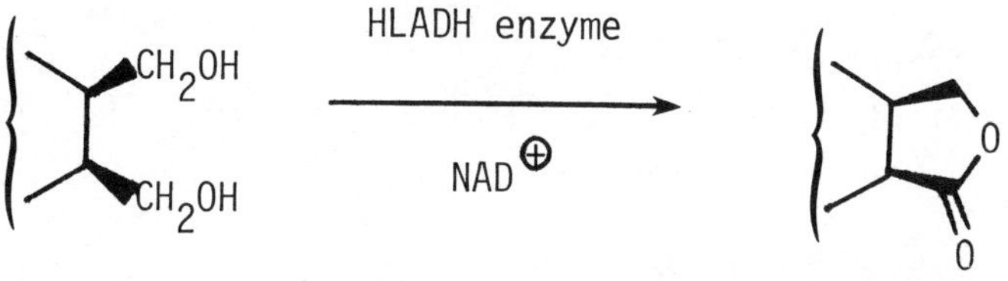

$$\text{diol} \xrightarrow[\text{NAD}^{\oplus}]{\text{HLADH enzyme}} \text{lactone}$$

68-90%
100%ee

II.A.2-4   S. O. Nwaukwa and P. M. Keehn, Tetrahedron Lett., **23**, 3131 (1982).

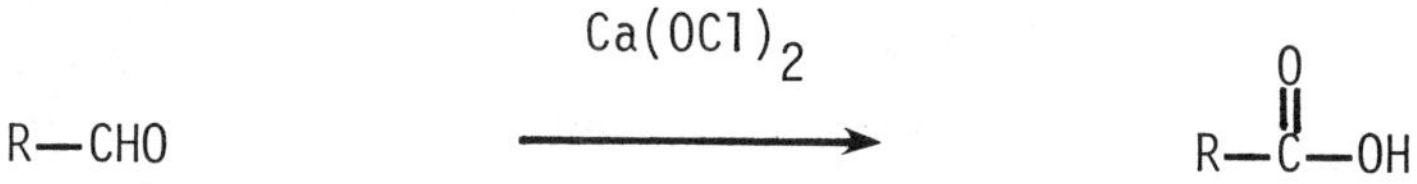

$$R\text{—CHO} \xrightarrow{Ca(OCl)_2} R\text{—C(=O)—OH}$$

60-93%

R = subst. Ph, alkyl, cycloalkyl

II.A.2-5 S. R. Wilson, S. Tofigh, and R. N. Misra, J. Org. Chem., 47, 1360 (1982).

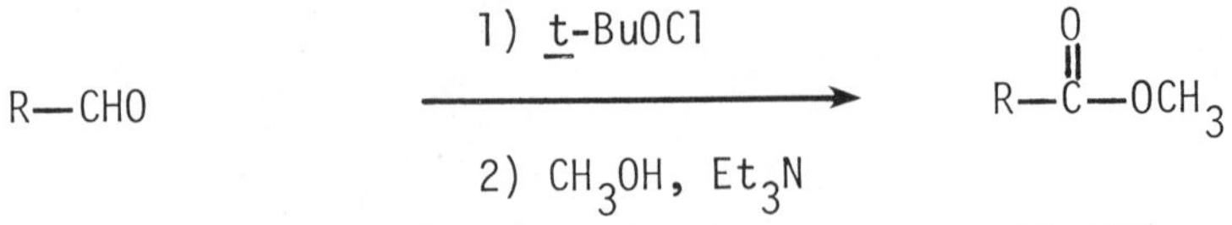

$$R\text{—CHO} \xrightarrow[\text{2) } CH_3OH,\ Et_3N]{\text{1) } \underline{t}\text{-BuOCl}} R\text{—C(=O)—OCH}_3$$

39-98%

R = Ph, cinnamyl, heterocyclic
Uses mildly oxidative conditions, no heavy metal.

II.A.2-6 T. Chiba et al., Bull. Chem. Soc. Japan, 55, 335 (1982).

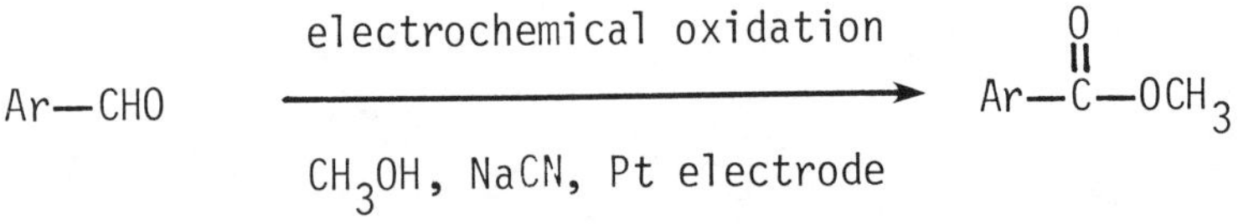

$$Ar\text{—CHO} \xrightarrow[CH_3OH,\ NaCN,\ Pt\ electrode]{electrochemical\ oxidation} Ar\text{—C(=O)—OCH}_3$$

48-83%

Ar = subst. Ph

II.A.2-7 G. Boche et al., Tetrahedron Lett., 23, 3255 (1982).

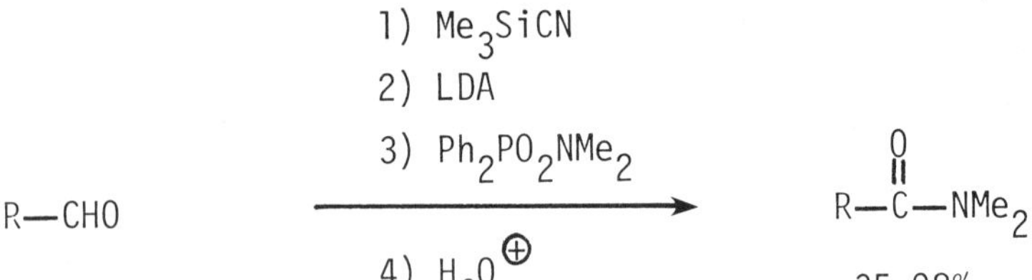

$$R\text{—CHO} \xrightarrow[\substack{\text{3) } Ph_2PO_2NMe_2 \\ \text{4) } H_3O^{\oplus}}]{\substack{\text{1) } Me_3SiCN \\ \text{2) } LDA}} R\text{—C(=O)—NMe}_2$$

35-98%

R = aryl, α,β-unsat., heterocyclic

II.B. C—H Oxidations

1. C—H ⟶ C—O

II.B.1-1 H. Shirahama et al., Chem. Lett., 1703 (1981).

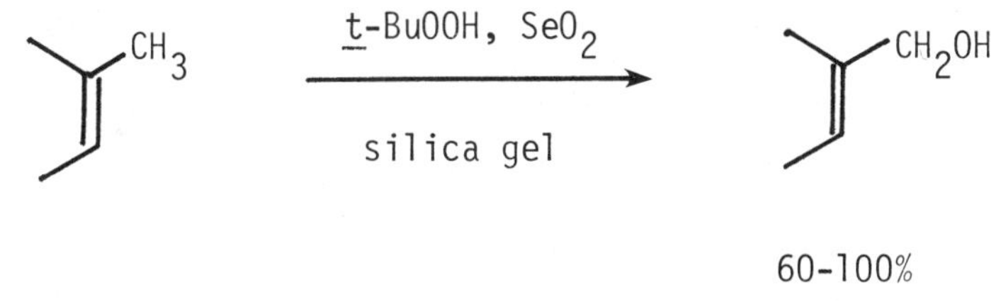

$$\text{alkene-CH}_3 \xrightarrow[\text{silica gel}]{\text{t-BuOOH, SeO}_2} \text{alkene-CH}_2\text{OH}$$

60-100%

II.B.1-2 B. Waegell et al., Angew. Chem. Int. Ed., 21, 366 (1982).

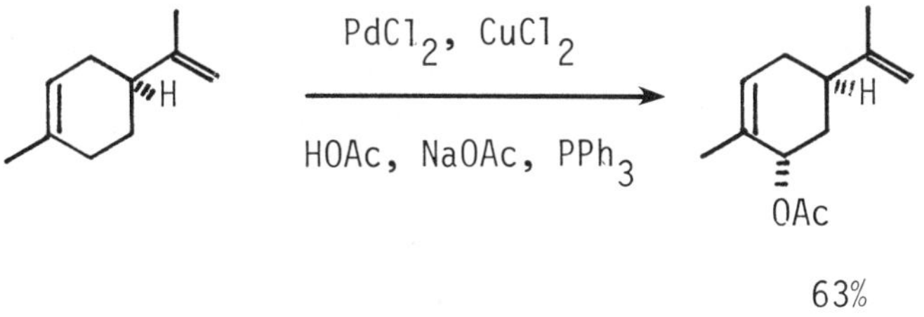

$$\xrightarrow[\text{HOAc, NaOAc, PPh}_3]{\text{PdCl}_2,\ \text{CuCl}_2}$$

63%

II.B.1-3 T. V. Lee and J. Toczek, Tetrahedron Lett., 23, 2917 (1982).

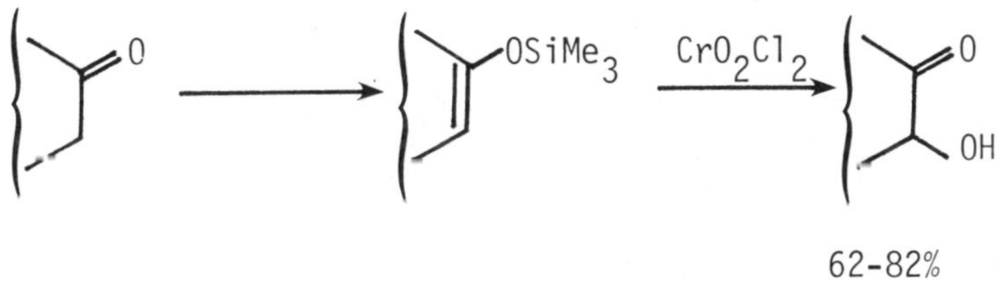

$$\text{C=O} \longrightarrow \text{C=C-OSiMe}_3 \xrightarrow{\text{CrO}_2\text{Cl}_2} \text{C(=O)-C-OH}$$

62-82%

II.B.1-4   I. Saito et al., Tetrahedron Lett., 23, 1717 (1982).

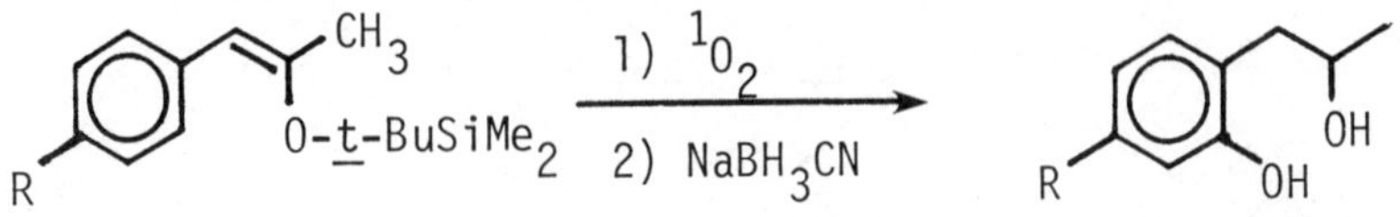

[Scheme: 4-R-C$_6$H$_4$-CH=C(CH$_3$)-O-$\underline{t}$-BuSiMe$_2$ →(1) ^{1}O$_2$; 2) NaBH$_3$CN) 2-hydroxyaryl isopropanol derivative]

~60%

R = H, OMe

II.B.1-5   M. K. Chaudhuri et al., Synthesis, 588 (1982).

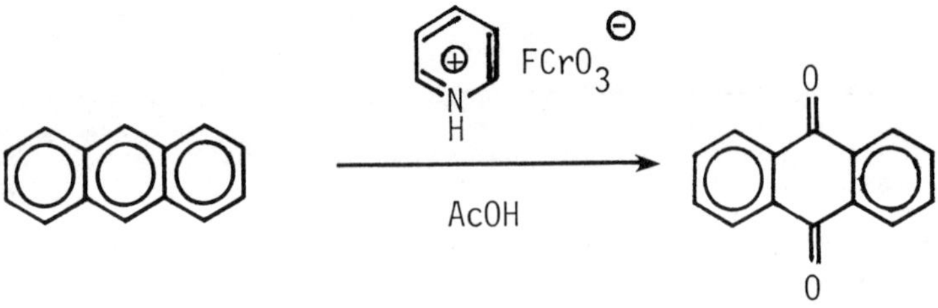

[Scheme: anthracene →(pyridinium FCrO$_3^-$, AcOH) anthraquinone]

98%

II.B.2. C—H ⟶ C—Hal

II.B.2-1 M. Ouertani, P. Girard, and H. B. Kagan, Bull. Soc. Chim. France II, 327 (1982).

$$Ar-CH_3 \xrightarrow[\text{La(OAc)}_3]{Br_2} ArCH_2Br$$

53-90%

Ar = subst. Ph

II.B.2-2 F. D. Marsh et al., J. Am. Chem. Soc., 104, 4680 (1982).

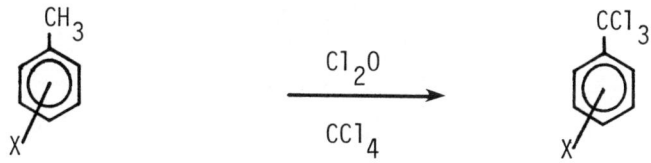

89-100%

X = -NO$_2$, -CN, -SO$_2$Me, etc

II.B.2-3 E. B. Merkushev and N. D. Yudina, J. Org. Chem. (USSR), 17, 2320 (1982).

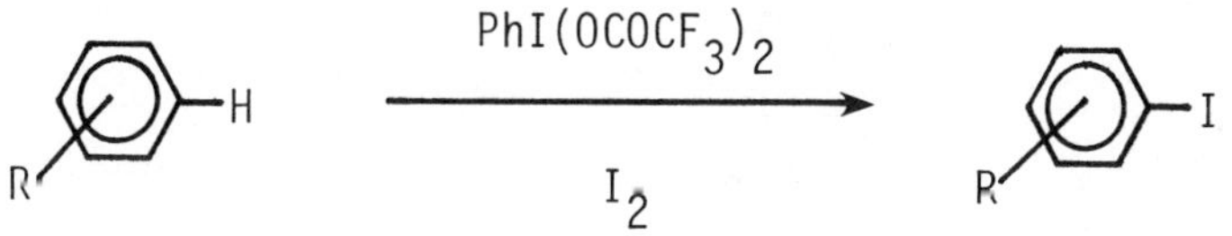

$$\underset{R}{\underset{|}{C_6H_4}}-H \xrightarrow[I_2]{PhI(OCOCF_3)_2} \underset{R}{\underset{|}{C_6H_4}}-I$$

R = H, alkyl, aryl, alkoxy, halo, etc.

II.B.2-4   T. Sugita et al., Chem. Lett., 1481 (1982).

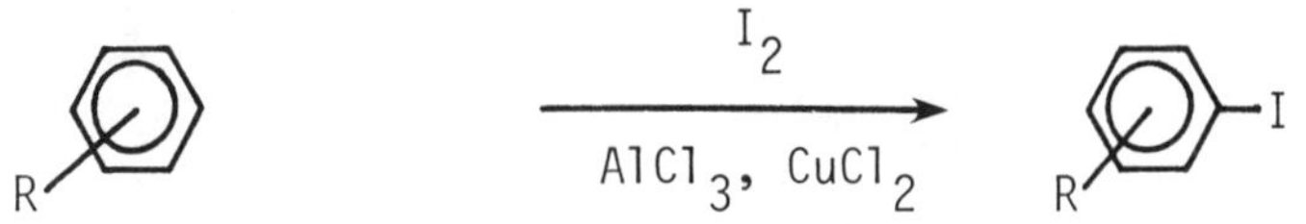

$$\text{R-C}_6\text{H}_5 \xrightarrow[\text{AlCl}_3,\ \text{CuCl}_2]{I_2} \text{R-C}_6\text{H}_4\text{-I}$$

widely varying yields

R = Me, OMe, Cl, Br, I

II.B.2-5   A. Guy, M. Lemaire, and J. -P. Guetté, Synthesis, 1018 (1982).

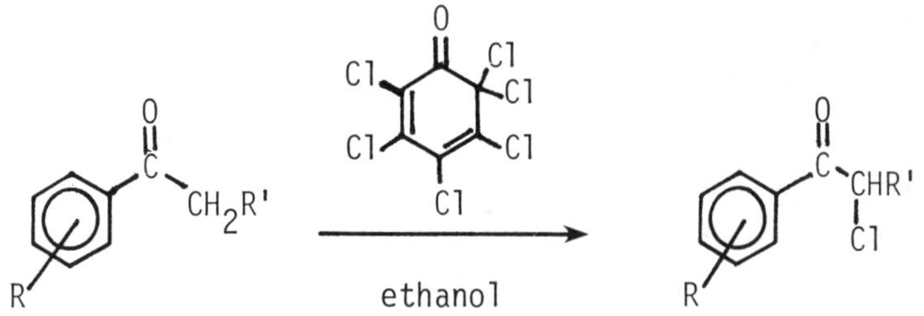

$$\text{R-C}_6\text{H}_4\text{-CO-CH}_2\text{R'} \xrightarrow[\text{ethanol}]{\text{C}_6\text{Cl}_4\text{O}_2} \text{R-C}_6\text{H}_4\text{-CO-CHR'Cl}$$

50-100%

R = -OH, -OMe

R' = H, alkyl

II.B.2-6 S. Motohashi et al., Synthesis, 1021 (1982).

$$\text{(cycloalkenyl-OR)} \xrightarrow{\text{Pb(OAc)}_4, \text{NaX, CH}_3\text{OH}} \text{(cycloalkanone-X)}$$

58-99%

R = Me, Et, Ac, SiMe$_3$
X = Cl, Br, I

II.B.2-7 S. Chandrasekaran et al., Synthesis, 309 (1982).

$$\underset{\text{R}-\overset{\text{O}}{\underset{\|}{\text{C}}}-\text{CH}_2-\text{R}'}{} \xrightarrow[\text{HOCH}_2\text{CH}_2\text{OH/THF}]{\overset{\oplus}{\text{PhNMe}}_3 \; \overset{\ominus}{\text{Br}_3}} \underset{\text{R}-\text{C}-\text{CH}-\text{R}'}{\overset{\text{O} \diagdown \diagup \text{O}}{}} \; \underset{\text{Br}}{}$$

74-90%

R, R' = alkyl, Ph

II.B.2-8 C. J. Kowalski, A. E. Weber, and K. W. Fields, J. Org. Chem., 47, 5088 (1982).

$$\text{(cyclohexenone)} \xrightarrow[\text{2) Et}_3\text{N}]{\text{1) Br}_2} \text{(2-bromocyclohexenone)}$$

up to ~90%

II.B.3. Other C—H Oxidations

II.B.3-1 N. A. Meanwell and C. R. Johnson, Synthesis, 283 (1982).

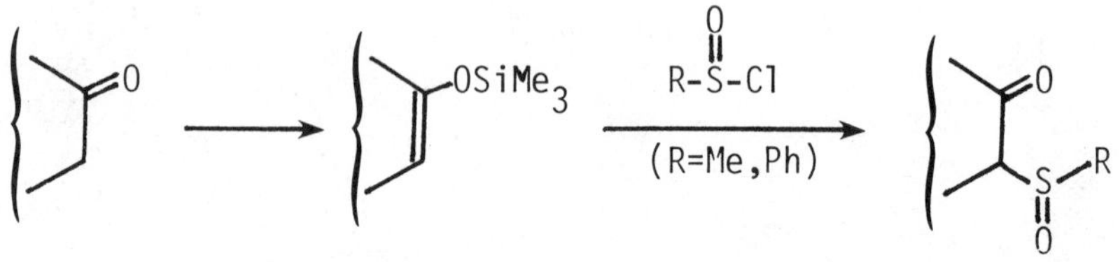

$$\text{cyclohexanone} \longrightarrow \text{enol-OSiMe}_3 \xrightarrow[\text{(R=Me,Ph)}]{\overset{O}{\underset{}{R-S-Cl}}} \text{α-sulfinyl ketone}$$

~80-90%

II.C. C—N Oxidations

II.C-1 T. F. Buckley and H. Rapoport, J. Am. Chem. Soc., 104, 4446 (1982).

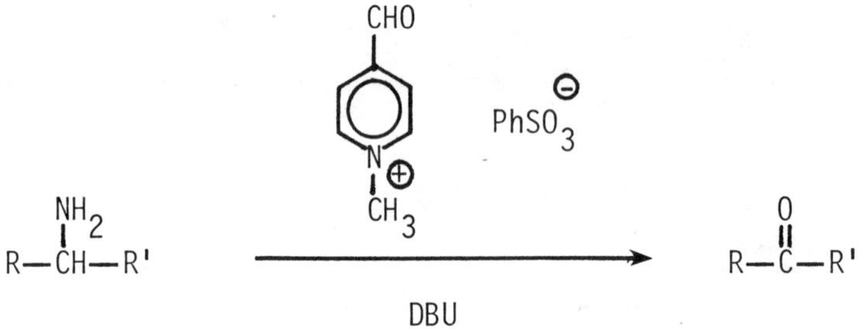

$$\underset{R-CH-R'}{\overset{NH_2}{|}} \xrightarrow[\text{DBU}]{\text{4-CHO-N-methylpyridinium PhSO}_3^{\ominus}} \underset{R-C-R'}{\overset{O}{\|}}$$

77-94%

R, R' = H, alkyl, aryl, protected amino acid, etc.

II.C-2   S. Ohta and M. Okamoto, Synthesis, 756 (1982).

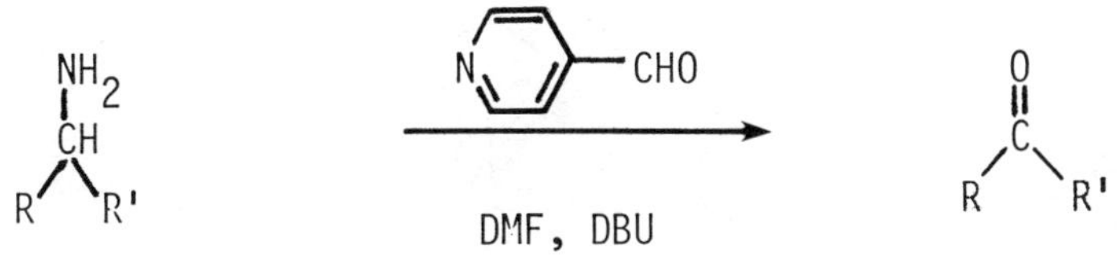

$$\underset{RR'}{\overset{NH_2}{\underset{|}{CH}}} \xrightarrow[\text{DMF, DBU}]{\text{4-pyridine-CHO}} \underset{RR'}{\overset{O}{\underset{\|}{C}}}$$

R, R' = H, alkyl, subst. Ph

II.C-3   N. Kornblum et al., J. Org. Chem., 47, 4534 (1982).

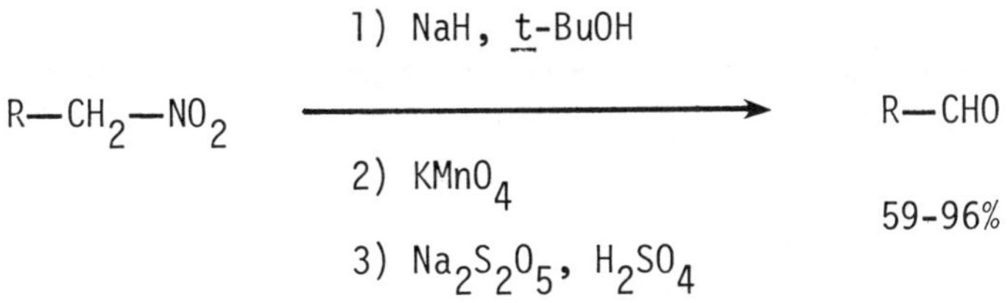

$$R-CH_2-NO_2 \xrightarrow[\substack{\text{2) KMnO}_4 \\ \text{3) Na}_2S_2O_5, H_2SO_4}]{\text{1) NaH, }t\text{-BuOH}} R-CHO \quad 59\text{-}96\%$$

R = 1°, 2°, 3° alkyl. May contain -CN, ester, etc.
Also works for ketones: $R_2CH-NO_2 \longrightarrow R_2C=O$, ~90%

II.C-4 A. R. Katritzky and J. M. Lloyd, J.C.S. Perkin I, 2347 (1982); J. Org. Chem., 47, 3506 (1982).

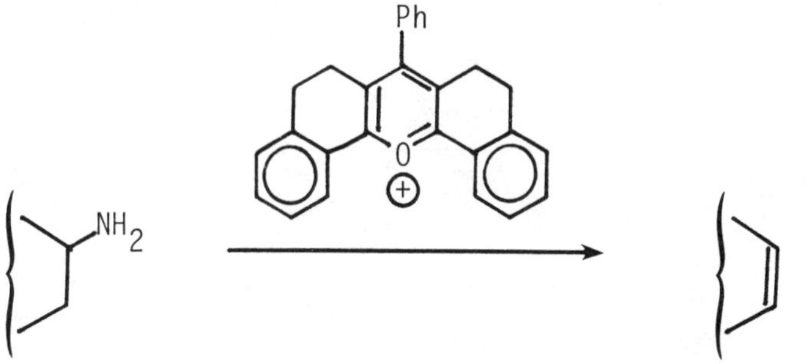

33-95%

II.E. Sulfur Oxidations

II.E-1 W. A. Pryor et al., J. Org. Chem., 47, 156 (1982).

$$2 \text{ R—SH} \xrightarrow[\text{H}_2\text{O/EtOH}]{\text{NO or NO}_2} \text{R—S—S—R}$$

>95%

II.E-2 R. G. Srivastiva and P. S. Venkataramani, Indian J. Chem., 20B, 996 (1981).

$$2 \text{ R—SH} \xrightarrow{\text{barium manganate}} \text{R—S—S—R}$$

∼80-90%

R = alkyl, aryl

II.E-3 X. Huang and C. -C. Chan, Synthesis, 1091 (1982).

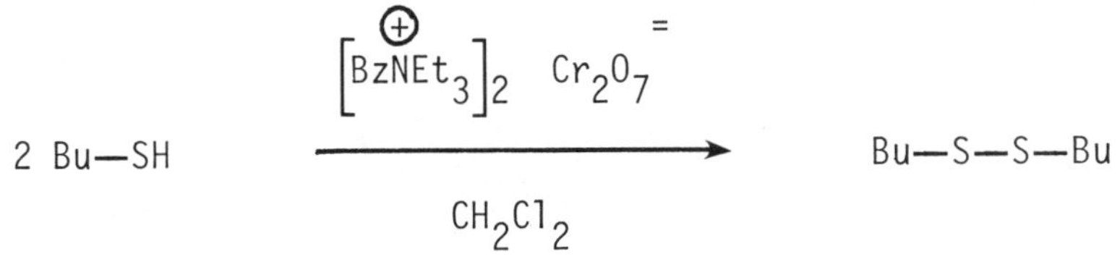

$$2\ Bu-SH \xrightarrow[CH_2Cl_2]{[BzNEt_3]_2^{\oplus}\ Cr_2O_7^{=}} Bu-S-S-Bu$$

II.E-4 F. Ogura et al., Bull. Chem. Soc. Japan, 55, 641 (1982).

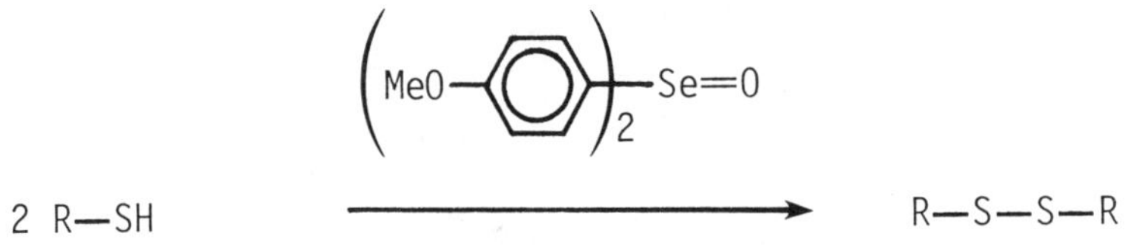

$$2\ R-SH \xrightarrow{(MeO-C_6H_4-)_2Se=O} R-S-S-R$$

~90%

R = alkyl, aryl

$$R-S-R' \xrightarrow{(MeO-C_6H_4-)_2Se=O} R-\overset{\overset{O}{\|}}{S}-R'$$

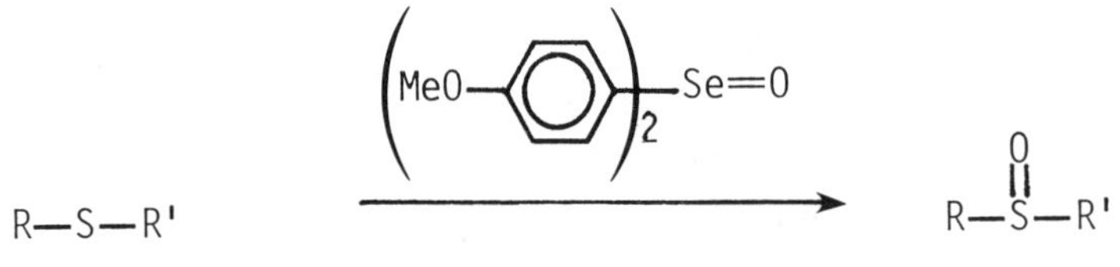

~90%

R, R' = alkyl, aryl

II.E-5 F. A. Davis et al., J. Am. Chem. Soc., 104, 5412 (1982).

$$Ar-S-R \xrightarrow{\text{camphor-SO}_2\text{-N-C(Ar)(H) with O}} Ar-\overset{O}{\underset{*}{S}}-R$$

Ar = Ph, p-Tol   ~80-90% yields
R = Me, t-Bu   up to 35% ee

II.E-6 C. G. Venier et al., J. Org. Chem., 47, 3773 (1982).

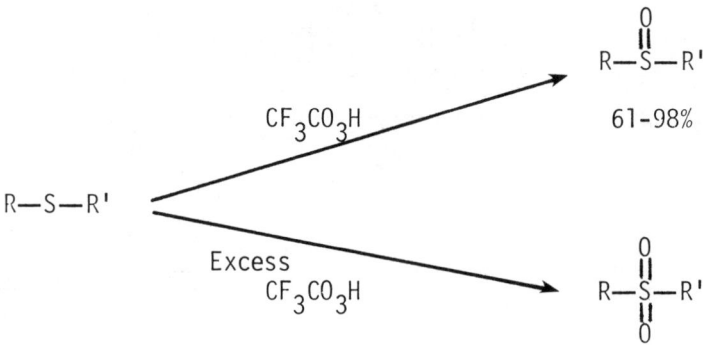

R, R' = alkyl, allyl, Ph;   58-99%
        also methionine, benzothiphene

II.F. Oxidative Additions to C—C Multiple Bonds

1. Epoxidations

II.F.1-1 S. Ito, K. Inoue, and M. Matsumoto, J. Am. Chem. Soc., 104, 6450 (1982).

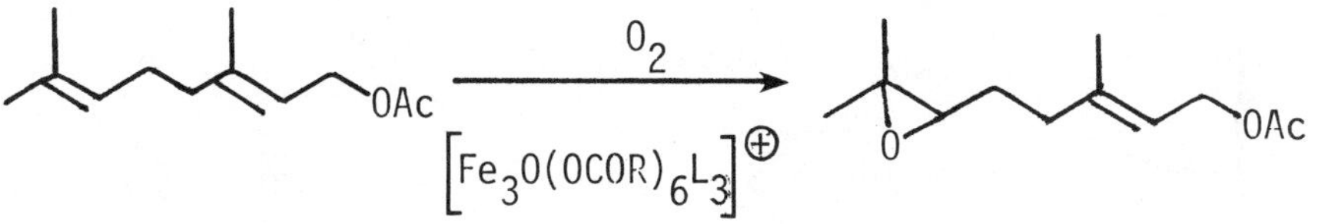

[geranyl acetate] $\xrightarrow[{[Fe_3O(OCOR)_6L_3]^{\oplus}}]{O_2}$ [6,7-epoxygeranyl acetate]

82% conversion
87% yield

Several additional examples

II.F.1-2 N. Kawabata et al., J. Org. Chem., 47, 3575 (1982).

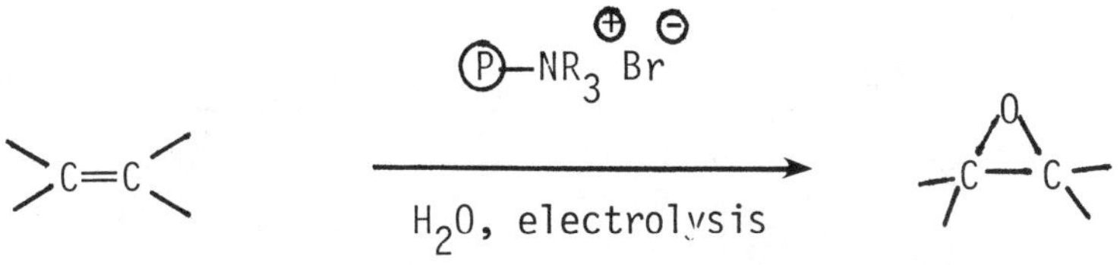

$>C=C<$ $\xrightarrow[{H_2O, \text{ electrolysis}}]{\text{P}-NR_3^{\oplus} Br^{\ominus}}$ epoxide

~60-80%

1-alkene, 2-alkenes, styrene, etc.

II.F.1-3 A. L. Baumstark and R. S. Pilcher, J. Org. Chem., 47, 1141 (1982).

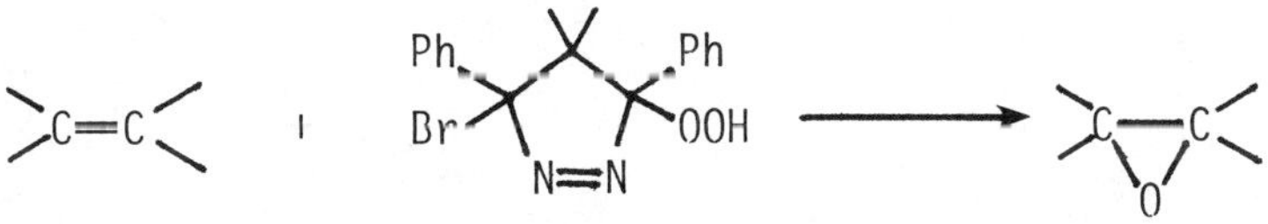

$>C=C<$ + [Ph, Br, Ph, OOH, N=N pyrazoline] ⟶ epoxide

19-84%

II.F.1-4   R. Curci et al., J. Org. Chem., 47, 2670 (1982).

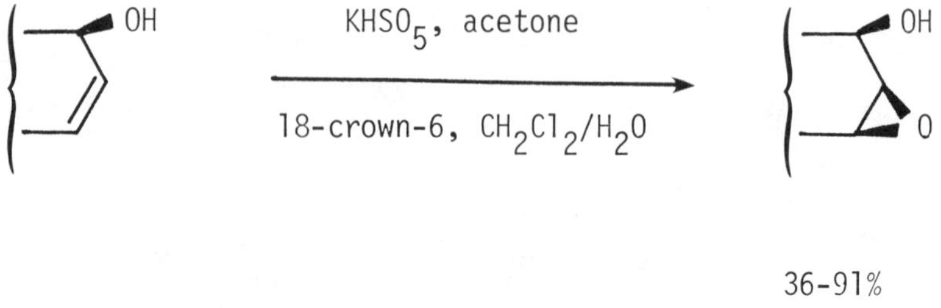

$$\text{allylic alcohol} \xrightarrow[\text{18-crown-6, CH}_2\text{Cl}_2/\text{H}_2\text{O}]{\text{KHSO}_5, \text{ acetone}} \text{epoxy alcohol}$$

36-91%

II.F.2. Hydroxylation

II.F.2-1   E. J. Corey and J. Das, Tetrahedron Lett., 23, 4217 (1982).

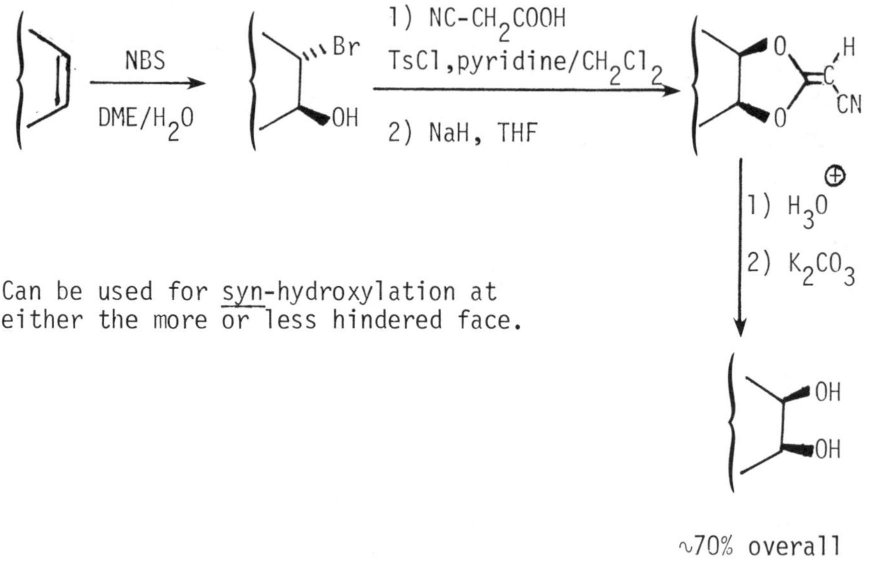

$$\text{cyclopentadiene} \xrightarrow[\text{DME/H}_2\text{O}]{\text{NBS}} \text{bromohydrin} \xrightarrow[\text{2) NaH, THF}]{\substack{\text{1) NC-CH}_2\text{COOH} \\ \text{TsCl,pyridine/CH}_2\text{Cl}_2}} \text{cyanomethylene acetal}$$

Can be used for syn-hydroxylation at either the more or less hindered face.

1) $H_3O^{\oplus}$
2) K_2CO_3

→ diol

∼70% overall

II.F.3. Other Oxidative Additions to C—C Multiple Bonds

II.F.3-1 J. Tsuji, H. Nagashima, and K. Hori, *Tetrahedron Lett.*, 23, 2679 (1982).

$$R\diagup\!\!\!\diagdown\!\!\!\diagup OR' \xrightarrow[DMF, O_2]{PdCl_2/CuCl} R\diagup\!\!\!\overset{O}{C}\!\!\!\diagdown\!\!\!\diagup OR'$$

R = alkyl
R' = Me, Bz, Ac

∼40-76%

II.F.3-2 H. Nagashima, K. Sakai, and J. Tsuji, *Chem. Lett.*, 859 (1982).

$$R\diagup\!\!\!\diagdown\!\!\!\diagup\overset{O}{C}\!\!\diagdown X \xrightarrow[H_2O/dioxane]{PdCl_2, CuCl, O_2} R\overset{O}{C}\!\!\!\diagup\!\!\!\diagdown\!\!\!\overset{O}{C}\!\!\diagdown X$$

X = Me, OMe
R = alkyl

45-61%

II.G. Phenol ⟶ Quinone Oxidations

II.G-1 C. R. Harrison and P. Hodge, *J.C.S. Perkin I*, 509 (1982).

hydroquinone—X $\xrightarrow{\text{polymer-bound periodate}}$ quinone—X

X = alkyl, acyl, benzo, Cl

∼90-100%

II.H. Oxidative Cleavages

II.H-1 J. E. Hernandez et al., Synth. Comm., 12, 833 (1982).

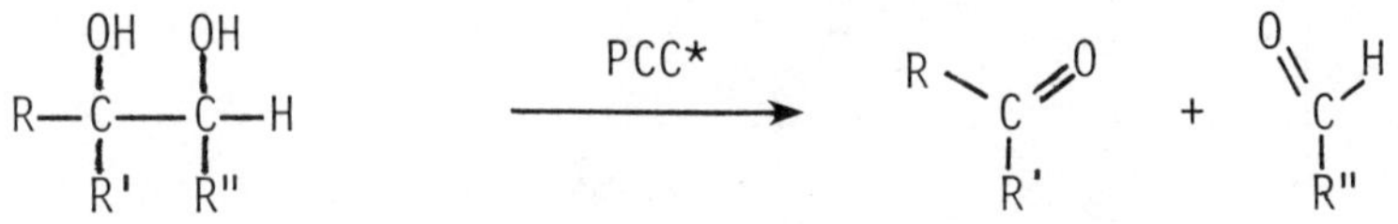

R-C(OH)(R')-C(OH)(R'')-H →[PCC*] R-C(=O)-R' + O=CH-R''

R's = alkyl, Ph, H, cyclic

PCC = pyridinium chlorochromate

II.H-2 C. R. Harrison and P. Hodge, J.C.S. Perkin I, 509 (1982).

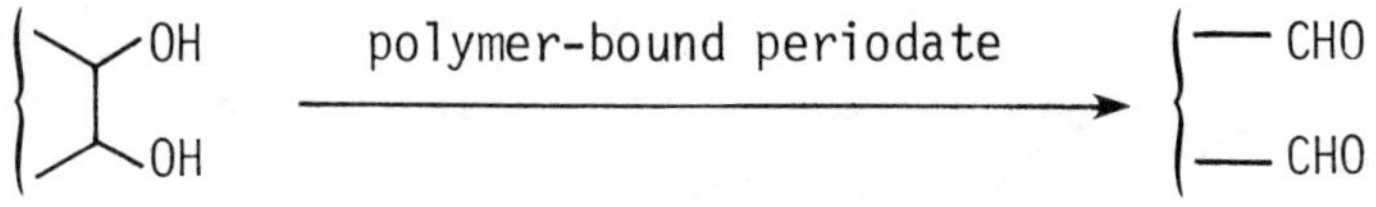

cyclic diol (OH, OH) →[polymer-bound periodate] dialdehyde (CHO, CHO)

∼90%

II.H-3 S. O. Nkwaukwa and P. M. Keehn, Tetrahedron Lett., 23, 3135 (1982).

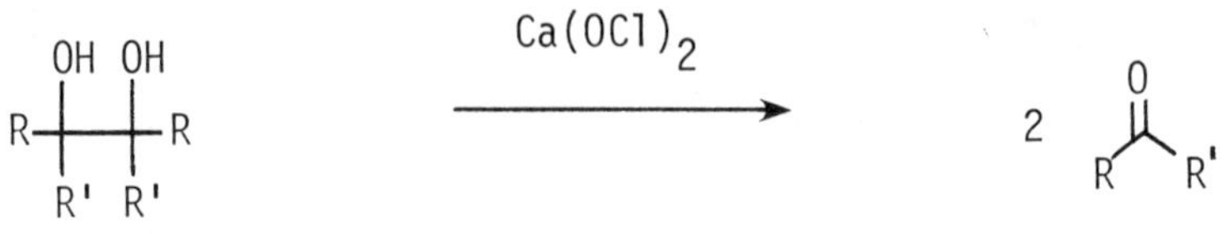

R-C(OH)(R')-C(OH)(R')-R →[Ca(OCl)$_2$] 2 R-C(=O)-R'

∼80-90%

R, R' = alkyl, aryl

Also cleaves α-diones, α-hydroxy ketones, α-hydroxy acids, and α-ketoacids.

II.H-4   D. Gupta, R. Soman, and S. Dev, <u>Tetrahedron</u>, <u>38</u>, 3013 (1982).

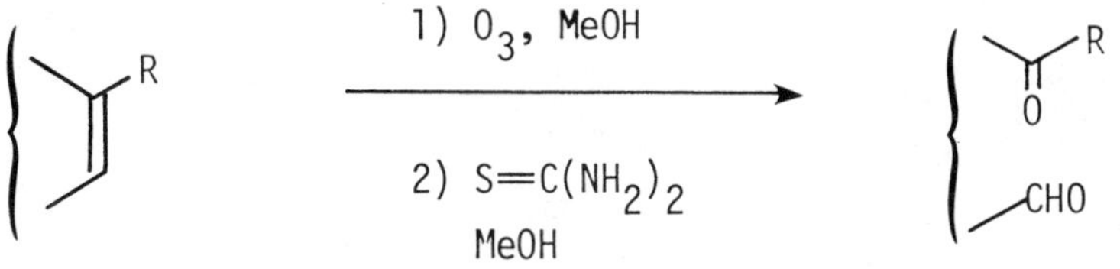

$$\text{alkene-R} \xrightarrow[\text{MeOH}]{\substack{1) \ O_3, \ \text{MeOH} \\ 2) \ S{=}C(NH_2)_2}} \text{R-C(=O)-, -CHO}$$

R = H, alkyl, cycloalkyl

(+ dimethyl acetal)

II.H-5   T. K. Chakraborty and S. Chandrasekaran, <u>Org. Prep. Proc. Int.</u>, <u>14</u>, 362 (1982).

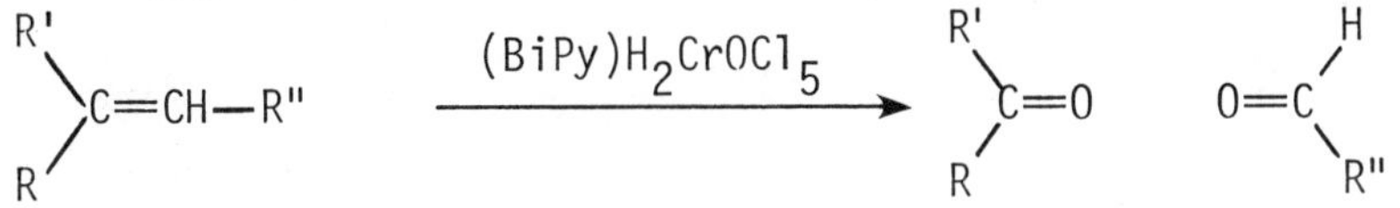

$$\underset{R}{\overset{R'}{>}}C{=}CH{-}R'' \xrightarrow{(BiPy)H_2CrOCl_5} \underset{R}{\overset{R'}{>}}C{=}O \quad O{=}C\underset{R''}{\overset{H}{<}}$$

R's = H, alkyl, aryl   70-96%

$$R{-}C{\equiv}C{-}R' \xrightarrow{(BiPy)H_2CrOCl_5} \underset{H}{\overset{R}{>}}C{=}O \quad O{=}C\underset{H}{\overset{R'}{<}}$$

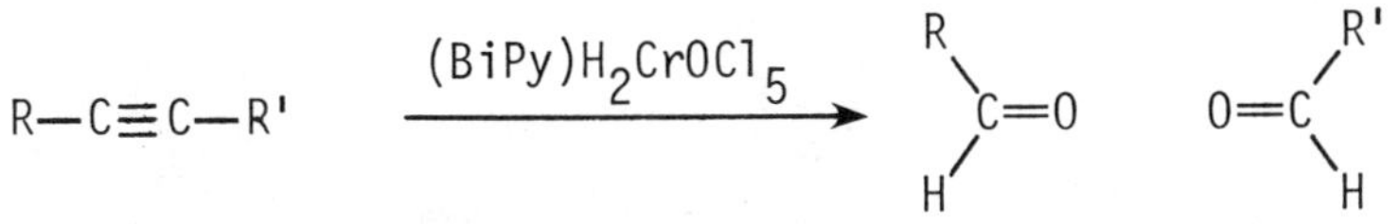

80-96%

R, R' = alkyl, aryl

II.H-6 T. R. Beebe et al., J. Org. Chem, 47, 3006 (1982).

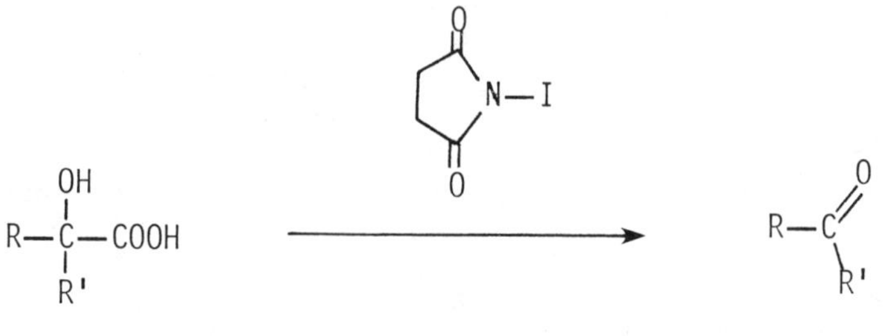

R, R' = H, alkyl, aryl

80-103%

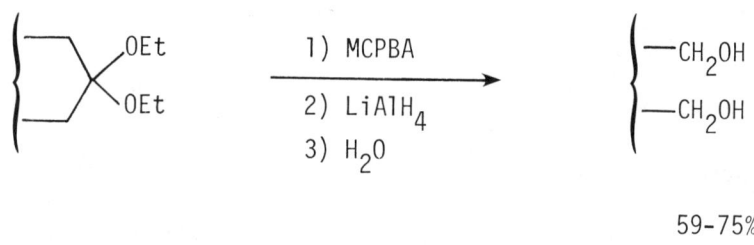

II.H-7 W. F. Bailey and M. -J. Shih, J. Am. Chem. Soc., 104, 1769 (1982).

$$\text{(cyclic)C(OEt)}_2 \xrightarrow{\text{1) MCPBA} \atop \text{2) LiAlH}_4 \text{ 3) H}_2\text{O}} \text{(cyclic with two -CH}_2\text{OH)}$$

59-75%

II.H-8 C. C. Fortes et al., J.C.S. Chem. Comm., 857 (1982).

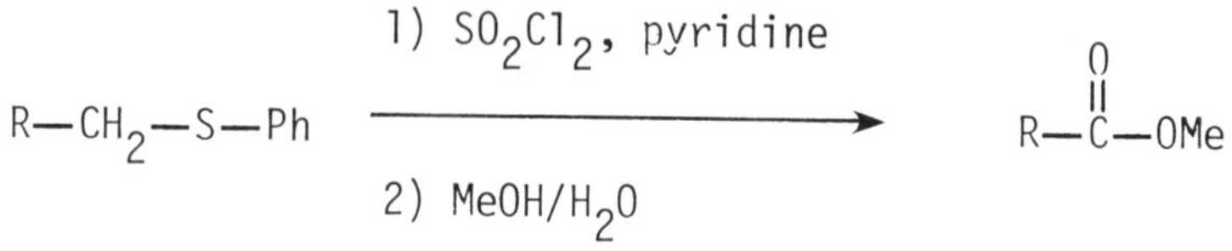

$$R-CH_2-S-Ph \xrightarrow{\text{1) SO}_2\text{Cl}_2, \text{ pyridine} \atop \text{2) MeOH/H}_2\text{O}} R-C(=O)-OMe$$

R = 1° alkyl

41-76%

II.H-9 S. L. Schreiber, R. E. Claus, and J. Reagan, Tetrahedron Lett., 23, 3867 (1982).

[Scheme: Ozonolysis of cyclic alkene $(CH_2)_n$ with O_3, ROH, $NaHCO_3$ gives $(CH_2)_n$ with CHO and CHOOH(OR) groups; then Ac_2O, Et_3N gives $(CH_2)_n$ with CHO and COOR groups, 47–96%.

Alternatively, O_3, ROH, TsOH gives $(CH_2)_n$ with $CH(OR)_2$ and CH(OR)OOH groups; then Me_2S, $NaHCO_3$ gives $(CH_2)_n$ with $CH(OR)_2$ and CHO groups, 48–95%; or Ac_2O, Et_3N gives $(CH_2)_n$ with $CH(OR)_2$ and C(O)OR groups, 72–100%.]

II.H-10 I. Shimizu and J. Tsuji, J. Am. Chem. Soc., 104, 5844, (1982).

[Scheme: α-allyloxycarbonyl cycloalkanone with R substituent, $Pd(OAc)_2$, $Ph_2PCH_2CH_2PPh_2$, CH_3CN gives α,β-unsaturated cycloalkenone with R substituent.]

R = alkyl, Bz   ~50–90%

II.I. Photosensitized Oxygenations

II.I-1 S. R. Byrn et al., J. Org. Chem., **47**, 2978 (1982).

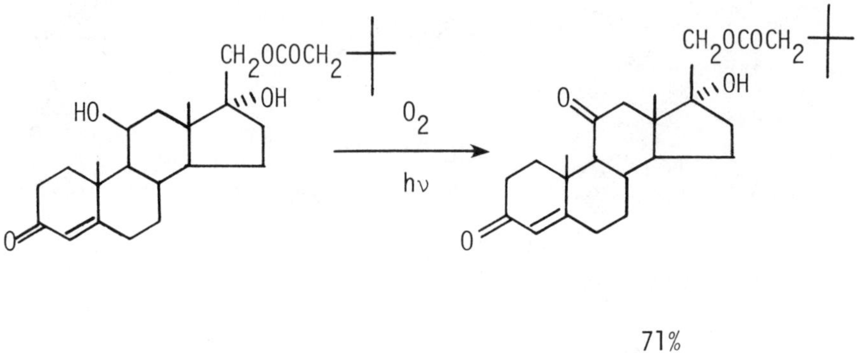

71%

II.J. Dehydrogenation

II.J-1 A. Toshimitsu et al., Tetrahedron Lett., **23**, 2105 (1982).

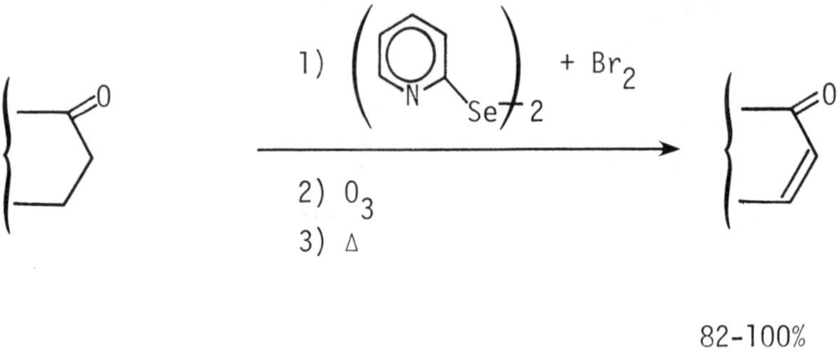

82-100%

Also works for α,β-unsaturated aldehydes.

II.J-2 S. Mashraqui and P. Keehn, Synth. Comm., 12, 637 (1982).

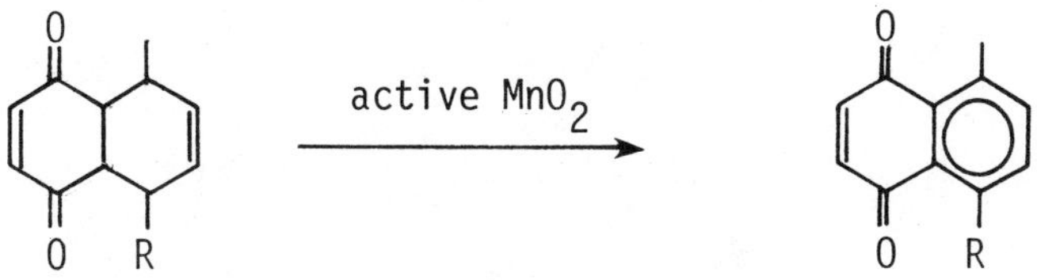

~60%

Many other oxidative aromatizations characteristic of DDQ etc. may be accomplished with MnO_2.

II.J-3 D. Cavalla and S. Warren, Tetrahedron Lett., 23, 4505 (1982).

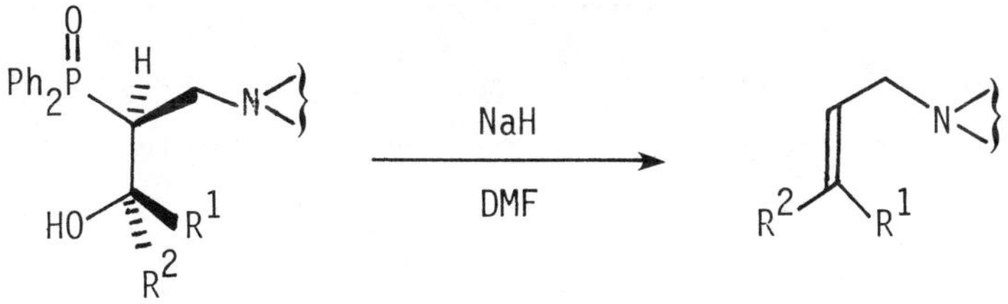

~60-80%

R^1, R^2 = H, alkyl, cyclic

II.K. Other Oxidations and Reviews

II.K-1   G. Piancatelli, A. Scettri, and M. D'Auria, Synthesis, 245 (1982).

  Review: "Pyridinium Chlorochromate: A Versatile Oxidant in Organic Synthesis"

II.K-2   V. N. Odinokov and G. A. Tolstikov, Russ. Chem. Rev., 50, 636 (1981).

  Review: "Ozonolysis--A Modern Method in the Chemistry of Olefins"

II.K-3   V. Karnojitzky, Russ. Chem. Rev., 50, 888 (1981).

  Review: "Oxidation of Ketones by Molecular Oxygen"

II.K-4   A. N. Kashin and I. P. Beletskaya, Russ. Chem. Rev., 51, 503 (1982).

  Review: "Oxidation of Organometallic Compounds by Transition Metal Salts"

III
REDUCTIONS

III.A. C=O Reductions

(Reductions of carboxylic acids and esters to aldehydes and alcohols are included in section III.F.1.)

III.A-1 S. Kim, S. J. Lee, and H. J. Kang, Synth.Comm., 12, 723 (1982).

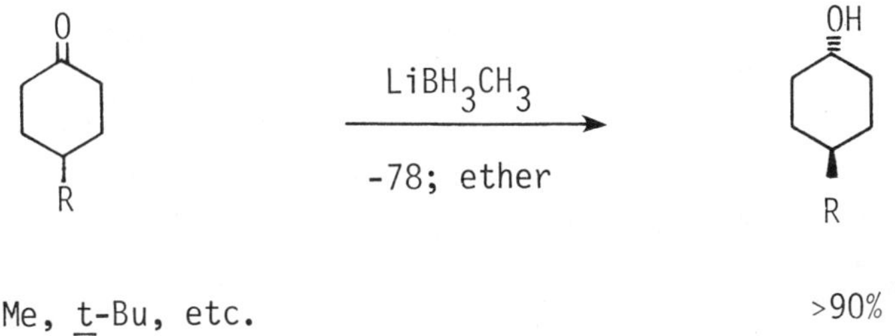

4-R-cyclohexanone $\xrightarrow[-78;\ \text{ether}]{\text{LiBH}_3\text{CH}_3}$ trans-4-R-cyclohexanol

R = Me, t-Bu, etc.

>90%

III.A-2 D. Nasipuri et al., Indian J. Chem., 21B, 212 (1982).

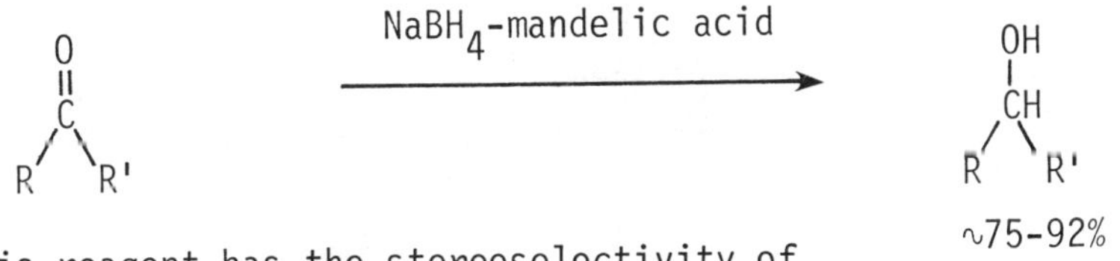

$$\text{R-CO-R'} \xrightarrow{\text{NaBH}_4\text{-mandelic acid}} \text{R-CH(OH)-R'}$$

This reagent has the stereoselectivity of LiAlH$_4$, but its reactivity is milder than NaBH$_4$.

~75-92%

Gives the more stable isomer.

III.A-3 M. P. Paradisi and G. P. Zecchini, Tetrahedron, 38, 1827 (1982).

[steroid with 3-oxo and 17-CHO]
1) t-BuNH$_2$ (protects the aldehyde)
2) Li(t-BuO)$_3$AlH
3) H$_2$O
4) Basic alumina

→ [3α-hydroxy steroid with 17-CHO] 83%

III.A-4 G. Gondos and J. C. Orr, J.C.S. Chem. Comm., 1238 and 1239 (1982).

Use of a chiral hydrosilane-rhodium phosphine reagent allows greater stereoselectivity of 17 α-alcohol formation than with other methods.

Potassium tri(R,S-s-butyl)borohydride reduces 3-oxo steroids to the axial alcohols, without affecting the 17- and 20-ketone groups.

III.A-5 A. M. Caporusso et al., J. Org. Chem., 47, 4640 (1982).

>C=C–C–
      ‖
      O

1) (i-Bu)$_3$Al
2) NH$_4$Cl, H$_2$O

→ >C=C–CH–
          |
          OH

23-100%

Substituents are H, Me, cyclic.

III.A-6 M. Yamashita et al., Bull. Chem. Soc. Japan, 55, 1329 (1982).

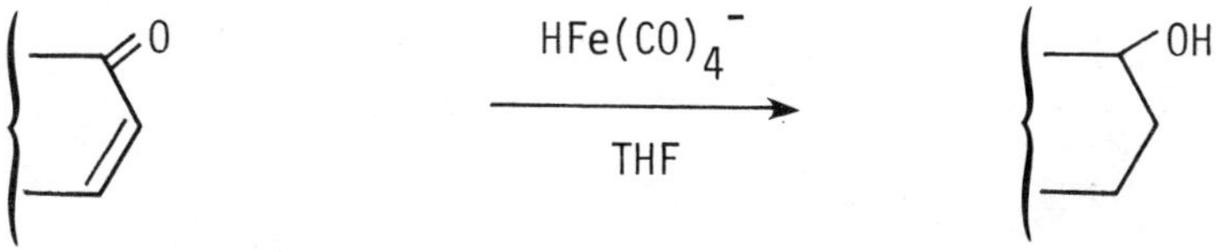

cyclohexenone → cyclohexanol

reagents: $HFe(CO)_4^-$, THF

>98%

III.A-7 S. Kim, Y. C. Moon, and K. H. Ahn, J. Org. Chem., 47, 3311 (1982).

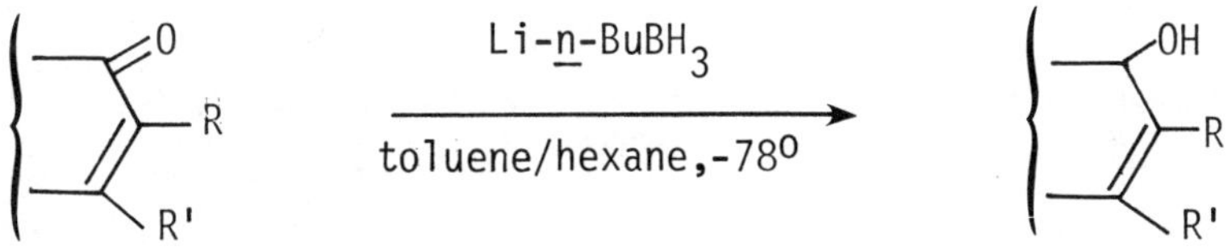

reagents: Li-$\underline{n}$-BuBH$_3$, toluene/hexane, $-78°$

R, R' = H, alkyl, vinyl

46-99%

III.A-8 Y. Watanabe et al., Bull. Chem. Soc. Japan, 55, 2441 (1982).

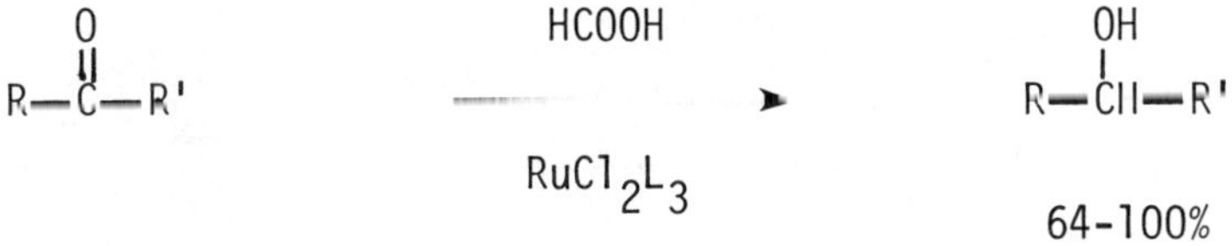

$$R-\overset{O}{\underset{\|}{C}}-R' \xrightarrow[RuCl_2L_3]{HCOOH} R-\overset{OH}{\underset{|}{C}H}-R'$$

64-100%

R, R' = 1° alkyl, Ph

III.A-9 A. Tai et al., Bull. Chem. Soc. Japan, 55, 2186 (1982).

$$CH_3(CH_2)_n\overset{O}{\underset{\|}{C}}-CH_2COOMe \xrightarrow[(H_2)]{\text{Ni catalyst*}} CH_3(CH_2)_n-\overset{OH}{\underset{*}{CH}}-CH_2COOMe$$

n = 0-12

70-82%
83-87% ee

* (R,R)-tartaric acid-NaBr-modified Raney nickel

III.A-10 M. Hojo et al., Tetrahedron Lett., 23, 4585 (1982).

$$CH_3-\overset{O}{\underset{\|}{C}}-(CH_2)_n-\overset{O}{\underset{\|}{C}}-OMe \xrightarrow[\text{ether}]{LiAlH_4-SiO_2} CH_3-\overset{OH}{\underset{|}{CH}}-(CH_2)_n-\overset{O}{\underset{\|}{C}}-OMe$$

n = 0-3   42-84%

III.A-11 T. Fujisawa et al., Tetrahedron Lett., 23, 4111 (1982).

$$\underset{Ar\quad R}{\overset{O}{\underset{\|}{C}}} \xrightarrow{Li^{\oplus}\left[\text{chiral Al-H complex}\right]^{\ominus}} \underset{Ar\quad R}{\overset{OH}{\underset{|}{C}\text{''}H}}$$

(with ligand: N-Me, N-Ph piperazine-Al-H)

Ar = Ph
R = alkyl, cyclic

(S)
84-93%
51-88% ee

III.A-12 H. C. Brown and G. G. Pai, *J. Org. Chem.*, **47**, 1606 (1982).

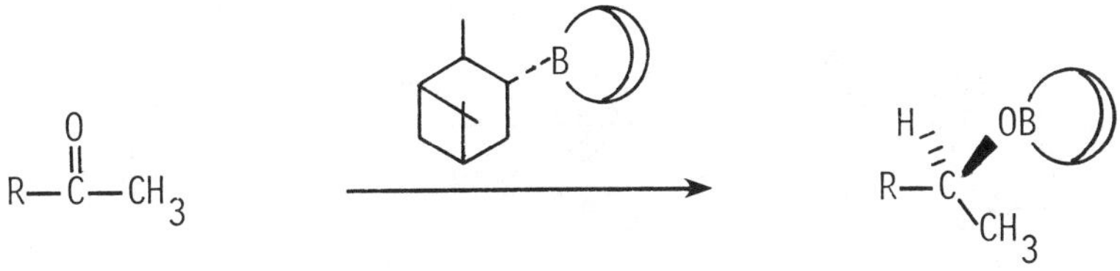

R = alkyl, Ph, vinyl, cinnamyl, alkynyl

∼50-90% ee

III.A-13 M. M. Midland and A. Kazubski, *J. Org. Chem.*, **47**, 2814 (1982).

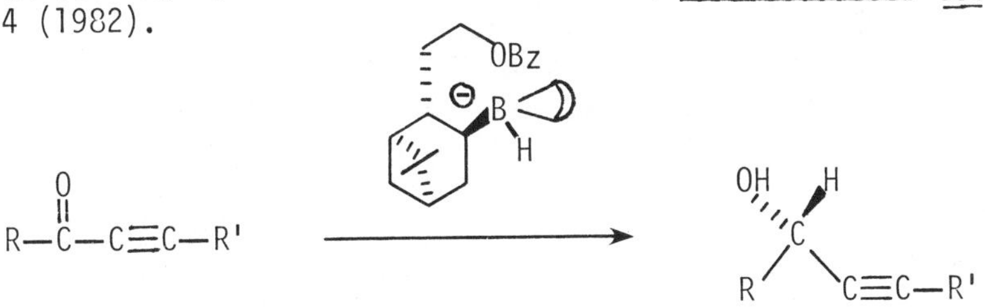

R = alkyl, cyclohexyl
R' = H, alkyl, Ph, -CO$_2$Et, TMS

74-87%
86-96% ee

III.A-14 M. M. Midland and A. Kazubski, *J. Org. Chem.*, **47**, 2496 (1982).

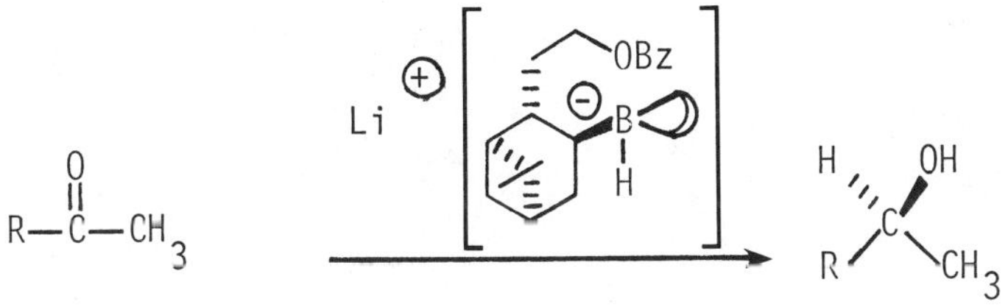

R = alkyl, Ph

up to 79% ee (S)

III.A-15 M. F. Semmelhack and R. N. Misra, J. Org. Chem., 47, 2469 (1982).

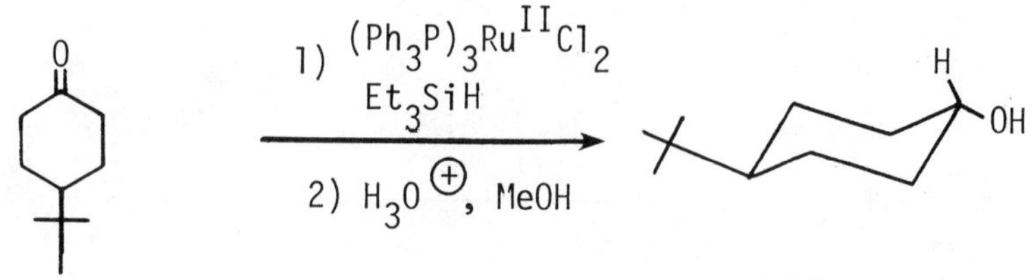

4-tert-butylcyclohexanone →
1) $(Ph_3P)_3Ru^{II}Cl_2$, Et_3SiH
2) $H_3O^{\oplus}$, MeOH
→ 4-tert-butylcyclohexanol (H, OH equatorial)

95% equatorial

III.A-16 I. Ojima and T. Kogure, Organometallics, 1, 1390 (1982).

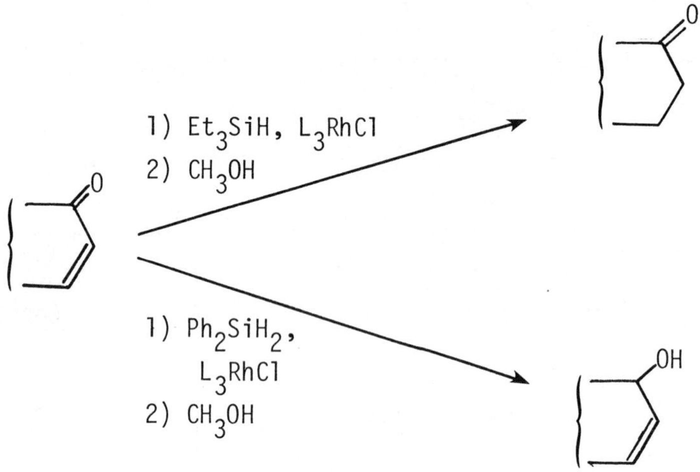

cyclohexenone:

1) Et_3SiH, L_3RhCl
2) CH_3OH
→ cyclohexanone

1) Ph_2SiH_2, L_3RhCl
2) CH_3OH
→ cyclohexenol

yields >90%

III.A-17   V. B. Jigajinni and R. H. Wightman, Tetrahedron Lett., 23, 117 (1982).

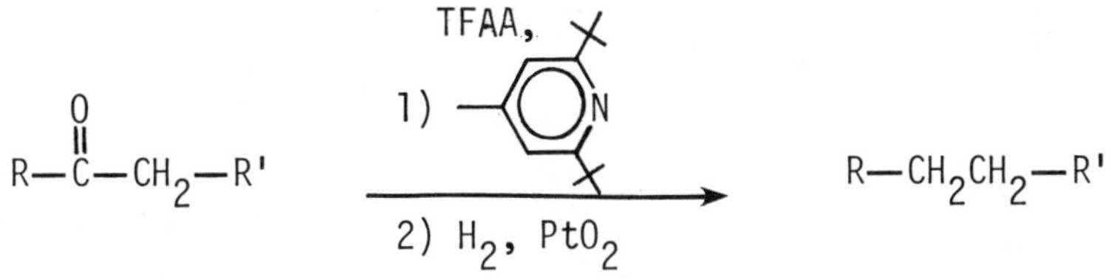

$$R-\overset{O}{\underset{\|}{C}}-CH_2-R' \xrightarrow[2)\ H_2,\ PtO_2]{1)\ \text{TFAA, 2,6-lutidine}} R-CH_2CH_2-R'$$

R, R' = alkyl, vinyl, cyclic

III.B.   Nitrile Reductions

III.B-1   G. R. Brown and A. J. Foubister, Synthesis, 1036 (1982).

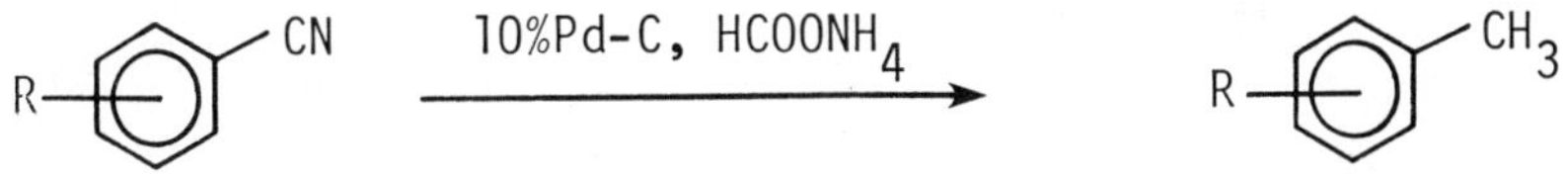

$$R-C_6H_4-CN \xrightarrow{10\%Pd-C,\ HCOONH_4} R-C_6H_4-CH_3$$

42-100%

R = OH, OMe, benzo-

III.C.   Reductions of Sulfur Compounds

III.C-1 S. -K. Chung and G. Han, Synth. Commun., 12, 903 (1982).

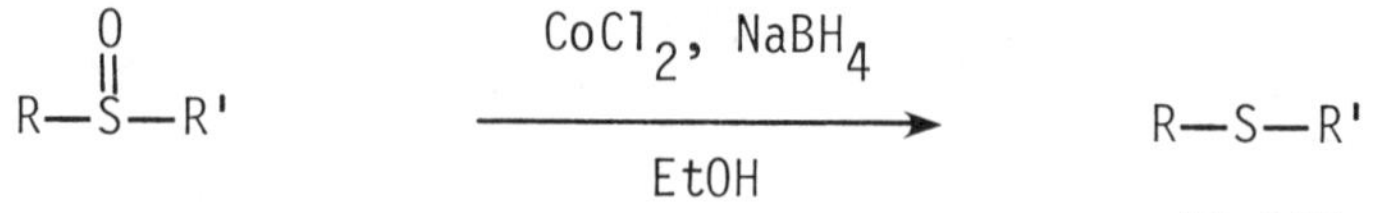

$$R-\underset{\underset{O}{\|}}{S}-R' \xrightarrow[\text{EtOH}]{CoCl_2, NaBH_4} R-S-R'$$

R, R' = alkyl, subst. Ph

56-96%

does not reduce sulfones.

III.C-2 H. -J. Liu and H. Wynn, Tetrahedron Lett., 23, 3151 (1982).

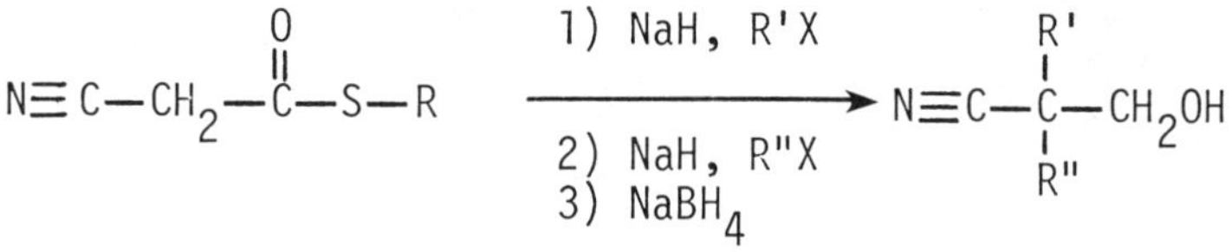

$$N\equiv C-CH_2-\underset{\underset{O}{\|}}{C}-S-R \xrightarrow[\substack{\text{2) NaH, R''X} \\ \text{3) NaBH}_4}]{\text{1) NaH, R'X}} N\equiv C-\underset{\underset{R''}{|}}{\overset{\overset{R'}{|}}{C}}-CH_2OH$$

R = Bz, t-Bu
R', R'' = H, 1°, 2° alkyl, Bz

∼70-90%

III.D. N—O Reductions

III.D-1 S. Oae et al., Bull. Chem. Soc. Japan, 55, 3000 (1982).

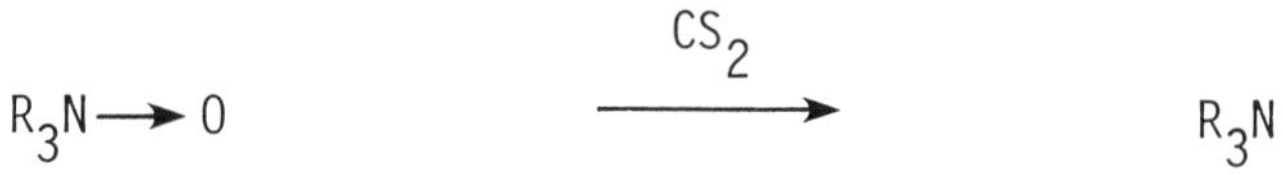

$$R_3N \rightarrow O \xrightarrow{CS_2} R_3N$$

R = alkyl, aryl

69-92%

III.D-2 F. Yuste, M. Saldana, and F. Walls, <u>Tetrahedron Lett.</u>, 23, 147 (1982).

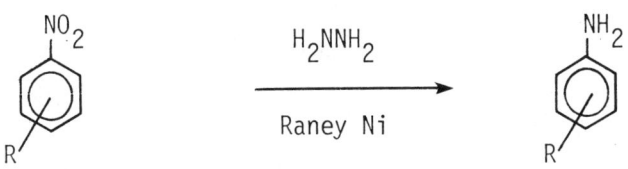

R = OPh, Cl, NHPh

40-96%

III.D-3 A. P. Krapcho and T. A. Collins, <u>Synth. Comm.</u>, 12, 293 (1982).

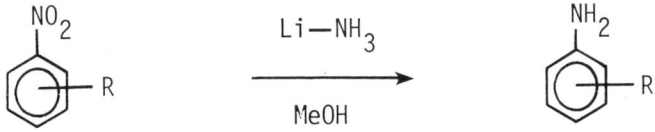

R = H, alkyl

81-95%

III.E. <u>C—C Multiple Bond Reductions</u>

1. <u>C=C Reductions</u>

(Reductions to form amino acids are included in section VI.A.6.)

III.E.1-1 P. A. Wade and N. V. Amin, Synth. Comm., 12, 287 (1982).

$$R-CH=CH-R' \xrightarrow[DMF]{NH_2OH,\ CH_3\overset{O}{\underset{\|}{C}}-OEt} R-CH_2-CH_2-R'$$

67-96%

R = alkyl, Ph
R' = H, CH_2OH, CH_2NO_2, COOH

III.E.1-2 I. Ojima and T. Kogure, Organometallics, 1, 1390 (1982).

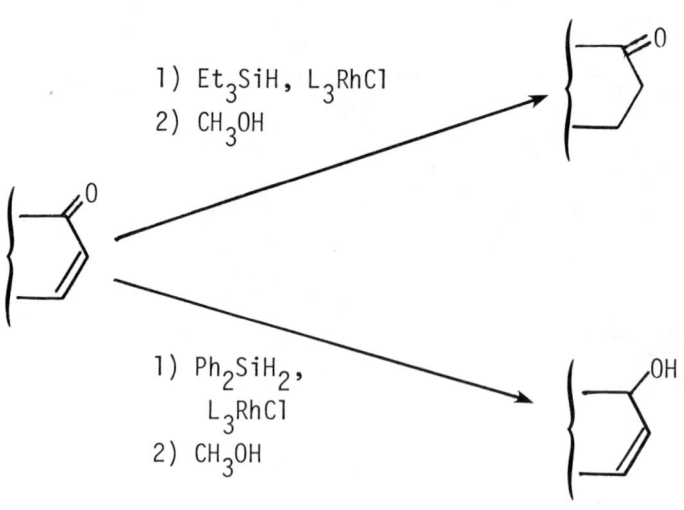

yields >90%

III.E.1-3 E. Keinan and P. A. Gleize, Tetrahedron Lett., 23, 477 (1982).

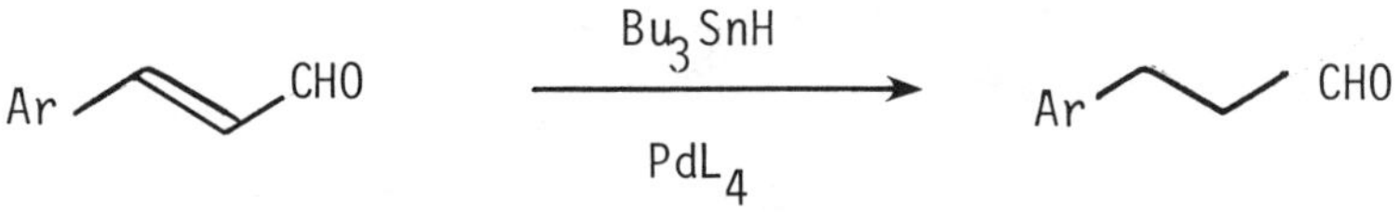

$$Ar\text{—CH=CH—CHO} \xrightarrow[PdL_4]{Bu_3SnH} Ar\text{—CH}_2\text{—CH}_2\text{—CHO}$$

Ar = subst. Ph

>99%

III.E.1-4 M. Sakai et al., Bull. Chem. Soc. Japan, 55, 343 (1982).

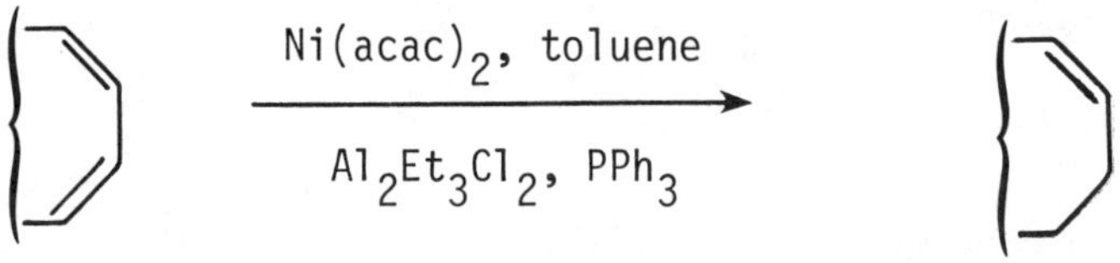

$$\text{cyclic diene} \xrightarrow[Al_2Et_3Cl_2,\ PPh_3]{Ni(acac)_2,\ toluene} \text{cyclic monoene}$$

(conjugated or non-conjugated diene)

~70-90%

III.E.1-5 F. Camps et al., Chem. Lett., 715 (1982).

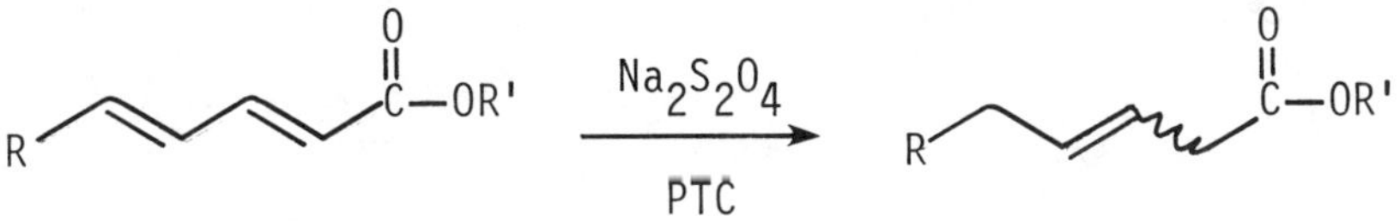

$$R\text{—CH=CH—CH=CH—C(O)—OR'} \xrightarrow[PTC]{Na_2S_2O_4} R\text{—CH}_2\text{—CH=CH—CH}_2\text{—C(O)—OR'}$$

R = alkyl
R' = H, Me, Et

~40-80%

III.E.1-6 G. Descotes et al., J. Chem. Research (S), 117 (1982).

$$\underset{\underset{O}{\overset{\|}{NHC-R^2}}}{\overset{\overset{O}{\overset{\|}{C-OR^3}}}{R^1}}\!\!\!C=C \quad \xrightarrow[\text{Rh catalyst}^*]{H_2} \quad R^1-CH_2-\overset{*}{C}H(NHCOR^2)(CO_2R^3)$$

~78-86%

R^1 = H, subst. Ph
R^2 = Me, Ph
R^3 = H, Me

* Rhodium complex with (S)-1,2-O-isopropylideneglycerol

III.E.2. C≡C Reductions

III.E.2-1 M. Sato and K. Oshima, Chem. Lett., 157 (1982).

$$R-C\equiv C-R' \xrightarrow{NbCl_5/NaAlH_4} \underset{R'}{\overset{H}{>}}C=C\underset{R'}{\overset{H}{<}}$$

R, R' = alkyl, Ph

III.E.2-2 H. C. Brown et al., J. Org. Chem., 47, 171 (1982).

$$R-C\equiv C-R \xrightarrow[\text{2) NaOMe, }I_2]{\text{1) }R_2'BX,\ LiAlH_4} \underset{R'}{\overset{R}{>}}C=C\underset{R}{\overset{H}{<}}$$

69-76%

REDUCTIONS

III.E.3. Reduction of Aromatic Rings

III.E.3-1 T. Okano et al., Chem. Lett., 603 (1982).

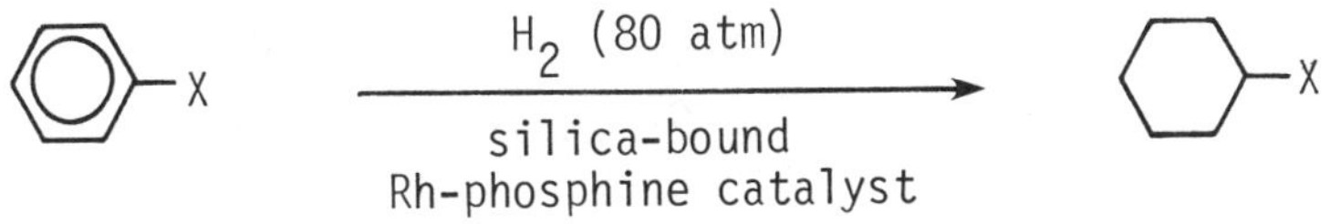

Ph–X $\xrightarrow[\text{silica-bound Rh-phosphine catalyst}]{H_2 \text{ (80 atm)}}$ Cy–X

widely varying yields

X = alkyl, -OMe, -NH$_2$

III.E.3-2 R. H. Fish, A. D. Thormodsen, and G. A. Cremer, J. Am. Chem. Soc., 104, 5234 (1982).

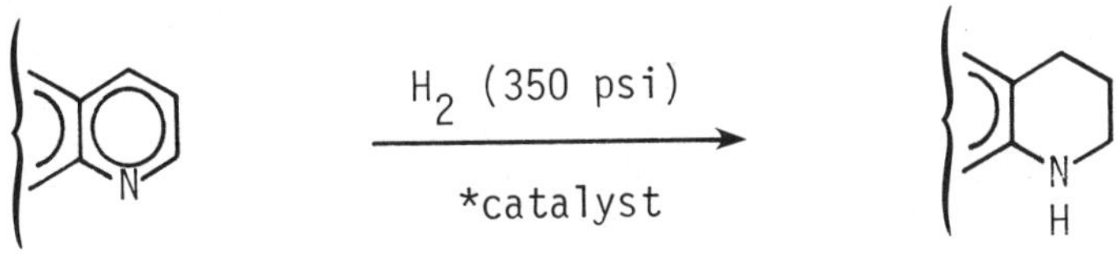

quinoline $\xrightarrow[\text{*catalyst}]{H_2 \text{ (350 psi)}}$ 1,2,3,4-tetrahydroquinoline

yields up to 100%

acridine $\xrightarrow{\text{similar conditions}}$ 9,10-dihydroacridine

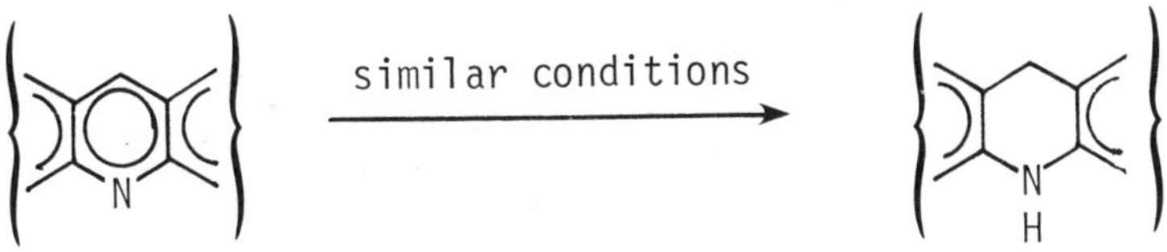

yields up to 100%

*catalyst = various Fe, Mn, Co, Ru carbonyl phosphines

III.F. Hydrogenolysis of Hetero Bonds

1. C—O ⟶ C—H

III.F.1-1 R. O. Hutchins and K. Learn, J. Org. Chem., 47, 4380 (1982).

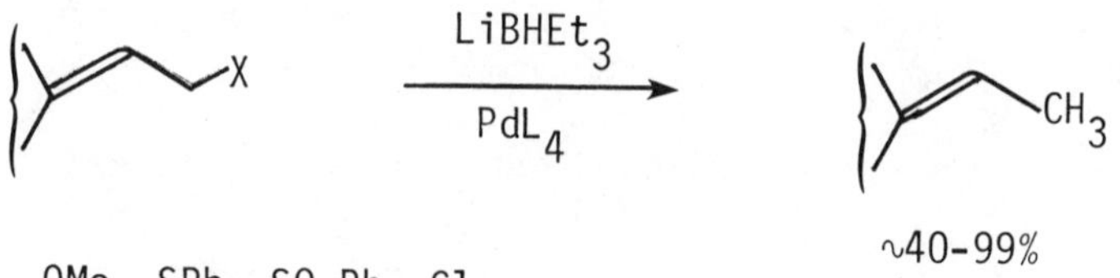
X
$LiBHEt_3$
PdL_4
CH_3
~40-99%

X = OPh, OMe, SPh, SO_2Ph, Cl

III.F.1-2 V. B. Jigajinni and R. H. Wightman, Tetrahedron Lett., 23, 117 (1982).

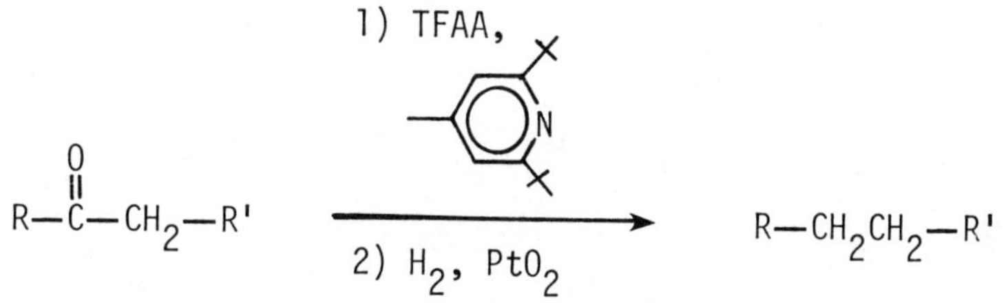
1) TFAA,
N
R—C(=O)—CH_2—R'
2) H_2, PtO_2
R—CH_2CH_2—R'

R, R' = alkyl, vinyl, cyclic

III.F.1-3 N. M. Yoon and B. T. Cho, Tetrahedron Lett., 23, 2475 (1982).

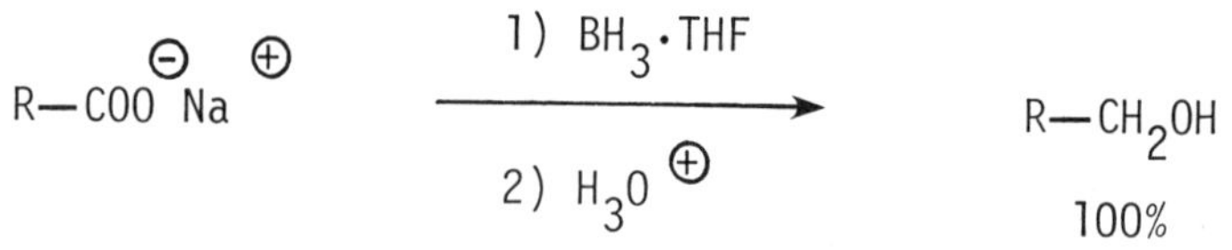
R—$COO^{\ominus}$ $Na^{\oplus}$
1) BH_3·THF
2) $H_3O^{\oplus}$
R—CH_2OH
100%

R = alkyl, subst. Ph

III.F.1-4 H. C. Brown, Y. M. Choi, and S. Narasimhan, J. Org. Chem., 47, 3153 (1982).

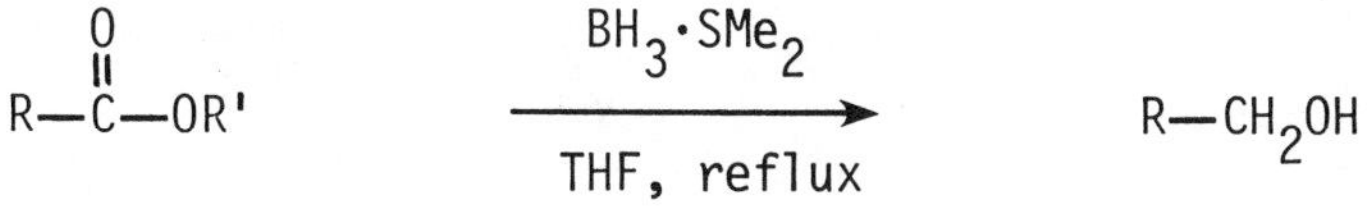

$$R-\underset{\underset{O}{\|}}{C}-OR' \xrightarrow[\text{THF, reflux}]{BH_3 \cdot SMe_2} R-CH_2OH$$

~90%

III.F.1-5 H. C. Brown, S. Narasimhan, J. Org. Chem., 47, 1604 (1982).

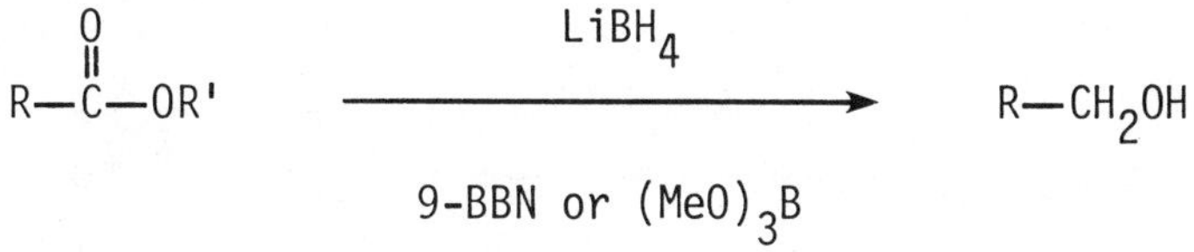

$$R-\underset{\underset{O}{\|}}{C}-OR' \xrightarrow[\text{9-BBN or } (MeO)_3B]{LiBH_4} R-CH_2OH$$

~80-90%

R = alkyl, aryl; may contain Cl, NO_2
R' = Me, Et

III.F.1-6 K. Soai et al., Synth. Comm., 12, 463 (1982).

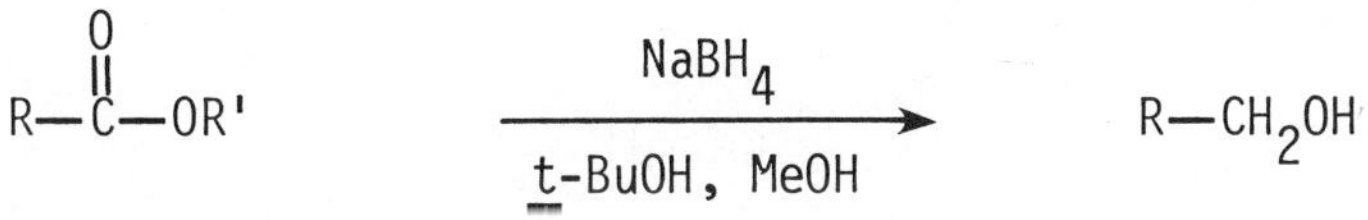

$$R-\underset{\underset{O}{\|}}{C}-OR' \xrightarrow[\underline{t}\text{-BuOH, MeOH}]{NaBH_4} R-CH_2OH$$

79-91%

R = alkyl, Ph, 3-pyridyl
R' = Me, Et

III.F.1-7   J. M. Finian and Y. Kishi, Tetrahedron Lett., 23, 2719 (1982).

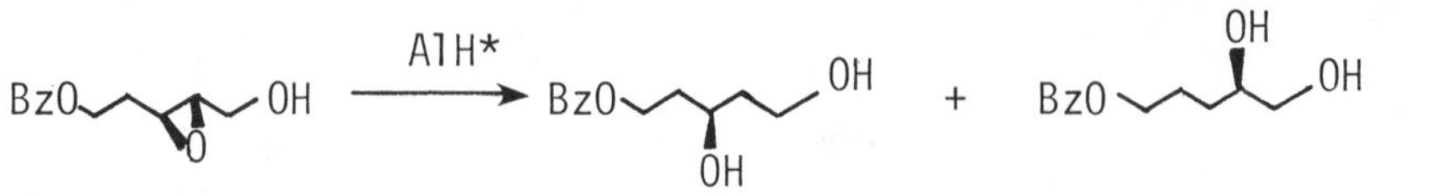

BzO−CH(−O−)−CH−OH →[AlH*] BzO−CH₂−CH(OH)−CH₂−CH₂−OH + BzO−CH₂−CH₂−CH(OH)−CH₂−OH

                                           A   B

*AlH	Ratio A:B
Red-Al	150:1
DIBAL	1:13

III.F.1-8   S. M. Viti, Tetrahedron Lett., 23, 4541 (1982).

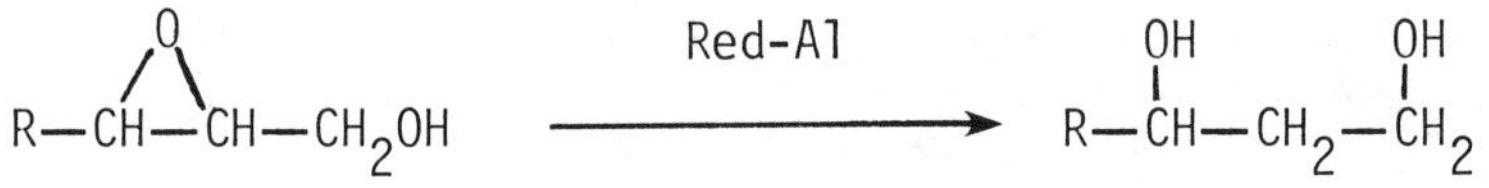

R−CH(−O−)CH−CH₂OH   →[Red-Al]   R−CH(OH)−CH₂−CH₂(OH)

R = alkyl   70-95%

III.F.1-9/III.F.2-1   E. Fujita et al., Tetrahedron Lett., 23, 689 (1982).

Ar−Y   →[CH₃CH₂SH / AlCl₃]   Ar−H

Ar = polynuclear benzenoid aromatic   ~80-100%
Y = −OR, −SR, F, Br

III.F.2. C—Hal ⟶ C—H

III.F.2-2 B. H. Han and P. Boudjouk, Tetrahedron Lett., 23, 1643 (1982).

$$Ar-X \xrightarrow[\text{ultrasound}]{\text{LiAlH}_4} Ar-H$$

70-99%

Ar = subst. Ph, naphthyl
X = Br, I (does not reduce Cl)

III.F.2-3 P. N. Pandey and M. L. Purkayastha, Synthesis, 876 (1982).

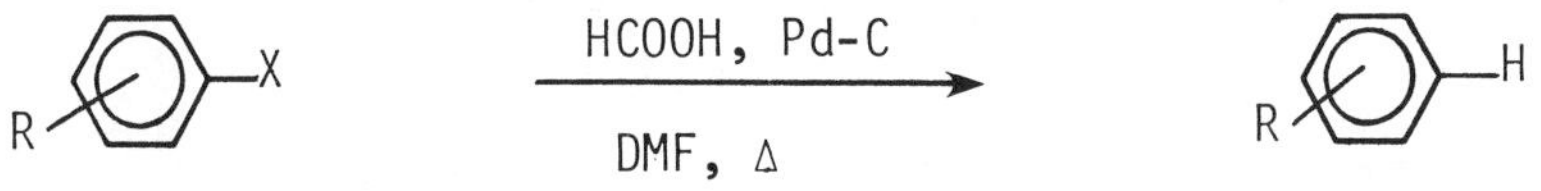

$$R-C_6H_4-X \xrightarrow[\text{DMF, }\Delta]{\text{HCOOH, Pd-C}} R-C_6H_4-H$$

80-95%

R = H, NH_2, OH, NO_2, $-\overset{O}{\underset{\|}{C}}-R$, $-CH_2CH_2Cl$
X = Cl, Br, I

III.F.2-4 I. Colon, J. Org. Chem., 47, 2622 (1982).

$$R-X \xrightarrow[\text{DMF/H}_2\text{O}]{\text{Ni, NiCl}_2\text{, NaI, Ph}_3\text{P}} R-H$$

46-99%

R = alkyl, subst. Ph
X = halide

III.F.2-5   S. -K. Chung and Q. -Y. Hu, <u>Synth. Comm.</u>, 12, 261 (1982).

$$R-\overset{O}{\underset{}{C}}-\underset{X}{CH}-R' \xrightarrow[H_2O, DMF]{Na_2S_2O_4, 90°} R-\overset{O}{\underset{}{C}}-CH_2-R'$$

R = Ph, cyclic
R' = H, Me, cyclic
X = Br, Cl

Up to ~90%

III.F.2-6   D. L. J. Clive and P. L. Beaulieu, <u>J. Org. Chem.</u>, 47, 1124 (1982).

$$\underset{R}{\overset{O}{\underset{}{C}}}\underset{\underset{X}{CH}}{}R' \xrightarrow[EtOH]{(EtO)_2\overset{O}{\underset{}{P}}Te^{\ominus} \ Na^{\oplus}} \underset{R}{\overset{O}{\underset{}{C}}}CH_2 R'$$

~50-90%

X = Cl, Br
R, R' = alkyl, aryl

III.F.2-7   A. U. Ronchi et al., <u>J. Org. Chem.</u>, 47, 876 (1982).

$$\text{(cyclic ketone with Br, H)} \xrightarrow[THF/D_2O]{\text{Iron-graphite}} \text{(cyclic ketone with D, H)}$$

75-96%

III.F.2-8   J. H. Babler, Synth. Comm., 12, 839 (1982).

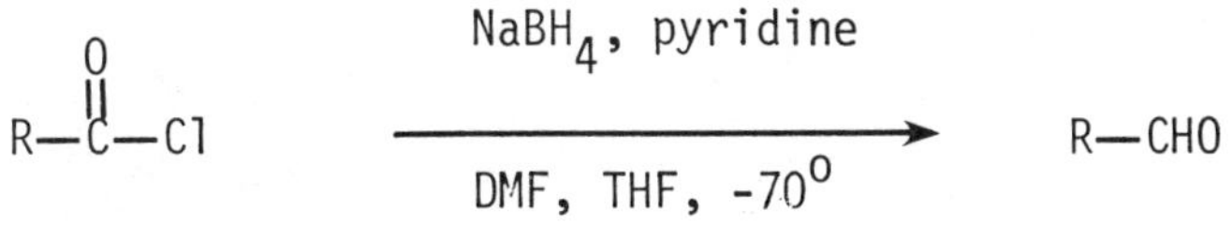

$$R-\underset{\underset{O}{\|}}{C}-Cl \xrightarrow[DMF, THF, -70°]{NaBH_4, \text{ pyridine}} R-CHO$$

R = alkyl, subst. Ph

III.F.2-9   S. Krishnamurthy and H. C. Brown, J. Org. Chem., 47, 276 (1982).

A thorough study of the use of $LiAlH_4$ in THF to reduce alkyl halides.

III.F.3.   C—S ⟶ C—H

III.F.3-1   E. Fujita et al., Tetrahedron Lett., 23, 689 (1982).

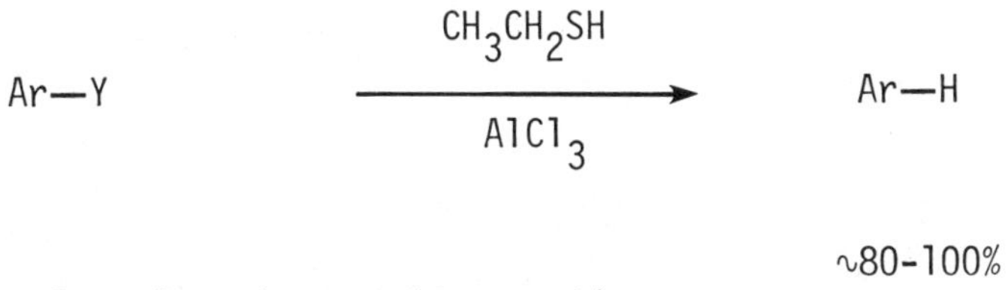

$$Ar-Y \xrightarrow[AlCl_3]{CH_3CH_2SH} Ar-H$$

∼80-100%

Ar = polynuclear benzenoid aromatic
Y = -OR, -SR, F, Br

III.F.3-2 R. O. Hutchins and K. Learn, J. Org. Chem., 47, 4380 (1982).

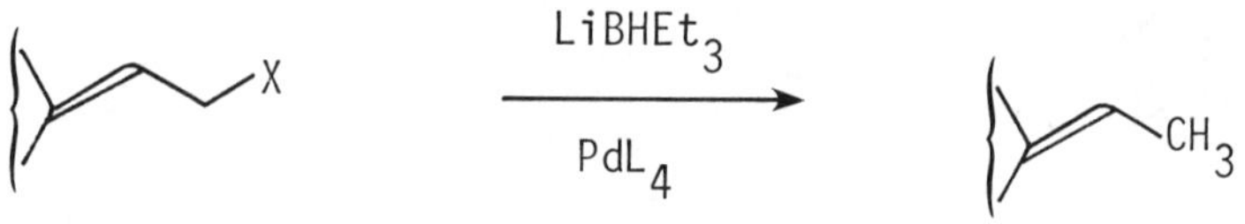

$$\text{allyl-X} \xrightarrow[\text{PdL}_4]{\text{LiBHEt}_3} \text{allyl-CH}_3$$

X = OPh, OMe, SPh, SO$_2$Ph, Cl

~40-99%

III.F.3-3 M. Julia et al., Tetrahedron Lett., 23, 3265 (1982).

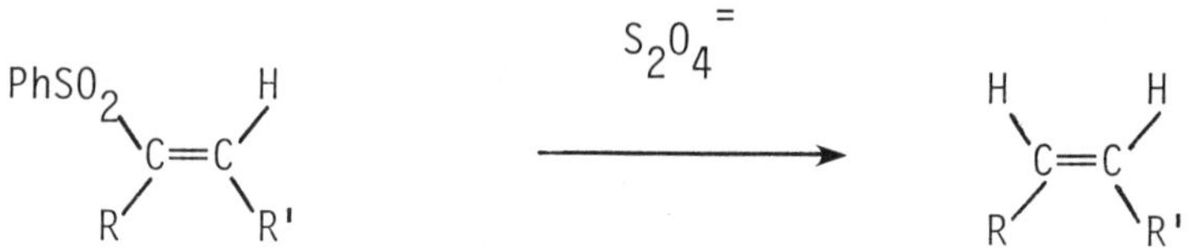

$$\underset{R}{\overset{PhSO_2}{\diagdown}}C=C\underset{R'}{\overset{H}{\diagup}} \xrightarrow{S_2O_4^=} \underset{R}{\overset{H}{\diagdown}}C=C\underset{R'}{\overset{H}{\diagup}}$$

R, R' = n-alkyl

52-88%
(trans product is formed from trans reactants)

III.G. Reductive Eliminations

III.G-1 N. C. Barua and R. P. Sharma, Tetrahedron Lett., 23, 1365 (1982).

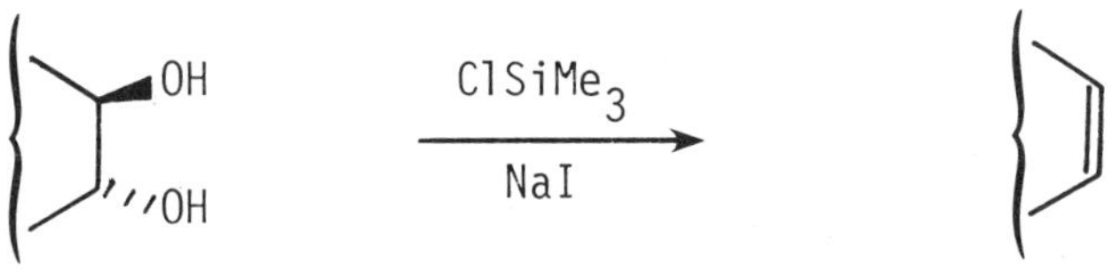

[cis-diol] →(ClSiMe$_3$ / NaI)→ [alkene]

80-98%

III.G-2 E. J. Corey and P. B. Hopkins, Tetrahedron Lett., 23, 1979 (1982).

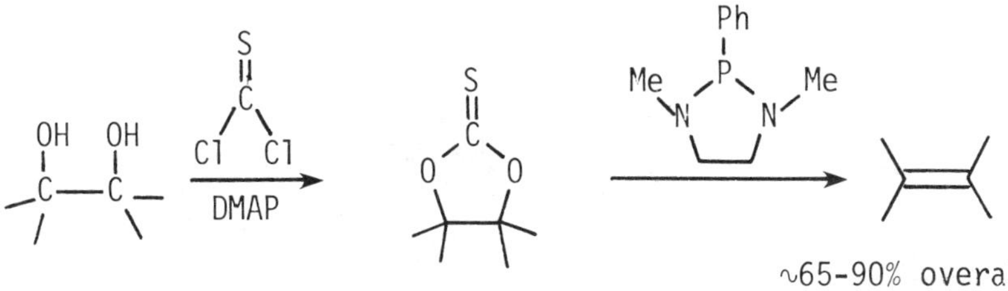

[diol] →(S=C(Cl)Cl, DMAP)→ [thiocarbonate] →(Me-N-P(Ph)-N-Me diazaphospholidine)→ [alkene]

~65-90% overall.
Stereospecific.

Subst. by alkyl, aryl, cyclic, macrocyclic groups.

III.G-3 H. M. Walborsky and H. H. Wüst, J. Am. Chem. Soc., 104, 5807 (1982).

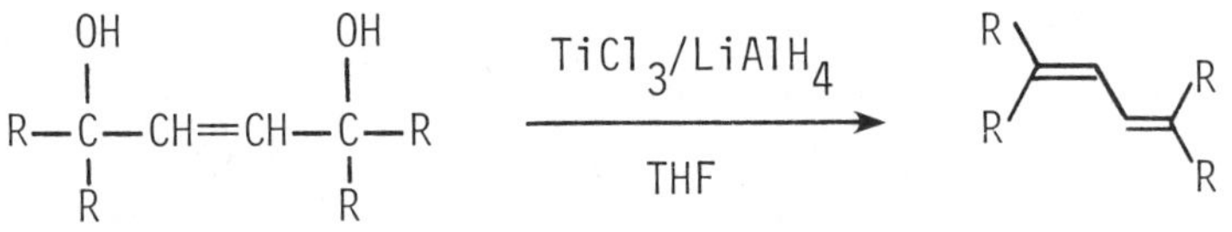

$$R-\underset{R}{\underset{|}{C}}(OH)-CH=CH-\underset{R}{\underset{|}{C}}(OH)-R \xrightarrow[\text{THF}]{TiCl_3/LiAlH_4} R_2C=CR-CR=CR_2$$

42-83%

R = Me, Ph, H, -(CH$_2$)$_5$-

(E or Z isomer)

III.G-4 M. Sato and K. Oshima, <u>Chem. Lett.</u>, 157 (1982).

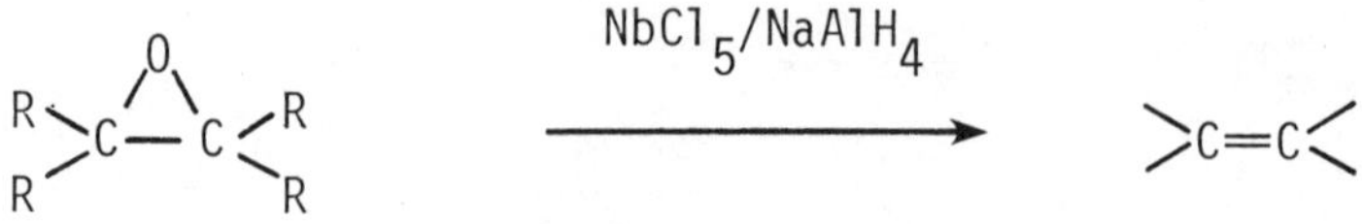

$$\underset{R}{\overset{R}{>}}C\underset{}{\overset{O}{-}}C\underset{R}{\overset{R}{<}} \xrightarrow{NbCl_5/NaAlH_4} >C=C<$$

R's = H, alkyl, aryl

50-75%

III.G-5 G. W. Gribble, W. J. Kelly, and M. P. Sibi, <u>Synthesis</u>, 143 (1982).

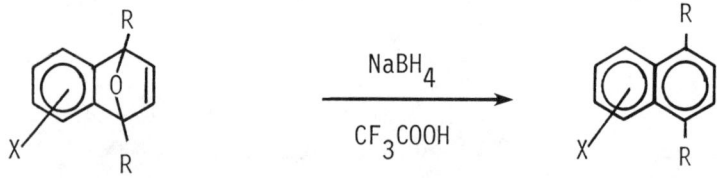

X = H, F, Cl, polyhalogenated
R = H, Me

57-97%

III.G-6 F. Sato <u>et al.</u>, <u>Synthesis</u>, 1025 (1982).

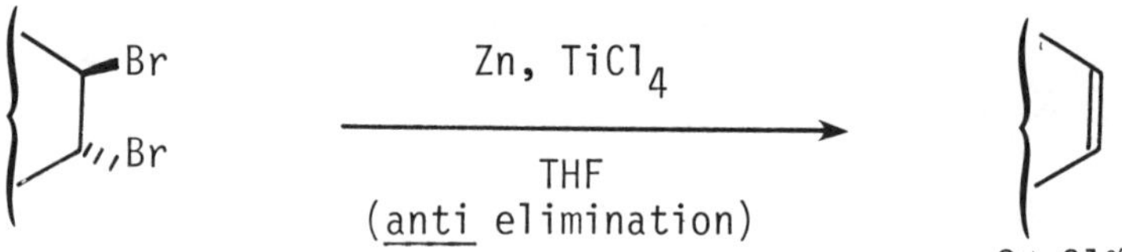

Zn, TiCl$_4$

THF
(<u>anti</u> elimination)

82-91%

III.G-7   A. U. Ronchi et al., J. Org. Chem., 47, 876 (1982).

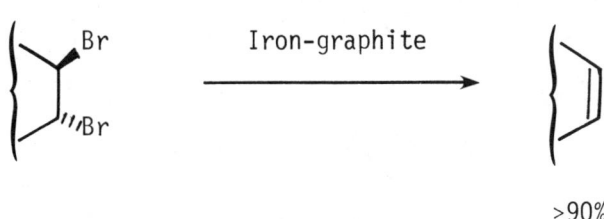

>90%

III.G-8   L. Engman, Tetrahedron Lett., 23, 3601 (1982).

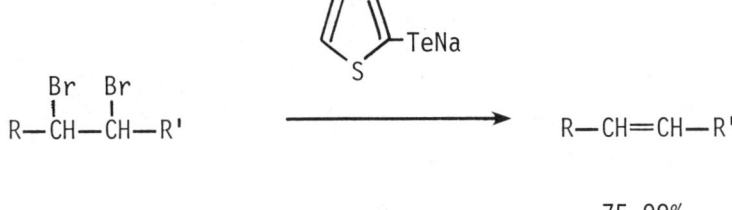

75-99%

Anti elimination, threo— cis, erythro— trans.

III.G-9   J. Halpern, Accounts Chem. Res., 15, 332 (1982).

Review: "Formation of Carbon-Hydrogen Bonds by Reductive Elimination"

III.H. Reductive Cleavages

III.H-1 Y. Sato et al., Synthesis, 141 (1982).

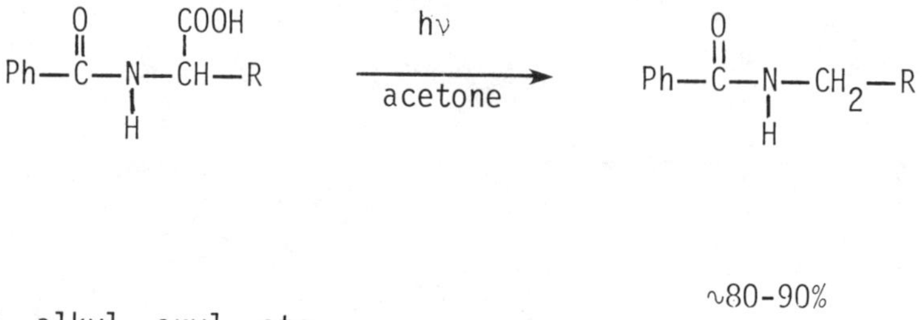

$$Ph-\underset{\underset{H}{|}}{\overset{\overset{O}{\|}}{C}}-N-\underset{}{\overset{COOH}{\underset{|}{C}H}}-R \xrightarrow[\text{acetone}]{h\nu} Ph-\underset{\underset{H}{|}}{\overset{\overset{O}{\|}}{C}}-N-CH_2-R$$

R = H, alkyl, aryl, etc.

∼80-90%

III.H-2 H.-P. Husson et al., Tetrahedron Lett., 23, 3369 (1982).

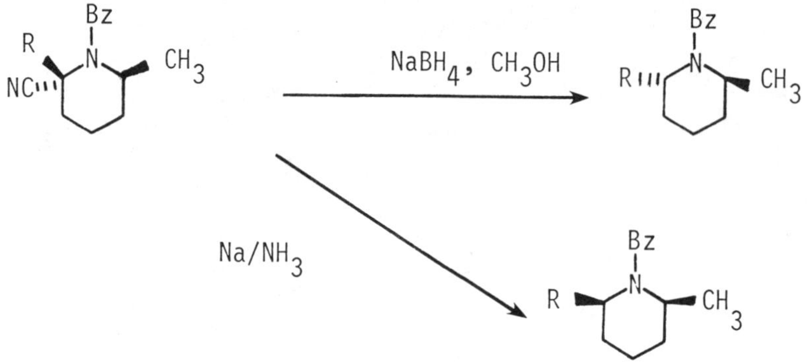

R = n-alkyl

III.I. Hydroboration (Reduction only)

III.I-1 M. M. Midland and A. Kazubski, <u>J. Org. Chem.</u>, **47**, 2496 (1982).

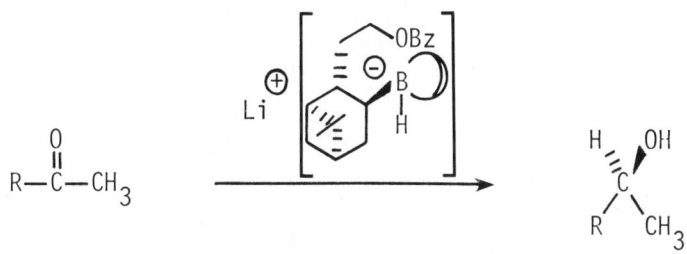

R = alkyl, Ph

up to 79% ee (<u>S</u>)

III.I-2 H. C. Brown, Y. M. Choi, and S. Narasimhan, <u>J. Org. Chem.</u>, **47**, 3153 (1982).

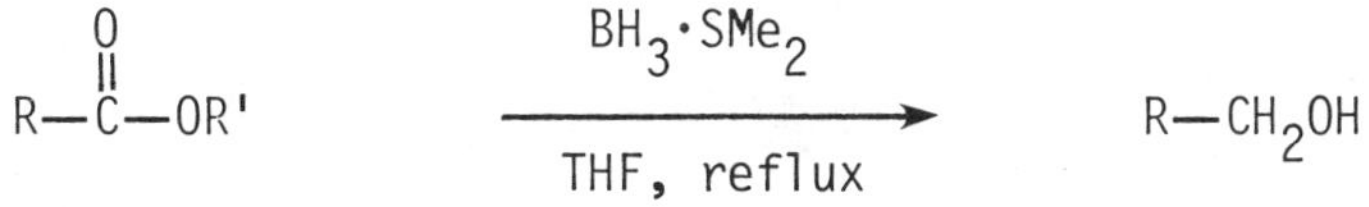

$$R-\overset{O}{\underset{\|}{C}}-OR' \xrightarrow[\text{THF, reflux}]{BH_3 \cdot SMe_2} R-CH_2OH$$

∼90%

III.I-3 H. C. Brown and S. Narasimhan, J. Org. Chem., 47, 1604 (1982).

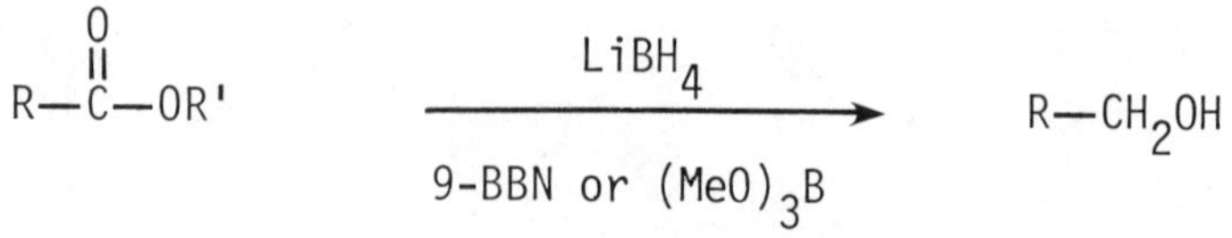
R—C(=O)—OR'
LiBH4
9-BBN or (MeO)3B
R—CH2OH

~80-90%

R = alkyl, aryl; may contain Cl, NO_2
R' = Me, Et

III.I-4 H. C. Brown and G. G. Pai, J. Org. Chem., 47, 1606 (1982).

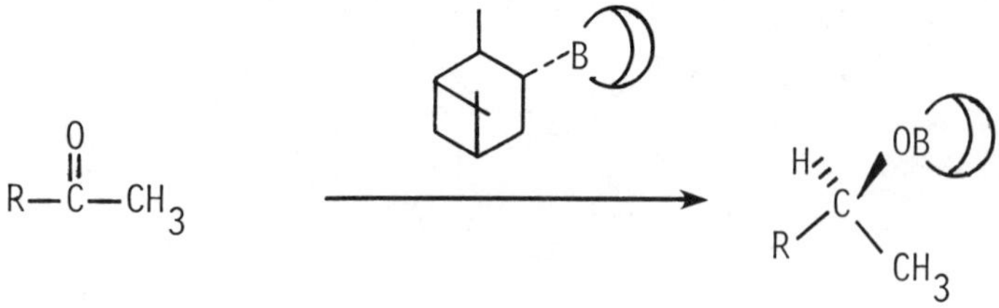
R—C(=O)—CH3
B
H
OB
C
R
CH3

~50-90% ee

R = alkyl, Ph, vinyl, cinnamyl, alkynyl

III.J. Other Reductions and Reviews

III.J-1   F. Rolla, J. Org. Chem., 47, 4327 (1982).

$$RN_3 \xrightarrow[C_{16}H_{33}Bu_3P^{\oplus} Br^{\ominus}]{NaBH_4, H_2O/toluene} RNH_2$$

∼90%

R = alkyl, aryl, Bz, Ts

III.J-2   T. H. Black, Aldrichimica Acta, 15, 13 (1982).

Review: "Recent Applications of Homogeneous Catalysis to Organic Synthesis"

IV
SYNTHESIS OF HETEROCYCLES

IV.A. Aziridines

IV.A-1 S. Zbaida and E. Breuer, J. Org. Chem., 47, 1073 (1982).

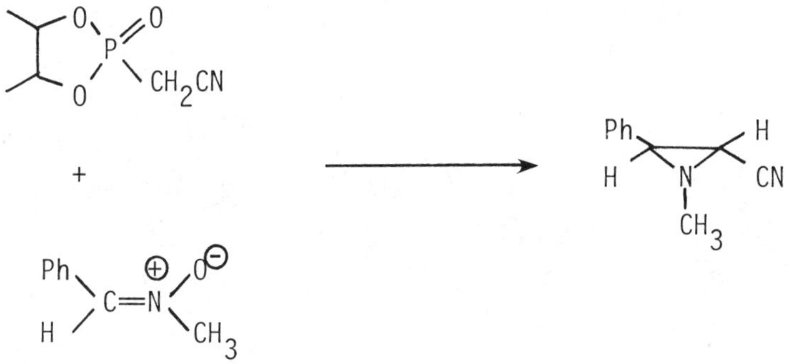

IV.A-2 F. D'Angeli et al., Synthesis, 586 (1982).

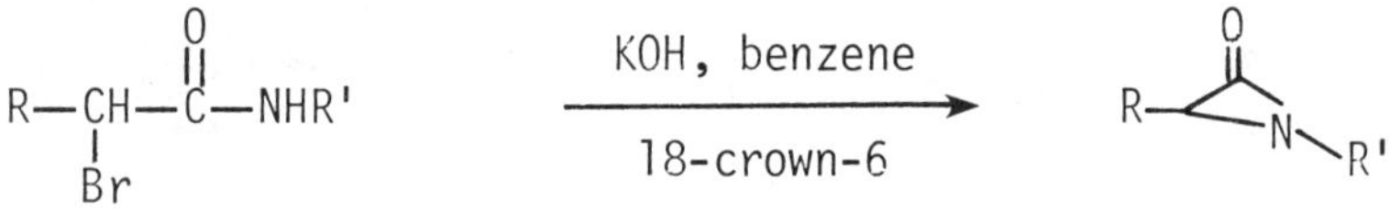

R, R' = t-Butyl, 1-adamantyl

IV.B. Furans, etc.

IV.B-1 F. Yuste and R.S. Obregon, *J. Org. Chem.*, **47**, 3665 (1982).

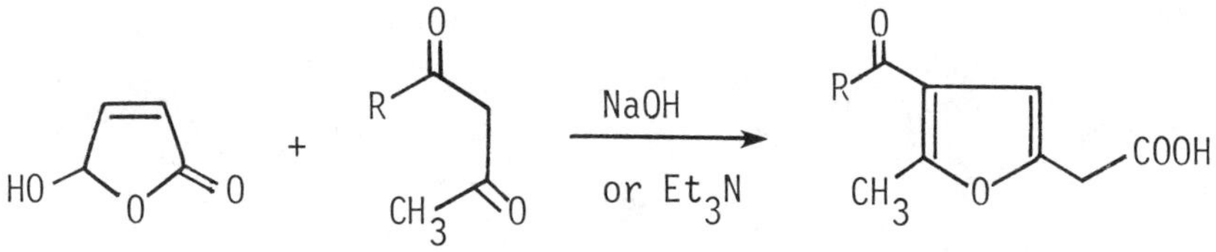

[Reaction scheme: 5-hydroxy-2(5H)-furanone + R-CO-CH$_2$-CO-CH$_3$ (R = Me, OEt), with NaOH or Et$_3$N, gives 3-acyl-5-(carboxymethyl)-2-methylfuran, ~60-80%]

IV.B-2 D. Couturier *et al.*, *Synth. Comm.*, **12**, 647 (1982).

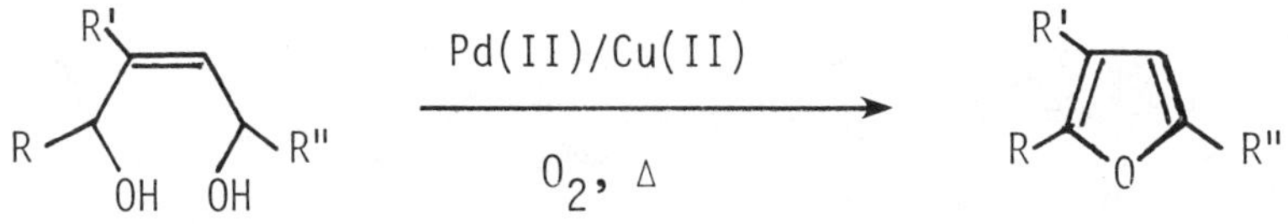

[Reaction scheme: R-CH(OH)-C(R')=CH-CH(OH)-R'' with Pd(II)/Cu(II), O$_2$, Δ gives 2,3,5-trisubstituted furan]

R's = H, alkyl   22-77%

IV.B-3 H. Yamamoto *et al.*, *Chem. Lett.*, 1029 (1982)

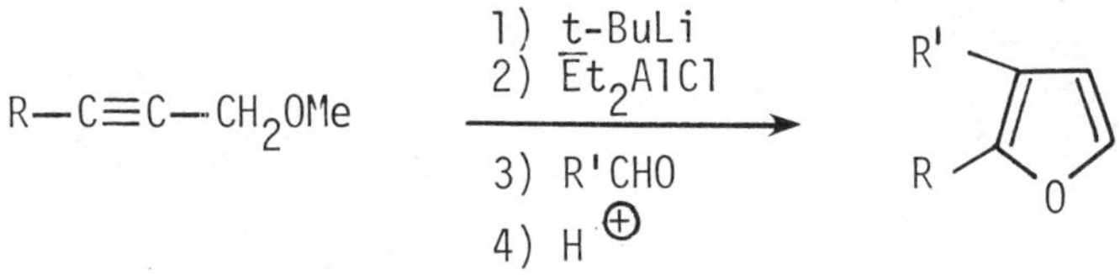

R—C≡C—CH$_2$OMe

1) t-BuLi
2) Et$_2$AlCl
3) R'CHO
4) H$^\oplus$

[gives 2,3-disubstituted furan]

R = Me, Me$_3$Si
R' = 1°, 2° alkyl, Ph, geranyl   30-89%

IV.B-4   H. Kinoshita et al., Bull. Chem. Soc. Japan, 55, 3225 (1982).

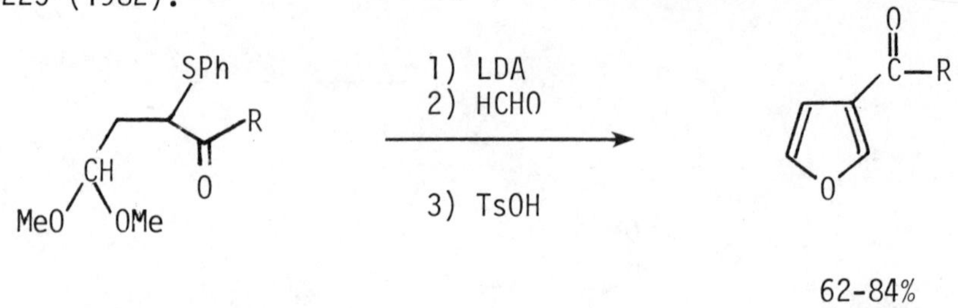

[Structure: CH(OMe)(OMe)-CH2-CH(SPh)-C(=O)-R]   1) LDA   2) HCHO   3) TsOH   →   [3-acyl furan: furan-C(=O)-R]

R = alkyl

62-84%

IV.B-5   J. A. Ballesteros et al., Bull. Soc. Chim. France II, 176 (1982).

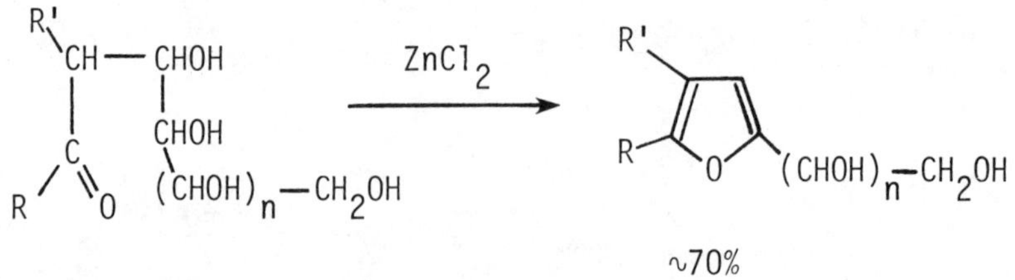

[R-C(=O)-CH(R')-CH(OH)-CH(OH)-(CHOH)$_n$-CH$_2$OH]   ZnCl$_2$ →   [2,3-disubstituted furan with R at 2, R' at 3, and -(CHOH)$_n$-CH$_2$OH at 5]

~70%

n = 2, 3
R = Me, Ph
R' = -COOH, -C(=O)-Me, -COOMe, -C(=O)-NH$_2$

IV.B-6   S. P. Tanis, Tetrahedron Lett., 23, 3115 (1982).

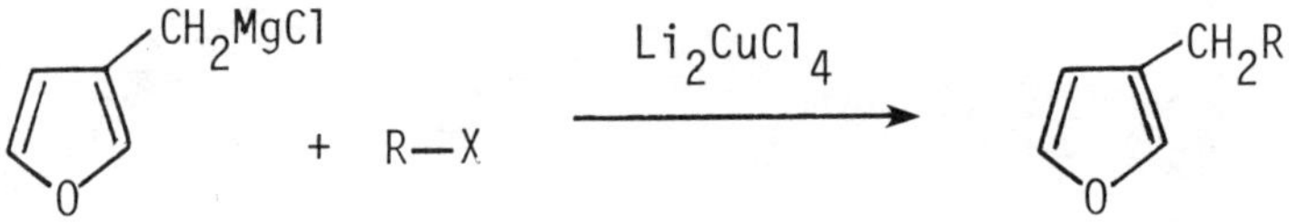

[3-(CH$_2$MgCl)-furan]   +   R—X $\xrightarrow{\text{Li}_2\text{CuCl}_4}$ [3-(CH$_2$R)-furan]

R = 1°, 2° alkyl, allylic

IV.B-7   D. Seebach et al., Helv. Chim. Acta, 65, 419 (1982).

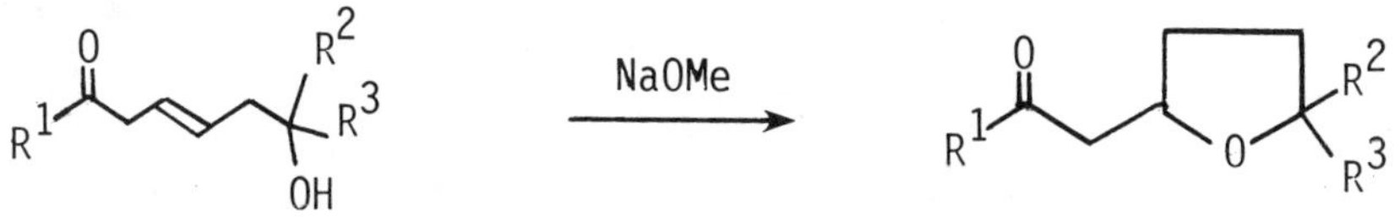

R^1, R^2 = alkyl, Ph, vinyl, etc.
R^3 = H, alkyl

62-94%

Tetrahydropyrans may also be synthesized by this method.

IV.B-8   Y. Ueno et al., J. Am. Chem. Soc., 104, 5564 (1982).

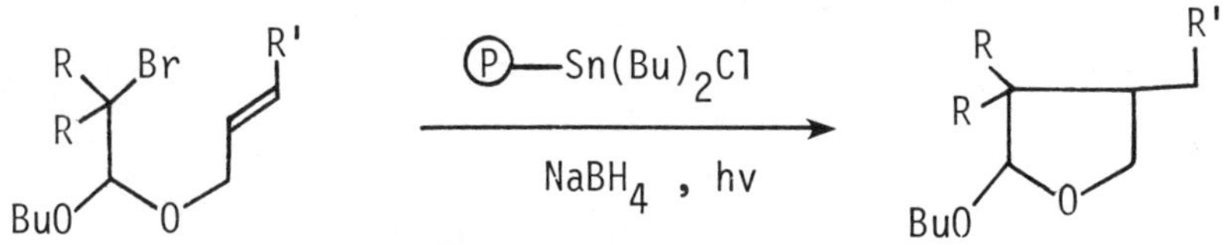

R = H, —(CH$_2$)$_{\overline{5}}$—
R' = H, alkyl, —CH$_2$SPh

73-91%

IV.B-9/IV.C-1   Y. Ueno, K. Chino, and M. Okawara, Tetrahedron Lett., 23, 2575 (1982).

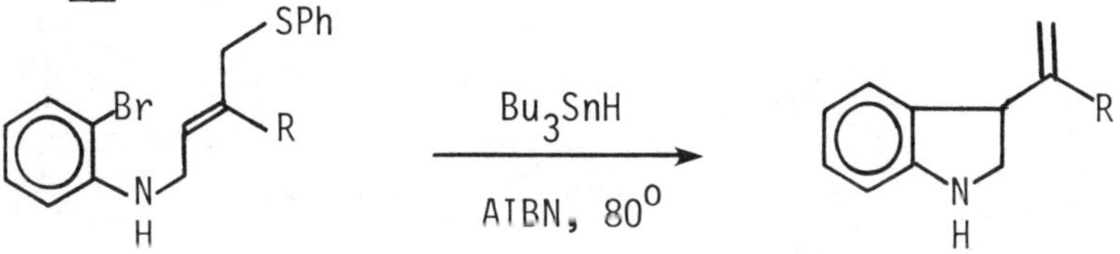

56% (R = Me)
96% (R = H)

IV.C. Indoles

IV.C-2   R. B. Perni and G. W. Gribble, Org. Prep. Proc. Int., **14**, 343 (1982).

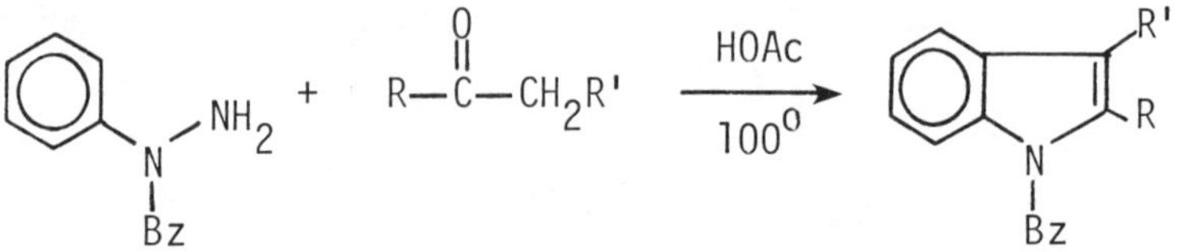

PhN(Bz)NH$_2$ + R—C(=O)—CH$_2$R' →(HOAc, 100°)→ 1-Bz-2-R-3-R'-indole

62-91%

R = H, alkyl,
R' = alkyl,] cyclic

IV.C-3   D. H. R. Barton et al., Tetrahedron Lett., **23**, 4949 (1982).

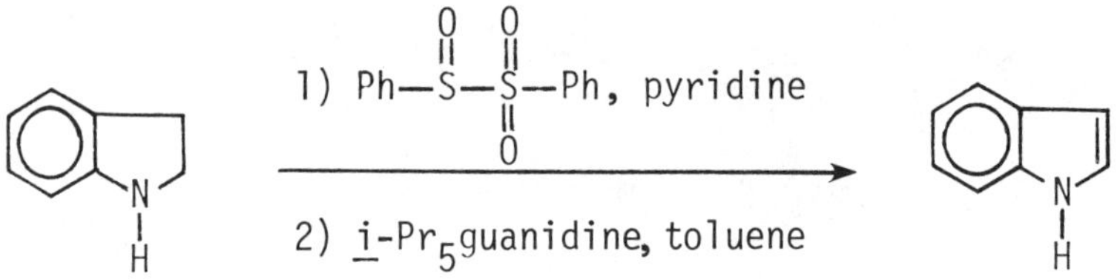

indoline → 1) Ph—S(=O)—S(=O)$_2$—Ph, pyridine; 2) $\underline{i}$-Pr$_5$guanidine, toluene → indole

~90%

IV.C-4   T. Itahara, Chem. Lett., 1151 (1982).

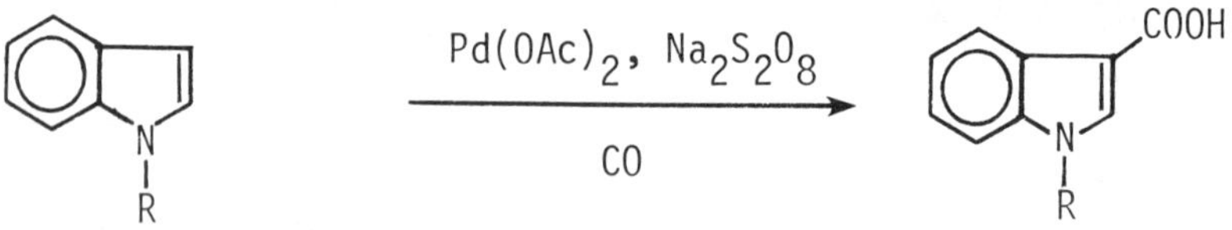

1-R-indole →(Pd(OAc)$_2$, Na$_2$S$_2$O$_8$, CO)→ 1-R-indole-3-COOH

R = H, —C(=O)—Me, —C(=O)—Ph

~30-60%

IV.C-5   V. Bocchi and G. Palla, Synthesis, 1096 (1982).

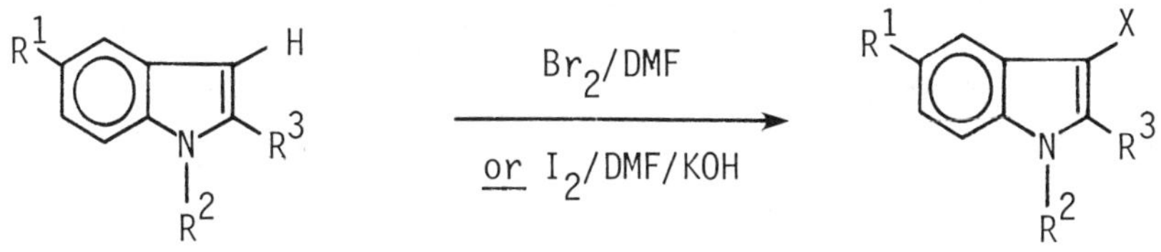

R^1 = H, Cl, OMe
R^2 = H, Me
R^3 = H, Me, Ph

Reagents: Br_2/DMF or I_2/DMF/KOH (X = Br or I), >90%

IV.C-6   A. J. Elliott and H. Guzik, Tetrahedron Lett., 23, 1983 (1982).

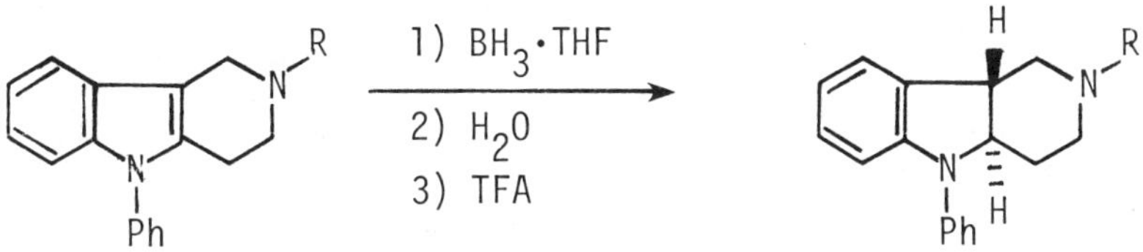

R = H, Me

1) BH_3·THF
2) H_2O
3) TFA

>80%

IV.C-7   G. Nechvatal and D. A. Widdowson, J.C.S. Chem. Comm., 467 (1982).

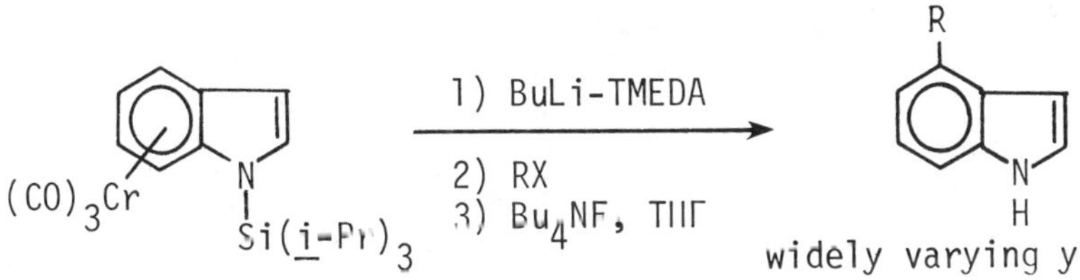

$(CO)_3Cr$, Si($\underline{i}$-Pr)$_3$

1) BuLi-TMEDA
2) RX
3) Bu_4NF, THF

RX = Me_3SiCl, EtO_2CCl, PhSCl, $Me_2C{=}CHCH_2Br$

widely varying yields

IV.C-8   M. Lounasmaa and Andras Nemes, Tetrahedron, 38, 223 (1982).

Review: "The Synthesis of Bis-indole Alkaloids and their Derivatives"

IV.C-9   F. S. Babichev et al., Russ. Chem. Rev., 50, 1087 (1981).

Review: "Advances in the Chemistry of Isoindole:

IV.D. Lactams

IV.D-1   F. D'Angeli et al., Synthesis, 586 (1982).

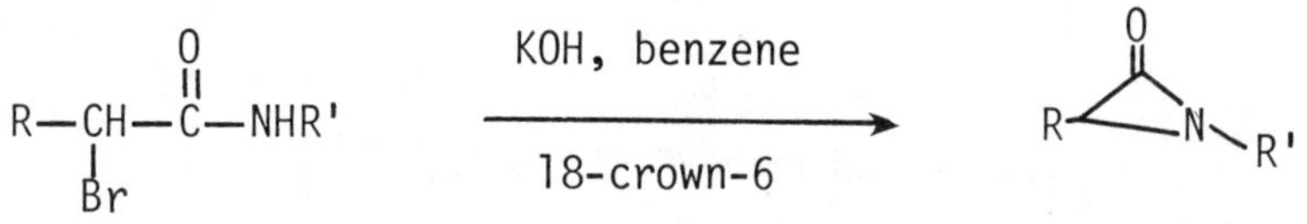

$$R-\underset{\underset{Br}{|}}{CH}-\overset{\overset{O}{\|}}{C}-NHR' \xrightarrow[\text{18-crown-6}]{\text{KOH, benzene}} R\overset{O}{\underset{}{\triangle}}N{-}R'$$

80-90%

R, R' = t-Butyl, 1-adamantyl

IV.D-2 M. A. McGuire and L. S. Hegedus, J. Am. Chem. Soc., 104, 5538 (1982).

$(CO)_5Cr=C\begin{smallmatrix}OMe\\R^1\end{smallmatrix}$ + $\begin{smallmatrix}R^2\\ \ \ \ C\\R^3-N\end{smallmatrix}\begin{smallmatrix}H\\ \ \end{smallmatrix}$ $\xrightarrow{h\nu}$ [β-lactam with R^1, OMe, R^2, R^3]

R^1 = Me, Ph
R^2 = Me, Ph, ⎰—S—CH$_2$
R^3 = Me, Ph, ⎱——CH$_2$

38-81%

IV.D-3 A. J. Biloski, R. D. Wood, and B. Ganem, J. Am. Chem. Soc., 104, 3233 (1982).

[alkene-NHSO$_2$R^1 starting material] $\xrightarrow[\text{2) Bu}_3\text{SnH}]{\text{1) X}_2\text{, NaHCO}_3}$ [β-lactam product]

(X = Br, I)

R^1 = H, alkoxy
R^2, R^3 = H, Me

IV.D-4 M. A. L. Santiago et al., Synthesis, 989 (1982).

$R^1-\overset{O}{\underset{\underset{R^1}{|}}{C}}-C=N-R^2$ $\xrightarrow[\text{or } R^3_{R^4}\!\!>C=C=O]{R^3_{R^4}\!\!>CH-\overset{O}{C}-Cl,\ Et_3N}$ [β-lactam product]

R^1 = Me, Ph
R^2 = Bz, subst. Ph
R^3 = Me, Cl, Ph
R^4 = H, Cl, Ph

40-85%

IV.D-5 M. S. Manhas et al., Synthesis, 407 (1982).

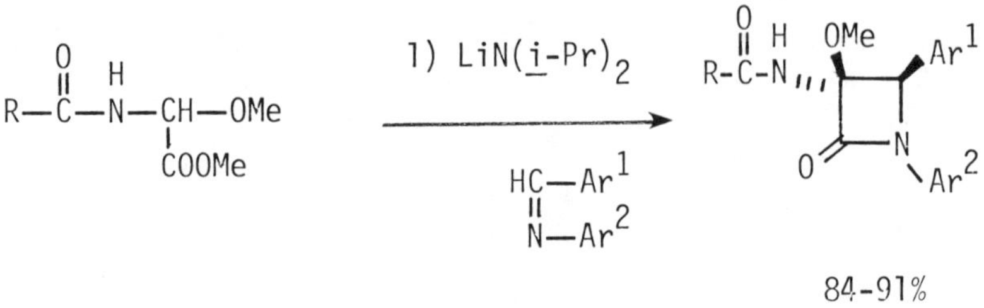

$$R-\underset{O}{\overset{\parallel}{C}}-N-\underset{\underset{COOMe}{|}}{\overset{H}{C}H}-OMe \quad \xrightarrow[\underset{N-Ar^2}{\overset{HC-Ar^1}{\parallel}}]{1)\ LiN(i\text{-}Pr)_2} \quad \text{β-lactam product}$$

84-91%

R = Ph, OBz
Ar's = Ph, α-naphthyl, —C₆H₄—Cl

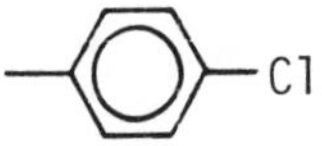

IV.D-6 N. Tokutake et al., Synthesis, 1053 (1982).

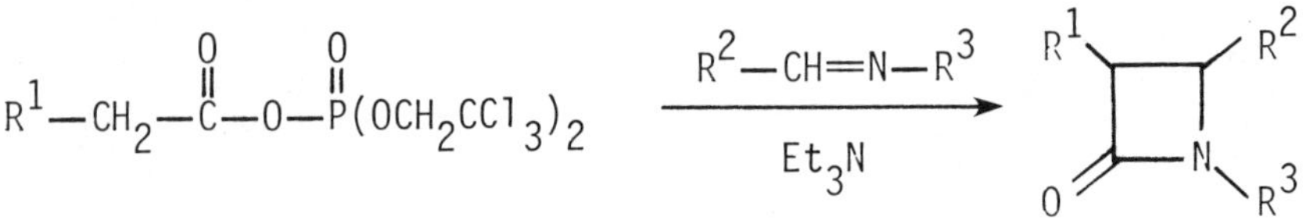

$$R^1-CH_2-\underset{O}{\overset{\parallel}{C}}-O-\underset{O}{\overset{\parallel}{P}}(OCH_2CCl_3)_2 \quad \xrightarrow[Et_3N]{R^2-CH=N-R^3} \quad \text{β-lactam}$$

43-59%

R^1 = OMe, OPh, phthalimide
R^2 = Ph, styryl
R^3 = Ph, Bz

IV.D-7 D. R. Shridhar et al., Synthesis, 63 (1982).

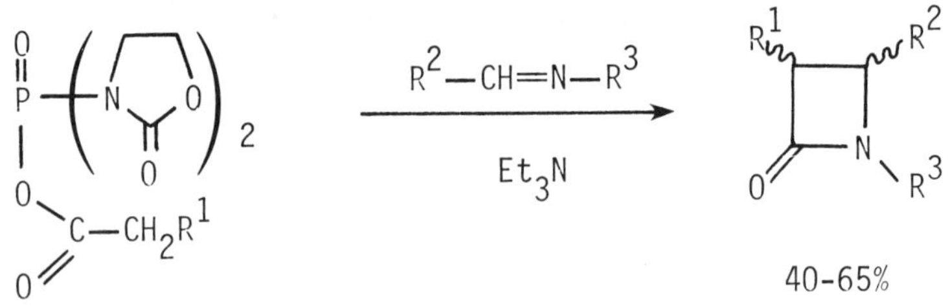

$$\xrightarrow[Et_3N]{R^2-CH=N-R^3}$$

40-65%

R's = subst. Ph, —OPh, —OBz

IV.D-8   T. Okawara et al., Chem. Pharm. Bull., 30, 1574 (1982).

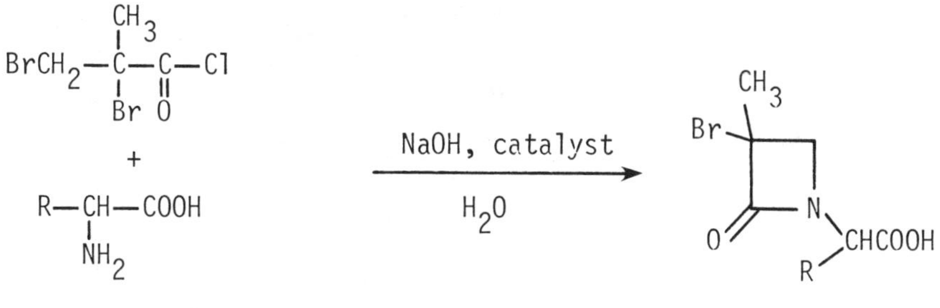

$BrCH_2-\underset{\underset{Br}{|}}{\overset{\overset{CH_3}{|}}{C}}-\underset{\overset{||}{O}}{C}-Cl$

+

$R-\underset{\underset{NH_2}{|}}{CH}-COOH$

$\xrightarrow[H_2O]{NaOH, catalyst}$

[β-lactam product with CH₃, Br substituents and N-CHCOOH-R group]

43-91%

IV.D-9   S. Torii et al., Bull. Soc. Chim. Belges, 91, 951 (1982).

Review: "Prominent Aspects of Electroorganic Synthesis in β-lactam Chemistry

---

IV.D-10   E. Schmitz and S. Schramm, J. Prakt. Chem., 324, 82 (1982).

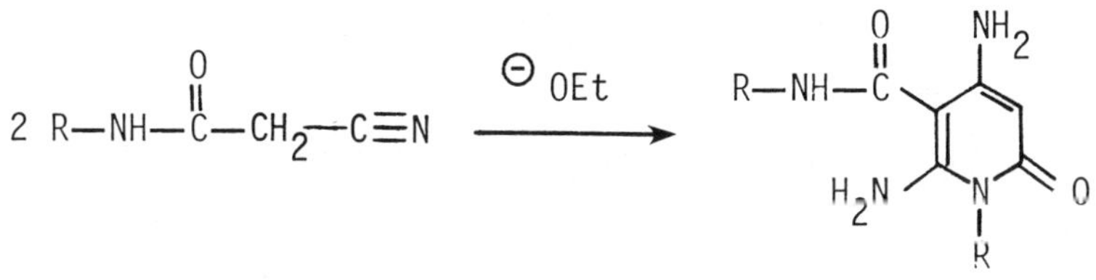

$2\ R-NH-\overset{\overset{O}{||}}{C}-CH_2-C\equiv N$ $\xrightarrow{\ominus OEt}$ [pyridinone product]

57%, R = Bz
71%, R = Bu

IV.D-11 L. Ghosez et al., J. Am. Chem. Soc., 104, 1428 (1982).

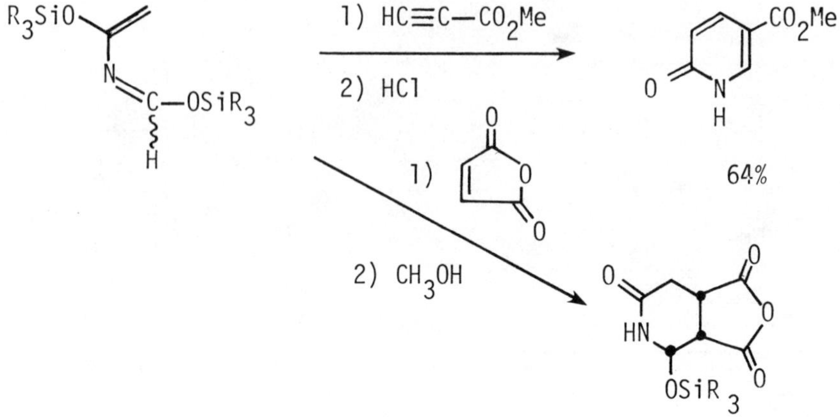

R_3Si = $\underline{t}$-$BuMe_2Si$

64%

82%

IV.D-12 G. S. Poindexter, J. Org. Chem., 47, 3787 (1982).

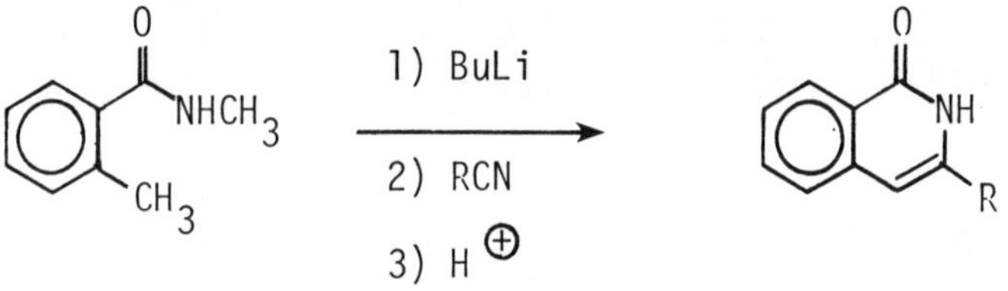

R = alkyl, subst. Ph, thienyl

42-87%

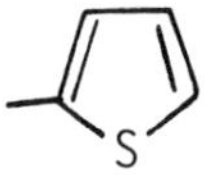

IV.D-13 T. Shono et al., Tetrahedron Lett., 23, 97 (1982).

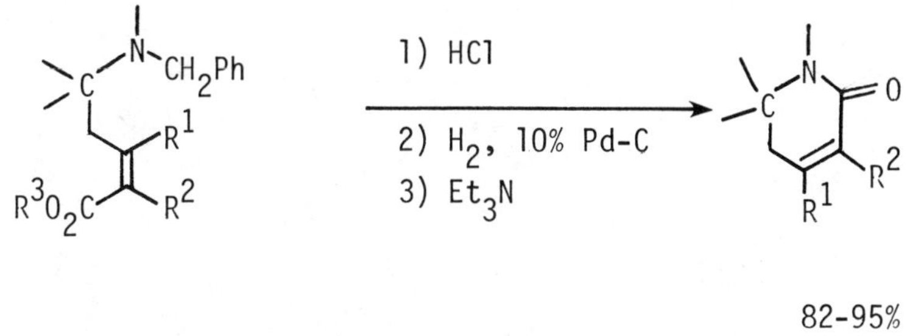

1) HCl
2) H$_2$, 10% Pd-C
3) Et$_3$N

82-95%

IV.D-14 R. Wälchli and M. Hesse, Helv. Chim. Acta, 65, 2299 (1982).

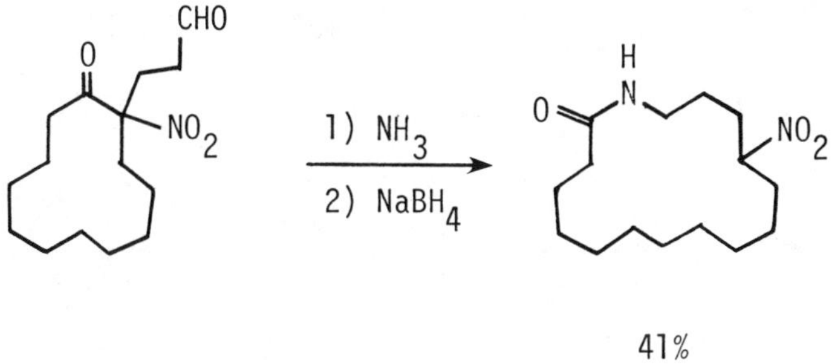

1) NH$_3$
2) NaBH$_4$

41%

IV.E. Lactones

IV.E-1   A. Takeda et al., Chem. Lett., 1909 (1982).

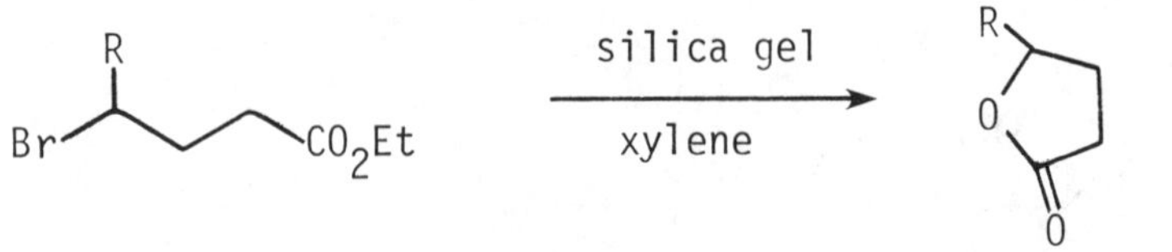

$$\text{Br-CHR-CH}_2\text{-CH}_2\text{-CO}_2\text{Et} \xrightarrow[\text{xylene}]{\text{silica gel}} \text{R-substituted } \gamma\text{-butyrolactone}$$

R = H, alkyl, etc.

∼50-80%

IV.E-2   P. T. Lansbury et al., Tetrahedron Lett., 23, 2623 and 2627 (1982).

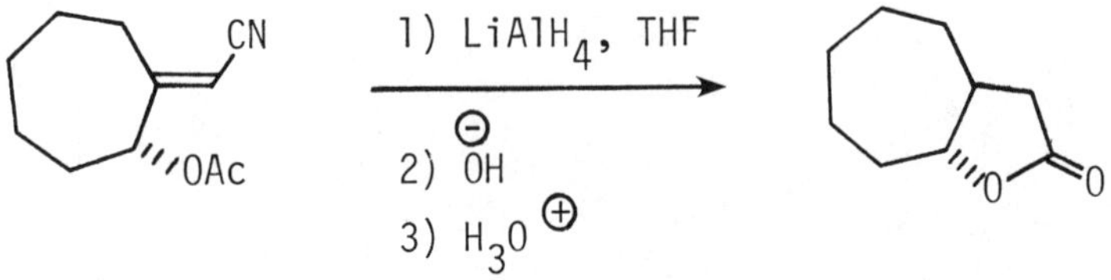

cycloheptane with =CHCN and ''''OAc substituents

1) LiAlH$_4$, THF
2) $\overset{\ominus}{\text{OH}}$
3) H$_3$O$^{\oplus}$

→ bicyclic lactone

∼70%

IV.E-3   L. Jalander and M. Broms, Acta Chem. Scand. B, 36, 371 (1982).

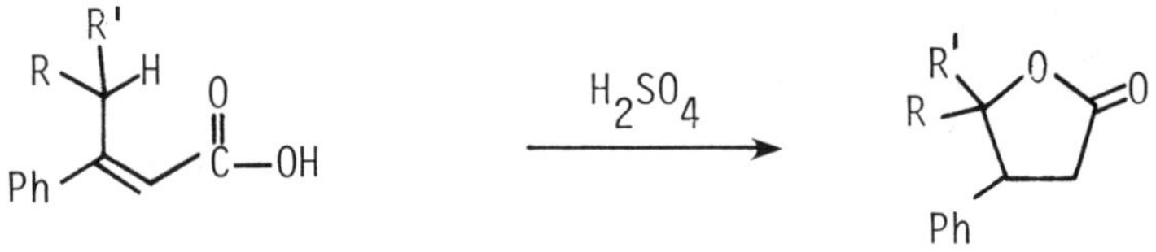

$$\text{R,R',H,Ph-substituted acrylic acid} \xrightarrow{\text{H}_2\text{SO}_4} \text{substituted } \gamma\text{-butyrolactone with Ph}$$

R = H, alkyl,
R' = alkyl,] cyclic

64-93%

IV.E-4   T. -L. Ho, Synth. Comm., 12, 53 (1982).

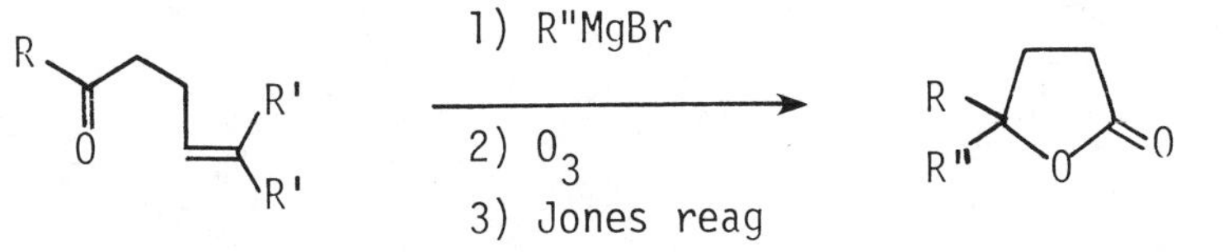

[Reaction scheme: R-C(=O)-CH2-CH2-C(R')=CHR' with 1) R"MgBr, 2) O3, 3) Jones reag → γ-butyrolactone with R, R" substituents]

R = H, Me
R' = H, Me
R" = n-alkyl

~60-75% overall

IV.E-5   J. B. Jones et al., J. Am. Chem. Soc., 104, 4659 (1982).

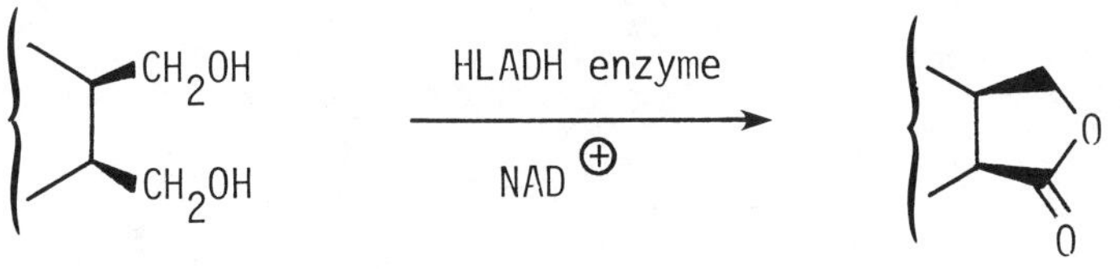

[Reaction scheme: bicyclic diol with two CH2OH groups → bicyclic lactone, using HLADH enzyme, NAD⊕]

68-90%
100% ee

IV.E-6   Y. Ito, H. Kato, and T. Saegusa, J. Org. Chem., 47, 741 (1982).

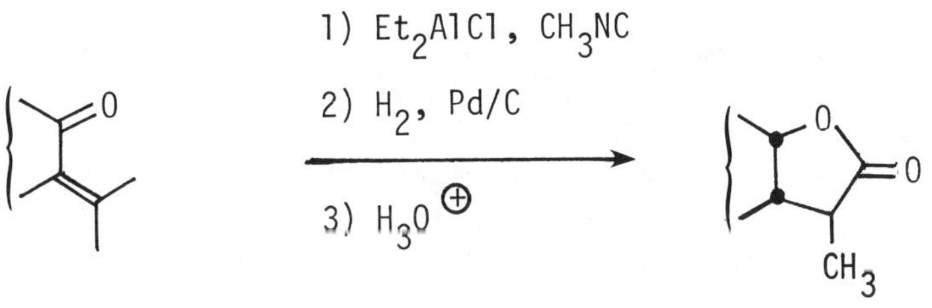

[Reaction scheme: α,β-unsaturated ketone → lactone with CH3, using 1) Et2AlCl, CH3NC, 2) H2, Pd/C, 3) H3O⊕]

IV.E-7   L. D. Martin and J. K. Stille, J. Org. Chem., 47, 3630 (1982).

$$\underset{R', OH}{\overset{R}{\underset{Br}{\diagup\!\!\!\!\diagdown}}} \xrightarrow[CH_3CN, K_2CO_3, 70^0]{Pd(Ph_3P)_4, CO} \text{(lactone product)}$$

R, R' = H, Me, Et

62-93%

IV.E-8   M. Okabe and M. Tada, J. Org. Chem., 47, 5382 (1982).

$$\underset{R'}{\overset{R}{\diagup}}CH-CHO \xrightarrow[\substack{3) \text{Cobaloxime, NaBH}_4 \\ 4) \text{CrO}_3, H^\oplus}]{\substack{1) Br_2 \\ 2) H^\oplus, HC\equiv C-CH_2OH, \\ (HC\equiv C-CH_2O)_3CH}} \text{(product)}$$

∼50% overall

IV.E-9   K. Tanaka, M. Terauchi, and A. Kaji, Chem. Lett., 351 (1982).

$$\underset{MeS}{\diagup}C=C\underset{O^\ominus}{\overset{O^\ominus}{\diagup}} \xrightarrow[\text{several steps}]{E^\oplus} \text{(product with E)}$$

$E^\oplus$ = alkyl halides, aldehydes

∼70% overall

IV.E-10 F. M. Araujo and J. Gore, <u>Tetrahedron</u>, <u>38</u>, 2897 (1982).

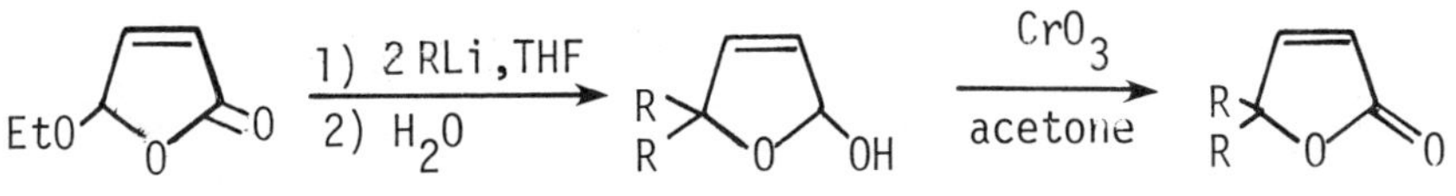

21-68% >90%

R = 1°, 2° alkyl, Ph

IV.E-11 A. Pelter, R. Al-Bayati, and W. Lewis, <u>Tetrahedron Lett.</u>, <u>23</u>, 353 (1982).

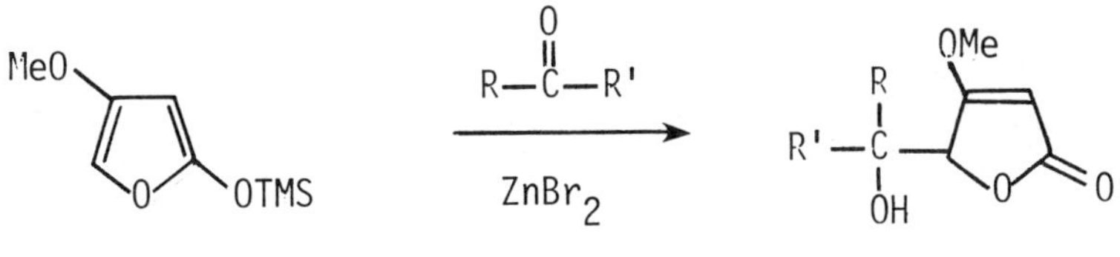

IV.E-12 F. Kido, Y. Noda, and A. Yoshikoshi, <u>J. Am. Chem. Soc.</u>, <u>104</u>, 5509 (1982).

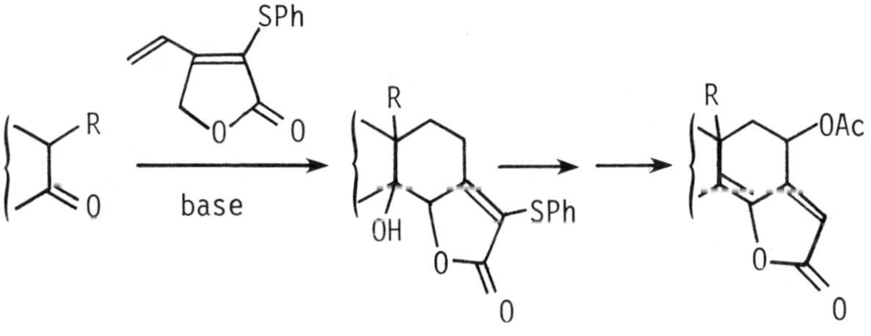

R = Me, CN, —COOEt 53-80%

IV.E-13   B. M. Trost and B. P. Coppola, J. Am. Chem. Soc., 104, 6879 (1982).

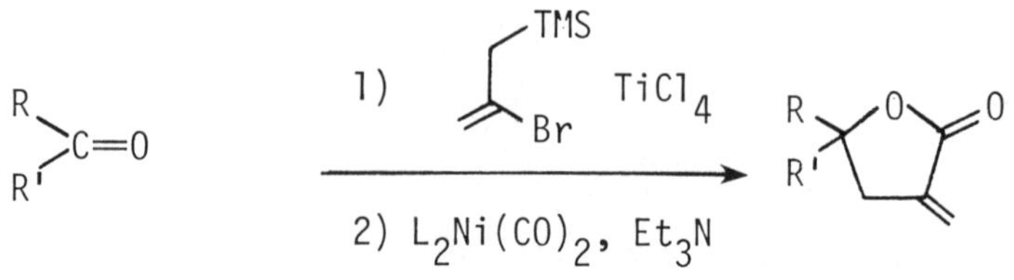

R, R' = H, alkyl, cyclic

~80% overall

IV.E-14   H. A. Khan and I. Paterson, Tetrahedron Lett., 23, 5083 (1982).

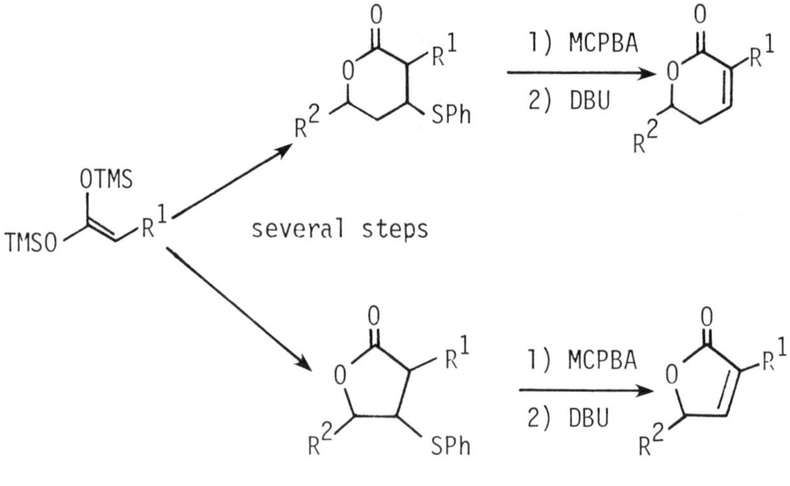

~70-80% overall

IV.E-15   R. C. Larock and C. A. Fellows, J. Am. Chem. Soc., 104, 1900 (1982).

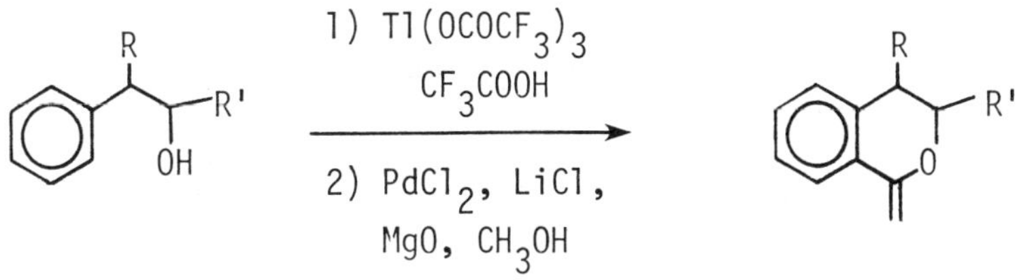

1) Tl(OCOCF$_3$)$_3$
   CF$_3$COOH
2) PdCl$_2$, LiCl, MgO, CH$_3$OH

R, R' = H, alkyl, cyclic

IV.E-16   P. Jarglis and F. W. Lichtenthaler, Tetrahedron Lett., 23, 3781 (1982).

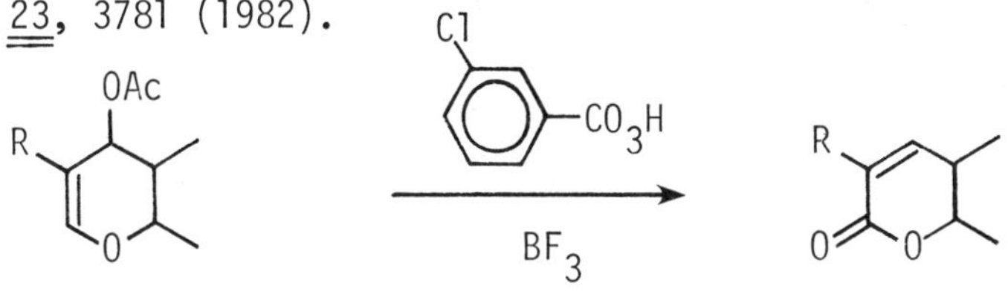

(glycal esters)

Reagent: m-Cl-C$_6$H$_4$-CO$_3$H, BF$_3$

IV.E-17   R. T. Taylor and R. A. Cassell, Synthesis, 672 (1982).

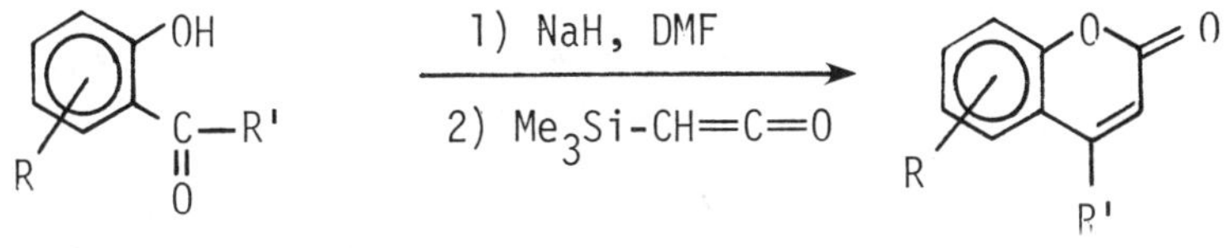

1) NaH, DMF
2) Me$_3$Si-CH=C=O

R = H, Cl, NO$_2$, OH, benzo—
R' = H, Me, Ph

60-98%

IV.E-18   M. Darbarwar and V. Sundarameurthy, Synthesis, 337 (1982).

Review: "Synthesis and Physiological Activity of Coumarins with 3:4-Fused Ring Systems"

IV.E-19   T. Fujisawa et al., Chem. Lett., 1891 (1982).

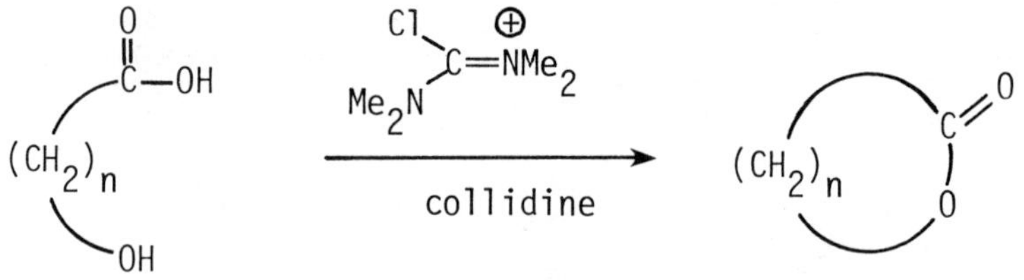

n = 11, 12, 14

54-90%

IV.E-20   K. Kostova et al., Helv. Chim. Acta, 65, 249 (1982).

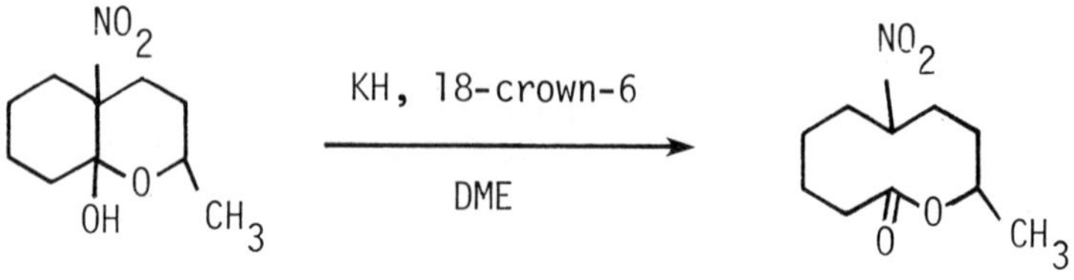

IV.E-21   M. Asaoka et al., Chem. Lett., 215 (1982).

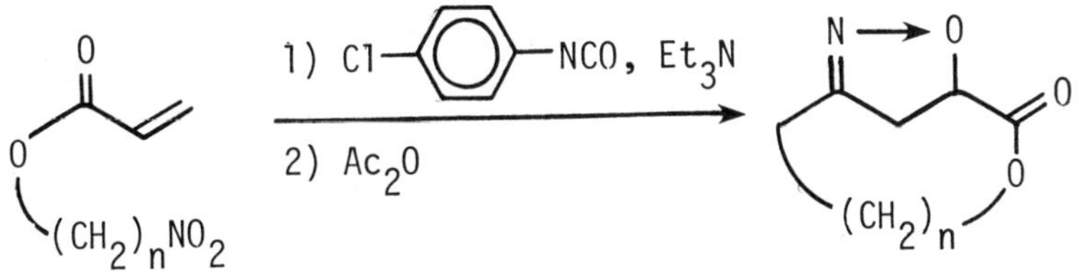

[Scheme: acrylate ester of $HO(CH_2)_n NO_2$ + 1) Cl–C$_6$H$_4$–NCO, Et$_3$N; 2) Ac$_2$O → bicyclic isoxazoline lactone with $(CH_2)_n$ tether]

widely varying yields

IV.F.   Pyridines, Quinolines, etc.

IV.F-1   M. Komatsu et al., Angew. Chem. Int. Ed., 21, 213 (1982).

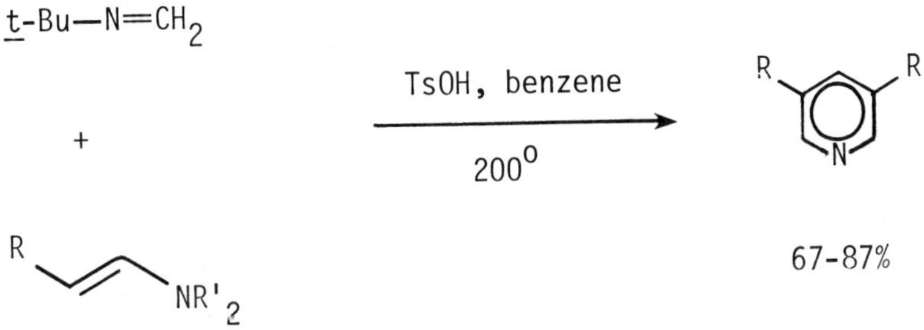

t-Bu—N=CH$_2$

+

R–CH=CH–NR'$_2$

$\xrightarrow{\text{TsOH, benzene}, 200°}$

3,5-R-disubstituted pyridine

67–87%

R = alkyl, cycloalkyl, Ph, PhS
NR'$_2$ = piperidino, morpholino, dimethylamino

IV.F-2 M. A. Tius et al., Tetrahedron Lett., 23, 2819 (1982).

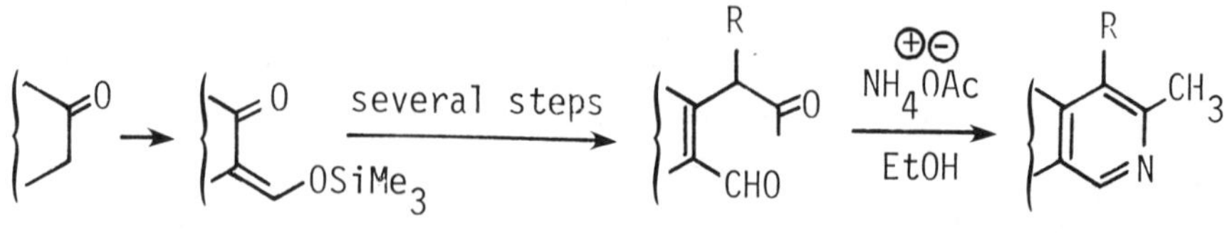

O
O
several steps
OSiMe3
R
O
CHO
NH4OAc
EtOH
R
CH3
N

49-98%
(R = H, Me)

IV.F-3 K. T. Potts, et al., J. Org. Chem., 47, 3027 (1982).

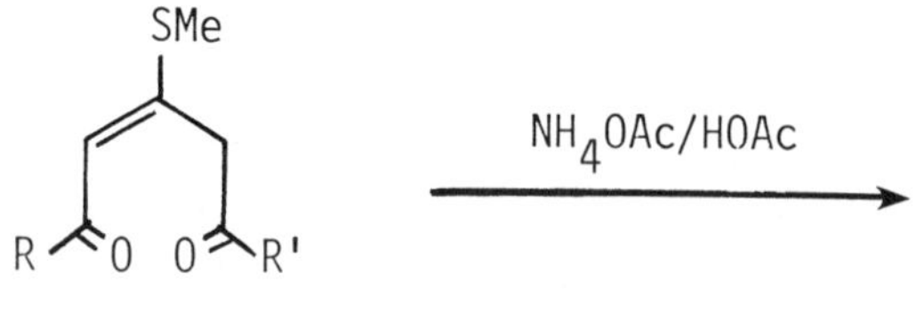

SMe
R
O
O
R'
NH4OAc/HOAc
SMe
R
N
R'

48-99%

R, R' = Me, Ph, thiophenyl, pyridyl, furyl

IV.F-4 K. Akiba, T. Kasai, and M. Wada, Tetrahedron Lett., 23, 1709 (1982).

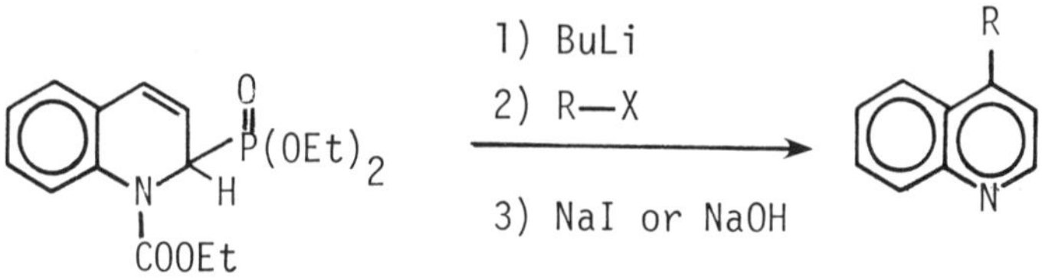

O
P(OEt)2
N
H
COOEt
1) BuLi
2) R—X
3) NaI or NaOH
R
N

67-93%

R = 1°, 2° alkyl, allyl, Bz

IV.F-5 S. M. M. Elshafie, Indian J. Chem., 21B, 586 (1982).

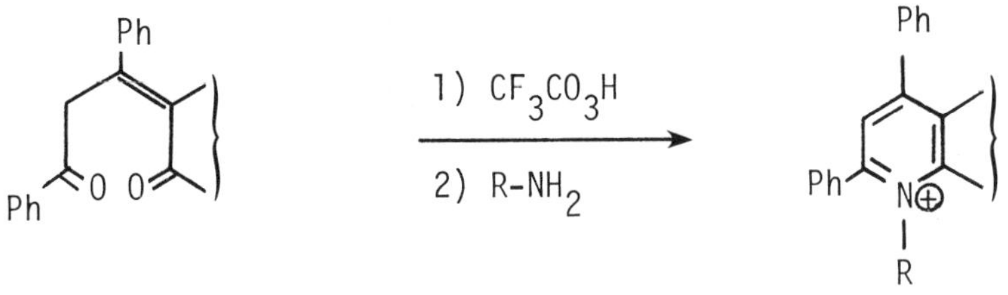

R = alkyl, aryl   45-96%

IV.F-6 D. L. Comins and A. H. Abdullah, J. Org. Chem., 47, 4315 (1982).

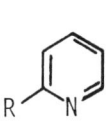

1) 5% CuI
2) EtOCOCl
3) R'MgX
4) S, Δ

R = H, Me
R' = alkyl, Ph

widely varying yields

IV.F-7 K. Akiba, Y. Iseki, and M. Wada, Tetrahedron Lett., 23, 429 (1982).

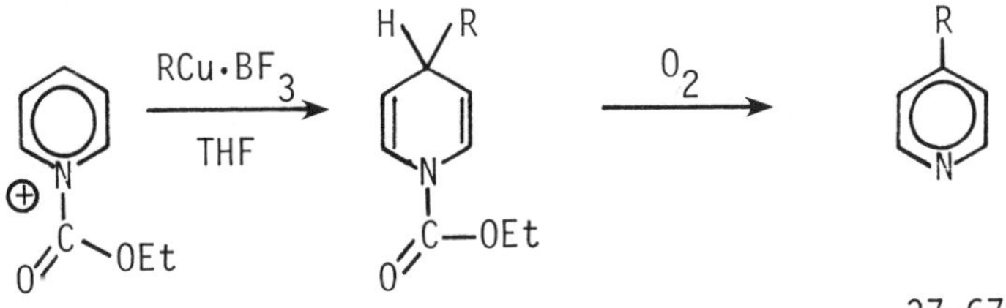

37-67%

R = alkyl, Ph

IV.F-8 K. Akiba, Y. Iseki, and M. Wada, Tetrahedron Lett., 23, 3935 (1982).

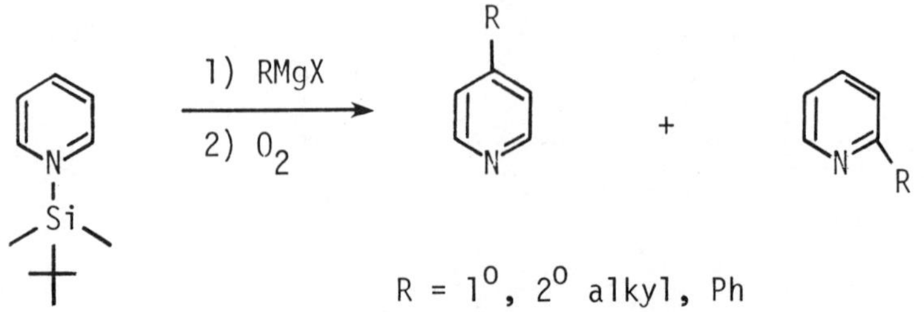

R = 1°, 2° alkyl, Ph

IV.F-9 G. Queguiner et al., Synthesis, 235 (1982).

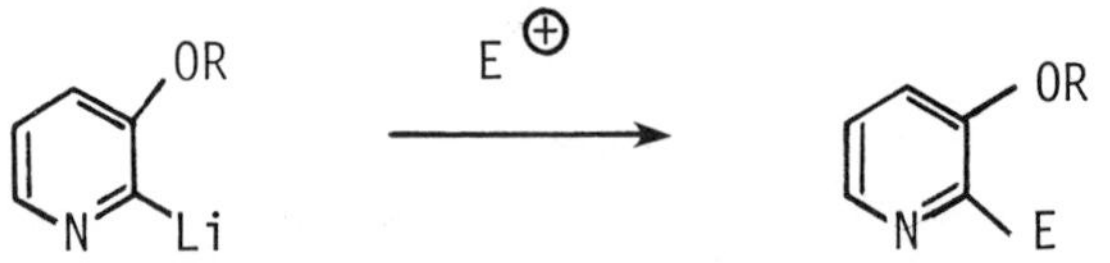

~50-80%

$$E^{\oplus} = R\text{-CHO}, \text{ClSiMe}_3, R\text{-}\underset{\underset{O}{\|}}{C}\text{-}R'$$

IV.F-10 A. I. Meyers and R. A. Gabel, J. Org. Chem., 47, 2634 (1982).

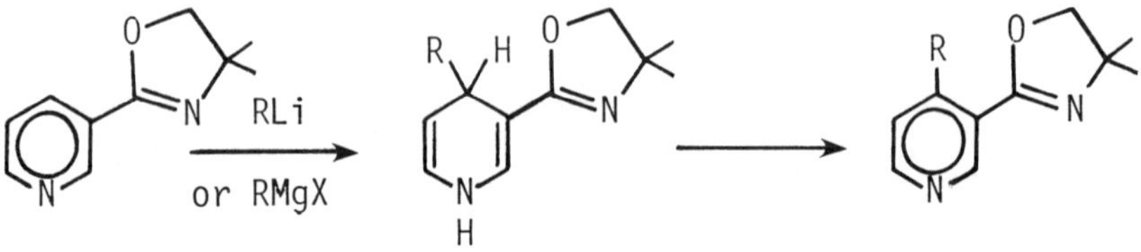

71-99%

R = alkyl, Ph, —CH$_2$C≡N

IV.F-11 D. D. Weller, G. R. Luellen, and D. L. Weller, J. Org. Chem., 47, 4803 (1982).

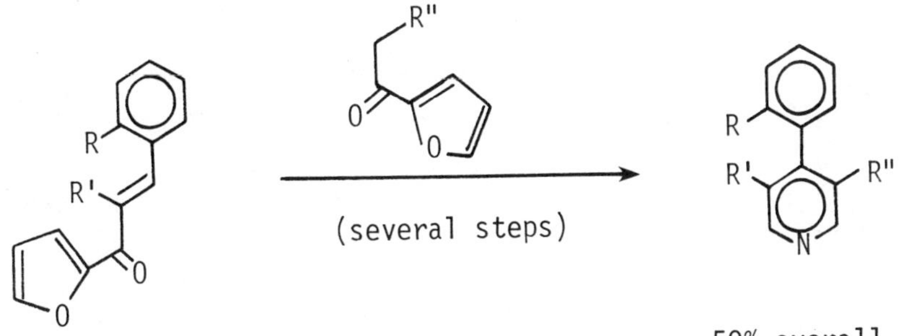

[Reaction scheme: cinnamoyl furan derivative (with substituents R, R') + acylfuran with R" substituent → (several steps) → pyridine product with substituents R, R', R" and ortho-phenyl/furyl groups, ~50% overall]

IV.F-12 W. Ando and H. Tsumaki, Synthesis, 263 (1982).

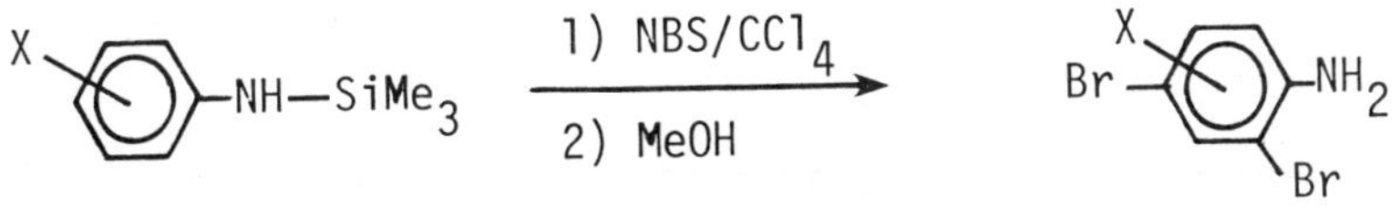

[Reaction: X-C$_6$H$_4$-NH-SiMe$_3$ → 1) NBS/CCl$_4$ 2) MeOH → 2,4-dibromoaniline derivative, 67-95%]

X = H

Monobrominated products are obtained if an _ortho_ or _para_ position is blocked, or if only one mole of NBS is used.

IV.F-13 C. -C. Cheng and S. -J. Yan, Org. React., 28, 37 (1982).

Review: "The Friedländer Synthesis of Quinolines"

IV.F-14 D. J. Hart and Y. -M. Tsai, J. Org. Chem., 47, 4403 (1982).

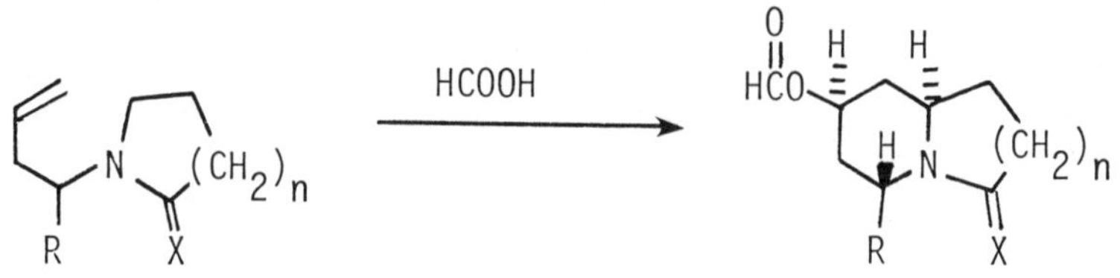

[Scheme: pyrrolidinone with allyl substituent + HCOOH → bicyclic formate ester product]

n = 1, 2
X = O, CHCO$_2$Et
R = alkyl, aryl

IV.F-15 D. M. Stout and A. I. Meyers, Chem. Rev., 82, 223 (1982).

Review: "Recent Advances in the Chemistry of Dihydropyridines"

IV.F-16 H. -P. Husson, Bull. Soc. Chim. Belges, 91, 985 (1982).

Review: "Dihydropyridine Equivalents as Intermediates for the Synthesis of Alkaloids"

IV.G. Pyrroles, etc.

IV.G-1 R. A. Jones et al., Synth. Comm., 12, 231 (1982).

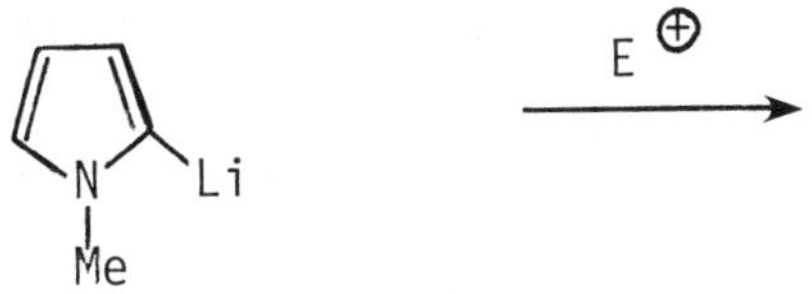

[Reaction: N-methyl-2-lithiopyrrole + E⊕ → N-methyl-2-E-pyrrole]

~60-90%

E = COOH
    COOEt
    COPh
    COMe
    CHO
    Me
    Et
    PhCH$_2$

IV.G-2 S. E. Korostova et al., J. Org. Chem. (USSR), 18, 460 (1982).

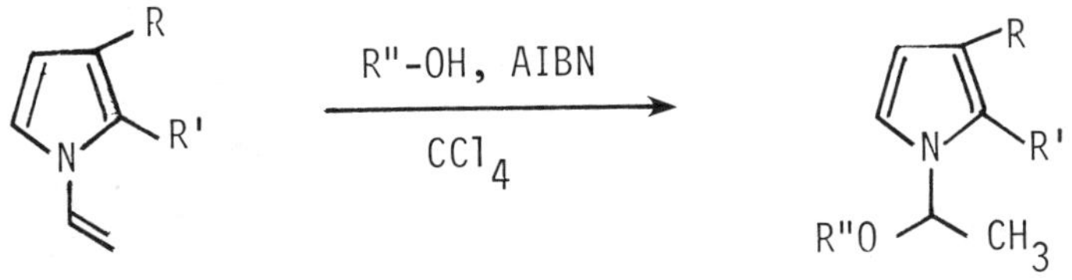

[Reaction: N-vinyl pyrrole with R, R' substituents + R"-OH, AIBN, CCl$_4$ → N-CH(OR")CH$_3$ pyrrole]

widely varying yields

R, R' = H, alkyl, aryl
R" = Et, Pr, i-Pr, propargyl

IV.G-3 F. Yuste and R. S. Obregón, J. Org. Chem., **47**, 3665 (1982).

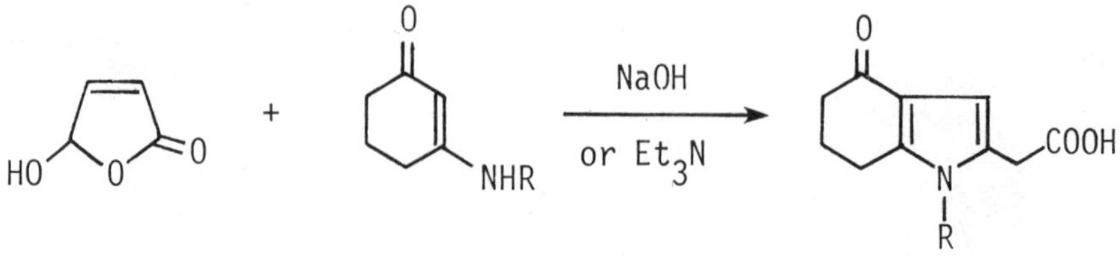

R = H, Bz

~60%

IV.G-4 L. S. Hegedus and J. M. McKearin, J. Am. Chem. Soc., **104**, 2444 (1982).

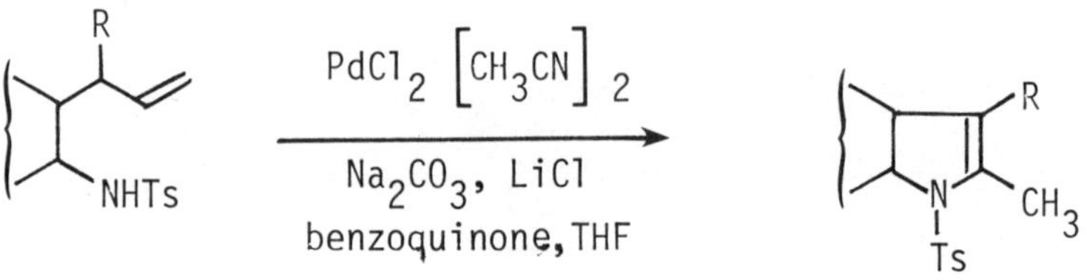

R = H, CH_3

~50-80%

IV.G-5 K. Achiwa and M. Sekiya, Tetrahedron Lett., **23**, 2589 (1982).

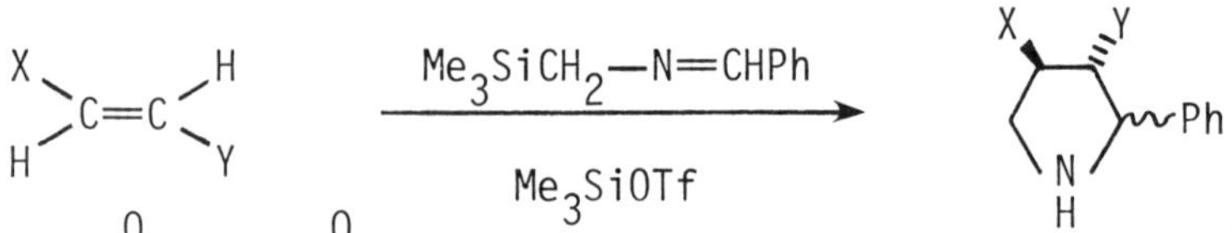

$$X = H, -\overset{O}{\underset{\|}{C}}-Me, -\overset{O}{\underset{\|}{C}}-OMe$$

$$Y = -\overset{O}{\underset{\|}{C}}-Me, -\overset{O}{\underset{\|}{C}}-OMe$$

83-92%

SYNTHESIS OF HETEROCYCLES

IV. H. Other Heterocycles with One Heteroatom

(see also: II.F.1, VI.A.9.)

IV.H-1   Z. M. Ismail and H. M. R. Hoffman, *Angew. Chem. Int. Ed.*, **21**, 859 (1982).

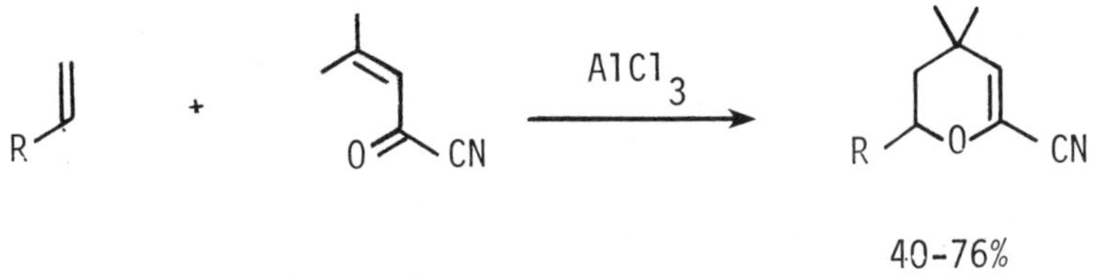

$$R-CH=CH_2 \;+\; \text{(dimethylacryloyl cyanide)} \xrightarrow{AlCl_3} \text{dihydropyran product}$$

40-76%

R = -O-i-Pr, -CH$_2$TMS, Ph, -CH=CHMe

IV.H-2   E. Fujita *et al.*, *J.C.S. Chem. Comm.*, 1108 (1982).

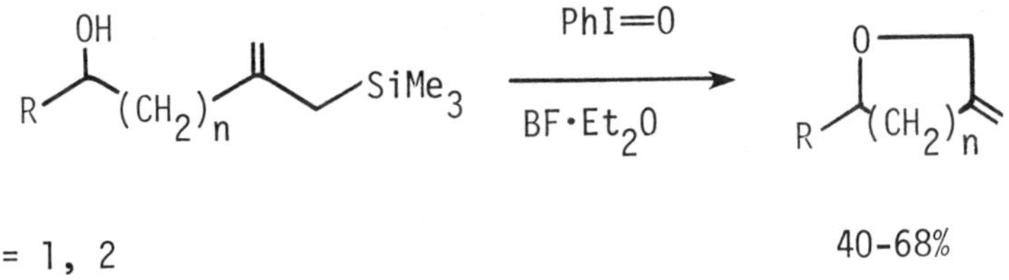

$$\underset{OH}{R-CH}-(CH_2)_n-C(=CH_2)-CH_2-SiMe_3 \xrightarrow[BF \cdot Et_2O]{PhI=O} \text{cyclic ether product}$$

n = 1, 2
R = 1° alkyl

40-68%

IV.H-3   H. -J. Kabbe and A. Widdig, *Angew. Chem. Int. Ed.*, **21**, 247 (1982).

Review: "Synthesis and Reactions of 4-Chromanones"

IV.H-4   W. T. Brady and M. O. Agho, Synthesis, 500 (1982).

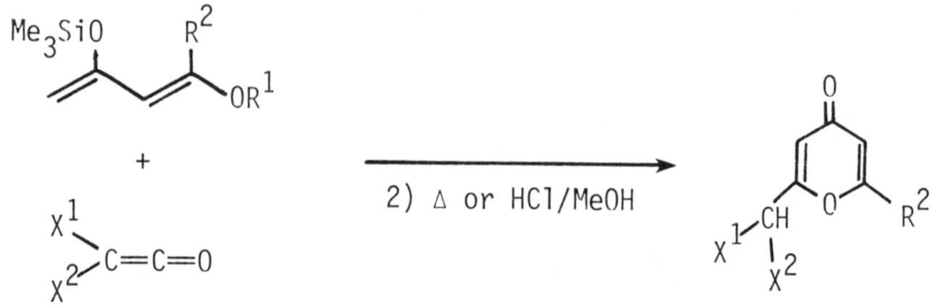

R^1 = Me, SiMe$_3$
R^2 = H, Me
X^1, X^2 = H, Cl, Ph

48-70%

IV.H-5   S. Murata and R. Noyori, Tetrahedron Lett., 23, 2601 (1982).

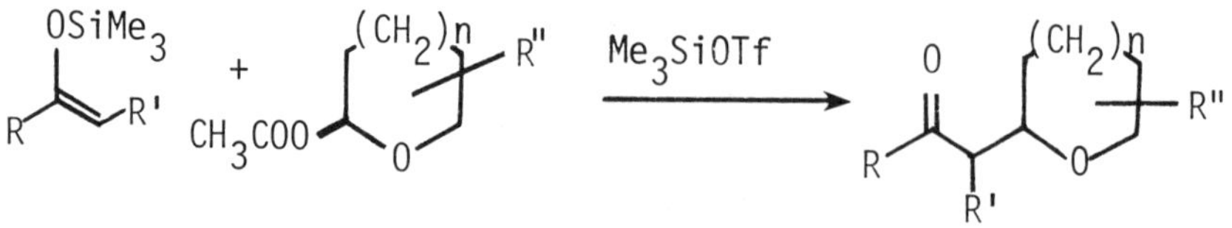

R = H, Ph, alkyl, thioalkyl
R' = H, Me
n = 0, 1

78-96%

IV.H-6 P. H. Lambert, M. Vaultier, and R. Carrié, J.C.S. Chem. Comm., 1224 (1982).

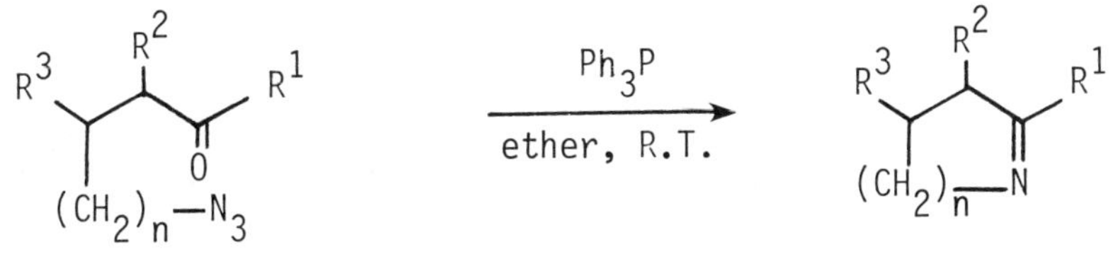

$$R^3\text{-CH}(CH_2)_n\text{-}N_3\text{-CHR}^2\text{-C(O)}R^1 \xrightarrow{Ph_3P, \text{ ether, R.T.}} \text{cyclic imine}$$

60-92%

n = 1, 2, 3
R^1 = Me, p-BrPh
R^2 = H, Me, Et
R^3 = H, SPh

IV.H-7 D. R. Shridhar et al., Synthesis, 1061 (1982).

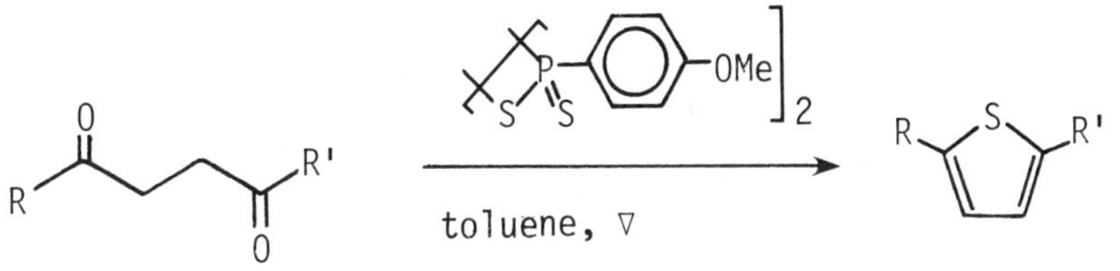

$$R\text{-C(O)-CH}_2\text{CH}_2\text{-C(O)-}R' \xrightarrow{[\text{Ar-P(S)S}]_2, \text{ toluene, }\nabla} \text{2,5-disubstituted thiophene}$$

62-98%

R, R' = Me, subst. Ph

IV.H-8 E. Vedejs, T. H. Eberlein, and D. L. Varie, J. Am. Chem. Soc., 104, 1445 (1982).

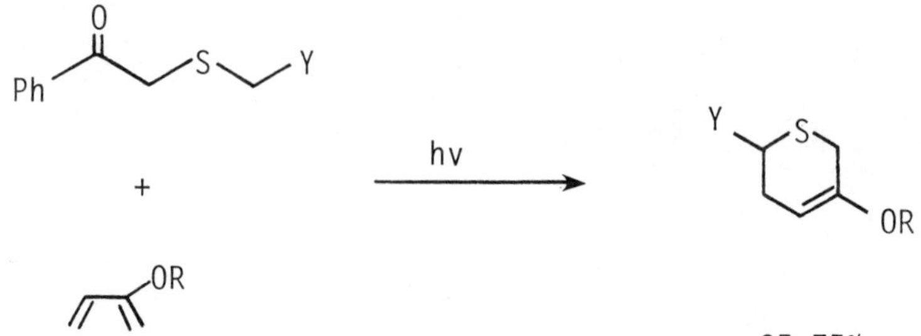

∿35-75%

Y = —C≡N, —C(=O)—R, —C(=O)—OR

R = Et, t-$BuMe_2Si$

IV.H-9 D. N. Reinhoudt, Rec. Trav. Chim. Pays-Bas, 101, 277 (1982).

Review: "Thiepins and Benzothiepins: The Conquest of Elusive Sulfur Heterocycles"

IV.I. Heterocycles with Two or More Heteroatoms

1.a. 5-Membered Heterocycles with 2 N's

IV.I.1.a-1   R. P. Soni, Aust. J. Chem., 35, 1493 (1982).

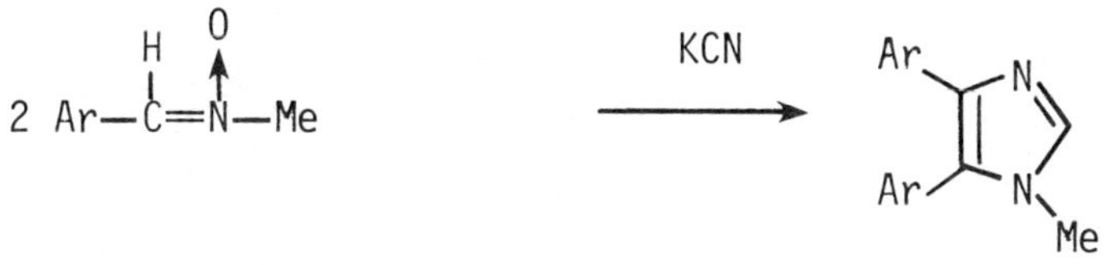

$$2\ Ar-\overset{H}{\underset{\|}{C}}=\overset{O}{\overset{\uparrow}{N}}-Me \xrightarrow{KCN} \text{imidazole}$$

Ar = subst. Ph, naphthyl, pyridyl

37-72%

IV.I.1.a-2   M. Casey, C. J. Moody, and C. W. Rees, J.C.S. Chem. Comm., 714 (1982).

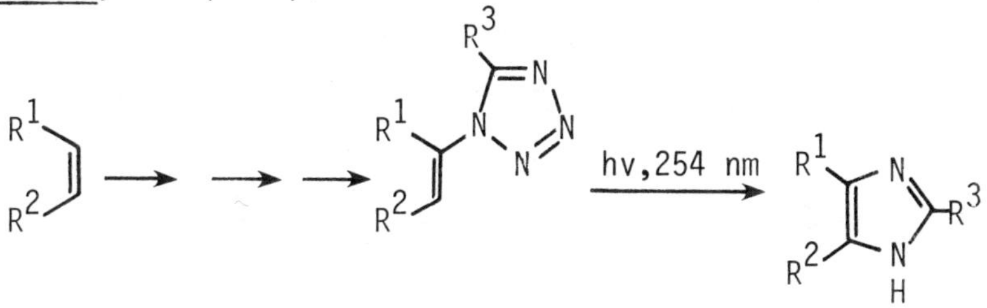

R^1 = H, Ph,
R^2 = H, Me, Ph,] $(CH_2)_4$
R^3 = H, Me, Ph

32-73% (last step)

IV.I.1.a-3   R. L. Webb and C. S. Labaw, J. Het. Chem., 19, 1205 (1982).

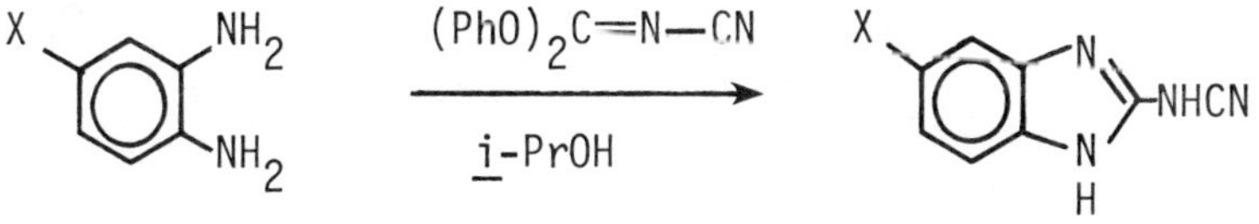

reagent: $(PhO)_2C=N-CN$, i-PrOH

X = H, Cl

88-92%

IV.I.1.a-4   M. P. Mahajan et al., Can. J. Chem., 60, 1122 (1982).

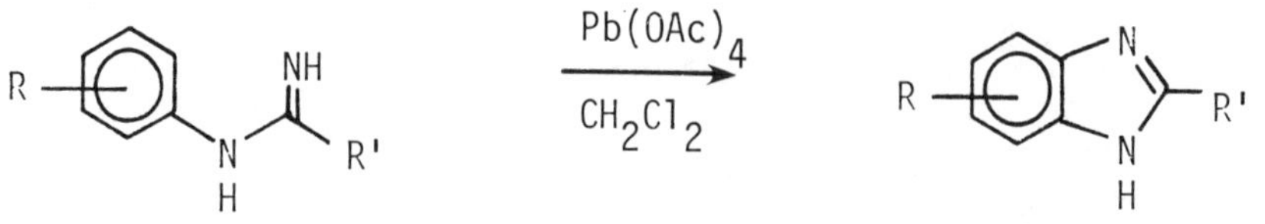

[Reaction: R-substituted phenyl amidine + Pb(OAc)$_4$ / CH$_2$Cl$_2$ → 2-R'-benzimidazole]

R = H, Cl
R' = Ph, Bz

77-98%

IV.I.1.a-5   H. C. Ooi and H. Suschitzky, J.C.S. Perkin I, 2871 (1982).

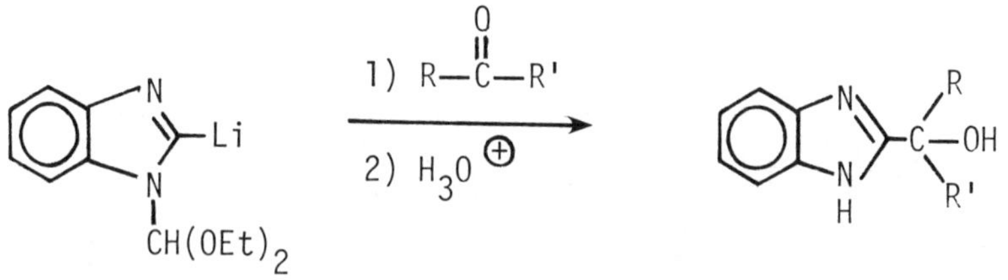

[Reaction: 2-lithio-1-(CH(OEt)$_2$)benzimidazole + 1) R–C(O)–R'; 2) H$_3$O$^\oplus$ → 2-(C(R)(R')OH)benzimidazole]

R, R' = H, Ph, alkyl, heterocyclic

widely varying yields

IV.I.1.a-6   P. Plath and W. Rohr, Synthesis, 318 (1982).

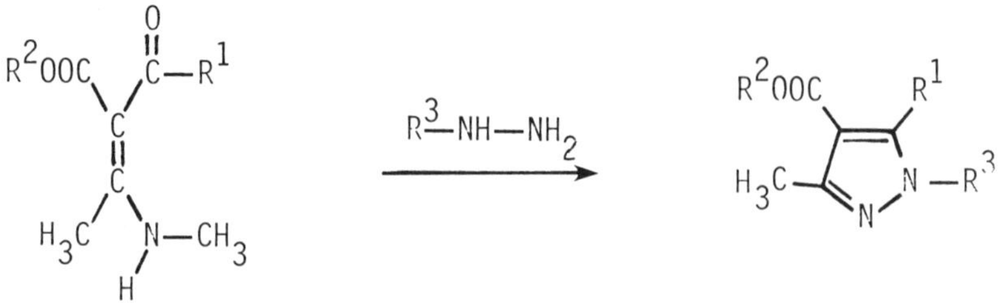

[Reaction: R^{2}OOC-C(=C(N(CH$_3$)H)CH$_3$)-C(O)-R^1 + R^3-NH-NH$_2$ → pyrazole with R^{2}OOC, R^1, H$_3$C, N-R^3 substituents]

R^1 = subst. Ph, heterocyclic
R^2 = Me, Et, i-Pr
R^3 = H, Me

7-91%

IV.I.1.a-7 G. Seitz et al., Angew. Chem. Int. Ed., 21, 284 (1982).

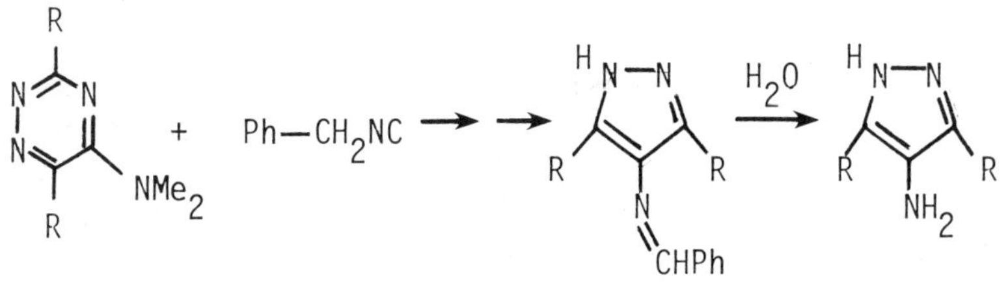

R = $-CO_2CH_3$, Ph, CF_3

~70%

IV.I.1.a-8 K. Takada, T. K. Woon, and A. J. Boulton, J. Org. Chem., 47, 4323 (1982).

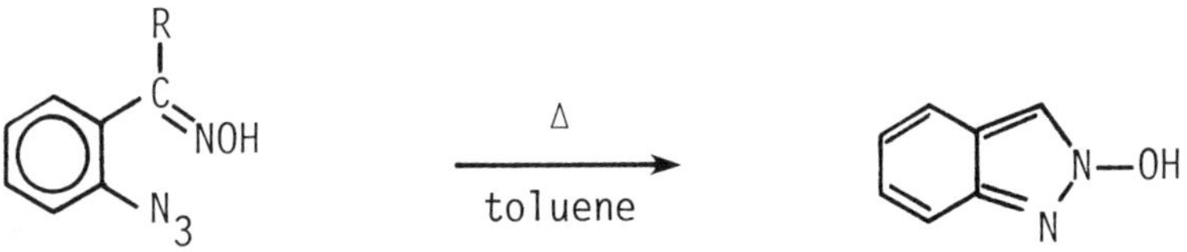

R = Me, Ph

60%

IV.I.1.a-9/IV.I.1.b-1 H. Ila et al., Synthesis, 792 (1982).

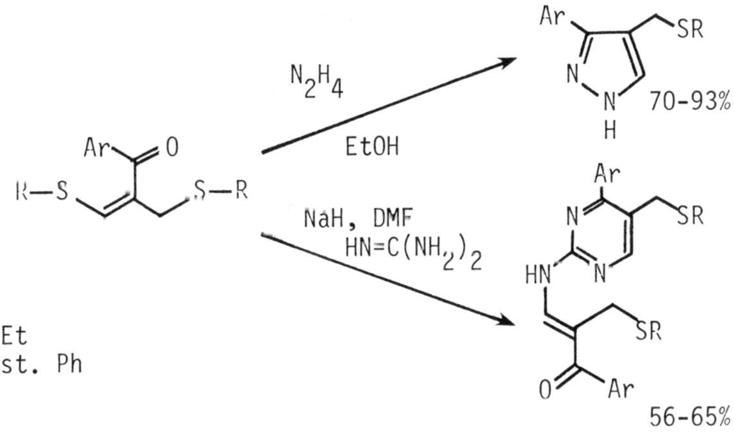

R = Me, Et
Ar = subst. Ph

70-93%

56-65%

IV.I.1.b. 6-Membered Heterocycles with 2 N's

(see also: VI.A.15.)

IV.I.1.b-2 M. H. Elnagdi et al., J.C.S. Perkin I, 2667 (1982).

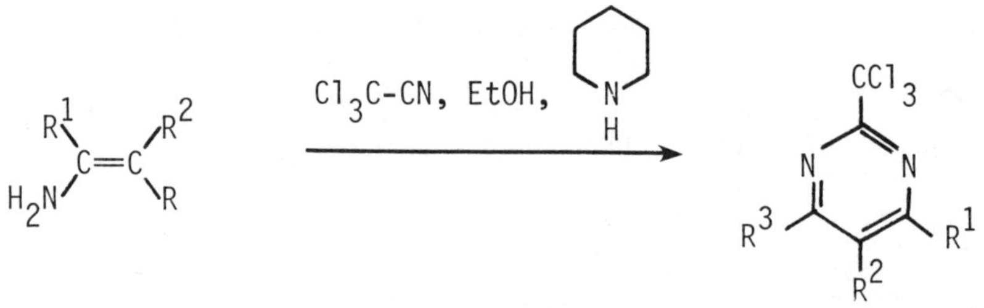

R, R^2 = CN, COOEt
R^1 = CH_2CN, CCl_3, COOEt

55-95%

R^3 = NH_2, OH

IV.I.1.b-3 D. L. Boger et al., J. Org. Chem., 47, 2673 (1982).

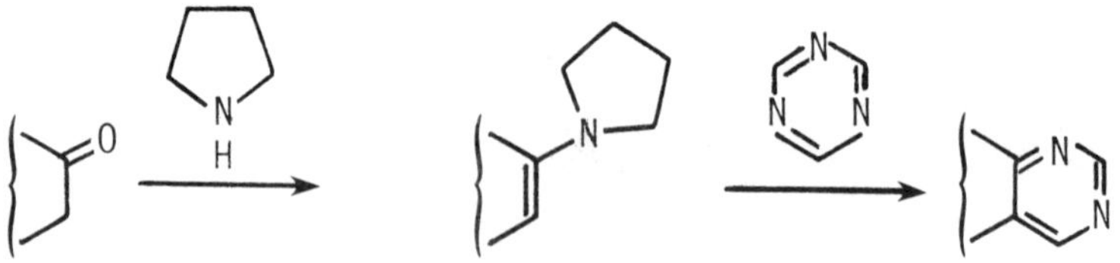

50-80%

IV.I.1.b-4 K. -D. Kampe, Angew. Chem. Int. Ed., 21, 540 (1982).

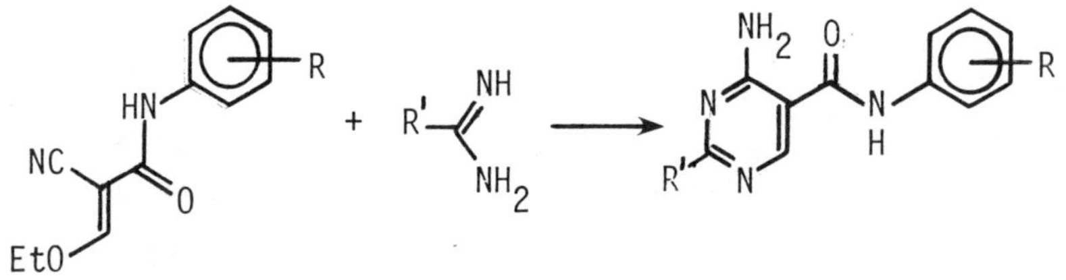

R = Cl, CF_3
R' = H, Ph, $-NR_2$, $-NH-\overset{O}{\underset{\|}{C}}-R$

45-93%

IV.I.1.c. Other Heterocycles with 2 N's

IV.I.1.c-1 T. Tsuchiya et al., Chem. Pharm. Bull., 30, 3757 and 3764 (1982).

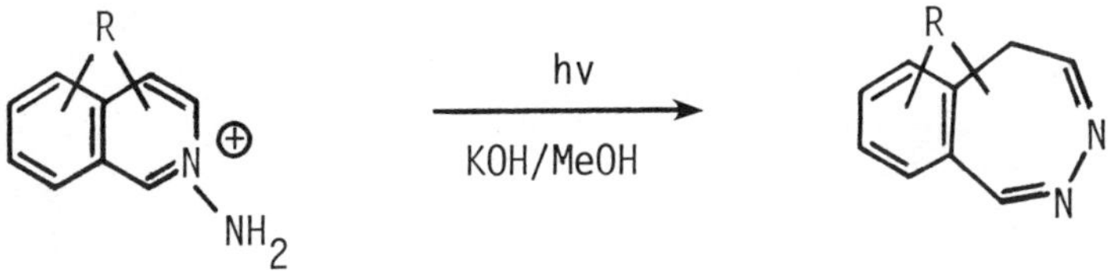

25-60%

R = H, Me, OMe

IV.I.1.c-2/IV.I.2-1   W. Müller and U. Stauss, Helv. Chim. Acta, 65, 2118 (1982).

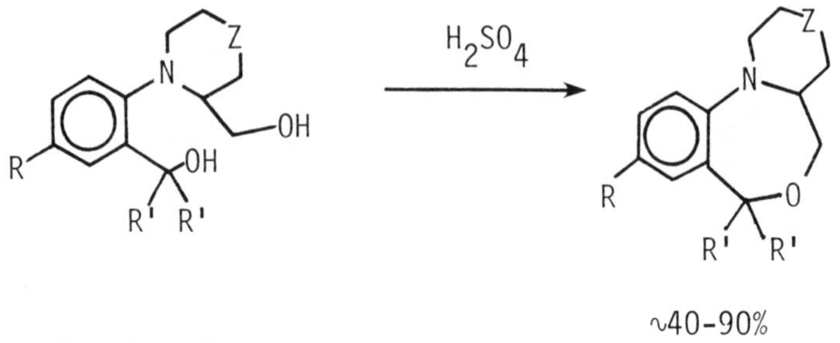

R = H, Cl, NO_2, NH_2
R' = H, Me, Ph
Z = NMe, CH_2

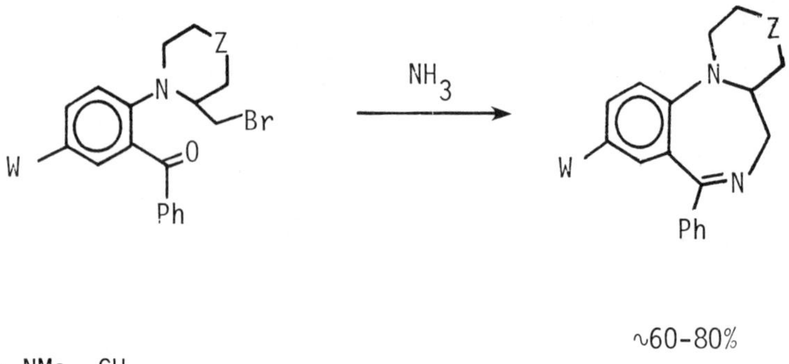

~40-90%

Z = NMe, CH_2
W = $-NO_2$, $-SO_2Me$

~60-80%

IV.I.2.   Heterocycles with 1 N and 1 O

IV.I.2-2 P. G. Gassman and T. L. Guggenheim, J. Am. Chem. Soc., 104, 5849 (1982).

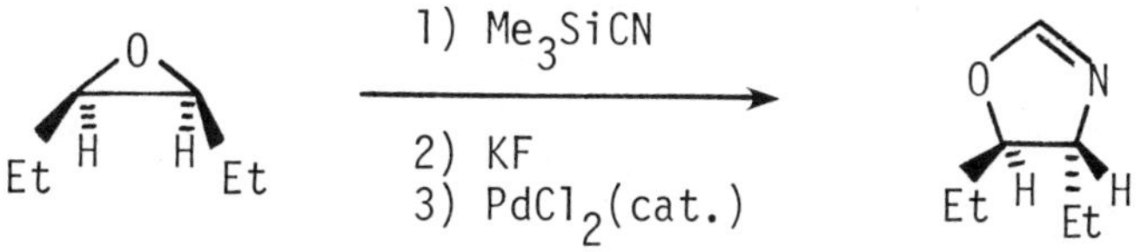
1) Me_3SiCN
2) KF
3) $PdCl_2$(cat.)
Et
H
O
N

49% overall

IV.I.2-3 R. L. Webb and C. S. Labaw, J. Het. Chem., 19, 1205 (1982).

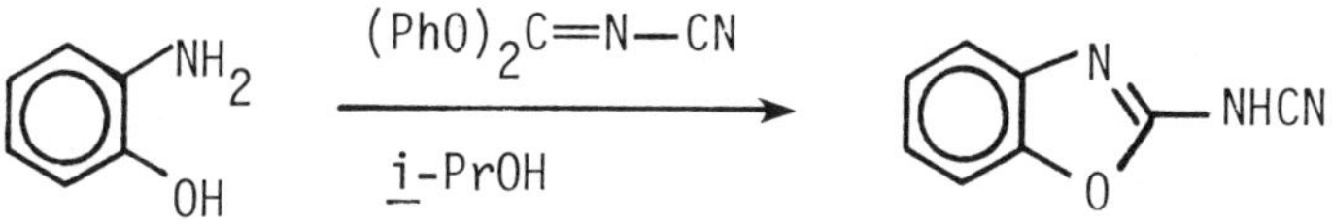
NH_2
OH
$(PhO)_2C=N-CN$
i-PrOH
N
O
NHCN

74%

IV.I.2-4 L. N. Pridgen, J. Org. Chem., 47, 4319 (1982).

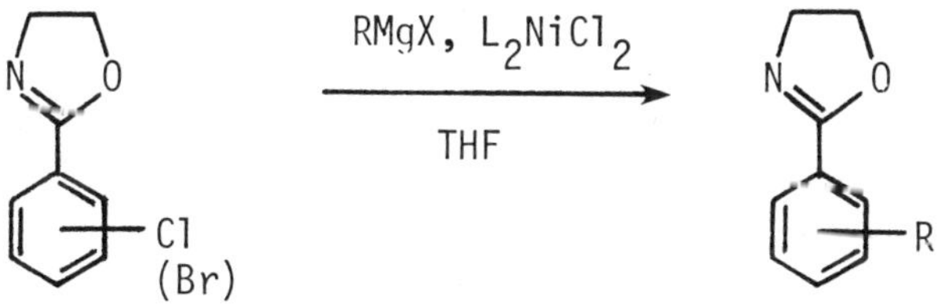
RMgX, L_2NiCl_2
THF
N
O
Cl
(Br)
R

56-95%

R = alkyl, Bz, subst. Ph

IV.I.2-5   Y. Kanaoka et al., Synthesis, 484 (1982).

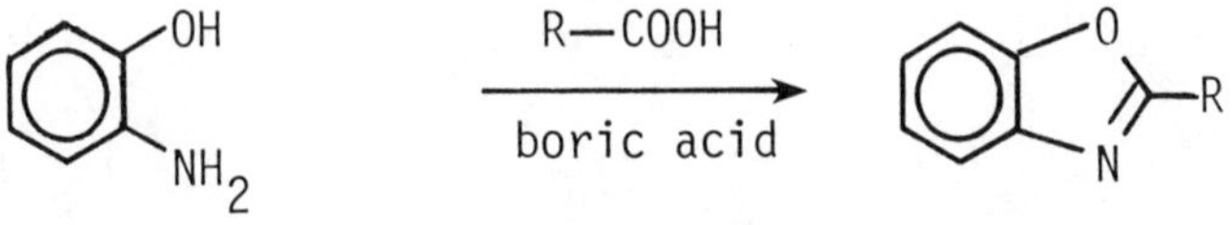

R = alkyl, styryl, subst. Ph, heterocyclic   34-68%

IV.I.2-6   S. Fujita et al., Synthesis, 68 (1982).

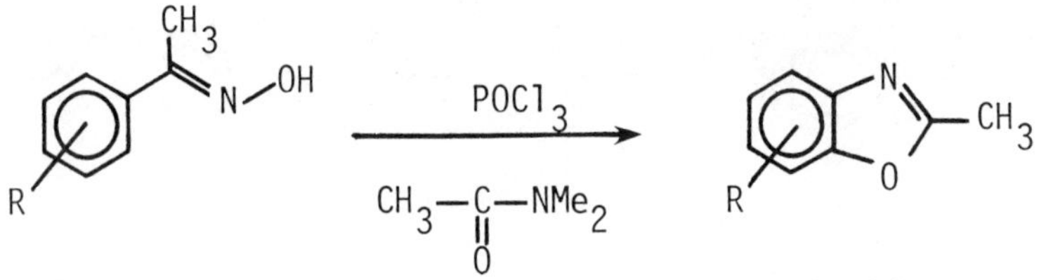

62-92%

R = alkyl, OH, alkoxy

IV.I.2-7   G. Prasad and K. N. Mehrotra, J. Org. Chem., 47, 2806 (1982).

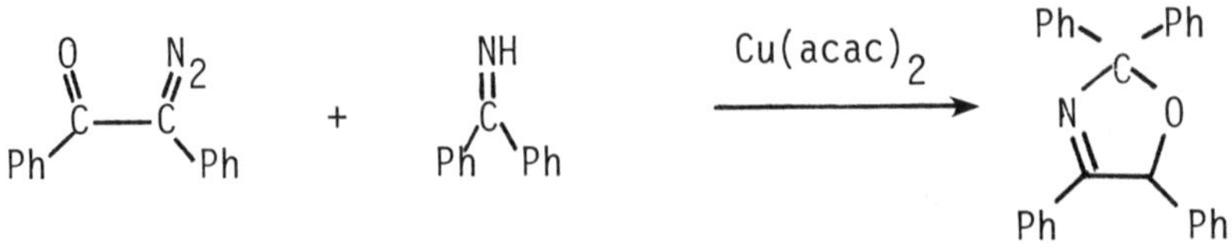

36%

IV.I.2-8   C. Kashima et al., Chem. Lett., 1455 (1982).

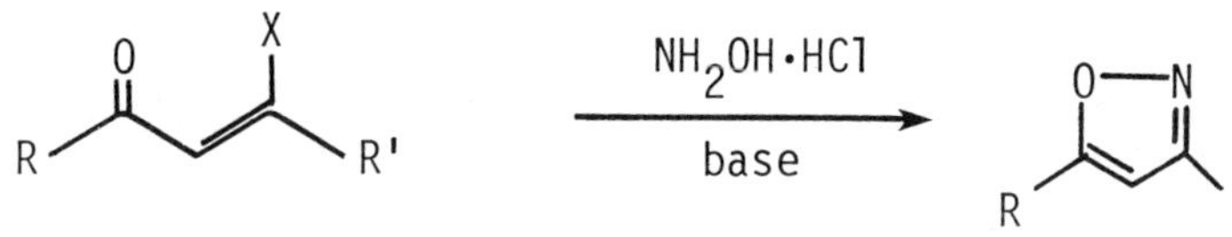

R, R' = alkyl, Ph
X = alkoxy, aryloxy, SR, NHR, etc.

∼50-80%

IV.I.2-9   A. P. Kozikowski and A. K. Ghosh, J. Am. Chem. Soc., 104, 5788 (1982).

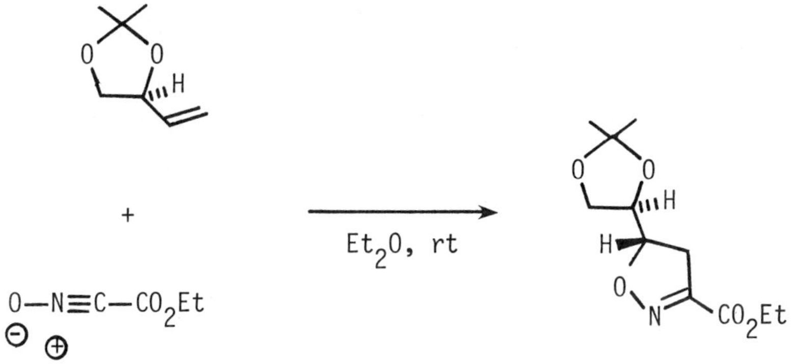

IV.I.2-10   K. Yordanova et al., Chem. Ber., 115, 2635 (1982).

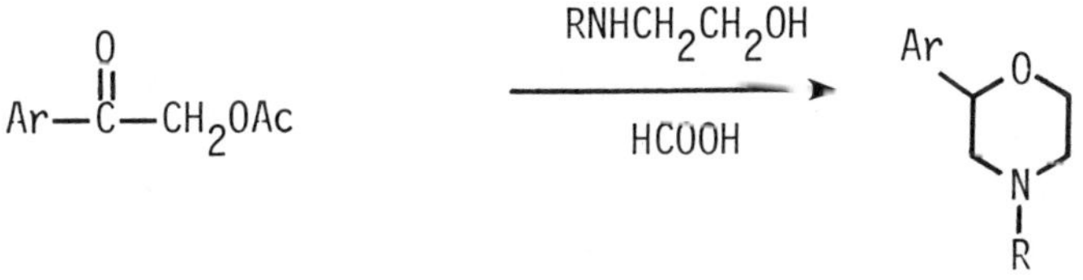

Ar = subst. Ph
R = alkyl, Bz

∼50-70%

IV.I.2-11   T. Kametani et al., Tetrahedron, 38, 2489 (1982).

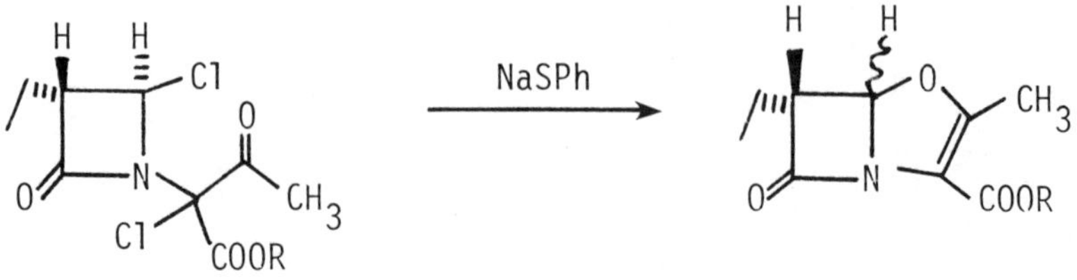

R = Me, PNB

~80-90%

IV.I.3. Heterocycles with 1 N and 1 S

IV.I.3-1   G. Purrello et al., Synth. Comm., 12, 865 (1982).

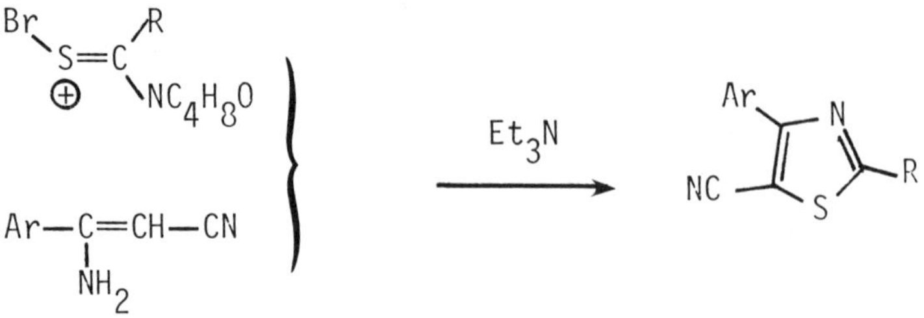

R = alkyl, subst. Ph
Ar = subst. Ph

58-69%

IV.I.3-2   T. Papenfuhs, *Angew. Chem. Int. Ed.*, **21**, 541 (1982).

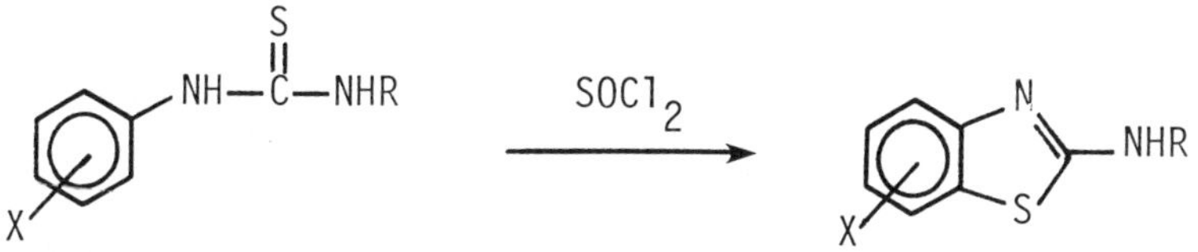

X = H, Me, OEt
R = H, Me, Ph, c-Hex

86-99%

IV.I.3-3   M. Ngounda, H. LeBozec, and P. Dixneuf, *J. Org. Chem.*, **47**, 4000 (1982).

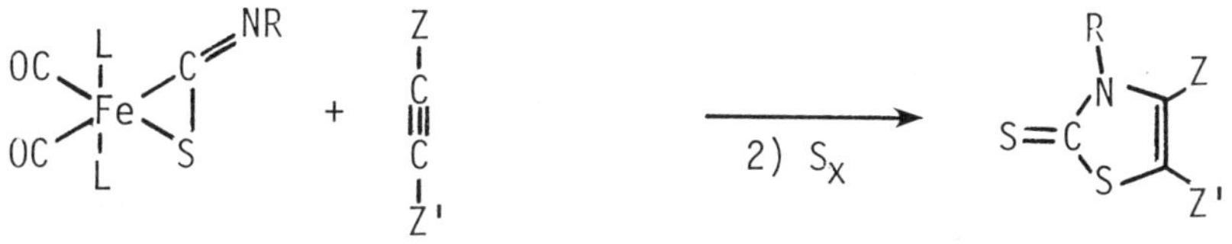

Z = -COOR, Ph
Z' = -COOR, CHO

18-32%

IV.I.3-4   J. E. Arrowsmith and C. W. Greengrass, *Tetrahedron Lett.*, **23**, 357 (1982).

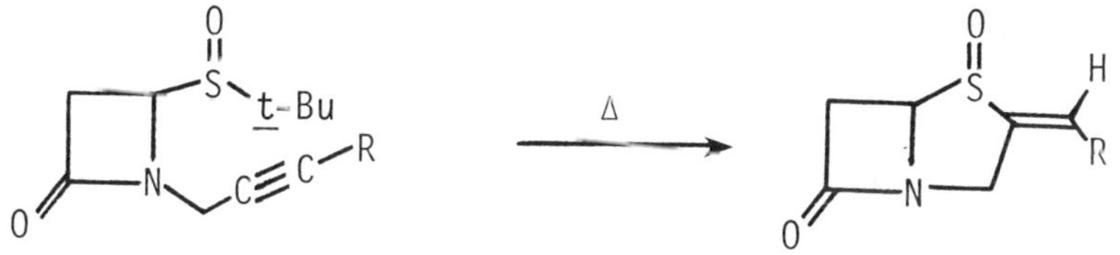

R = H, subst. Ph, CH_2OH

∼50%

IV.I.4. Heterocycles with 1 S and 1 O

IV.I.4-1   C. C. Lee et al., J. Het. Chem., 19, 801 (1982).

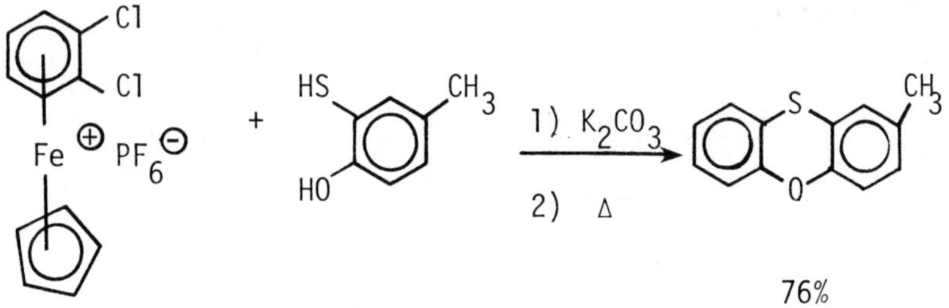

76%

IV.I.4-2   P. Schenone et al., J. Het. Chem., 19, 1031 and 1227 (1982).

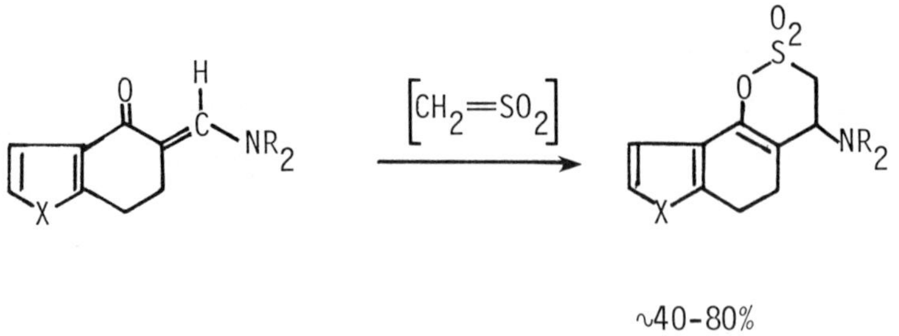

∼40-80%

X = NMe or O
NR_2 = morpholino, pyrrolidino, piperidino, NMe_2, NEt_2

IV.I.5. Heterocycles with 3 N's

IV.I.5-1 N. R. Smyrl and R. W. Smithwick III, *J. Het. Chem.*, **19**, 493 (1982).

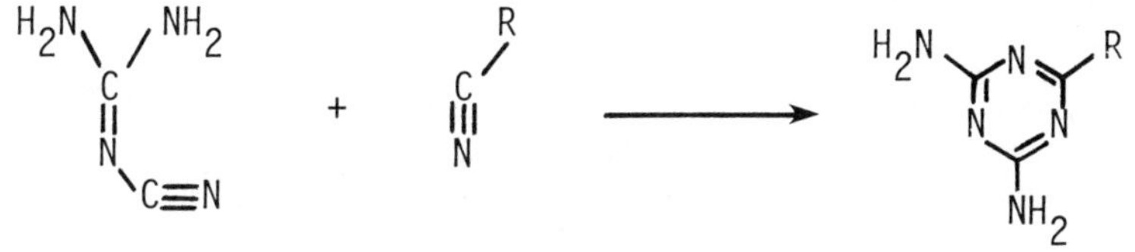

R = Me, Et, Ph

52-85%

IV.I.5-2/IV.I.6-1 S. K. Robev, *Tetrahedron Lett.*, **23**, 2903 (1982).

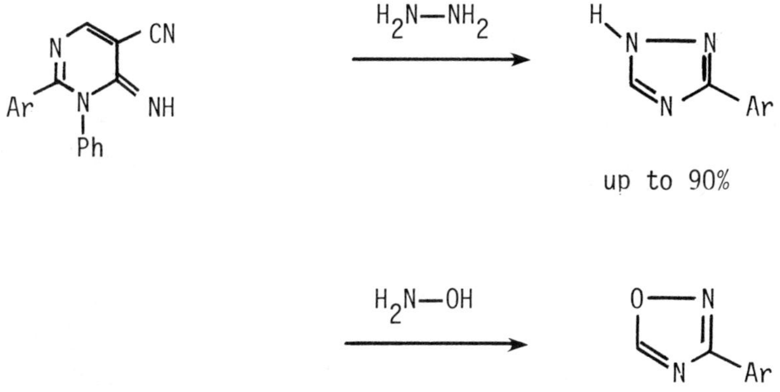

up to 90%

up to 90%

Ar = subst. Ph

IV.I.6. Other Heterocycles with Two or More Heteroatoms

IV.I.6-2 W. Steglich and T. van Ree, Synth. Comm., 12, 457 (1982).

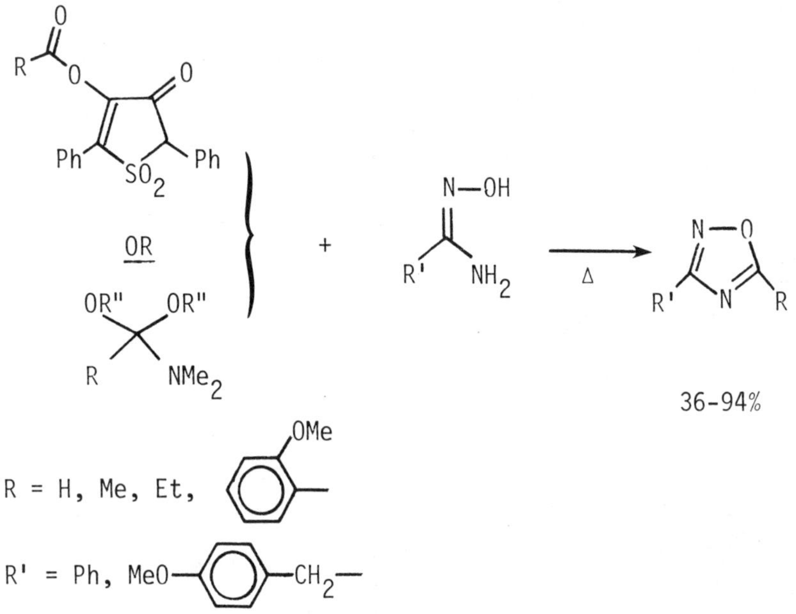

R = H, Me, Et,

R' = Ph, MeO—C₆H₄—CH₂—

36-94%

IV.I.6-3 G. W. Gokel et al., Synthesis, 997 (1982).

Review: "Synthesis of Aliphatic Azacrown Compounds"

IV.I.6-4 C. Westerlund, Tetrahedron Lett., 23, 4835 (1982).

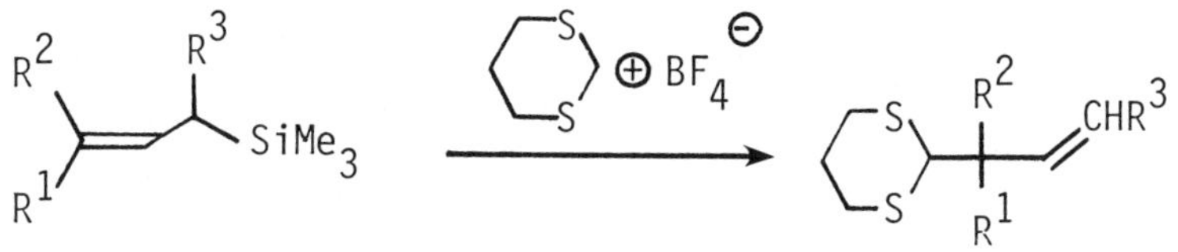

R's = H, Me, cyclic, Ph

60-79%

IV.I.6-5 M. Ngounda, H. LeBozec, and P. Dixneuf, J. Org. Chem., 47, 4000 (1982).

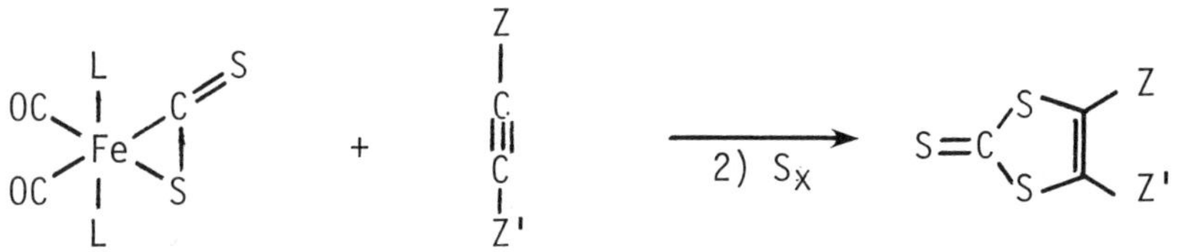

Z, Z' = -COOR, Ph, -CHO, -COCH$_3$

22-64%

IV.J. General Heterocyclic Reviews

IV.J-1   I. A. Maretina et al., Russ. Chem. Rev., 50, 657
(1981).

Review: "The Synthesis of Heterocycles from Vinyl-
         acetylenes or Diacetylenes and Nitrogen-
         containing Dinucleophiles"

IV.J-2   V. V. Korshak et al., Russ. Chem. Rev., 50, 1177
(1981).

Review: "Reductive Polyheterocyclization: A New Method
         For Preparation of Polyheteroarylenes"

IV.J-3   G. Descotes, Bull. Soc. Chem. Belges, 91, 973 (1982).

Review: "Acetalic Photoreactivity in Heterocyclic and
         Carbohydrate Series"

IV.J-4   C. G. Newton and C. A. Ramsden, Tetrahedron, 38, 2965 (1982).

Review: "Meso-ionic Heterocycles"

IV.J-5   M. G. Reinecke, Tetrahedron, 38, 427 (1982).

Review: "Hetarynes"

V
PROTECTING GROUPS

V.A. Hydroxyl Protecting Groups

(see also: VI.A.10., VI.A.11.)

V.A-1   T. P. Mawhinney and M. A. Madson, J. Org. Chem., 47, 3336 (1982).

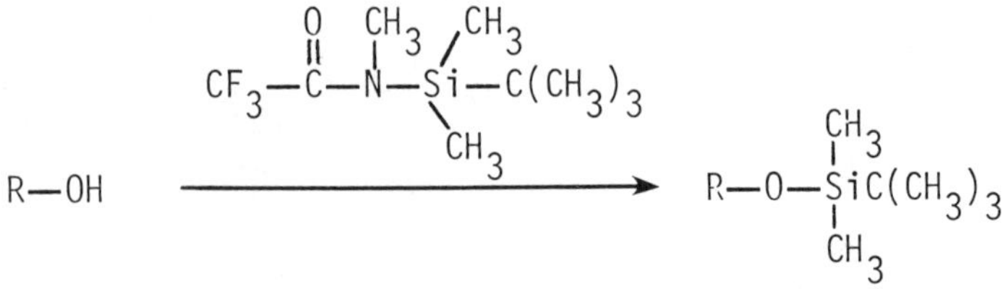

$$R-OH \xrightarrow{CF_3-\underset{\underset{}{}}{\overset{O}{\overset{\|}{C}}}-\underset{\underset{CH_3}{|}}{N}-\underset{\underset{CH_3}{|}}{\overset{CH_3}{\overset{|}{Si}}}-C(CH_3)_3} R-O-\underset{\underset{CH_3}{|}}{\overset{CH_3}{\overset{|}{Si}}}C(CH_3)_3$$

96-100%

V.A-2   Y. Oikawa et al., Tetrahedron Lett., 23, 885 and 889 (1982).

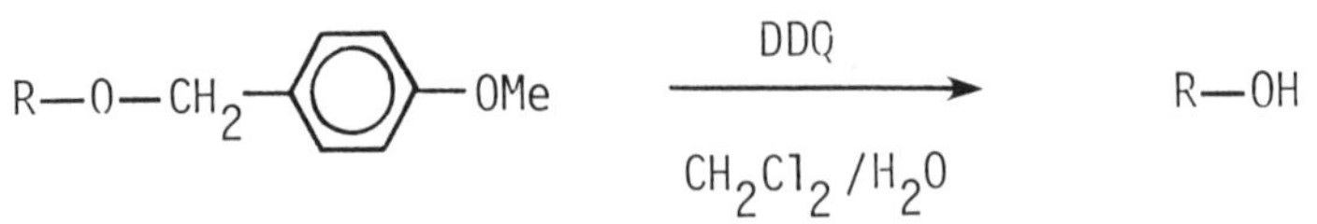

$$R-O-CH_2-\underset{}{\bigcirc}-OMe \xrightarrow[CH_2Cl_2/H_2O]{DDQ} R-OH$$

R = alkyl, aryl, cyclic. Isopropylidene, MEM, THP, TMS, etc. groups are unaffected.

V.A-3   R. Davis and J. M. Muchowski, Synthesis, 987 (1982).

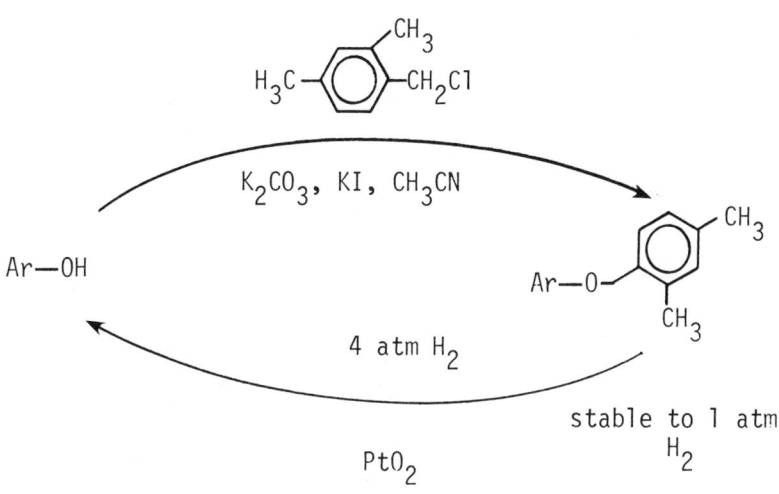

Ar = subst. Ph

V.A-4   M. V. Bhatt and S. S. El-Morey, Synthesis, 1048 (1982).

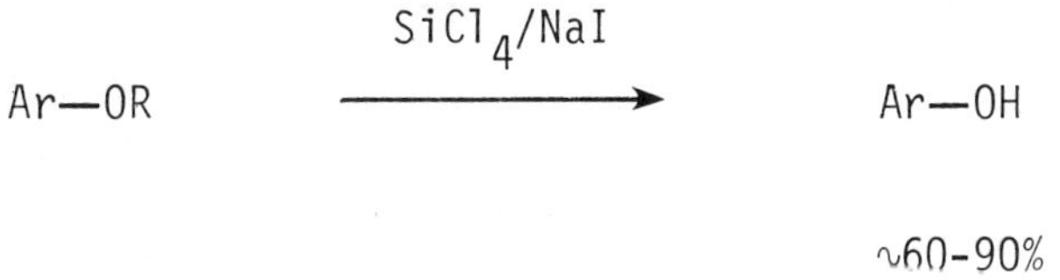

$$\text{Ar—OR} \xrightarrow{\text{SiCl}_4/\text{NaI}} \text{Ar—OH}$$

~60-90%

Ar = subst. Ph
R = Me, alkyl, allyl

V.A-5 A. Oku et al., Tetrahedron Lett., 23, 681 (1982).

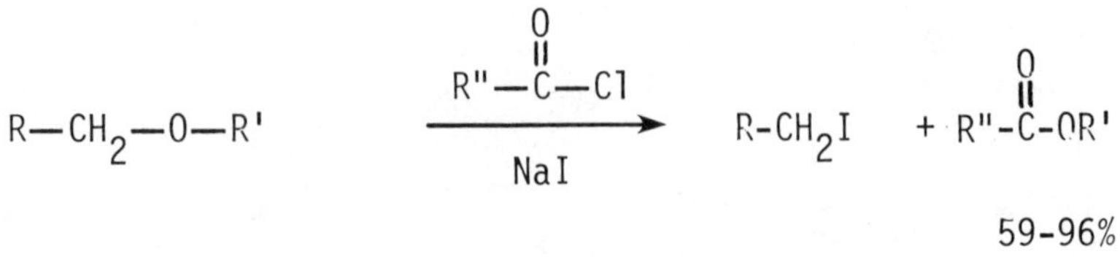

$$R-CH_2-O-R' \xrightarrow[NaI]{R''-\underset{\underset{O}{\|}}{C}-Cl} R-CH_2I + R''-\underset{\underset{O}{\|}}{C}-OR'$$

59-96%

R, R' = alkyl, cyclic
R'' = t-Bu, Me, Ph

V.A-6 A. Liptak et al., Synthesis, 421 (1982).

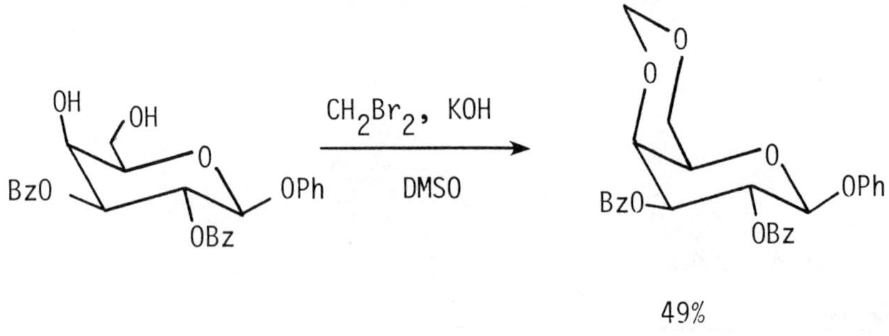

49%

V.A-7 E. J. Corey and P. B. Hopkins, Tetrahedron Lett., 23, 4871 (1982).

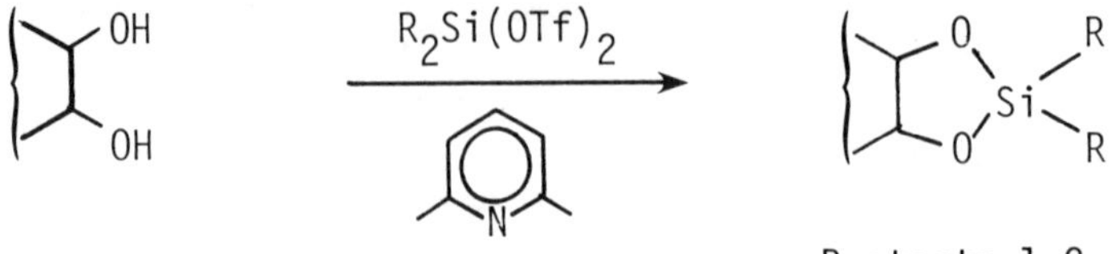

R = i-Pr, t-Bu

Protects 1,2-, 1,3-, and 1,4-diols

Deprotected by 48% aqueous HF in CH_3CN (1:7).

V.A-8   H. Köster and N. D. Sinha, Tetrahedron Lett., 23, 2641 (1982).

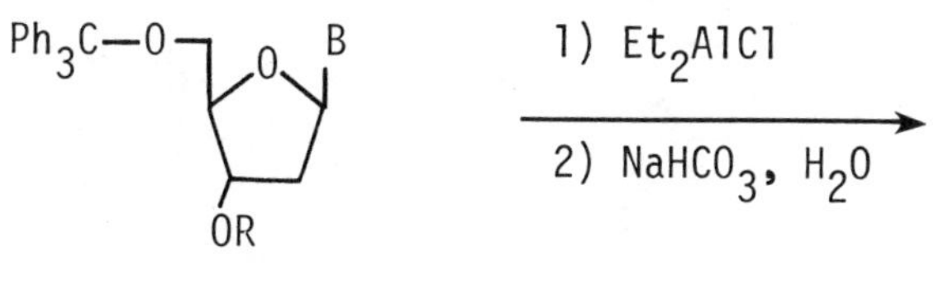

$$Ph_3C-O\text{-furanose(B)(OR)} \xrightarrow[\text{2) } NaHCO_3, H_2O]{\text{1) } Et_2AlCl} HO\text{-furanose(B)(OR)}$$

100%

V.A-9/V.B-1   T. Ohsawa et al., Chem. Pharm. Bull., 30, 3178 (1982).

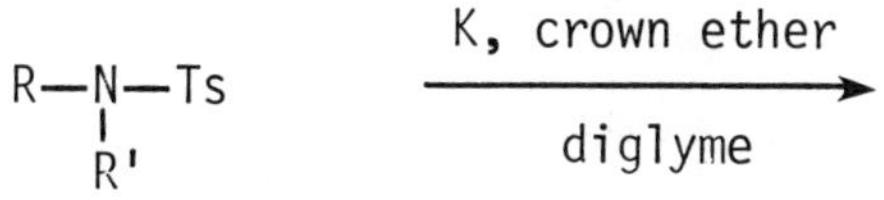

$$R-\underset{R'}{N}-Ts \xrightarrow[\text{diglyme}]{K, \text{ crown ether}} R-\underset{R'}{NH}$$

R, R' = H, alkyl, cyclic

$$R-\underset{R'}{CH}-OTs \xrightarrow[\text{diglyme}]{K, \text{ crown ether}} R-\underset{R'}{CHOH}$$

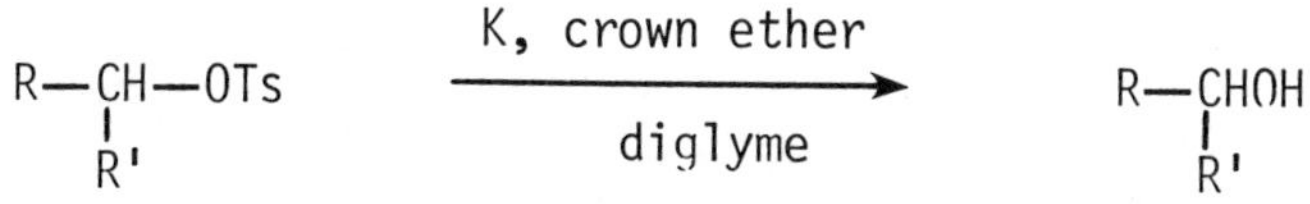

R, R' = H, alkyl, cyclic

V.B.   Amine Protecting Groups

(see also: VI.A.4.)

V.B-2 Y. Tamura et al., J. Org. Chem., **47**, 2697 (1982).

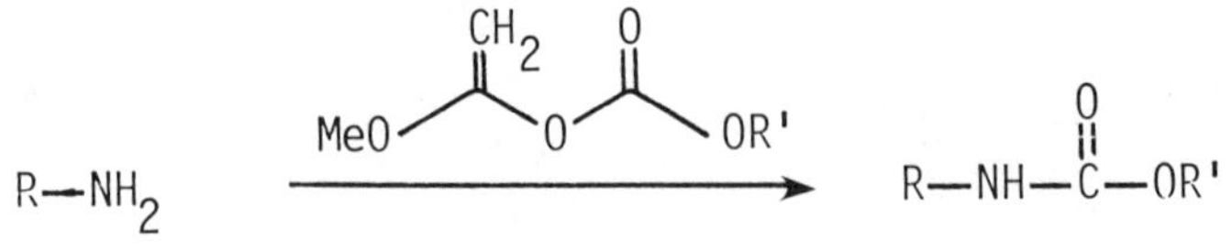

$$R-NH_2 \xrightarrow{\text{MeO}-\overset{CH_2}{\underset{\|}{C}}-O-\overset{O}{\underset{\|}{C}}-OR'} R-NH-\overset{O}{\underset{\|}{C}}-OR'$$

~70-90%

R = alkyl, aryl, heterocyclic, alcohol, amino acid, etc.

R' = t-Bu, Bz, $-CH_2CH_2-TMS$

V.B-3 M. J. O'Donnell and R. L. Polt, J. Org. Chem., **47**, 2663 (1982).

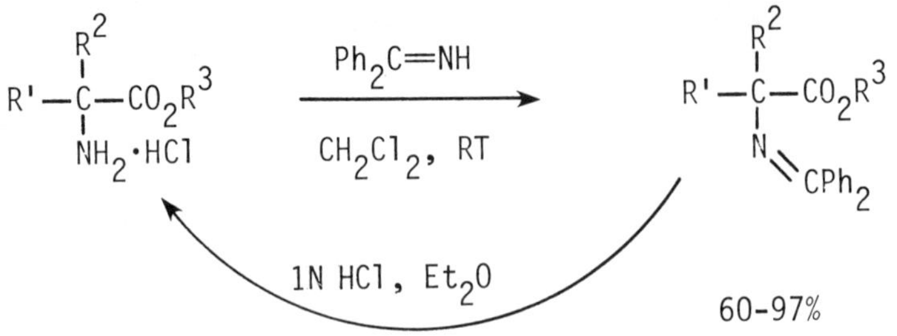

$$\underset{NH_2 \cdot HCl}{\overset{R^2}{\underset{|}{R'-C-CO_2R^3}}} \xrightarrow[CH_2Cl_2, \; RT]{Ph_2C=NH} \underset{N=CPh_2}{\overset{R^2}{\underset{|}{R'-C-CO_2R^3}}}$$

1N HCl, Et_2O

60-97%

V.B-4   D. Theodoropoulos et al., J. Org. Chem., 47, 1324 (1982).

$$\underset{H_3\overset{\oplus}{N}-\underset{R}{CH}-COO^{\ominus}}{} \xrightarrow[\text{2) Et}_3N]{\text{1) Me}_3SiCl} H_2N-\underset{R}{CH}-\overset{O}{\underset{\|}{C}}OSiMe_3$$

1) Et$_3$N 2) Ph$_3$CCl 3) MeOH

$$Ph_3C-\underset{H}{\overset{}{N}}-\underset{R}{\overset{}{CH}}-\overset{O}{\underset{\|}{C}}-OH$$

75-100%

V.B-5   R. Barthels and H. Kunz, Angew. Chem. Int. Ed., 21, 292 (1982).

Use of the Dmoc group for protection of the amino function in peptide synthesis, allowing peptide synthesis to be carried out by the carbodiimide method or the mixed anhydride method. Stable to acids, bases, TFA, etc; removed by peracetic acid.

$$\underline{Dmoc} = \underset{S}{\overset{S}{\diagup\!\!\!\diagdown}}\!\!\!\!\!\rangle-CH_2-O-\underset{\underset{O}{\|}}{C}-\underset{H}{N}-\underset{R}{CH}-COOH$$

V.B-6   W. F. Heath, J. P. Tam, and R. B. Merrifield, J.C.S. Chem. Comm., 896 (1982).

The N^i-formyl protecting group of tryptophan in solid-phase peptide synthesis is removed by $HF/Me_2S/\underline{p}$-thiocresol/$\underline{p}$-cresol.

V.B-7   M. Fujino et al., Chem. Pharm. Bull., 30, 2825 (1982).

Use of the 2,4,6-trimethoxybenzenesulfonyl protecting group for the indole N-H group of tryptophan in peptide synthesis. Protection is effected using the sulfonyl chloride. The protected indole is stable to TFA, but it is cleaved by HF or CH_3SO_3H.

V.B-8   T. Brown, J. H. Jones, and J. D. Richards, J.C.S. Perkin I, 1553 (1982).

Use of the π-benzyloxymethyl protecting group for histidine side chains in peptide synthesis prevents side-chain induced racemization and gives derivatives with convenient physical properties.

PROTECTING GROUPS

V.B-9 A. Kume, M. Sekine, and T. Hata, Tetrahedron Lett., 23, 4365 (1982).

Use of the phthaloyl group to protect the N^6-amino group of deoxyadenosine. Protected by silylation followed by acylation. Deprotected by hydrazine in pyridine/HOAc.

V.B-10 B. E. Watkins, J. S. Kiely, and H. Rapoport, J. Am. Chem. Soc., 104, 5702 (1982).

Protection of the exo amino groups of 2'-deoxyadenosine and 2'-deoxycytidine as the benzyl carbamates. 2'-deoxyguanosine is protected as its 2-N-(benzyloxycarbonyl)carbamate. Removed by transfer hydrogenation using cyclohexadiene and Pd/C.

V.C. Sulfhydryl Protecting Groups

(see also: VI.A.19.)

V.C-1 J. P. Tam, W. F. Heath, and R. B. Merrifield, Tetrahedron Lett., 23, 2939 (1982).

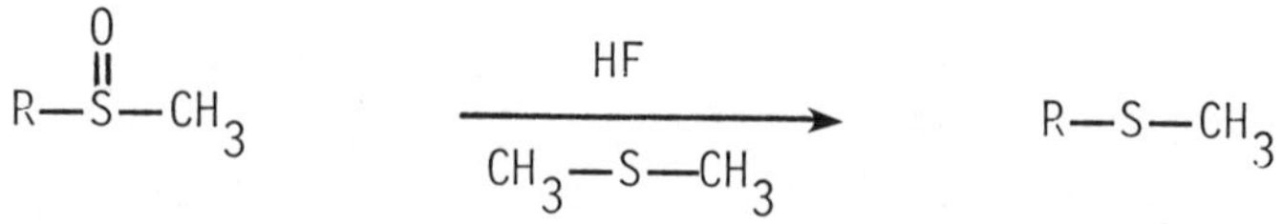

$$R-\overset{O}{\underset{\|}{S}}-CH_3 \xrightarrow[CH_3-S-CH_3]{HF} R-S-CH_3$$

methionine sulfoxide residues → methionine residues "quantitative"

V.C-2 O. S. Papsuevich et al., J. Gen. Chem. (USSR), 52, 404 (1982).

Use of the Pym group to protect the mercapto group of cysteine.   Pym = -CH$_2$-N⟩=O (pyrrolidinone)

$$\underset{H_2N-CH-COOH}{CH_2SH} \xrightleftharpoons[I_2,\ CH_3OH]{HO-CH_2-N\text{(pyrrolidinone)},\ H^{\oplus}} \underset{H_2N-CH-COOH}{CH_2-S-CH_2-N\text{(pyrrolidinone)}}$$

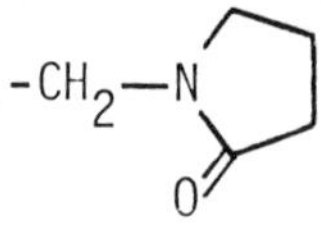

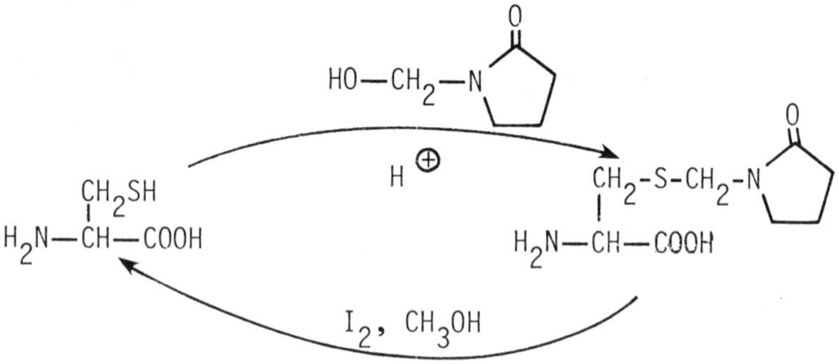

V.C-3   R. Matsueda et al., Chem. Lett., 921 (1982).

Conventional S-protecting groups of cysteine may be activated by treating them with Npys chloride to convert them to the 3-nitro-2-pyridine sulfenyl (Npys) group.

Npys chloride = (3-nitro-2-pyridinesulfenyl chloride structure: pyridine ring with NO_2 at 3-position and SCl at 2-position)

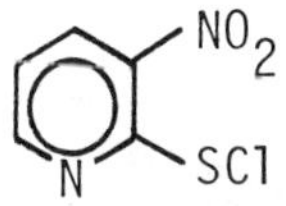

V.D.   Carboxyl Protecting Groups

(see also: VI.A.4., VI.A.10.)

V.D-1   M. J. Kukla, Tetrahedron Lett., 23, 4539 (1982).

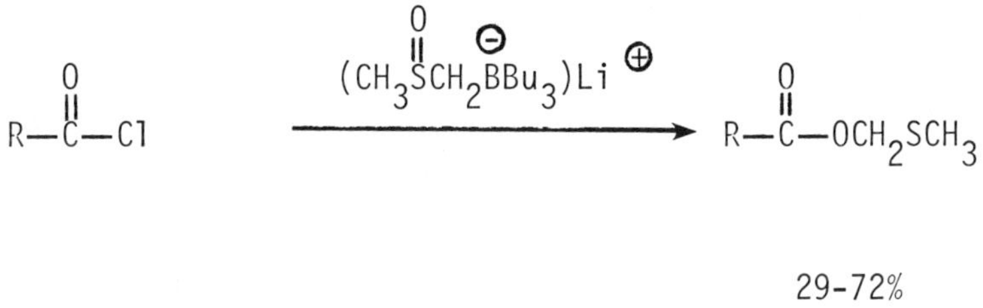

$$R-\overset{O}{\underset{\|}{C}}-Cl \quad \xrightarrow{(CH_3\overset{O}{\underset{\|}{S}}CH_2BBu_3)^{\ominus} Li^{\oplus}} \quad R-\overset{O}{\underset{\|}{C}}-OCH_2SCH_3$$

29-72%

R = alkyl, subst. Ph, $-CH_2OBz$

V.D-2 P. D. Jeffrey and S. W. McCombie, J. Org. Chem., 47, 587 (1982).

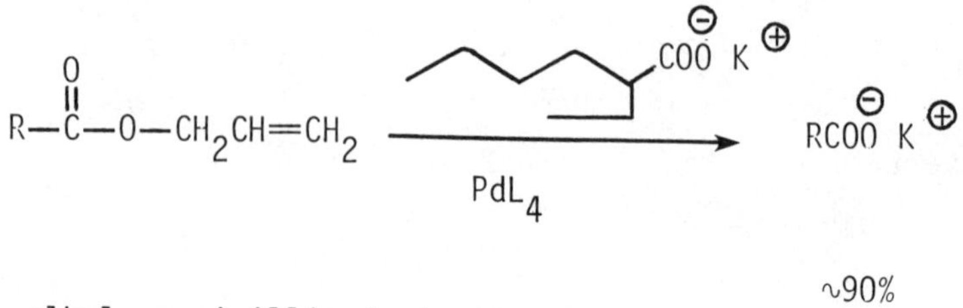

$$R-\overset{O}{\underset{\|}{C}}-O-CH_2CH=CH_2 \xrightarrow[PdL_4]{\text{CH}_3CH_2CH_2CH_2CH(COO^-K^+)CH_3} RCOO^-K^+$$

~90%

R = alkyl, penicillin derivatives

V.D-3 D. C. Tabor and S. A. Evans, Jr., Synth. Comm., 12, 855 (1982).

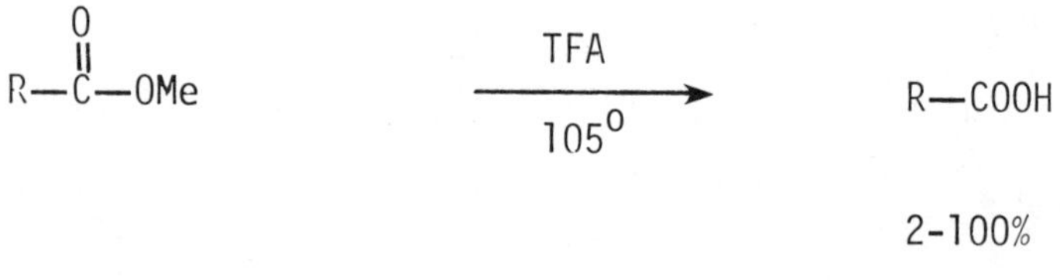

$$R-\overset{O}{\underset{\|}{C}}-OMe \xrightarrow[105°]{TFA} R-COOH$$

2-100%

R = alkyl, subst. Ph

V.D-4 E. G. Jampel and M. Wakselman, Synth. Comm., 12, 219 (1982).

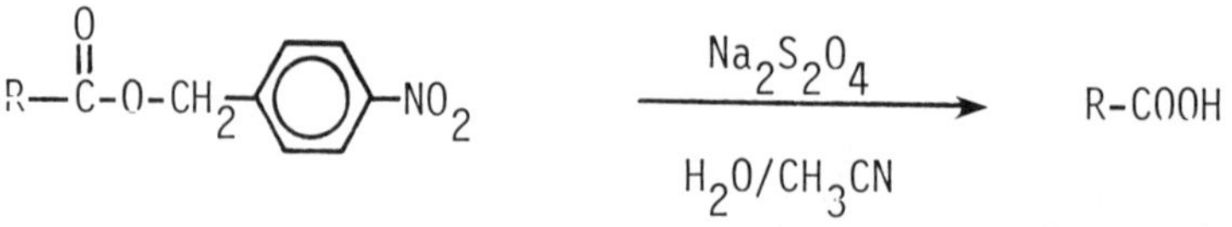

$$R-\overset{O}{\underset{\|}{C}}-O-CH_2-C_6H_4-NO_2 \xrightarrow[H_2O/CH_3CN]{Na_2S_2O_4} R-COOH$$

Used with protected amino acids.   85-95%

V.D-5 D. Landini and F. Rolla, J. Org. Chem., 47, 154 (1982).

Use of a two-phase system to hydrolyze carboxylic esters. Acids used are H_2SO_4, HCl, and HBr. Phase-transfer catalysts such as hecadecyltributylphosphonium bromide are used, and yields are >90%.

V.D-6 S. Dapperheld and E. Steckhan, Angew. Chem. Int. Ed., 21, 780 (1982).

4-methoxybenzyl esters are selectively deblocked by triarylamine cation radicals.

$$R-\overset{O}{\underset{\|}{C}}-O-\!\!\!\left\langle\bigcirc\right\rangle\!\!\!-OMe \quad \xrightarrow{[Ar_3N]^{+\cdot}} \quad R-\overset{O}{\underset{\|}{C}}-OH$$

V.D-7 L. G. Wade, Jr. and W. B. Silvey, Org. Prep. Proc. Int., 14, 357 (1982).

$$R-\overset{O}{\underset{\|}{C}}-NH_2 \quad \xrightarrow[H_2O]{HOSO_2ONO} \quad R-\overset{O}{\underset{\|}{C}}-OH$$

82-99%

R = alkyl, aryl, styryl

V.D-8 K. Narasaka et al., Chem. Lett., 991 (1982).

The 5,6-dihydrophenanthridine protecting group may be activated and removed by oxidation:

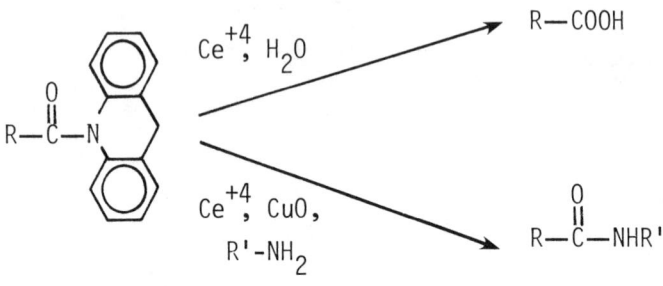

V.D-9 S. S. Isied, A. Vassilian, and J. M. Lyon, J. Am. Chem. Soc., 104, 3910 (1982).

Use of pentaamminecobalt(III) as a C-terminal group for sequential peptide synthesis.

V.E. Protecting Groups for Ketones and Aldehydes

(see also: VI.A.18.)

V.E-1 C. Stelin, B. deJeso, and J. C. Pommier, Synth. Comm., 12, 495 (1982).

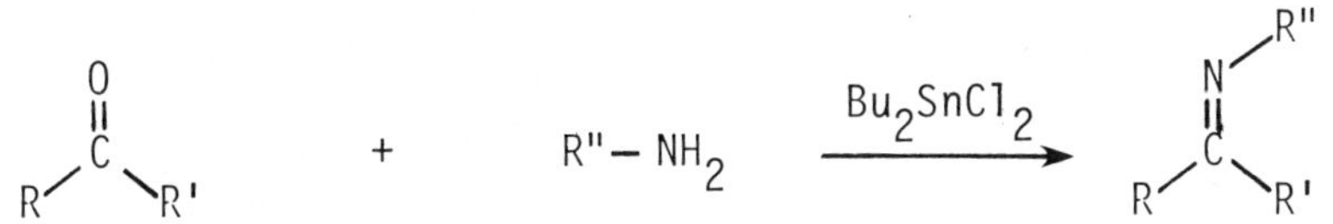

$$\underset{R}{\overset{O}{\underset{\|}{C}}}\underset{R'}{} + R''-NH_2 \xrightarrow{Bu_2SnCl_2} \underset{R}{\overset{N-R''}{\underset{\|}{C}}}\underset{R'}{}$$

R, R' = alkyl

\>80%

V.E-2 G. A. Olah and A. K. Mehrotra, Synthesis, 962 (1982).

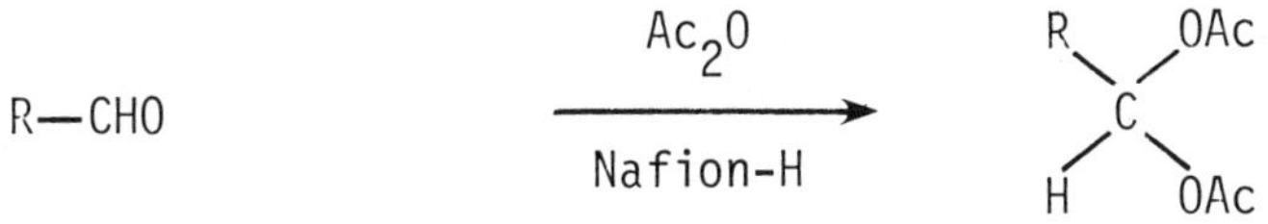

$$R-CHO \xrightarrow[\text{Nafion-H}]{Ac_2O} \underset{H}{\overset{R}{\underset{}{}}}\overset{OAc}{\underset{OAc}{C}}$$

50-99%

R = subst. Ph, 2-furyl, c-hexyl, Me, Cl_3C-, styryl

V.E-3   B. Burczyk and Z. Kortylewicz, Synthesis, 831 (1982).

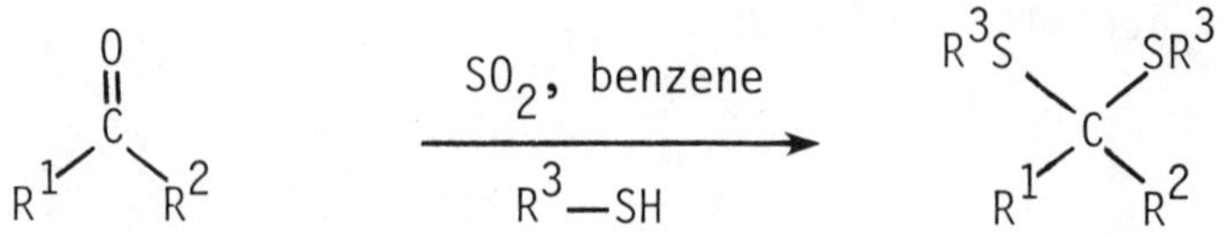

R^1, R^2 = H, alkyl, Ph

R^3 = alkyl, cyclic   54-81%

R^1, R^2 = H, alkyl, Ph

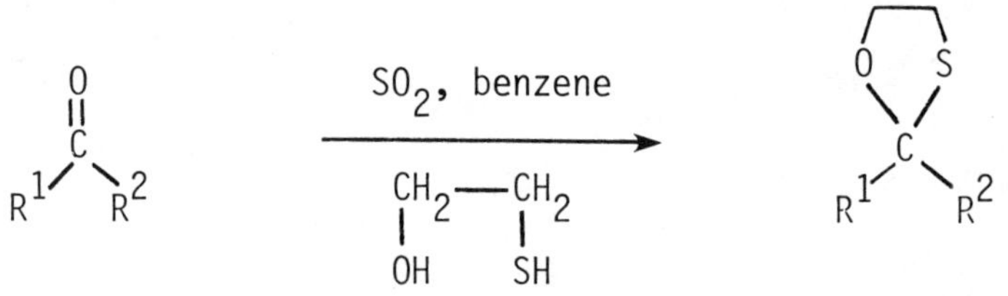

52-83%

V.E-4   S. A. Patwardhan, Indian J. Chem., 21B, 358 (1982).

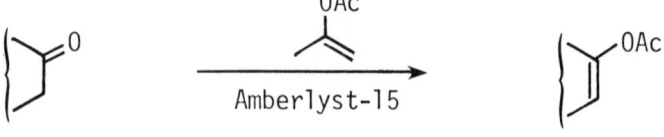

68-98%

V.E-5 R. E. Gawley and E. J. Termine, Synth. Comm., 12, 15 (1982).

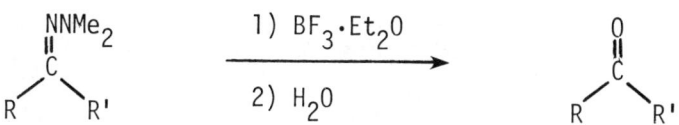

R, R' = alkyl, one with an enol acetate

65-73%

V.E-6 B. H. Lipshutz and D. F. Harvey, Synth. Comm., 12, 267 (1982).

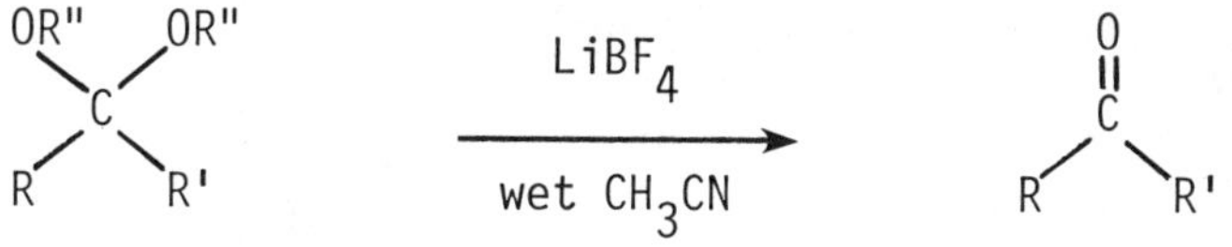

~90%

R, R' = H, alkyl, aryl
R" = Me, Et, —$(CH_2)_n$—
n = 2, 3

V.E-7 J. -M. Conia et al., J. Chem. Research(S), 248 (1982).

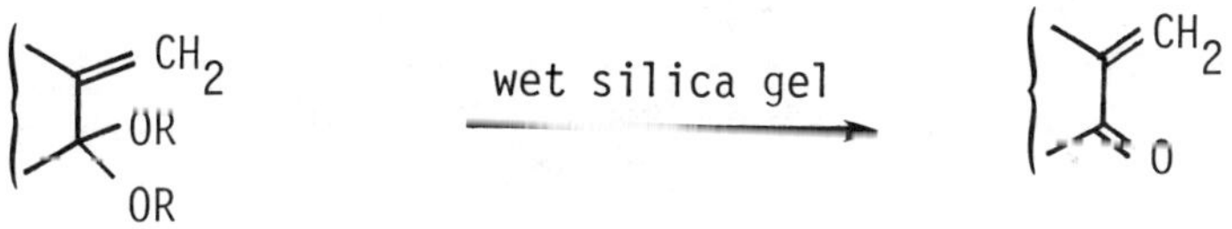

~90-100%

R = Me, Et, —$(CH_2)_2$—

V.E-8 Y. Tamura et al., Synthesis, 1089 (1982).

$$R-\underset{\underset{CH_2R'}{}}{\overset{O}{\overset{\|}{C}}} \xrightarrow[Bu_4N^{\oplus} F^{\ominus}]{Me-CH=C(OSiMe_3)(OMe)} R-\underset{CHR'}{\overset{OSiMe_3}{\overset{|}{C}}}= \xrightarrow[H^{\oplus}]{HXCH_2CH_2XH} R-\underset{CH_2R'}{\overset{X\frown X}{\overset{|}{C}}}$$

70-87%   (X = O, S)   43-66%

R, R' = alkyl, Ph, cyclic

V.E-9 D. Ghiringhelli, Synthesis, 580 (1982).

$$\underset{R\diagup \diagdown R'}{\overset{S\frown S}{C}} \xrightarrow[BF_3 \cdot THF]{PbO_2, H_2O} R-\overset{O}{\overset{\|}{C}}-R'$$

80-96%

R, R' = H, alkyl, subst. Ph, cyclic

V.E-10 G. Scorrano et al., Synthesis, 679 (1982).

$$\underset{R\diagup \diagdown R'}{\overset{S\frown S}{C}} \xrightarrow[\text{or } Me-\overset{\oplus}{S}(SMe)_2 \ SbCl_6^{\ominus}]{DMSO/HCl/H_2O/dioxane} R-\overset{O}{\overset{\|}{C}}-R'$$

>95%

R, R' = H, alkyl, aryl

V.E-11 G. A. Olah et al., Synthesis, 965 (1982).

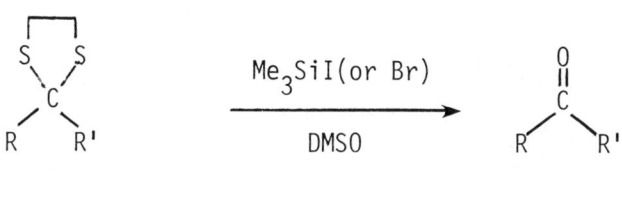

R, R' = H, alkyl, aryl, cyclic

65-99%

V.E-12 V. Janout and S. L. Regen, J. Org. Chem., 47, 2212 (1982).

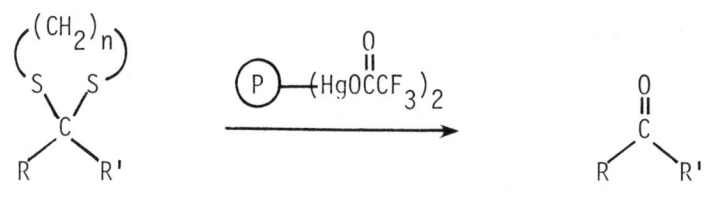

R, R' = H, alkyl, aryl, cyclic

65-92%

V.E-13 M. A. Nashed and L. Anderson, J.C.S. Chem. Comm., 1274 (1982).

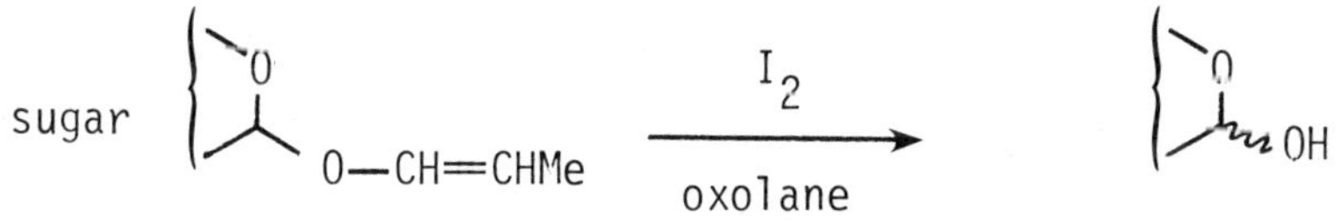

sugar $\begin{Bmatrix} \text{O} \\ \text{O—CH=CHMe} \end{Bmatrix}$ $\xrightarrow[\text{oxolane}]{I_2}$ $\begin{Bmatrix} \text{O} \\ \text{OH} \end{Bmatrix}$

V.F. Phosphate Protecting Groups

V.F-1 M. Sekine, H. Mori, and T. Hata, Bull. Chem. Soc. Japan, 55, 239 (1982).

The ethoxycarbonyl group may be used to protect either
$$H-\underset{|}{\overset{\overset{O}{\|}}{P}}-$$
groups or
$$HO-\underset{|}{\overset{\overset{O}{\|}}{P}}-$$
groups. Protection is accomplished using $EtO-\overset{\overset{O}{\|}}{C}-Cl$ in pyridine. Deprotection occurs under mildly acidic conditions. Alternatively, the protected derivative may be treated with 1M NaOH, followed by trimethylsilylation to give a highly reactive bis(trimethylsilyl) nucleoside phosphite intermediate

---

V.F-2 R. L. Letsinger, E. P. Groody, and T. Tanaka, J. Am. Chem. Soc., 104, 6805 (1982).

Protection of P—O internucleoside links may be accomplished by the use of the 2,2,2-trichloro-1,1-dimethylethyl group. Protected using $Cl_3CC(CH_3)_2OPCl_2$ and pyridine in CH_2Cl_2 or THF. Deprotected by tributylphosphine.

V.G. Pi-Bond Protecting Groups

V.G-1 F. Sato et al., Synthesis, 1025 (1982); A. U. Ronchi et al., J. Org. Chem., 47, 876 (1982); L. Engman, Tetrahedron Lett., 23, 3601 (1982).

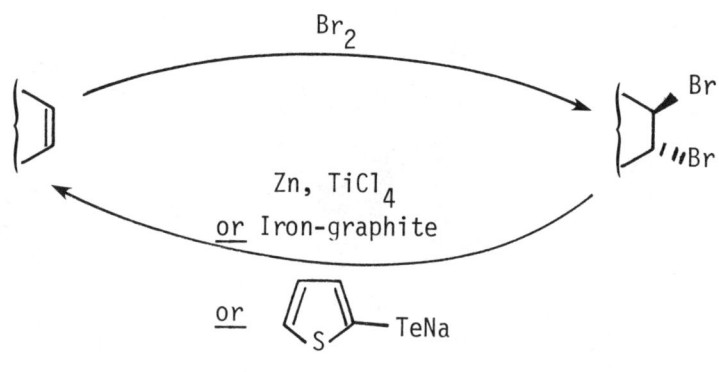

V.H. Miscellaneous Protecting Groups

V.H-1 H. Emde et al., Synthesis, 1 (1982).

Review: "Trialkylsilyl Perfluoroalkanesulfonates: Highly Reactive Silylating Agents and Lewis Acids in Organic Synthesis"

VI
USEFUL SYNTHETIC PREPARATIONS

VI.A. Functional Group Preparations

    1. Acids, Acid Halides, etc.

    (see also: II.A.2.)

VI.A.1-1 L. G. Wade, Jr. and W. B. Silvey, Org. Prep. Proc. Int., 14, 357 (1982).

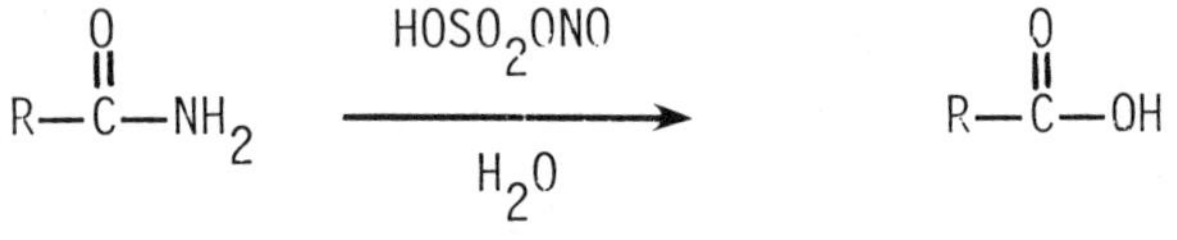

$$R-\overset{O}{\underset{\|}{C}}-NH_2 \xrightarrow[H_2O]{HOSO_2ONO} R-\overset{O}{\underset{\|}{C}}-OH$$

82-99%

R = alkyl, aryl, styryl

VI.A.1-2 R. K. Haynes and M. Holden, Aust. J. Chem., 35, 517 (1982).

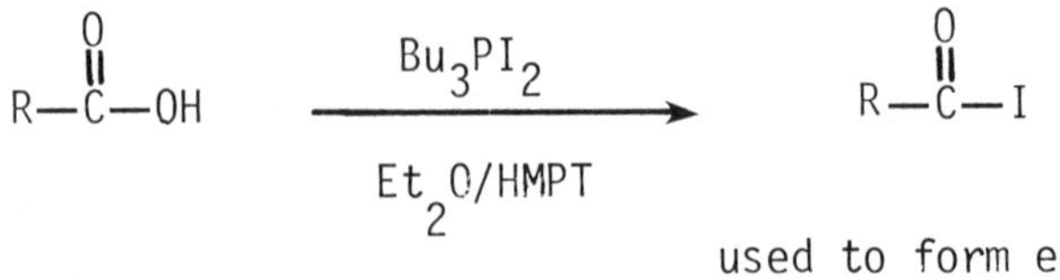

$$R-\overset{O}{\underset{\|}{C}}-OH \xrightarrow[Et_2O/HMPT]{Bu_3PI_2} R-\overset{O}{\underset{\|}{C}}-I$$

used to form esters

R = alkyl, aryl

VI.A.1-3   J. M. Aizpurua and C. Palomo, Synthesis, 684 (1982).

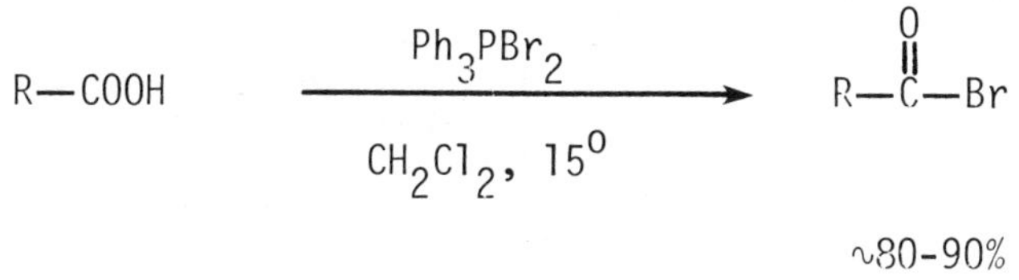

$$R-COOH \xrightarrow[CH_2Cl_2,\ 15°]{Ph_3PBr_2} R-\overset{O}{\underset{\|}{C}}-Br$$

∼80-90%

VI.A.1-4   H. M. R. Hoffman et al., Synthesis, 237 (1982).

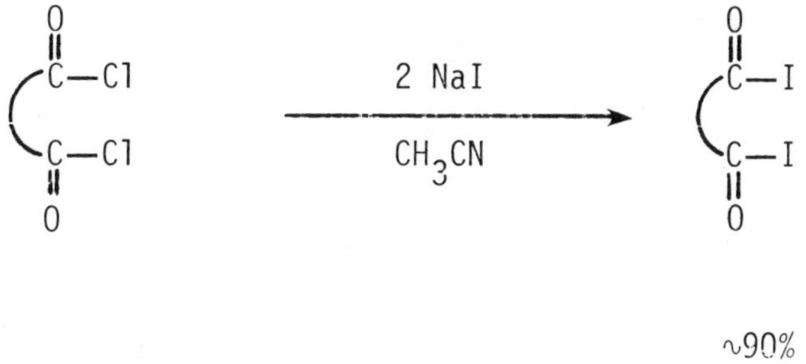

$$\begin{matrix} \overset{O}{\underset{\|}{C}}-Cl \\ \underset{\|}{\overset{}{C}}-Cl \\ O \end{matrix} \xrightarrow[CH_3CN]{2\ NaI} \begin{matrix} \overset{O}{\underset{\|}{C}}-I \\ \underset{\|}{\overset{}{C}}-I \\ O \end{matrix}$$

∼90%

VI.A.1-5   K. S. Keshavamurthy et al., Synthesis, 506 (1982).

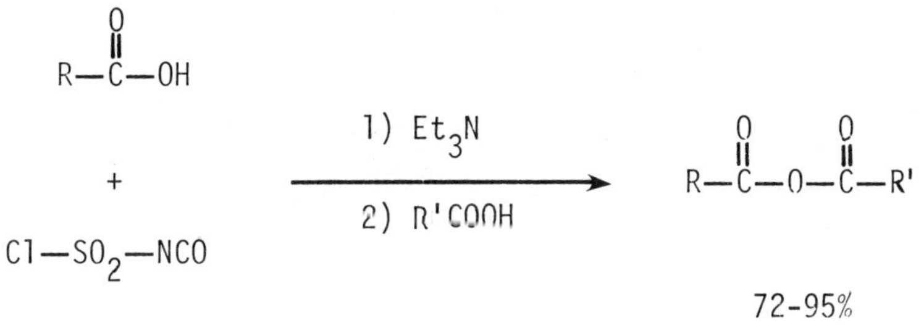

$$R-\overset{O}{\underset{\|}{C}}-OH$$

$$+$$

$$Cl-SO_2-NCO$$

$$\xrightarrow[2)\ R'COOH]{1)\ Et_3N} R-\overset{O}{\underset{\|}{C}}-O-\overset{O}{\underset{\|}{C}}-R'$$

72-95%

R = alkyl, aryl, etc.

VI.A.1-6   S. M. Rosenfeld, <u>Org. Prep. Proc. Int.</u>, **14**, 249 (1982).

Review: "Synthesis and Uses of β-Keto Acids"

VI.A.1-7   L. N. Pridgen, <u>J. Org. Chem.</u>, **47**, 4319 (1982).

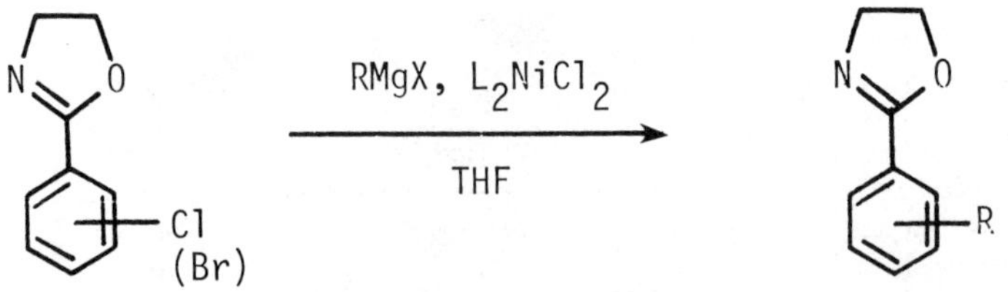

[Oxazoline-Ar-Cl(Br)] + RMgX, L_2NiCl_2, THF → [Oxazoline-Ar-R]

56-95%

R = alkyl, Bz, subst. Ph

VI.A.1-8   Y. Thebtaranouth et al., <u>Synthesis</u>, 579 (1982).

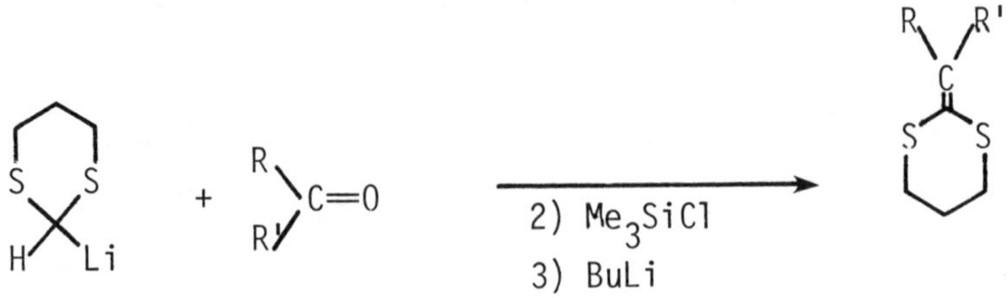

[dithiane-H,Li] + $\begin{matrix}R\\R'\end{matrix}$C=O → 2) Me_3SiCl 3) BuLi → [dithiane=CRR']

57-97%

R, R' = H, alkyl, aryl, cyclic

VI.A.2. Alcohols and Phenols

(see also: II.B.1, III.A., III.F.1)

VI.A.2-1 M. Numazawa and M. Nagaoka, J. Org. Chem., 47, 4024 (1982).

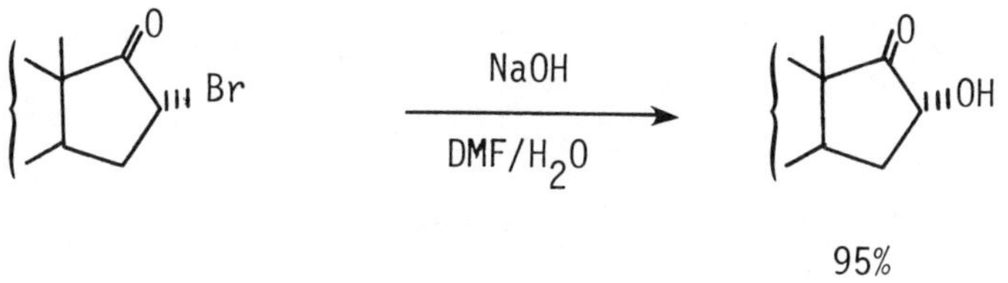

95%

VI.A.2-2 J. K. Crandall and H. S. Magaha, J. Org. Chem., 47, 5368 (1982). Similar reaction to give an epoxide, page 5372

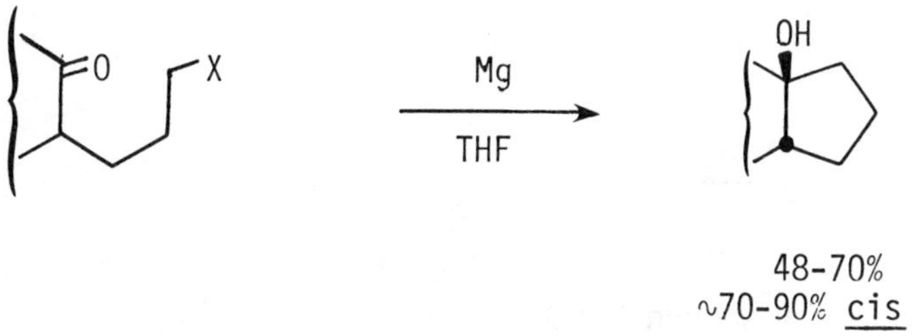

48-70%
~70-90% cis

X = Br, I

VI.A.2-3 H. Yamamoto et al., J. Am. Chem. Soc., 104, 7667 (1982).

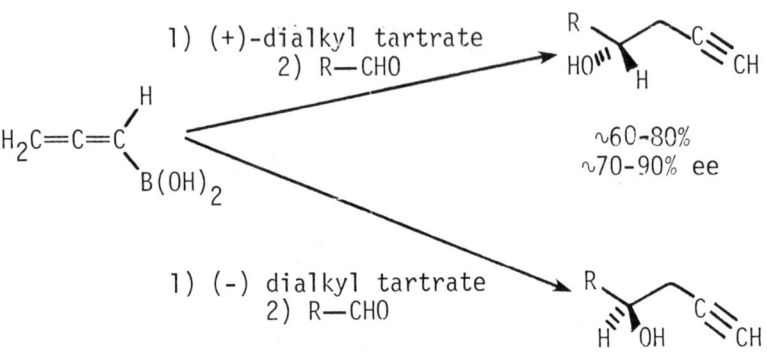

VI.A.2-4 M. Tramontini, Synthesis, 605 (1982).

Review: "Stereoselective Synthesis of Diastereomeric Amino Alcohols from Chiral Aminocarbonyl Compounds by Reduction or by Addition of Organometallic Reagents"

VI.A.2-5 S. Masamune and W. Choy, Aldrichimica Acta, 15, 47 (1982).

Review: "Advances in Stereochemical Control: The 1,2- and 1,3-Diol Systems"

VI.A.3. Alkyl and Aryl Halides
(see also: II.B.2.)

VI.A.3-1   J. Gloede, Z. Chem., 22, 126 (1982).

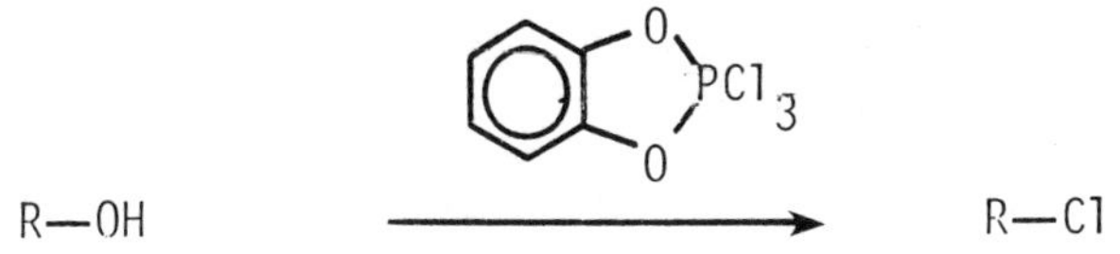

R—OH $\xrightarrow{\text{catecholyl-PCl}_3}$ R—Cl

R = 1°, 2° alkyl, Ph, Bz, etc.

55-90%

VI.A.3-2   R. K. Haynes and M. Holden, Aust. J. Chem., 35, 517 (1982).

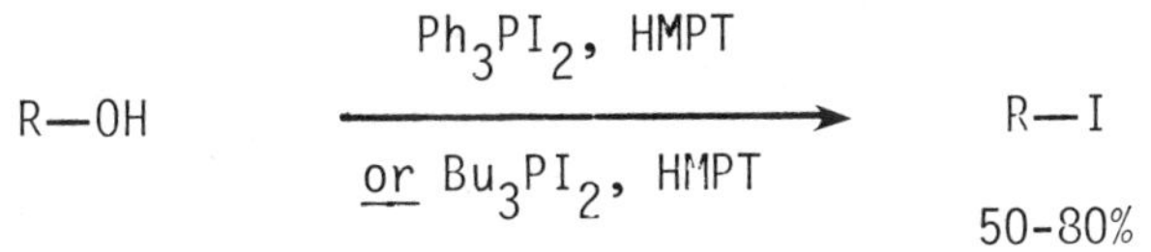

R—OH $\xrightarrow[\underline{\text{or}}\ Bu_3PI_2,\ HMPT]{Ph_3PI_2,\ HMPT}$ R—I

R = alkyl; may contain C=C, C≡C

50-80%

VI.A.3-3   I. Galynker and W. C. Still, Tetrahedron Lett., 23, 4461 (1982).

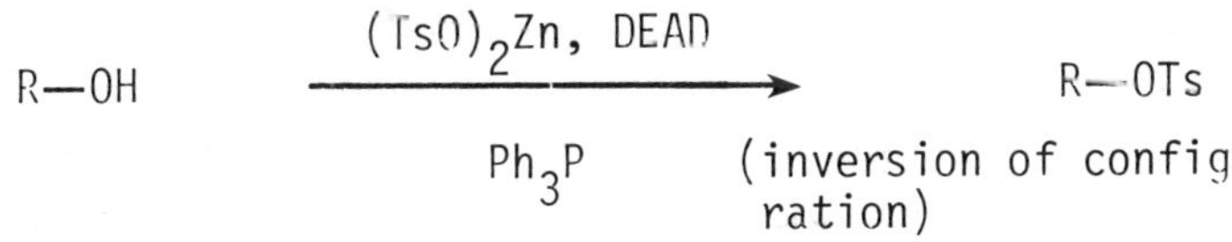

R—OH $\xrightarrow[Ph_3P]{(TsO)_2Zn,\ DEAD}$ R—OTs   (inversion of configuration)

R = 2° alkyl, cycloalkyl, steroidal

62-94%

VI.A.3-4   F. Ogura et al., Chem. Lett., 1081 (1982).

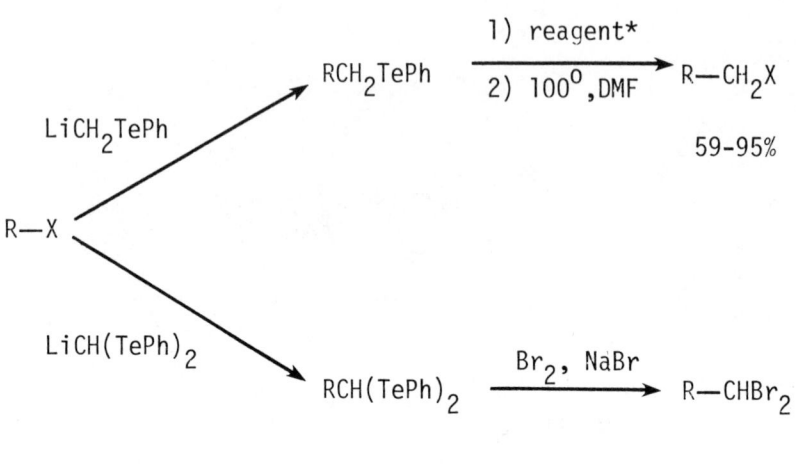

R = 1° alkyl

*Reagent = sulfuryl chloride, bromine, or iodine

VI.A.3-5   G. W. Kabalka et al., Org. Prep. Proc. Int., 14, 359 (1982).

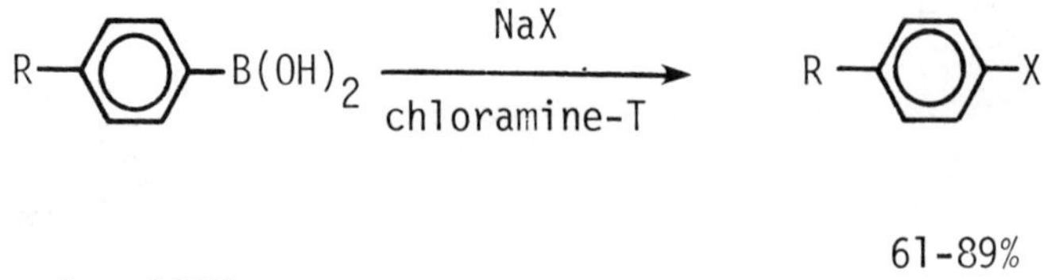

R—⟨C₆H₄⟩—B(OH)$_2$ $\xrightarrow[\text{chloramine-T}]{\text{NaX}}$ R—⟨C₆H₄⟩—X

61-89%

R = H, Me, Br, COOH
X = Br, I

VI.A.3-6   L. S. Levitt and R. Iglesias, *J. Org. Chem.*, **47**, 4770 (1982).

$$PhIO_3 \xrightarrow[H_2SO_4]{H_5IO_6} C_6I_6$$

48%

VI.A.3-7   R. H. Seevers and R. E. Counsell, *Chem. Rev.*, **82**, 575 (1982).

Review: "Radioiodination Techniques for Small Organic Molecules"

VI.A.4.   Amides

(see also: IV.D., VI.A.17.)

VI.A.4-1 I. Ganboa and C. Palomo, Bull. Soc. Chim. France
II, 167 (1982).

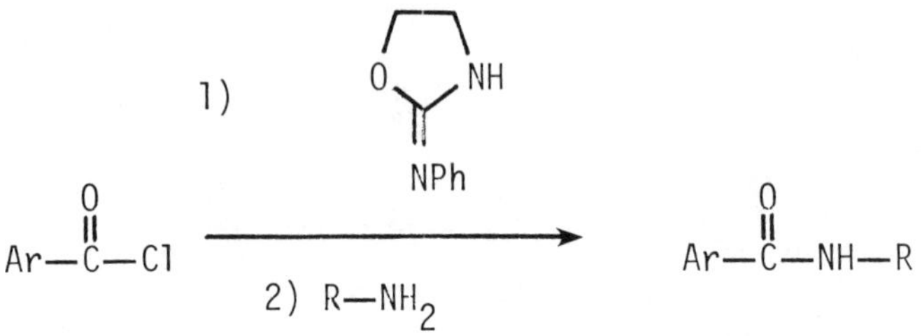

$$Ar-\underset{O}{\underset{\|}{C}}-Cl \xrightarrow[\text{2) R-NH}_2]{\text{1) oxazoline-NPh}} Ar-\underset{O}{\underset{\|}{C}}-NH-R$$

~50-75%

Ar = subst. Ph
R = subst. Ph, Bz, c-Hx

VI.A.4-2 M. Ueda and N. Kawaharsaki, Synthesis, 933 (1982).

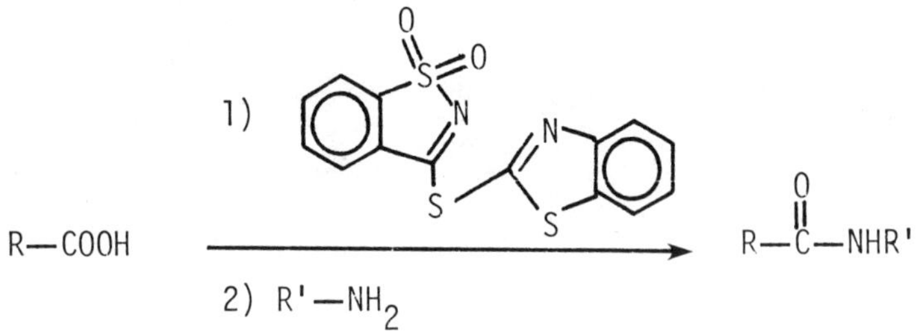

$$R-COOH \xrightarrow[\text{2) R'-NH}_2]{\text{1) benzisothiazole-benzothiazole reagent}} R-\underset{O}{\underset{\|}{C}}-NHR'$$

53-93%

R = Ph, n-C$_5$H$_{11}$
R' = Ph, Bz

VI.A.4-3 K. S. Keshavamurthy et al., Synthesis, 506 (1982).

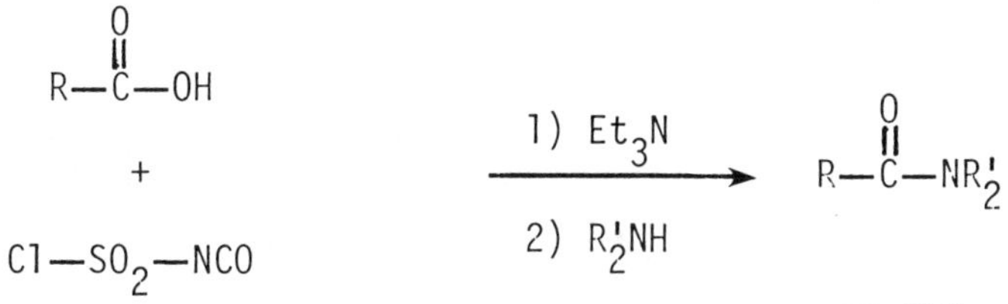

$$R-\underset{\underset{}{\overset{O}{\|}}}{C}-OH + Cl-SO_2-NCO \xrightarrow[\text{2) } R_2'NH]{\text{1) } Et_3N} R-\underset{\underset{}{\overset{O}{\|}}}{C}-NR_2'$$

68-90%

R = alkyl, aryl, etc.

VI.A.4-4 X. Huang, C. -C. Chan, and Q. -S. Zhou, Synth. Comm., 12, 709 (1982).

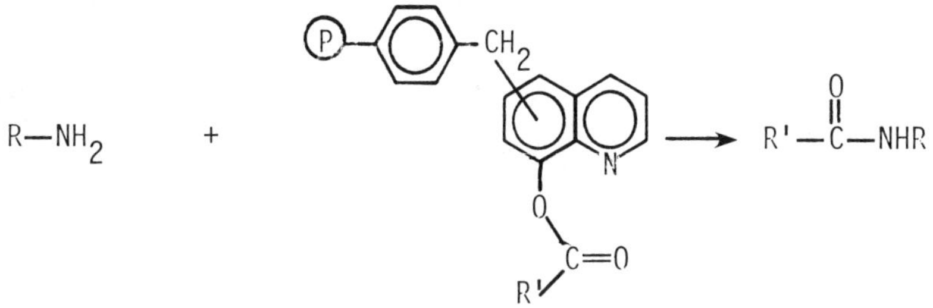

$$R-NH_2 \ + \ \text{[quinoline reagent]} \longrightarrow R'-\underset{\underset{}{\overset{O}{\|}}}{C}-NHR$$

R = alkyl, cycloalkyl, Ph, Bz
R = Me, Ph

VI.A.4-5 R. Mestres and C. Palomo, Synthesis, 288 (1982).

Use of $Ph-O-\underset{\underset{Cl}{}}{\overset{\overset{O}{\|}}{P}}-NHPh$ as a carbonyl-activating reagent for the synthesis of amides and anhydrides. Yields are generally >90%.

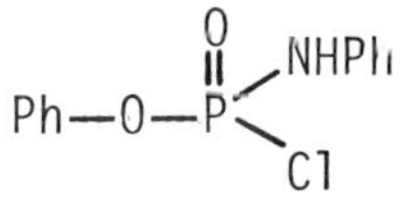

VI.A.4-6   M. Ravindranathan et al., J. Org. Chem., 47, 4812 (1982).

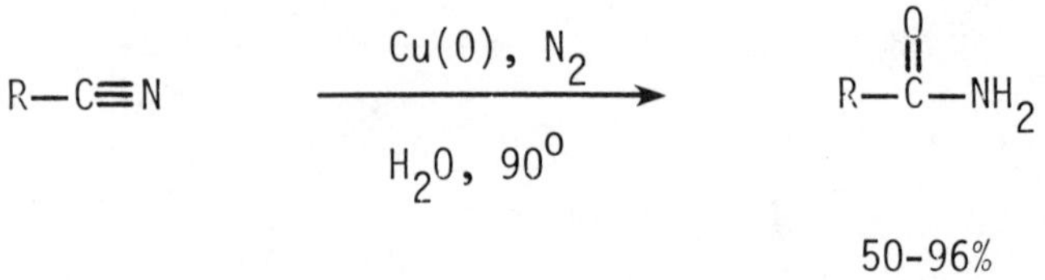

$$R-C\equiv N \xrightarrow[H_2O,\ 90°]{Cu(0),\ N_2} R-\underset{\underset{}{\|}}{\overset{\overset{}{O}}{C}}-NH_2$$

R = Me, vinyl, Ph, etc.

50-96%

VI.A.4-7   C. G. Rao, Synth. Comm., 12, 177 (1982).

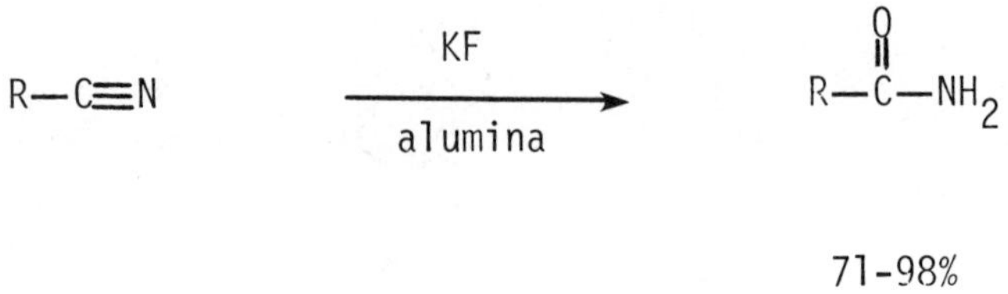

$$R-C\equiv N \xrightarrow[alumina]{KF} R-\underset{\underset{}{\|}}{\overset{\overset{}{O}}{C}}-NH_2$$

R = alkyl, aryl, Bz

71-98%

VI.A.4-8   G. Boche et al., Tetrahedron Lett., 23, 3255 (1982).

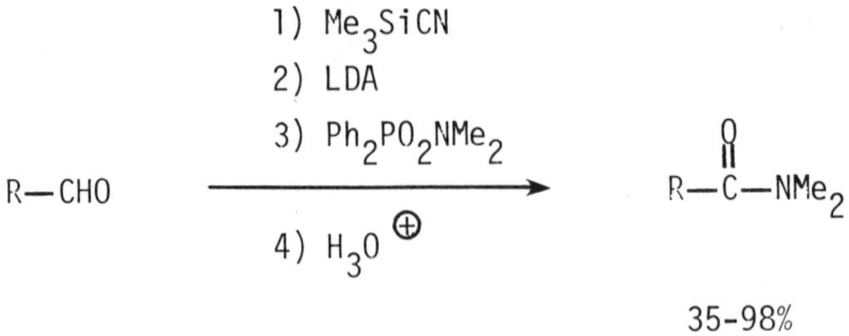

$$R-CHO \xrightarrow[\substack{3)\ Ph_2PO_2NMe_2 \\ 4)\ H_3O^{\oplus}}]{\substack{1)\ Me_3SiCN \\ 2)\ LDA}} R-\underset{\underset{}{\|}}{\overset{\overset{}{O}}{C}}-NMe_2$$

R = aryl, α,β-unsat., heterocyclic

35-98%

VI.A.4-9   P. Müller and J. Godoy, Tetrahedron Lett., 23, 3661 (1982).

$$R-C\equiv C-NR'_2 \xrightarrow[RuCl_2L_3]{Ph-I=O} R-\underset{\underset{O}{\|}}{C}-\underset{\underset{O}{\|}}{C}-NR'_2$$

R = alkyl, Ph
R' = alkyl

0-76%

VI.A.4-10   J. Garcia and J. Vilarrasa, Tetrahedron Lett., 23, 1127 (1982).

$$R-\underset{\underset{O}{\|}}{C}-NHR' \xrightarrow[\text{2) R"NH}_2]{\text{1) N}_2\text{O}_4\text{, AcONa}} R-\underset{\underset{O}{\|}}{C}-NHR"$$

65-98%

R = Me, Ph, n-octyl
R' = Me, Bu
R" = 1° alkyl, Bz, c-Hx, c-Pr

VI.A.4-11   G. Schmitt and W. Ebertz, Angew. Chem. Int. Ed., 21, 630 (1982).

$$R^1\underset{O}{\overset{N}{\diagup\!\!\!\diagdown}}\underset{R^3}{\overset{R^2}{\diagdown\!\!\!\diagup}} \xrightarrow{\text{t-BuOK, HMPT}} \left[R^1-\underset{\underset{O}{\|}}{C}-NH-CH=CR^2R^3\right]_n$$

R^1 = Me, t-Bu, subst. Ph, etc.   widely varying yields
R^2, R^3 = H, Me, Ph

VI.A.4-12 J. C. Gramain and R. Remuson, Synthesis, 264 (1982).

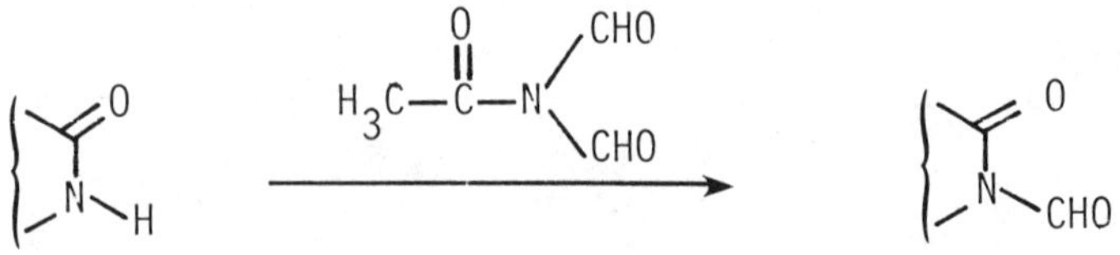

$$\text{lactam-NH} \xrightarrow{H_3C-\overset{O}{\underset{}{C}}-N(CHO)_2} \text{lactam-N-CHO}$$

52-86%

VI.A.4-13 Y. Sato et al., Synthesis, 141 (1982).

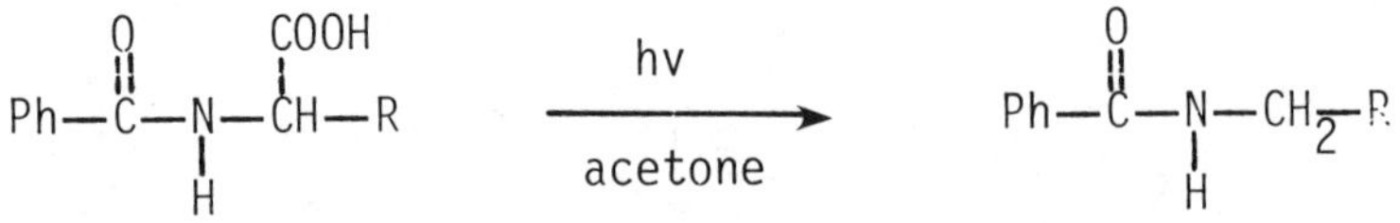

$$Ph-\overset{O}{\underset{}{C}}-\underset{H}{N}-\underset{COOH}{\overset{}{C}H}-R \xrightarrow[\text{acetone}]{h\nu} Ph-\overset{O}{\underset{}{C}}-\underset{H}{N}-CH_2-R$$

R = H, alkyl, aryl, etc.

~80-90%

VI.A.4-14 E. F. Novoselov et al., J. Org. Chem. (USSR), 17, 2284 (1982).

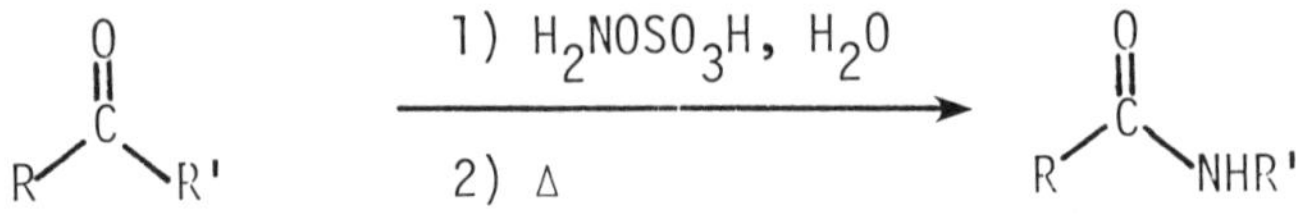

$$R-\overset{O}{\underset{}{C}}-R' \xrightarrow[\text{2) }\Delta]{\text{1) }H_2NOSO_3H,\ H_2O} R-\overset{O}{\underset{}{C}}-NHR'$$

R, R' = alkyl, aryl, cyclic

~20-60%

VI.A.5. Amines

(see also: III.D.)

VI.A.5-1 P. Beak and B. J. Kokko, J. Org. Chem., 47, 2822 (1982).

$$R-M \xrightarrow{CH_3Li,\ CH_3ONH_2} R-NH_2$$

R = alkyl, aryl
M = Li, MgBr

~50-90%
(isolated as the benzamides)

VI.A.5-2 F. Rolla, J. Org. Chem., 47, 4327 (1982).

$$R-N_3 \xrightarrow[\text{toluene, P.T.C.}]{NaBH_4,\ H_2O} R-NH_2$$

R = alkyl, aryl

~80-90%

VI.A.5-3 A. Hassner, P. Munger, and B. A. Belinka, Jr., Tetrahedron Lett., 23, 699 (1982).

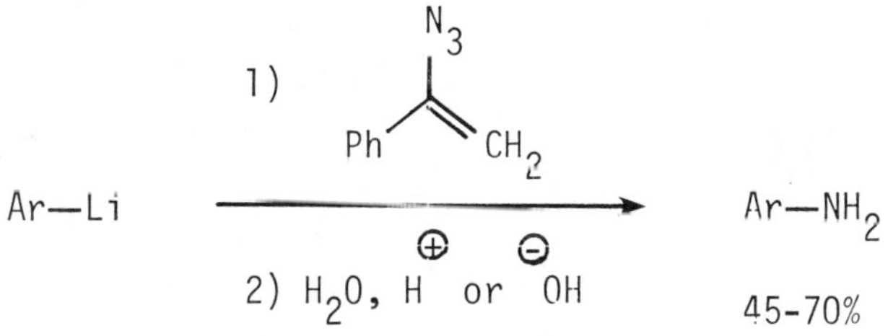

$$Ar-Li \xrightarrow[\text{2) } H_2O,\ H^\oplus \text{ or } OH^\ominus]{\text{1) } Ph\overset{N_3}{\underset{}{\diagup\!\!\diagdown}}CH_2} Ar-NH_2$$

45-70%

Ar = subst. Ph, pyridine, Bz, thiophene, imidazole, dithiane, etc.

VI.A.5-4 S. Krishnamurthy, Tetrahedron Lett., 23, 3315 (1982).

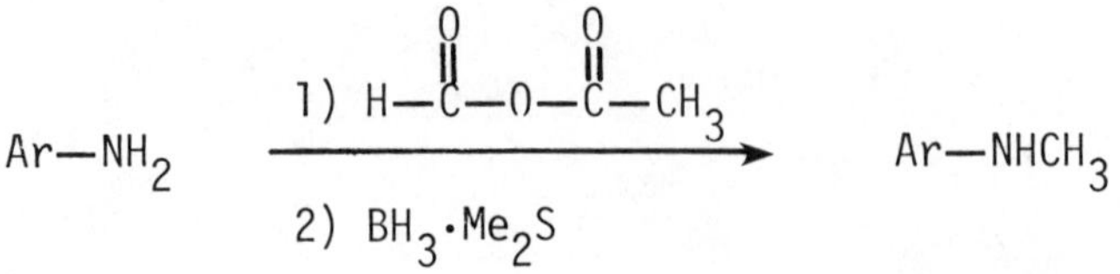

$$Ar-NH_2 \xrightarrow[\text{2) } BH_3 \cdot Me_2S]{\text{1) } H-\overset{O}{\overset{\|}{C}}-O-\overset{O}{\overset{\|}{C}}-CH_3} Ar-NHCH_3$$

85-98%

Ar = subst. Ph, pyridyl

VI.A.5-5 G. W. Kabalka et al., J.C.S. Chem. Comm., 62 (1982).

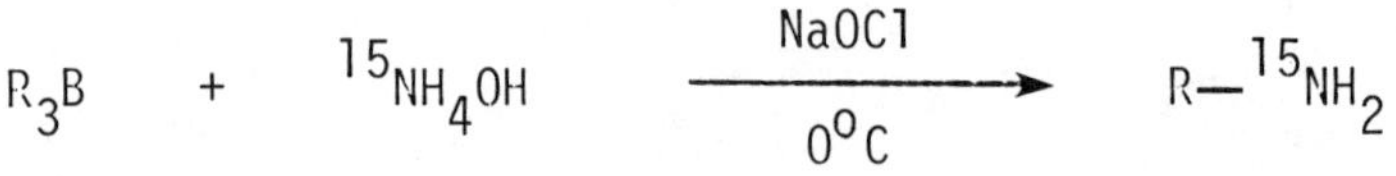

$$R_3B + {}^{15}NH_4OH \xrightarrow[0°C]{NaOCl} R-{}^{15}NH_2$$

66-85%
(based on ${}^{15}NH_4OH$)

R = 1°, 2° alkyl; may contain ester, sulfide

VI.A.5-6 G. Courtois and P. Miginiac, Bull. Soc. Chim. France II, 395 (1982).

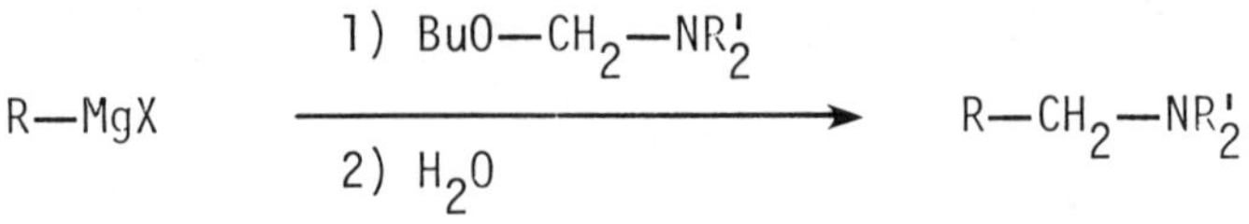

$$R-MgX \xrightarrow[\text{2) } H_2O]{\text{1) } BuO-CH_2-NR'_2} R-CH_2-NR'_2$$

~80%

R = alkyl, vinyl, -CH$_2$TMS, -CH$_2$OMe, -CH$_2$COOR, etc.
R' = Me, Et

VI.A.5-7 R. F. Smith and K. J. Coffman, Synth. Comm., 12, 801 (1982).

$$R\text{—}Br + Me_2NNH_2 \xrightarrow{\text{2) } HNO_2} Me_2NR$$

R = 1°, 2° alkyl, Bz, propargyl

59-96%

VI.A.5-8 A. I. Meyers and G. E. Jagdmann, Jr., J. Am. Chem. Soc., 104, 877 (1982).

$$\underset{Ar}{\overset{O}{\underset{\|}{C}}}\diagdown R \xrightarrow[\text{2) } NaBH_4, H^\oplus]{\text{1) BuLi, } CH_3\text{—}N(CH_2TMS)(CH=N\text{—}\underline{t}\text{-Bu})} \underset{Ar}{\overset{CH_2NHCH_3}{\underset{|}{CH}}}\diagdown R$$

Ar = Ph, 2-pyridyl
R = H, alkyl, cyclic

52-70%

VI.A.5-9 K. Soai, A. Ookawa, and K. Kato, Bull. Chem. Soc. Japan, 55, 1671 (1982).

$$\text{phthalimide-NK} + R\text{—}X \xrightarrow[\text{toluene}]{\text{18-crown-6}} \text{phthalimide-N-R}$$

84-100%

RX = 1° alkyl halide, BzCl, sulfonyl chloride, carbonyl chloride

VI.A.5-10 A. Zwierzak and S. Pilichowska, Synthesis, 922 (1982).

Use of

$$\text{t-Bu}-\underset{\underset{(\text{EtO})_2\text{P}=\text{O}}{|}}{\overset{\overset{O}{||}}{C}}-N^{\ominus} \, Na^{\oplus}$$

in a Gabriel-type synthesis of primary amines. Yields are ~70-90%

VI.A.5-11 A. Zwierzak et al., Synthesis, 918 (1982).

$$R-CH=CH-R' \xrightarrow[\substack{1) \, Hg(NO_3)_2, \, MeCHCl_2 \\ 2) \, NaBH_4, \, NaOH/H_2O \\ 3) \, HCl, \, Benzene}]{(EtO)_2\overset{\overset{O}{||}}{P}-NH_2} R-\underset{\underset{}{|}}{\overset{\overset{NH_3^{\oplus} \, Cl^{\ominus}}{|}}{CH}}-CH_2-R'$$

34-76%

R = alkyl, Ph, Bz, ⎤
R' = H, Et   ⎦ cyclic

VI.A.5-12 T. Shono et al., Chem. Lett., 565 (1982).

$$R-\overset{\overset{O}{||}}{C}-NH_2 \xrightarrow{\text{electrolysis}} [R-NCO] \xrightarrow{CH_3OH} R-NH\overset{\overset{O}{||}}{C}-OCH_3$$

22-92%

R = 1°, 2°, 3° alkyl, Bz

VI.A.5-13   D. Cavalla and S. Warren, Tetrahedron Lett., 23, 4505 (1982).

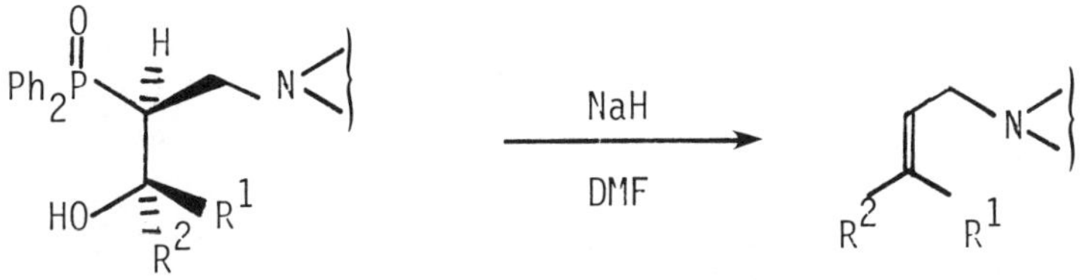

R^1, R^2 = H, alkyl, cyclic

~60-80%

VI.A.6.   Amino Acids and Derivatives

(see also: VI.A.4., VI.A.10.)

VI.A.6-1   H. Kuzuhara et al., Chem. Lett., 1765 and 1769 (1982).

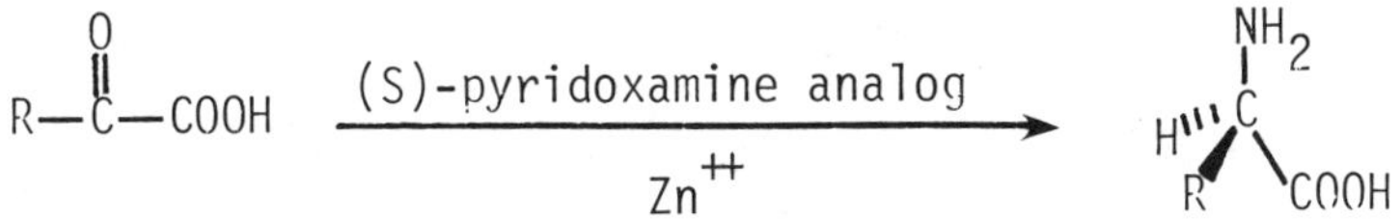

R = alkyl, Bz,

33-75%
60-96% ee

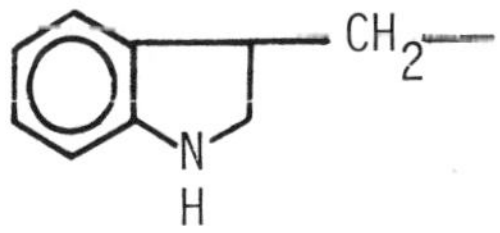

VI.A.6-2 U. Schöllkopf et al., Synthesis, 861 and 870 (1982).

$$\begin{bmatrix} \text{t-Bu} & \text{N} & \text{OMe} \\ \text{H} & \ominus & \\ \text{MeO} & \text{N} & \text{Li}^{\oplus} \end{bmatrix} \xrightarrow[\text{2) H}_3\text{O}^{\oplus}]{\text{1) R-Br, THF}} R-\overset{*}{C}H-COOMe$$
3) NH_3/H_2O 　　　　　　NH_2

~40-70%

R = alkyl, Bz, allyl, propargyl, etc.

Several additional methods are given for asymmetric synthesis of amino acids

---

VI.A.6-3 F. Effenberger and T. Beisswenger, Angew. Chem. Int. Ed., 21, 203 (1982).

$$R-CH_2-\underset{N_3}{CH}-C\overset{O}{\underset{OMe}{\diagdown}} \xrightarrow[(Re_2S_7)]{Ac_2O/AcOH} R-CH=C\overset{COOMe}{\underset{N(COCH_3)_2}{\diagdown}}$$

40-93%

R = H, Me, Pr, Ph

VI.A.6-4 G. Descotes et al., J. Chem. Research (S), 117 (1982).

$$\underset{R^1}{\overset{\overset{O}{\underset{\|}{C}}-OR^3}{\diagup}}\diagdown_{NHC-R^2}^{\|}_{O} \xrightarrow[\text{Rh catalyst*}]{H_2} R^1\diagdown\overset{*}{\diagup}\underset{NHC-R^2}{\overset{C-OR^3}{\|}}_{O}^{\|}$$

R^1 = H, subst. Ph 　　　　　　　　　~78-86%
R^2 = Me, Ph 　　　*Rhodium complex with
R^3 = H, Me 　　　(S)-1,2-O-isopropylideneglycerol

VI.A.6-5 W. Steglich et al., J.C.S. Chem. Comm., 1132 (1982).

NPS—NH—CH(R)—COOH →[DCC, R'OH] NPS—NH—CH(R)—C(=O)—OR'
        *   *

>90%
No racemization is observed

R' = Me, Bz

VI.A.6-6 M. J. O'Donnell et al., Tetrahedron Lett., 23, 4259 (1982).

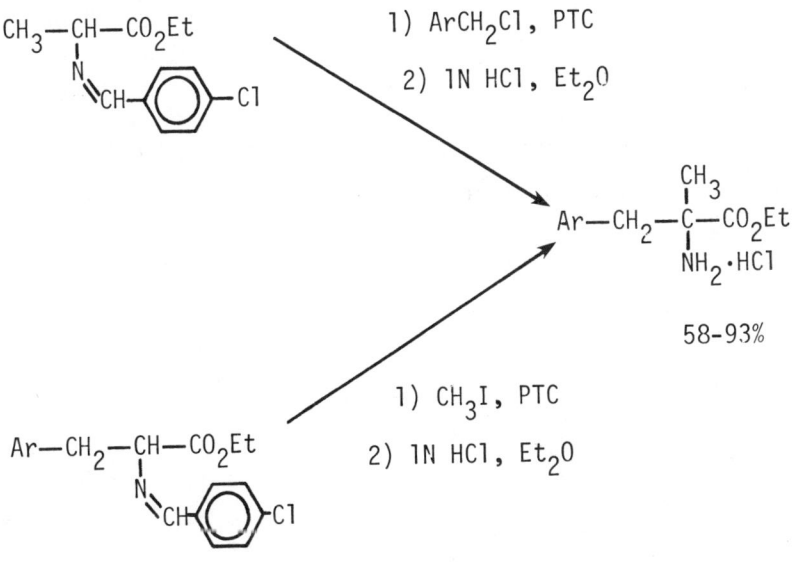

Ar = subst. Ph

VI.A.6-7   U. Schmidt et al., Angew. Chem. Int. Ed., 21, 776 (1982).

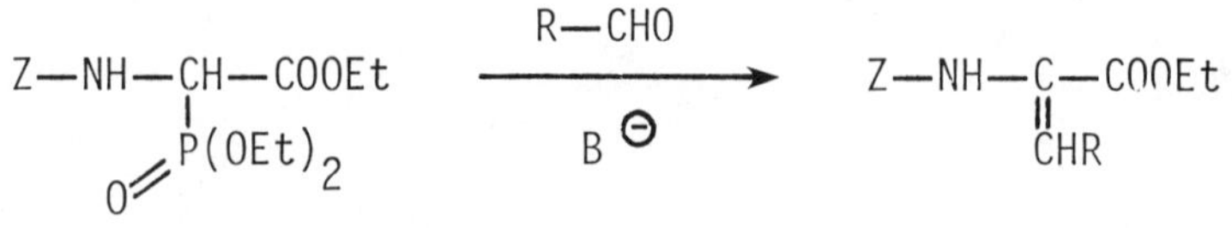

$$\underset{O\!\!\nearrow^{P(OEt)_2}}{Z-NH-CH-COOEt} \xrightarrow[B^{\ominus}]{R-CHO} \underset{CHR}{Z-NH-\overset{\|}{C}-COOEt}$$

73-85%

R = Pr, i-Pr, subst. Ph

VI.A.6-8   A. G. Agababyan et al., Russ. Chem. Rev., 51, 387 (1982).

Review: "Amino acids as the amine component in the Mannich reaction"

VI.A.7.   Carbenes

(see also: I.D.)

VI.A.7-1 J. A. Pincock and N. C. Mathur, *J. Org. Chem.*, **47**, 3699 (1982).

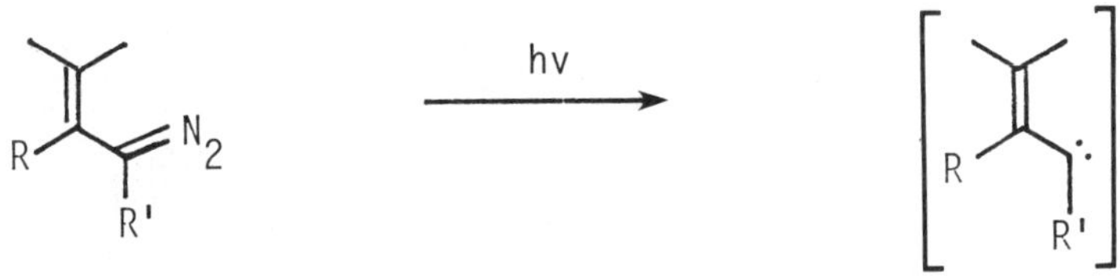

R, R' = Me, Ph

VI.A.7-2 U. R. Ghatak et al., *Indian J. Chem.*, **20B**, 911 (1981).

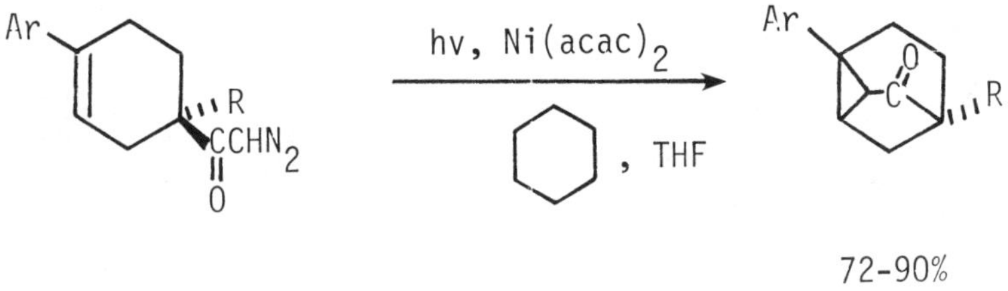

Ar = subst. Ph
R = H, Me

72-90%

VI.A.7-3 K. G. Taylor, *Tetrahedron*, **38**, 2751 (1982).

Review: "Carbenes and carbenoids with neighboring heteroatoms"

VI.A.7-4   P. J. Stang, Accounts Chem. Res., 15, 348 (1982).

Review: "Recent Developments in Unsaturated Carbenes and Related Chemistry"

VI.A.8.   Enamines

VI.A.8-1   P. W. Hickmott, Tetrahedron, 38, 1975 and 3363 (1982).

Review: "Enamines: Recent advances in synthetic, spectroscopic, mechanistic, and stereochemical aspects."

VI.A.8-2 L. Duhamel and J. -M. Poirer, Bull. Soc. Chim. France II, 297 (1982).

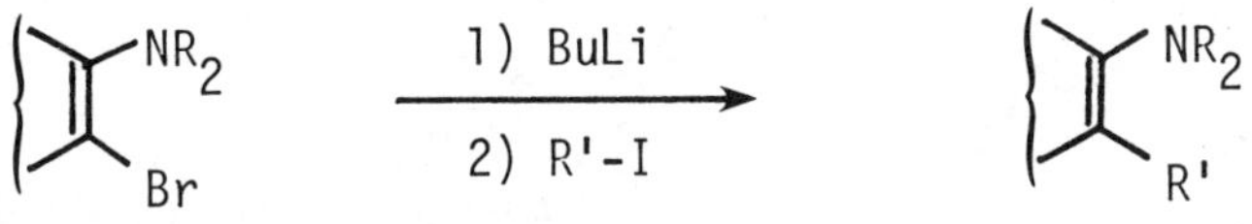
NR2
Br
1) BuLi
2) R'-I
NR2
R'

R' = Me, Et, Bu

widely varying yields

VI.A.8-3 W. Schroth *et al.*, Synthesis, 199 (1982).

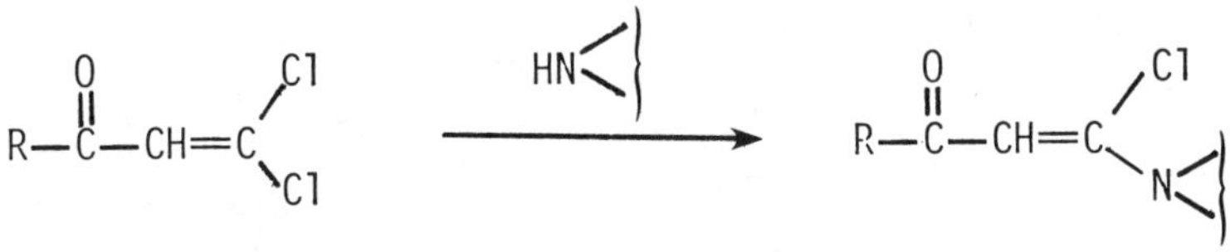
O
Cl
R—C—CH=C
Cl
HN
O
Cl
R—C—CH=C
N

~70-80%

R = Me, subst. Ph

VI.A.8-4 T. Shono *et al.*, Tetrahedron Lett., 23, 1201 (1982).

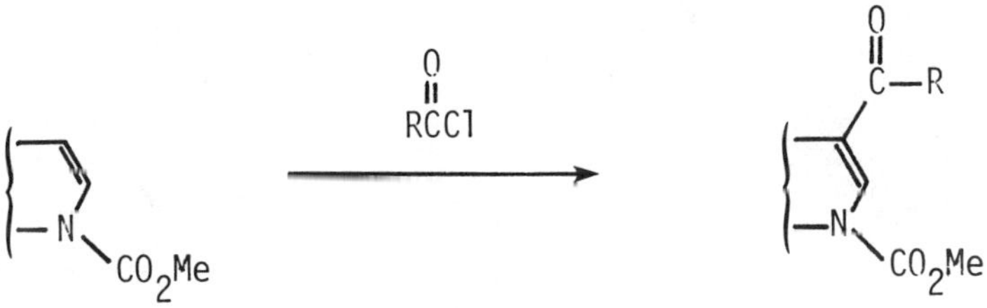
O
RCCl
N
CO2Me
O
C—R
N
CO2Me

32-85%

R = alkyl, c-Hx

VI.A.9. Epoxides

(see also: II.F.1.)

VI.A.9-1   E. Borredon et al., Tetrahedron Lett., 23, 5283 (1982).

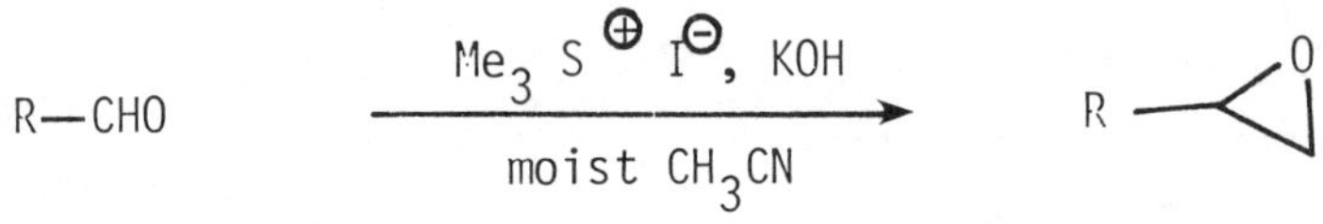

$$R-CHO \xrightarrow[\text{moist } CH_3CN]{Me_3S^{\oplus} I^{\ominus}, KOH} R-\triangleleft_O$$

95-98%

R = alkyl, aryl, heterocyclic

VI.A.9-2   V. Schurig et al., Synthesis, 316 (1982).

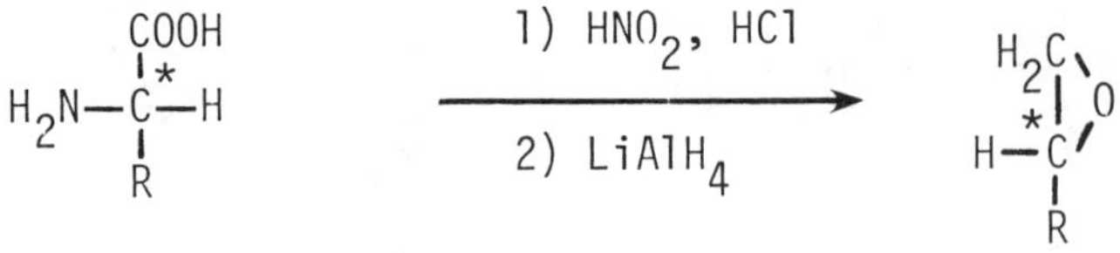

$$\underset{\text{(S) configuration}}{\overset{\underset{|}{COOH}}{H_2N-\overset{*}{C}-H}\atop\underset{|}{R}} \xrightarrow[\text{2) LiAlH}_4]{\text{1) HNO}_2, \text{HCl}} \underset{\text{(R) configuration}}{\overset{H_2C}{\underset{R}{\overset{|}{H-\overset{*}{C}}}}\diagdown_O\diagup}$$

~40-50% overall
~95% ee

R = alkyl

VI.A.9-3 G. Cardillo et al., J. Org. Chem., 47, 4626 (1982).

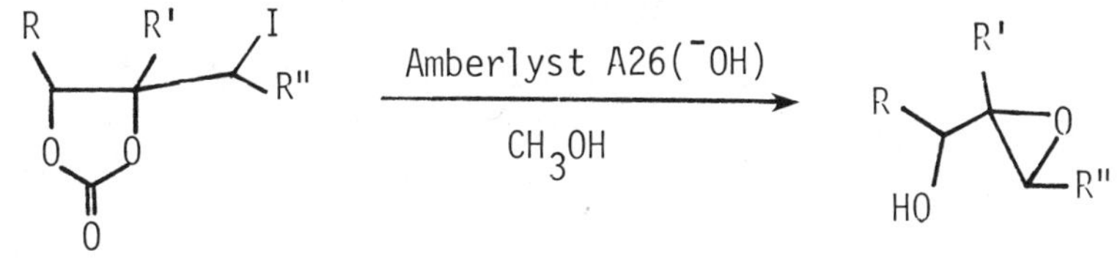

$$\text{cyclic carbonate with CHRR'I group} \xrightarrow[\text{CH}_3\text{OH}]{\text{Amberlyst A26(}^-\text{OH)}} \text{epoxide with CH(R)OH group}$$

R's = H, alkyl ∼90%

Full paper, many examples.

VI.A.10. Esters

(see also: IV.E, V.D.)

VI.A.10-1 T. Fujisawa et al., Chem. Lett., 1891 (1982).

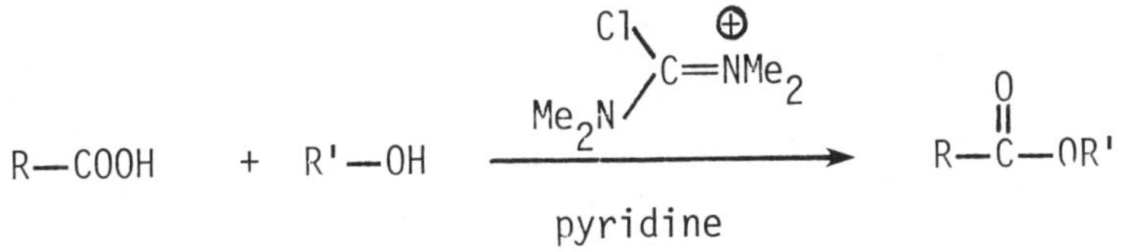

$$\text{R-COOH} + \text{R'-OH} \xrightarrow[\text{pyridine}]{\underset{\text{Me}_2\text{N}}{\overset{\text{Cl}}{>}}\text{C}=\overset{\oplus}{\text{NMe}_2}} \text{R-C(=O)-OR'}$$

∼80-90%

R, R' = alkyl, aryl; many examples

Also useful for forming macrocyclic lactones.

VI.A.10-2   S. Chandrasekaran and J. V. Turner, Synth. Comm., 12, 727 (1982).

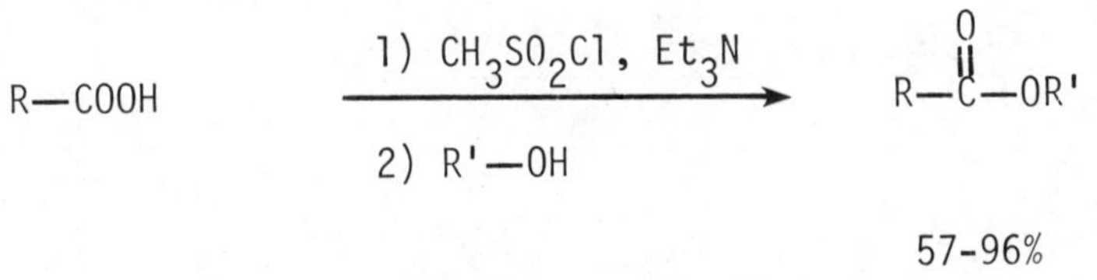

$$R-COOH \xrightarrow[\text{2) R'-OH}]{\text{1) CH}_3SO_2Cl, Et_3N} R-\overset{O}{\underset{\|}{C}}-OR'$$

57-96%

R = alkyl, aryl, cyclic, allylic, heterocyclic, etc.
R' = alkyl, Bz, cyclic, allylic

VI.A.10-3   K. S. Keshavamurthy et al., Synthesis, 506 (1982).

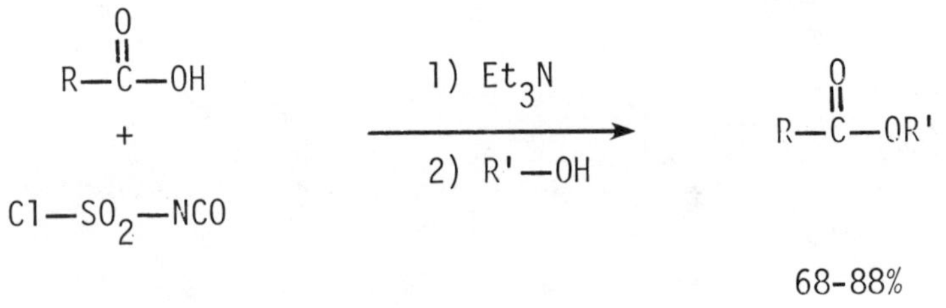

$$\begin{array}{c} R-\overset{O}{\underset{\|}{C}}-OH \\ + \\ Cl-SO_2-NCO \end{array} \xrightarrow[\text{2) R'-OH}]{\text{1) Et}_3N} R-\overset{O}{\underset{\|}{C}}-OR'$$

68-88%

R = alkyl, aryl, etc.

VI.A.10-4   V. Balasubramaniyan et al., Indian J. Chem., 21B, 259 (1982).

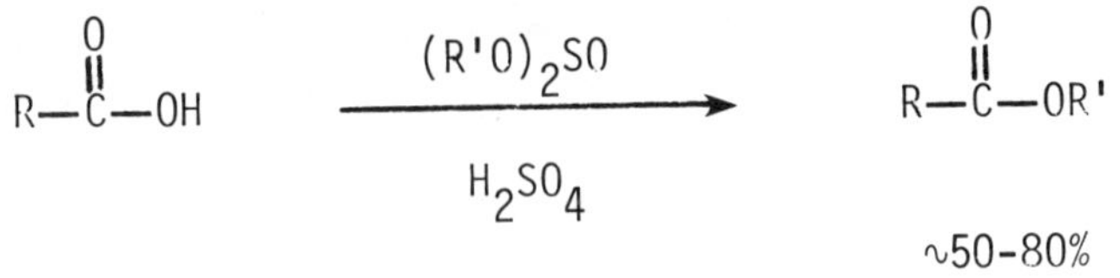

$$R-\overset{O}{\underset{\|}{C}}-OH \xrightarrow[H_2SO_4]{(R'O)_2SO} R-\overset{O}{\underset{\|}{C}}-OR'$$

∼50-80%

R = alkyl, aryl, alkenyl
R' = Me, Et

VI.A.10-5 H. Takaku et al., Chem. Pharm. Bull., 30, 2633 (1982).

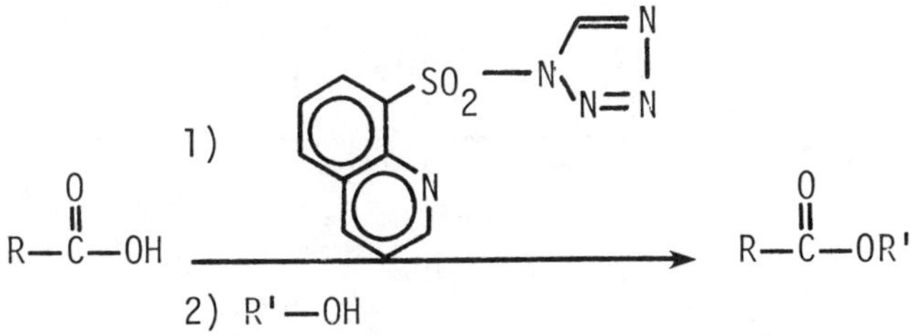

$$R-\underset{\underset{O}{\|}}{C}-OH \xrightarrow[\text{2) R'-OH}]{\text{1) 8-(1,2,4-triazolylsulfonyl)quinoline}} R-\underset{\underset{O}{\|}}{C}-OR'$$

74-93%

R = Ph, styryl, 1°, 2°, 3° alkyl
R' = Bz, Ph, 1°, 3° alkyl

VI.A.10-6 S. Ohta et al., Synthesis, 833 (1982).

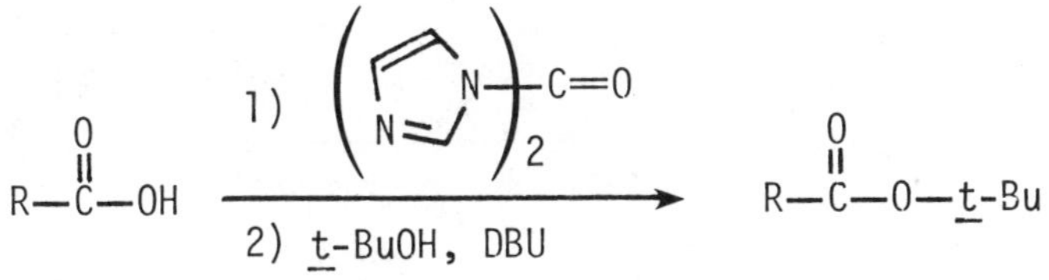

$$R-\underset{\underset{O}{\|}}{C}-OH \xrightarrow[\text{2) t-BuOH, DBU}]{\text{1) (Im)}_2C=O} R-\underset{\underset{O}{\|}}{C}-O-\underline{t}\text{-Bu}$$

54-91%

R = alkyl, aryl, vinyl, heterocyclic

VI.A.10-7 M. Dymicky, Org. Prep. Proc. Int., 14, 177 (1982).

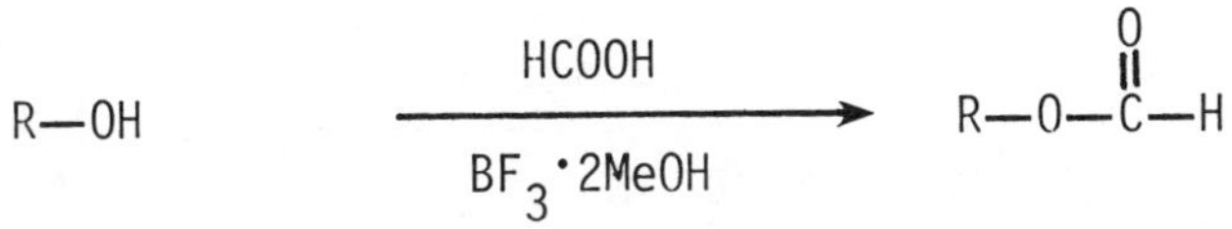

$$R-OH \xrightarrow[BF_3 \cdot 2MeOH]{HCOOH} R-O-\underset{\underset{O}{\|}}{C}-H$$

85-97%

R = 1°, 2° alkyl

VI.A.10-8 I. M. Downie et al., Tetrahedron, 38, 1457 (1982).

$$R-COOH \xrightarrow{(EtO)_2\overset{O}{\underset{\|}{P}}-CCl_3} R-\overset{O}{\underset{\|}{C}}-OEt$$

R = alkyl, aryl, haloalkyl

~70-90%

VI.A.10-9 T. Garcia, A. Arrieta, and C. Palomo, Synth. Comm., 12, 681 (1982).

$$R-COOH \xrightarrow[\text{2) R'OH, pyridine}]{\text{1) PhO}-\overset{O}{\underset{\|}{P}}Cl_2,\text{ DMF}} R-\overset{O}{\underset{\|}{C}}-OR'$$

R = alkyl, subst. Ph, vinyl
R' = alkyl, Bz, cinnamyl

72-99%

VI.A.10-10 M. K. Dhaon, R. K. Olsen, and K. Ramasamy, J. Org. Chem., 47, 1962 (1982).

$$\text{℗}-NH-CHR-COOH \xrightarrow[\text{DMAP, CH}_2Cl_2]{\text{R'OH, carbodiimide}} \text{℗}-NH-CHR-\overset{O}{\underset{\|}{C}}-OR'$$

P = Z, Boc
R' = t-Bu, Bz, Me

76-97%

very little racemization, except for Asp, Glu

VI.A.10-11   W. Steglich et al., J.C.S. Chem. Comm., 1132 (1982).

$$\text{NPS—NH—CH(R)—COOH} \xrightarrow[R'OH]{DCC} \text{NPS—NH—CH(R)—C(O)—OR'}$$

*   *

R' = Me, Bz

>90%
No racemization is observed.

VI.A.10-12   D. Seebach et al., Synthesis, 138 (1982).

$$R-\overset{O}{\underset{\|}{C}}-OR' \xrightarrow[R''OH]{Ti(OEt)_4} R-\overset{O}{\underset{\|}{C}}-OR''$$

50-99%

R = alkyl, aryl; subst. with Br, CN, NO_2
R" = alkyl, Bz, $-CH_2CH_2OCH_3$, $-CH_2CH_2TMS$

VI.A.10-13   E. Mohacsi, Synth. Comm., 12, 453 (1982).

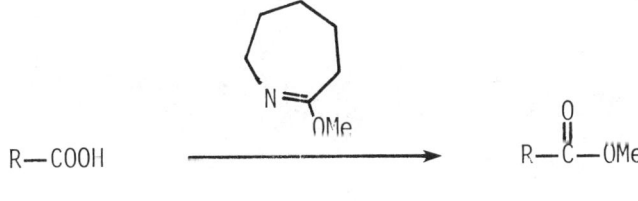

$$R-COOH \longrightarrow R-\overset{O}{\underset{\|}{C}}-OMe$$

72-96%

R = alkyl, aryl, vinyl

VI.A.10-14 I. Pri-Bar and J. K. Stille, *J. Org. Chem.*, **47**, 1215 (1982).

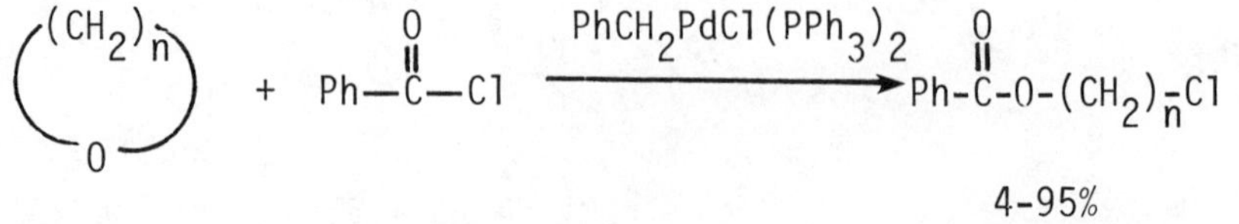

$$\text{cyclic ether }(CH_2)_n\text{-O} + Ph-\underset{\underset{O}{\|}}{C}-Cl \xrightarrow{PhCH_2PdCl(PPh_3)_2} Ph-\underset{\underset{O}{\|}}{C}-O-(CH_2)_n-Cl$$

4-95%

n = 4-5

VI.A.10-15 C. C. Fortes et al., *J.C.S. Chem. Comm.*, 857 (1982).

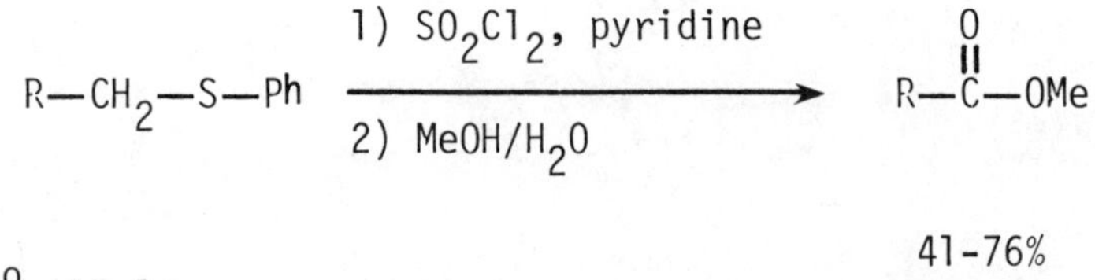

$$R-CH_2-S-Ph \xrightarrow[\text{2) MeOH/H}_2\text{O}]{\text{1) SO}_2\text{Cl}_2,\text{ pyridine}} R-\underset{\underset{O}{\|}}{C}-OMe$$

41-76%

R = 1° alkyl

VI.A.10-16 K. Fujii et al., *Synthesis*, 456 (1982).

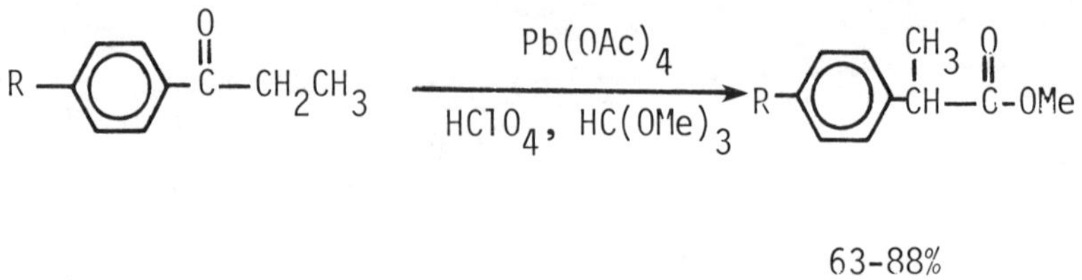

$$R-C_6H_4-\underset{\underset{O}{\|}}{C}-CH_2CH_3 \xrightarrow[HClO_4,\text{ HC(OMe)}_3]{Pb(OAc)_4} R-C_6H_4-\underset{CH_3}{\underset{|}{CH}}-\underset{\underset{O}{\|}}{C}-OMe$$

63-88%

R = H, alkyl, Ph, Br

VI.A.10-17 P. Müller and J. Godoy, Tetrahedron Lett., 23, 3661 (1982).

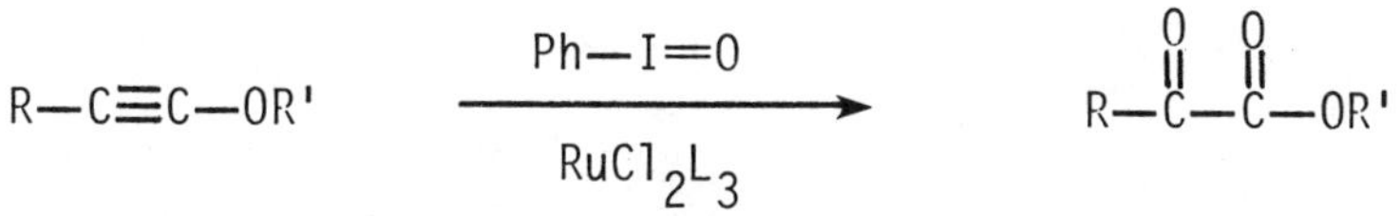

$$R-C\equiv C-OR' \xrightarrow[RuCl_2L_3]{Ph-I=O} R-\underset{O}{\underset{\|}{C}}-\underset{O}{\underset{\|}{C}}-OR'$$

R = alkyl, Ph
R' = alkyl

59-70%

$$R-C\equiv C-NR'_2 \xrightarrow[RuCl_2L_3]{Ph-I=O} R-\underset{O}{\underset{\|}{C}}-\underset{O}{\underset{\|}{C}}-NR'_2$$

R = alkyl, Ph
R' = alkyl

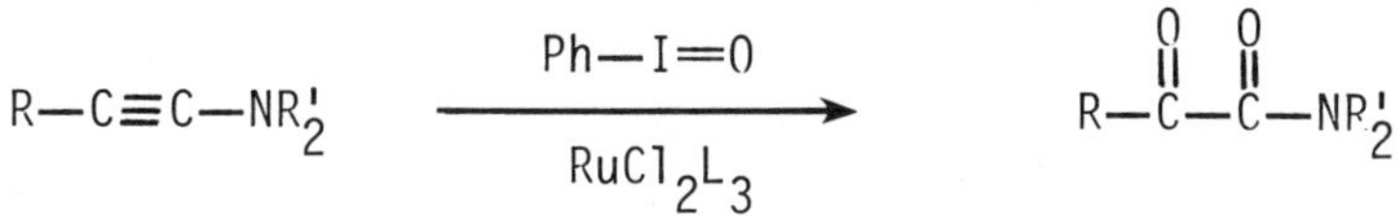

0-76%

VI.A.10-18 O. L. Mndzhoyan and V. O. Topuzyan, Russ. Chem. Rev., 50, 1151 (1981).

Review: "Methods of synthesis and properties of β-dimethylaminoethyl and choline esters of amino acids and peptides"

VI.A.11. Ethers

(see also: V.A.)

VI.A.11-1 T. Ando et al., Bull. Chem. Soc. Japan, 55, 2504 (1982).

$$R-OH \xrightarrow{MeI, \text{ KF-alumina}} R-OMe$$

R = alkyl, aryl

∼50-100%

VI.A.11-2 R. B. Bates and K. D. Janda, J. Org. Chem., 47, 4374 (1982).

$$Ar-OH \xrightarrow[\underline{t}-BuO^{\ominus} K^{\oplus}]{Me_2SO, \text{ PhI}} Ar-O-Ph$$

Ar = subst. Ph

∼40-80%

$$Ar-SH \xrightarrow[\underline{t}-BuO^{\ominus} K^{\oplus}]{Me_2SO, \text{ PhI}} Ar-S-Ph$$

50-100%

VI.A.11-3 S. K. Banerjee, B. D. Gupta, and K. Singh, J.C.S. Chem. Comm., 815 (1982).

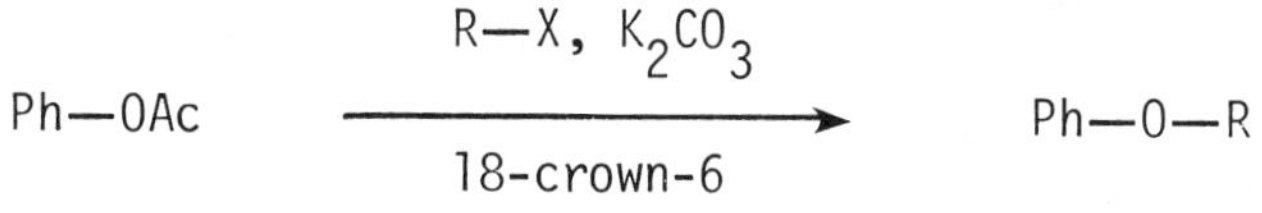

$$Ph-OAc \xrightarrow[\text{18-crown-6}]{R-X, K_2CO_3} Ph-O-R$$

R = alkyl, allylic, benzylic

VI.A.11-4 A. Ohta et al., Synthesis, 828 (1982).

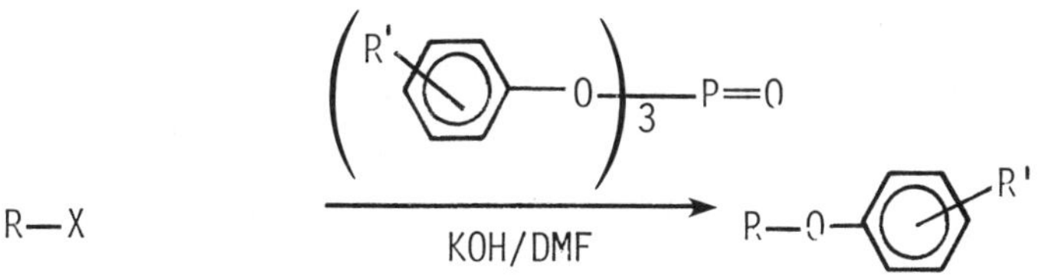

$$R-X \xrightarrow[\text{KOH/DMF}]{\left(R'\text{-C}_6H_4\text{-O}\right)_3 P=O} R-O-C_6H_4-R'$$

R = 1° alkyl, Bz, subst Ph, heterocyclic
X = Cl, Br
R' = H, Me, NO_2

48-98%

VI.A.11-5 F. Camps, J. Coll, and J. M. Moreto, Synthesis, 186 (1982).

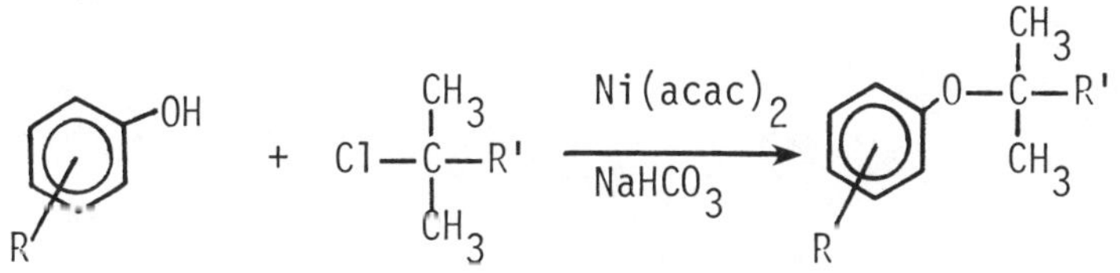

$$\text{R-C}_6H_4\text{-OH} + Cl-C(CH_3)_2-R' \xrightarrow[\text{NaHCO}_3]{Ni(acac)_2} \text{R-C}_6H_4\text{-O-C}(CH_3)_2\text{-R}'$$

R = H, Me, OMe, NO_2, F, Cl
R' = Me, Et

∼30%

VI.A.12. Ketones and Aldehydes

(see also: I.A.2., II.A.1., II.F.1., III.F.2.)

VI.A.12-1 S. Ohta and M. Okamoto, *Synthesis*, 756 (1982).

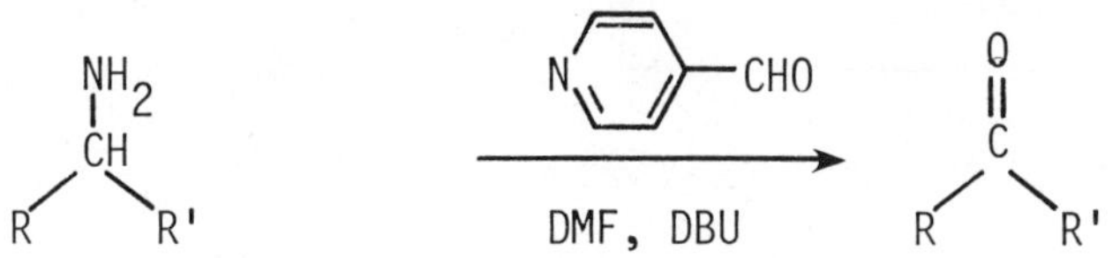

$$\underset{RR'}{\overset{NH_2}{\underset{|}{CH}}} \quad \xrightarrow[\text{DMF, DBU}]{\text{4-Py-CHO}} \quad \underset{RR'}{\overset{O}{\underset{\|}{C}}}$$

R, R' = H, alkyl, subst. Ph

VI.A.12-2 T. F. Buckley and H. Rapoport, *J. Am. Chem. Soc.*, **104**, 4446 (1982).

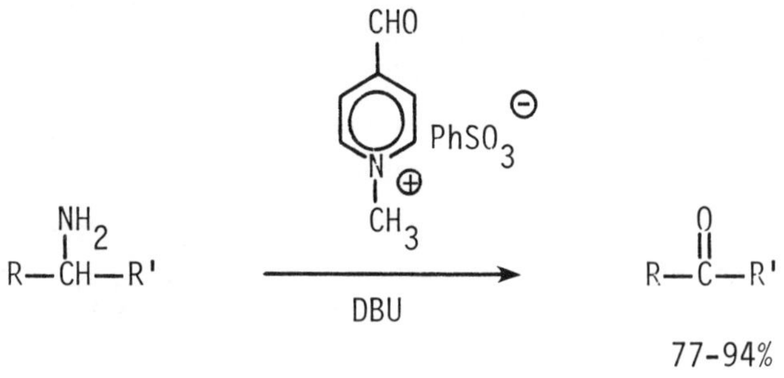

$$R-\underset{\underset{H}{|}}{\overset{NH_2}{\underset{|}{C}}}-R' \quad \xrightarrow[\text{DBU}]{\text{1-methyl-4-formylpyridinium PhSO}_3^-} \quad R-\overset{O}{\underset{\|}{C}}-R'$$

77-94%

R, R' = H, alkyl, aryl, protected amino acid, etc.

VI.A.12-3 M. Yamashita et al., Bull. Chem. Soc. Japan, 55, 1663 (1982).

$$R-MgBr \xrightarrow[\text{2) HOAc or DOAc}]{\text{1) Fe(CO)}_5} R-CHO \text{ or } R-CDO$$

40-99%

VI.A.12-4 T. Fujisawa, T. Mori, and T. Sato, Tetrahedron Lett., 23, 5059 (1982).

$$R-\overset{O}{\underset{\|}{C}}-OLi \xrightarrow{R'MgBr} R-\overset{O}{\underset{\|}{C}}-R'$$

(with reagent: 4-MeO-C$_6$H$_4$-C(Cl)=N$^{\oplus}$(Ph)(Ph) Cl$^{\ominus}$)

60-94%

R = 1°, 2°, 3° alkyl, Ph
R' = 2°, 3° alkyl, Ph, PhCH$_2$CH$_2$-

VI.A.12-5 N. Kornblum et al., J. Org. Chem., 47, 4534 (1982).

$$R-CH_2-NO_2 \xrightarrow[\text{2) KMnO}_4]{\text{1) NaH, }\underline{t}\text{-BuOH}} R-CHO$$
$$\text{3) Na}_2S_2O_5, H_2SO_4$$

59-96%

R = 1°, 2°, 3° alkyl. May contain -CN, ester, etc.
Also works for ketones: $R_2CH-NO_2 \longrightarrow R_2C=O$, ~90%

VI.A.12-6   T. R. Beebe et al., J. Org. Chem., 47, 3006 (1982).

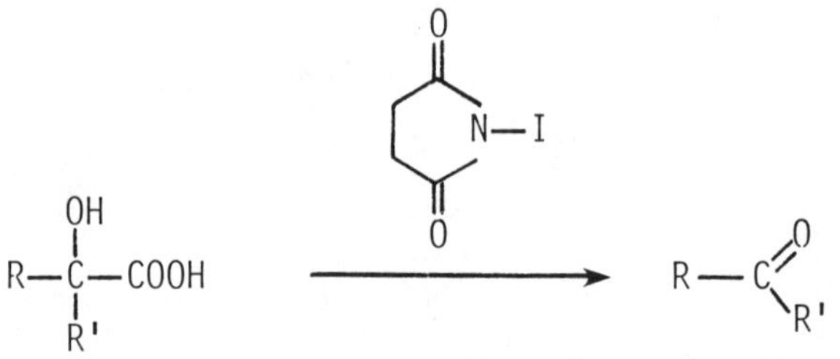

$$R-\underset{R'}{\underset{|}{\overset{OH}{\overset{|}{C}}}}-COOH \xrightarrow{\text{N-iodosuccinimide}} R-\overset{O}{\overset{\|}{C}}-R'$$

R, R' = H, alkyl, aryl   80-103%

VI.A.12-7   J. H. Babler, Synth. Comm., 12, 839 (1982).

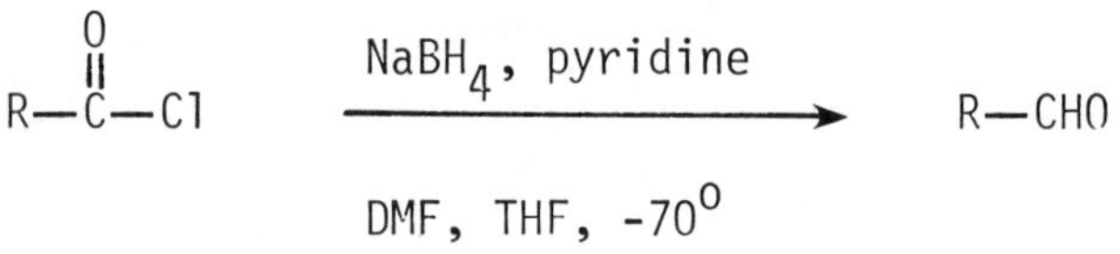

$$R-\overset{O}{\overset{\|}{C}}-Cl \xrightarrow[\text{DMF, THF, -70°}]{\text{NaBH}_4, \text{ pyridine}} R-CHO$$

R = alkyl, subst. Ph

VI.A.12-8   K. Ogura et al., Chem. Lett., 813 (1982).

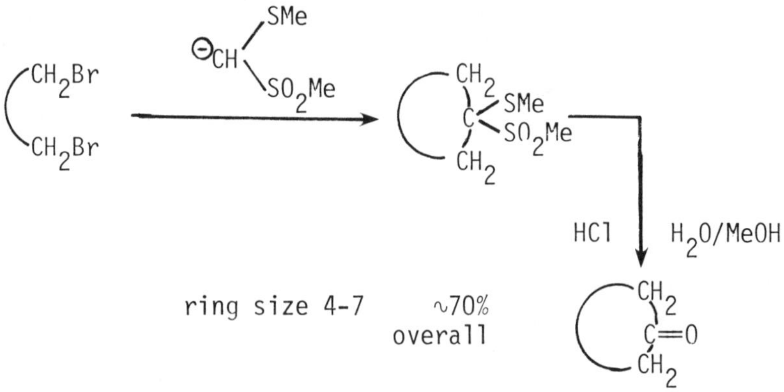

Reaction of α,ω-dibromide with $^{\ominus}CH(SMe)(SO_2Me)$ gives cyclic product with $C(SMe)(SO_2Me)$, then HCl, H$_2$O/MeOH gives cyclic ketone.

ring size 4-7   ~70% overall

VI.A.12-9 V. Janout and S. L. Regen, *J. Org. Chem.*, **47**, 3331 (1982).

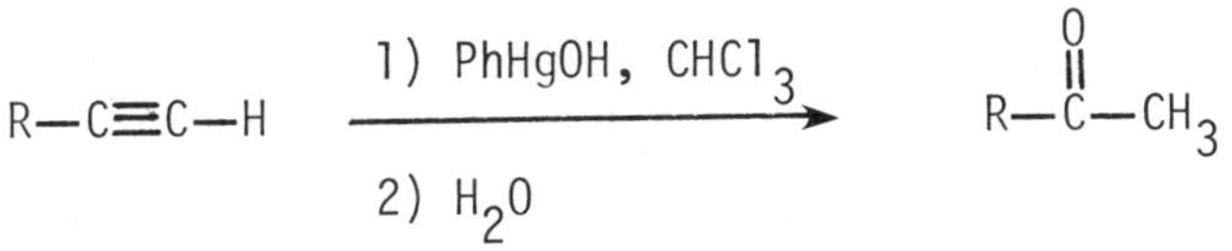

$$R-C\equiv C-H \xrightarrow[\text{2) } H_2O]{\text{1) PhHgOH, CHCl}_3} R-\overset{O}{\underset{\|}{C}}-CH_3$$

49-67%

R = alkyl

VI.A.12-10 G. A. Tolstikov et al., *J. Gen. Chem. (USSR)*, **52**, 1170 (1982).

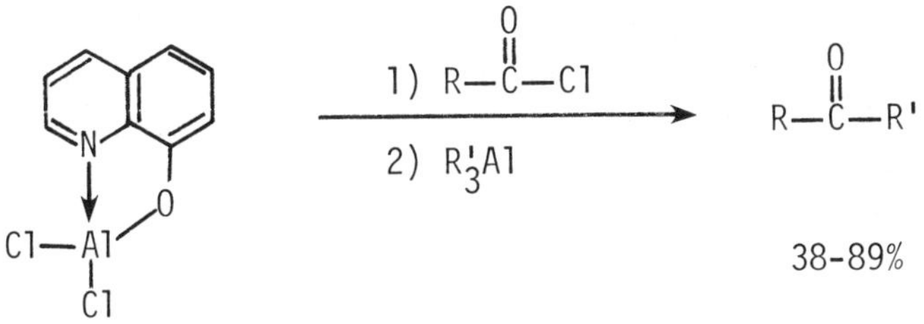

$$\underset{\underset{Cl}{\overset{|}{Al}}-Cl}{\text{(quinoline-8-olate complex)}} \xrightarrow[\text{2) } R'_3Al]{\text{1) } R-\overset{O}{\underset{\|}{C}}-Cl} R-\overset{O}{\underset{\|}{C}}-R'$$

38-89%

R = alkyl, aryl, vinyl, furyl
R' = alkyl

VI.A.12-11 N. Miyaura, K. Maeda, and H. Suginome, *J. Org. Chem.*, **47**, 2117 (1982).

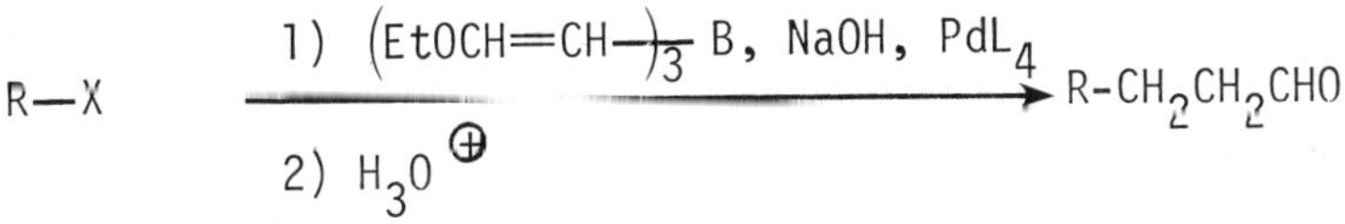

$$R-X \xrightarrow[\text{2) } H_3O^{\oplus}]{\text{1) } (EtOCH=CH)_3B, \text{ NaOH, PdL}_4} R-CH_2CH_2CHO$$

48-98%

R = Subst. Ph, Bz.
X = I, Cl, Br

VI.A.12-12   A. S. Rao et al., Indian J. Chem., 21B, 408 (1982).

$$R-CH_2X \xrightarrow[\substack{\text{2) NaOH, MeOH} \\ \text{3) NaBH}_4\text{, EtOH} \\ \text{4) Pd(OAc)}_4\text{, I}_2\text{, benzene}}]{\text{1) Ph-CO-CH}_2\text{-COOMe, NaH}} R-CH_2CH_2CHO$$

~50%

VI.A.12-13   M. W. Anderson, R. C. F. Jones, and J. Saunders, J.C.S. Chem. Comm., 282 (1982).

$$\text{imidazolinium salt (Bz, Me, I}^-\text{)} \xrightarrow{R''M} R''-\overset{O}{\underset{\|}{C}}-CHRR'$$

55-85%

R's = H, alkyl

VI.A.12-14   N. A. Bumagin, Bull. Acad. USSR Chem., 31, 211 (1982).

$$\begin{array}{c} Ar_2Hg \\ \text{or} \\ 2\ ArHgCl \end{array} \xrightarrow[\text{or CO, PhPdIL}_2\text{, HMPT}]{CO,\ [Rh(CO)_2Cl]_2,\ HMPT} Ar-\overset{O}{\underset{\|}{C}}-Ar$$

Ar = subst. Ph

~80-100% when optimized

VI.A.12-15 H. C. Brown et al., J. Org. Chem., 47, 754 (1982); Synthesis, 193 (1982).

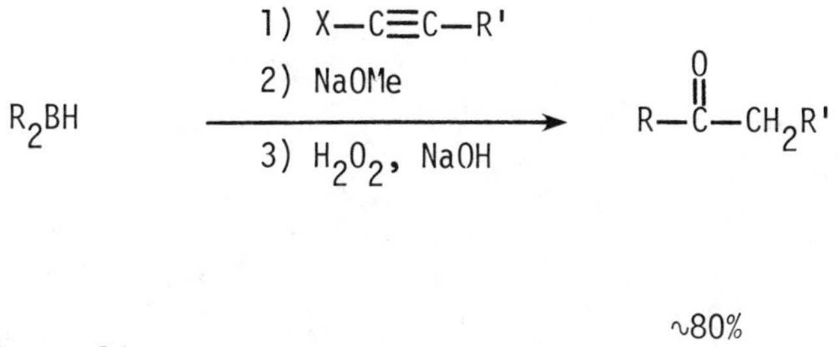

$$R_2BH \xrightarrow[\text{3) }H_2O_2,\text{ NaOH}]{\text{1) }X-C\equiv C-R' \quad \text{2) NaOMe}} R-\underset{\underset{O}{\|}}{C}-CH_2R'$$

~80%

R = alkyl, cyclic
R' = n-alkyl
X = Cl, Br, I

VI.A.12-16 I. K. Stamos, Tetrahedron Lett., 23, 459 (1982).

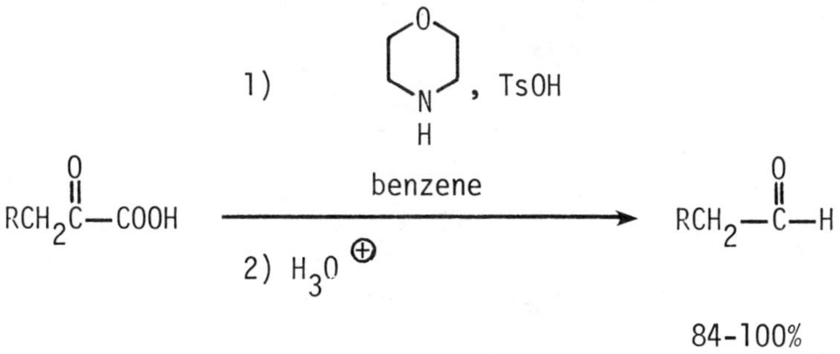

$$RCH_2\overset{O}{\underset{\|}{C}}-COOH \xrightarrow[\text{2) }H_3O^\oplus]{\text{1) morpholine, TsOH, benzene}} RCH_2-\overset{O}{\underset{\|}{C}}-H$$

84-100%

R = alkyl, subst. Ph

VI.A.12-17 N. Kornblum et al., J. Org. Chem., 47, 4534 (1982).

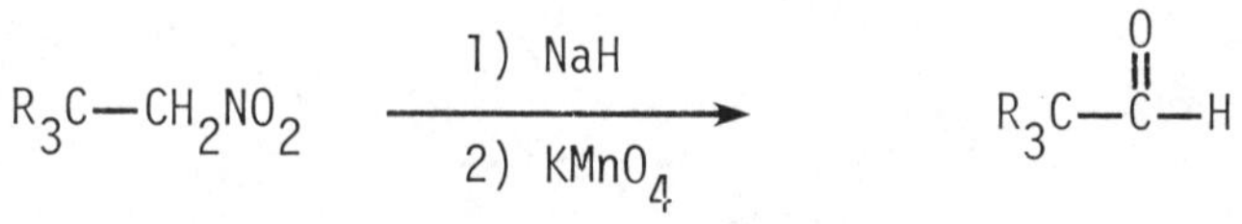

$$R_3C-CH_2NO_2 \xrightarrow[\text{2) KMnO}_4]{\text{1) NaH}} R_3C-\underset{\underset{O}{\|}}{C}-H$$

R = alkyl, aryl, H

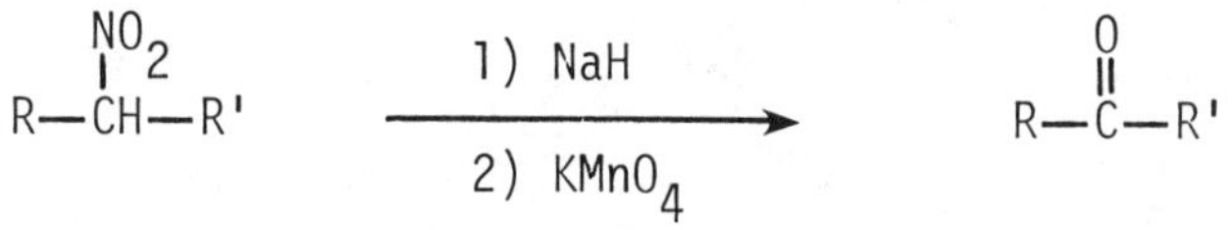

59-96%

$$R-\underset{\underset{NO_2}{|}}{CH}-R' \xrightarrow[\text{2) KMnO}_4]{\text{1) NaH}} R-\underset{\underset{O}{\|}}{C}-R'$$

R, R' = alkyl, aryl

90-91%

VI.A.12-18 J. Tsuji, H. Nagashima, and K. Hori, Tetrahedron Lett., 23, 2679 (1982).

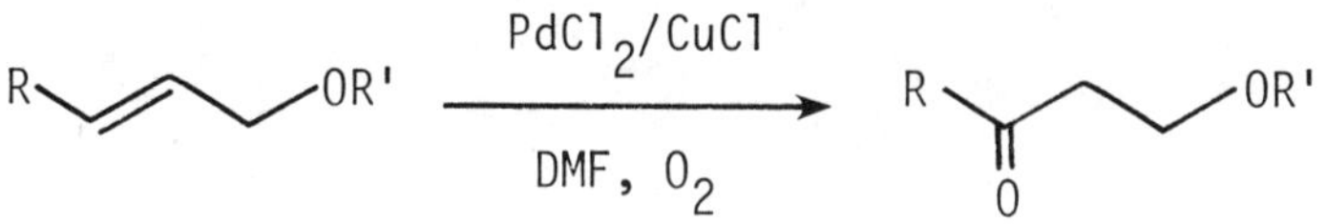

$$R\diagup\!\!\!\diagdown\!\!\!\diagup OR' \xrightarrow[\text{DMF, O}_2]{\text{PdCl}_2/\text{CuCl}} R\underset{\underset{O}{\|}}{\diagup\!\!\!\diagdown\!\!\!\diagup} OR'$$

∼40-76%

R = alkyl
R' = Me, Bz, Ac

VI.A.12-19   H. Nagashima, K. Sakai, and J. Tsuji, Chem. Lett., 859 (1982).

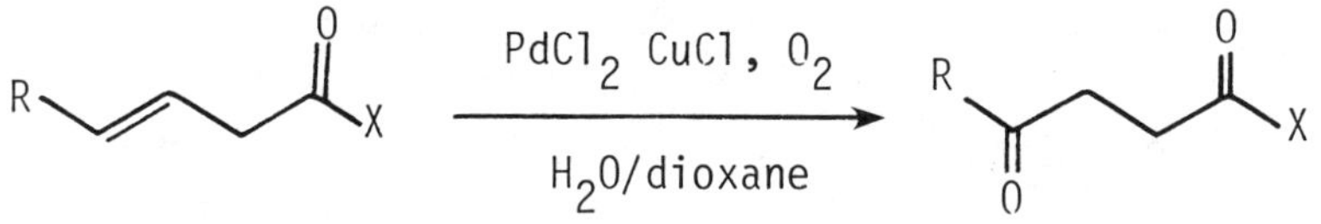

R–CH=CH–CH$_2$–C(=O)–X $\xrightarrow[\text{H}_2\text{O/dioxane}]{\text{PdCl}_2 \text{ CuCl, O}_2}$ R–C(=O)–CH$_2$–CH$_2$–C(=O)–X

X = Me, OMe
R = alkyl

45-61%

VI.A.12-20   T. Hirao et al., Chem. Lett., 1997 (1982).

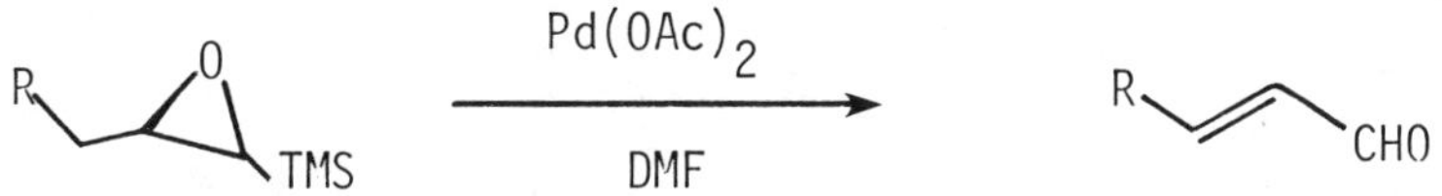

R–CH$_2$–(epoxide)–TMS $\xrightarrow[\text{DMF}]{\text{Pd(OAc)}_2}$ R–CH=CH–CHO

R = alkyl

widely varying yields

VI.A.12-21   K. Takabe et al., Chem. Lett., 1987 (1982).

RR'C=CHCH$_2$NMe$_2$ $\xrightarrow[\text{2) Ac}_2\text{O}]{\text{1) H}_2\text{O}_2}$ RR'C=CHCHO

R, R' = H, alkyl

∼70%

VI.A.12-22 D. L. Comins, J. D. Brown, and N. B. Mantlo, Tetrahedron Lett., 23, 3979 (1982).

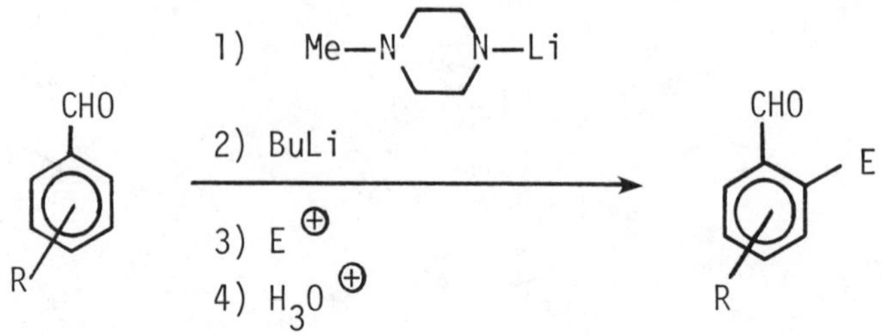
CHO
R
1) Me—N N—Li
2) BuLi
3) E ⊕
4) H_3O ⊕
CHO
E
R

47-76%

R = H, Cl, benzo-
E ⊕ = MeI, BuI, Me_3SiCl

VI.A.12-23 A. Rahm et al., Synth. Comm., 12, 485 (1982).

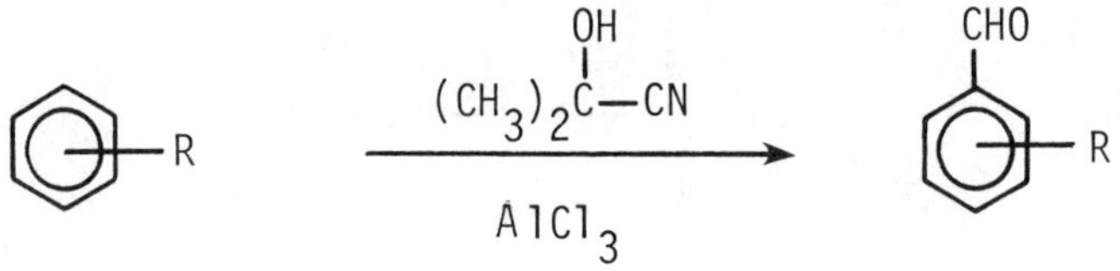
R
OH
$(CH_3)_2C$—CN
$AlCl_3$
CHO
R

(expected o,m,p distribution)

R = H, Me, -OMe, benzo- 40-83%

VI.A.12-24 A. P. Kozikowski and M. Adamczyk, Tetrahedron Lett., 23, 3123 (1982).

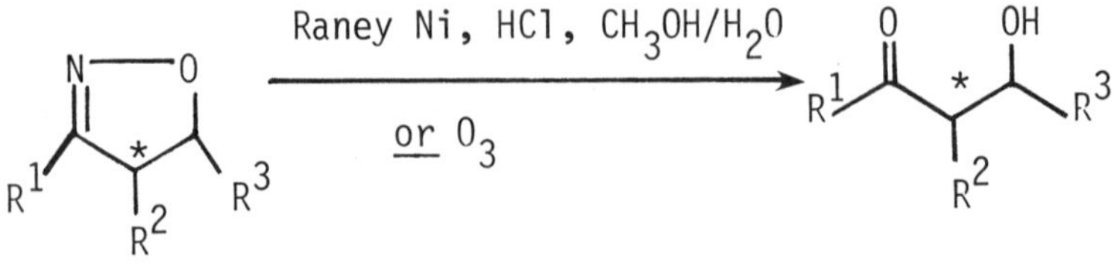
N O
*
R^1 R^2 R^3
Raney Ni, HCl, CH_3OH/H_2O
or O_3
O OH
*
R^1 R^3
R^2

VI.A.12-25   H. Wynberg and E. W.Meijer, Org. React., 28, 1 (1982).

Review: "The Reimer-Tiemann Reaction"

VI.A.12-26   G. Consiglio and P. Pino, Topics in Current Chem., 105, 77 (1982).

Review: "Asymmetric Hydroformylation"

VI.A.12-27   M. T. Reetz, Angew. Chem. Int. Ed., 21, 96 (1982).

Review: "Lewis Acid Induced α-Alkylation of Carbonyl Compounds"

VI.A.13. Nitriles

VI.A.13-1 U. Feldhues and H. J. Schäfer, Synthesis, 145 (1982).

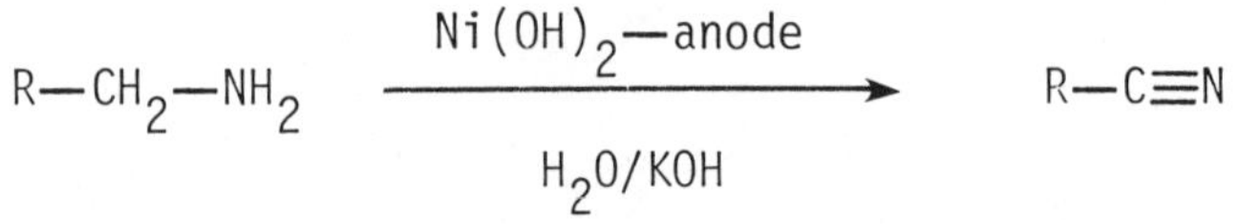

$$R-CH_2-NH_2 \xrightarrow[H_2O/KOH]{Ni(OH)_2-\text{anode}} R-C\equiv N$$

72-97%

R = alkyl, Bz, -CH$_2$-(furyl), -(CH$_2$)$_5$-COOH

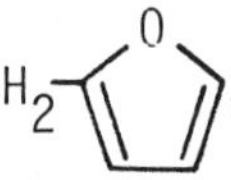

VI.A.13-2 A. D. Dunn, M. J. Mills, and W. Henry, Org. Prep. Proc. Int., 14, 396 (1982).

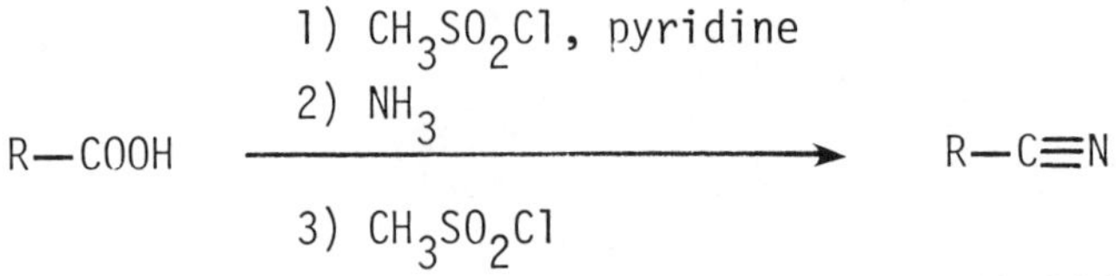

$$R-COOH \xrightarrow[\substack{2)\ NH_3 \\ 3)\ CH_3SO_2Cl}]{1)\ CH_3SO_2Cl,\ \text{pyridine}} R-C\equiv N$$

63-82%

R = alkyl, aryl, heterocyclic

VI.A.13-3 C. Bolleghi et al., Synth. Comm., 12, 25 (1982).

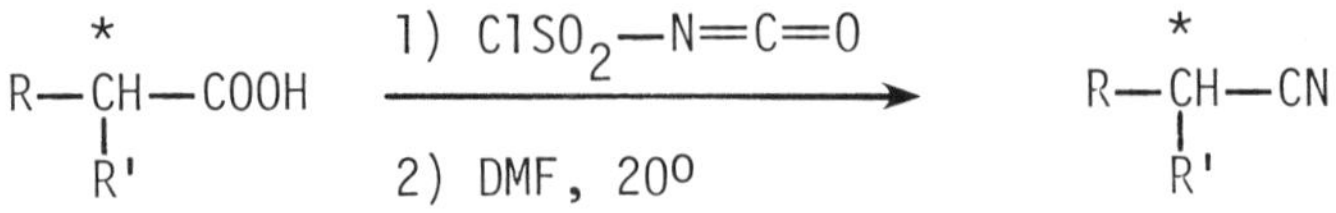

$$\overset{*}{R}-\underset{R'}{CH}-COOH \xrightarrow[2)\ DMF,\ 20°]{1)\ ClSO_2-N=C=O} \overset{*}{R}-\underset{R'}{CH}-CN$$

∼60%

>90% retention of configuration

R, R' = alkyl, Ph

VI.A.13-4   A. Hulkenberg and J. J. Troost, Tetrahedron Lett., 23, 1505 (1982).

$$R-\underset{\underset{O}{\|}}{C}-Cl \xrightarrow[120°]{H_2N-SO_2-NH_2} R-C\equiv N$$

62-97%

R = alkyl, aryl, vinyl, heterocyclic

This reaction may use the acid as a starting material in some cases, although the yields are slightly lower.

VI.A.13-5   M. Yokoyama et al., Synthesis, 591 (1982).

$$R-\underset{\underset{O}{\|}}{C}-NH_2 \xrightarrow{\left[\begin{array}{c}\underset{\underset{OSiMe_3}{|}}{\overset{\overset{O}{\|}}{P}}-O\end{array}\right]_n} R-C\equiv N$$

23-97%

R = subst. Ph, alkyl, heterocyclic

VI.A.13-6   M. -I. Lim, W. -Y. Ren, and R. S. Klein, J. Org. Chem., 47, 4594 (1982).

$$R-\underset{\underset{S}{\|}}{C}-NH_2 \xrightarrow[\underline{or}(Bu_3Sn)_2O/benzene]{Bu_2SnO/MeOH} R-CN$$

R = alkyl, aryl, pyridyl, thienyl, pyrrolyl

VI.A.13-7   A. Saednya, Synthesis, 190 (1982).

$$R-CHO \xrightarrow[\text{pyridine/toluene}]{NH_2OH \cdot HCl} R-C\equiv N$$

50-89%

R = alkyl, subst. Ph, thienyl

VI.A.13-8   P. Molina et al., Synthesis, 1016 (1982).

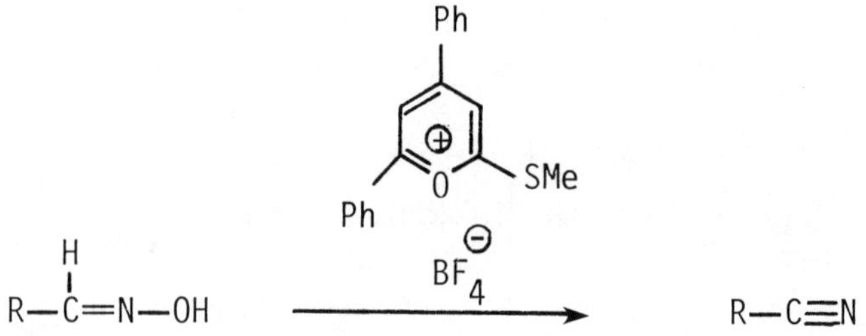

$$R-\underset{H}{C}=N-OH \xrightarrow{\text{[2,6-diphenyl-4-(methylthio)pyrylium } BF_4^-\text{]}} R-C\equiv N$$

75-93%

R = n-alkyl, subst. Ph, styryl, furyl

VI.A.13-9   H.-J. Liu and H. Wynn, Tetrahedron Lett., 23, 3151 (1982).

$$N\equiv C-CH_2-\underset{O}{\overset{O}{C}}-S-R \xrightarrow[\text{2) NaH, R''X}]{\text{1) NaH, R'X}} N\equiv C-\underset{R''}{\overset{R'}{C}}-CH_2OH$$
$$\text{3) NaBH}_4$$

R = Bz, t-Bu   ~70-90%
R', R'' = H, 1°, 2° alkyl, Bz

VI.A.13-10   T. Saegusa et al., J. Am. Chem. Soc., 104, 6449 (1982).

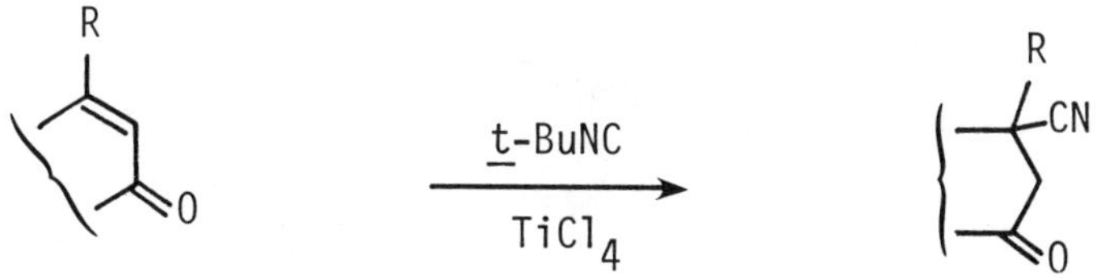

[reaction scheme: cyclohexenone derivative + t-BuNC / TiCl$_4$ → β-cyano ketone]

R = H, Me

63-87%

VI.A.13-11   T. Funabiki et al., J. Am. Chem. Soc., 104, 1560 (1982).

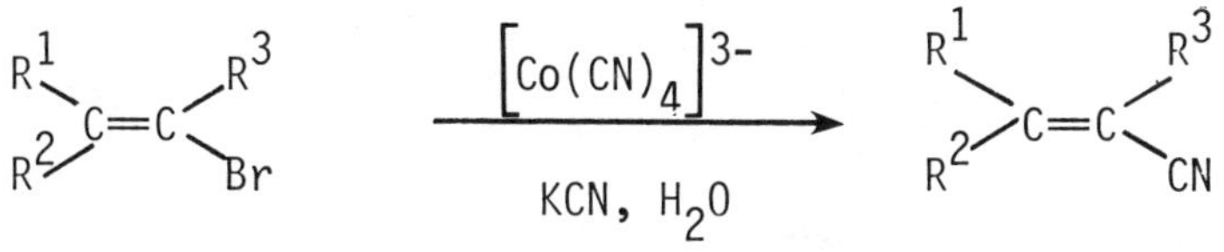

[reaction scheme: vinyl bromide $R^1R^2C=CR^3Br$ + [Co(CN)$_4$]$^{3-}$, KCN, H$_2$O → vinyl nitrile $R^1R^2C=CR^3CN$]

R's = H, Me, Ph, CO$_2$Me

∼50-90%

VI.A.13-12   Y. Sakakibara et al., Chem. Lett., 1565 (1982).

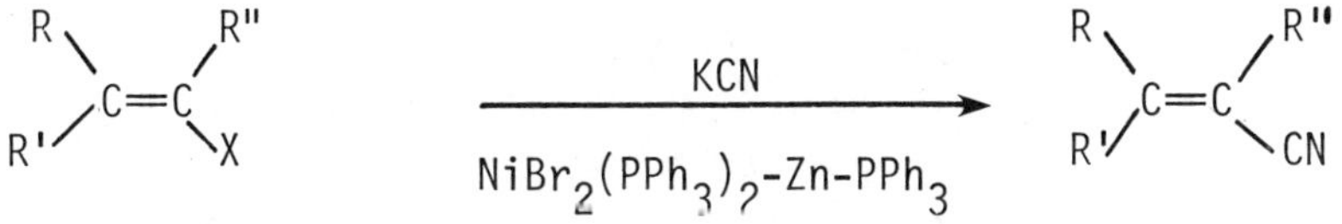

[reaction scheme: vinyl halide + KCN / NiBr$_2$(PPh$_3$)$_2$–Zn–PPh$_3$ → vinyl nitrile]

∼70-90%

X = Br, Cl
R's = monosub. alkyl, Ph

VI.A.13-13 Y. Sato and Y. Niinomi, J.C.S. Chem. Comm., 56 (1982).

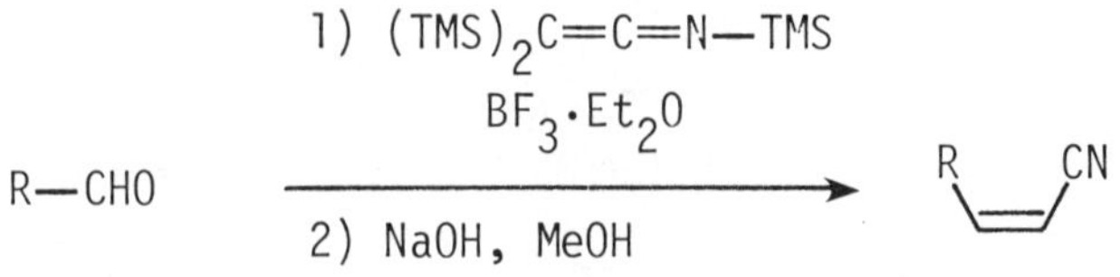

$$R-CHO \xrightarrow[\text{2) NaOH, MeOH}]{\text{1) (TMS)}_2C=C=N-TMS \quad BF_3 \cdot Et_2O} R\diagdown\diagup CN$$

R = alkyl, aryl

~50-85%

VI.A.13-14 S. Hünig and R. Schaller, Angew. Chem. Int. Ed., 21, 36 (1982).

Review: "The Chemistry of Acyl Cyanides"

VI.A.13-15 K. Haase and H. M. R. Hoffmann, Angew. Chem. Int. Ed., 21, 83 (1982).

$$R-\underset{\underset{O}{\|}}{C}-I \quad + \quad CuCN \quad \longrightarrow \quad R-\underset{\underset{O}{\|}}{C}-CN$$

R = alkyl, aryl, styryl

53-78%

VI.A.14. Nitro-compounds

VI.A.14-1 T. Miyakoshi et al., Chem. Lett., 1677 (1981).

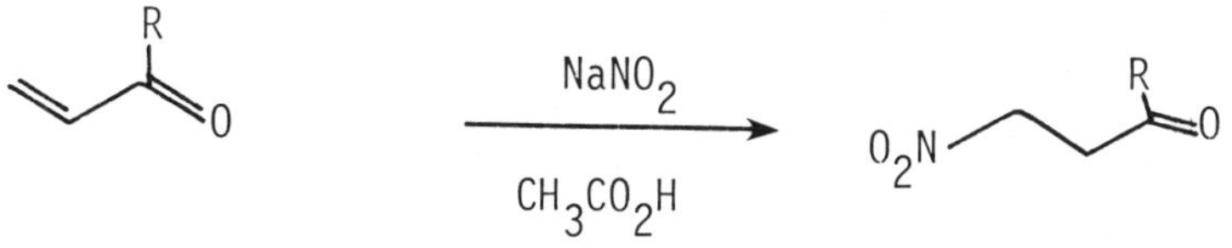

$$CH_2=CR-CO-R \xrightarrow[CH_3CO_2H]{NaNO_2} O_2N-CH_2-CHR-CO-R$$

R = alkyl

42-82%

VI.A.14-2 M. V. Prostenik and I. Butula, Angew. Chem. Int. Ed., 21, 139 (1982).

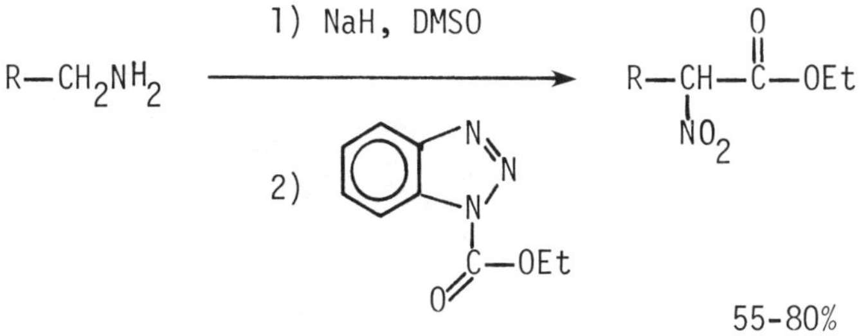

$$R-CH_2NH_2 \xrightarrow[\text{2) benzotriazole-CO-OEt}]{\text{1) NaH, DMSO}} R-CH(NO_2)-C(O)-OEt$$

55-80%

R = H, Me, Et

VI.A.14-3 S. Tomoda et al., Tetrahedron Lett., 23, 4733 (1982).

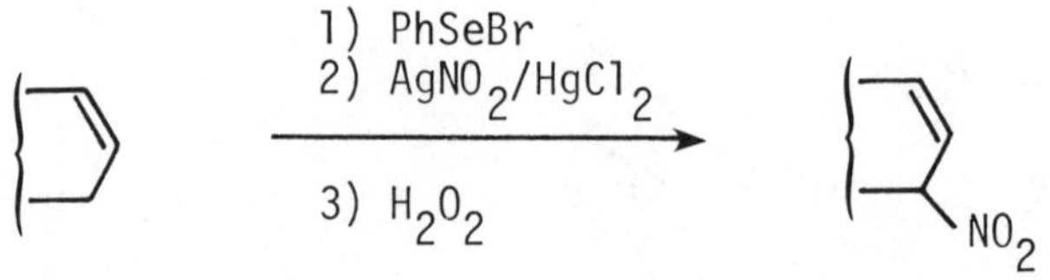

cyclopentadiene →(1) PhSeBr; 2) AgNO$_2$/HgCl$_2$; 3) H$_2$O$_2$)→ 3-nitrocyclopentene

58-83%

VI.A.14-4 S. Tomoda et al., Chem. Lett., 1109 (1982).

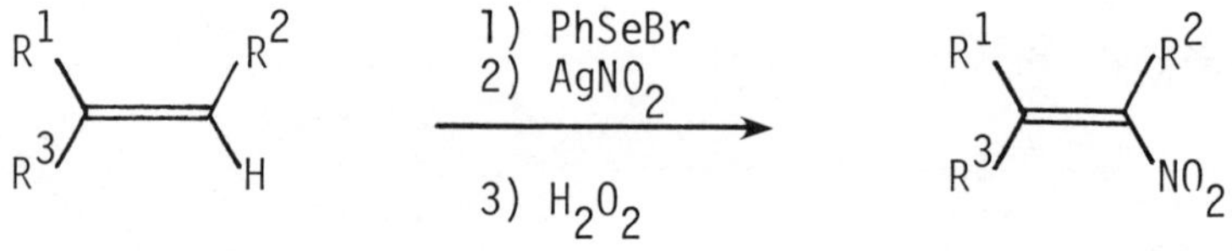

$R^1R^3C=CR^2H$ →(1) PhSeBr; 2) AgNO$_2$; 3) H$_2$O$_2$)→ $R^1R^3C=CR^2(NO_2)$

R's = H, alkyl, cyclic

VI.A.14-5 P. Knochel and D. Seebach, Synthesis, 1017 (1982).

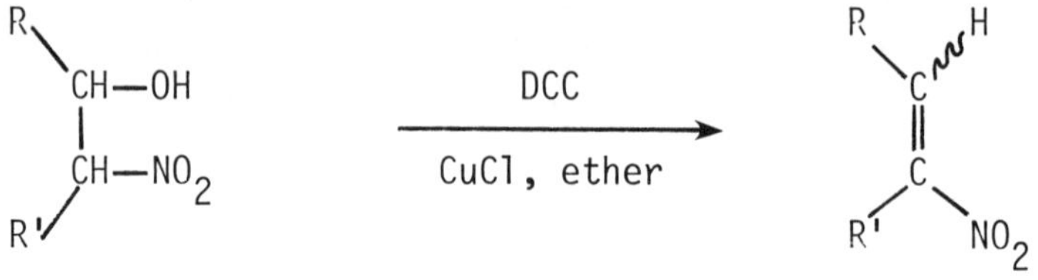

R–CH(OH)–CH(NO$_2$)–R' →(DCC, CuCl, ether)→ R(H)C=C(R')(NO$_2$)

45-99%

R, R' = H, alkyl, vinyl, furyl

USEFUL SYNTHETIC PREPARATIONS

VI.A.14-6 P. A. Wade, S. D. Morrow, and S. A. Hardinger, J. Org. Chem., **47**, 365 (1982).

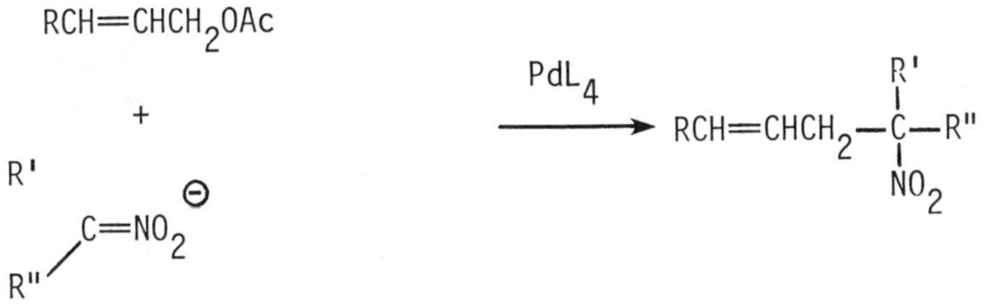

$$RCH=CHCH_2OAc + \underset{R''}{\overset{R'}{>}}C=NO_2^{\ominus} \xrightarrow{PdL_4} RCH=CHCH_2-\underset{NO_2}{\overset{R'}{\underset{|}{C}}}-R''$$

R = Ph, Me
R', R'' = H, alkyl, CO_2Et

VI.A.14-7 P. Dampawan and W. W. Zajac, Jr., Tetrahedron Lett., **23**, 135 (1982).

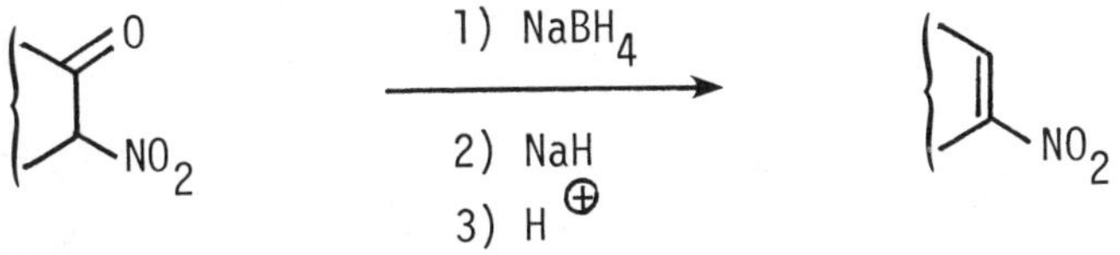

$$\text{cyclohexanone-}NO_2 \xrightarrow[\text{2) NaH}]{\text{1) NaBH}_4} \text{cyclohexene-}NO_2$$
3) H$^{\oplus}$

~20-70%

VI.A.14-8   M. Ouertani, P. Girard, and H. B. Kagan, Tetrahedron Lett., 23, 4315 (1982).

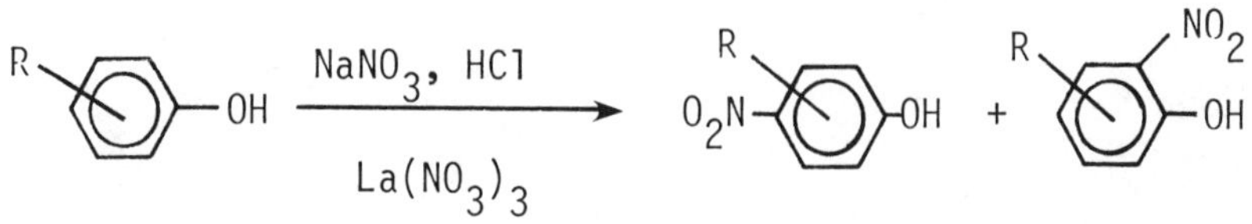

R–C₆H₄–OH →[NaNO₃, HCl / La(NO₃)₃] O₂N–C₆H₃(R)–OH + R–C₆H₃(NO₂)–OH

∼90% overall

VI.A.15. Nucleotides, etc.

(see also: IV.I.1.a, b; V.F.)

VI.A.15-1   V. Nair and S. G. Richardson, Synthesis, 670 (1982).

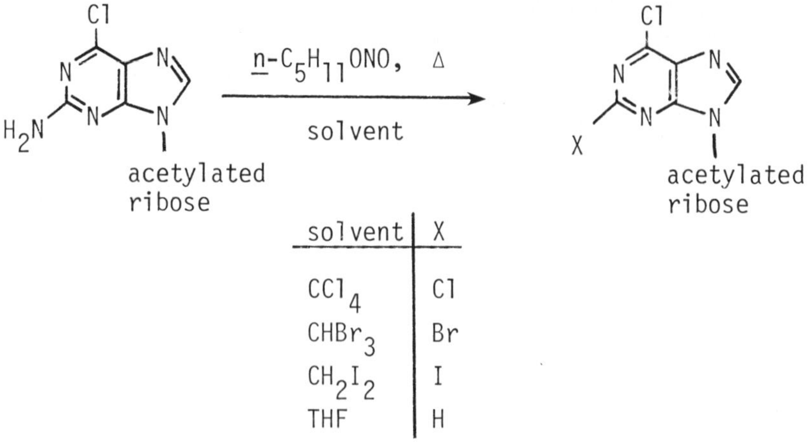

6-chloro-2-amino purine (acetylated ribose on N9) →[n-C_5H_{11}ONO, Δ, solvent] 6-chloro-2-X purine (acetylated ribose on N9)

solvent	X
CCl_4	Cl
$CHBr_3$	Br
CH_2I_2	I
THF	H

VI.A.15-2 N. S. Girgis and E. B. Pedersen, Synthesis, 480 (1982).

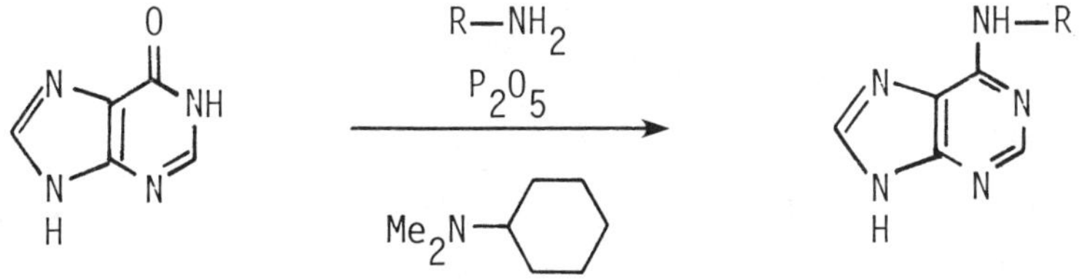

[Reaction: hypoxanthine + R–NH$_2$, P$_2$O$_5$, Me$_2$N–cyclohexyl → N6-substituted adenine]

21-83%

R = subst. Ph, -CH$_2$-het., Bz, etc.

VI.A.15-3 B. Classon et al., Acta Chem. Scand. B, 36, 251 (1982).

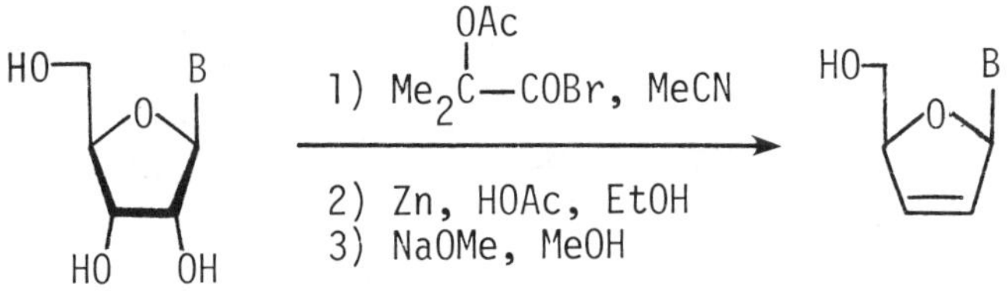

[Reaction: ribonucleoside →
1) Me$_2$C(OAc)–COBr, MeCN
2) Zn, HOAc, EtOH
3) NaOMe, MeOH
→ 2',3'-dideoxy-2',3'-didehydronucleoside]

~50-90%

VI.A.15-4   G. S. Ti, B. L. Gaffney, and R. A. Jones, J. Am. Chem. Soc., 104, 1316 (1982).

N-acyl deoxynucleosides may be obtained by protecting the hydroxyl groups with chlorotrimethylsilane in pyridine before the acylation step. Deprotection is accomplished by treatment with pyridine or dilute ammonia.

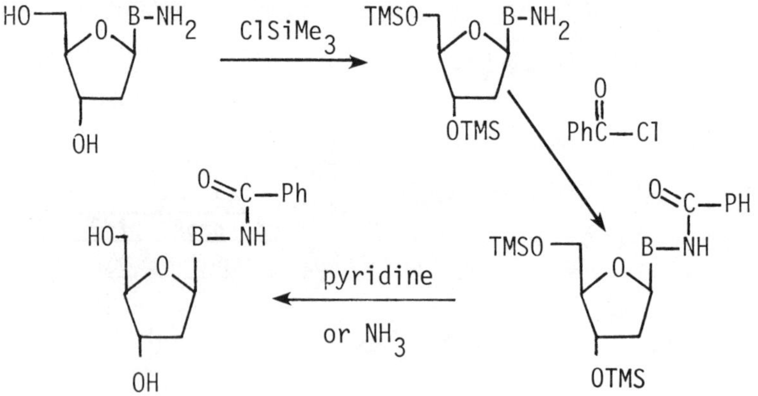

VI.A.16.   Olefins, Acetylenes

(see also: I.B., I.C., II.J., III.G.)

VI.A.16-1   F. Naso et al., J.C.S. Chem. Comm., 647 (1982).

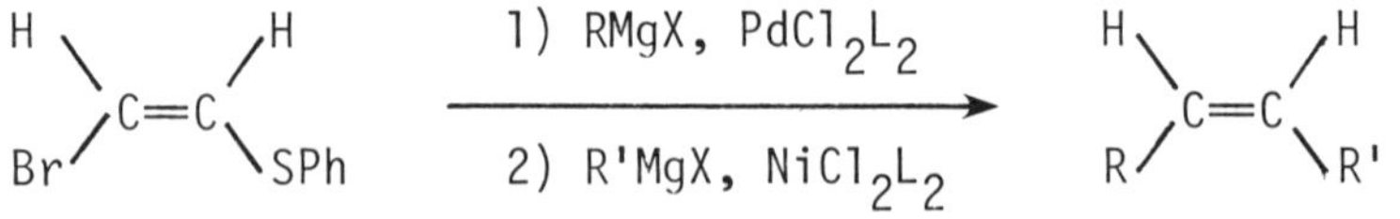

(E starting material produces E products)

53-100% overall

VI.A.16-2 J. Villieras and M. Rambaud, Comptes Rendus (C), 294, 37 (1982).

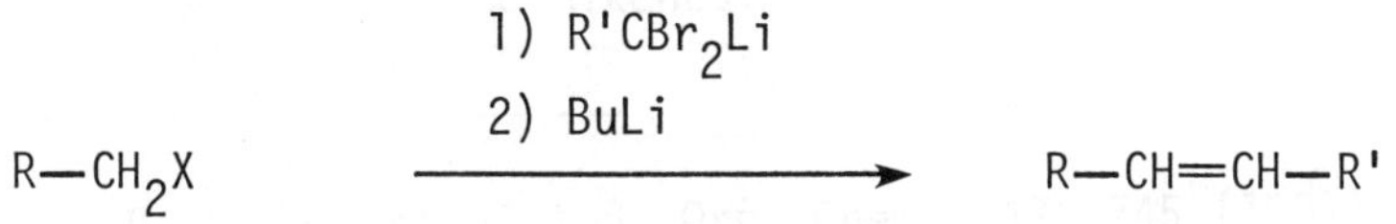

$$R-CH_2X \xrightarrow[\text{2) BuLi}]{\text{1) R'CBr}_2\text{Li}} R-CH=CH-R'$$

R = 1°, 2° alkyl, Ph
R' = H, 1° alkyl
X = I, Br

26-80% overall

VI.A.16-3 A. Suzuki et al., Synth. Comm., 12, 813 (1982).

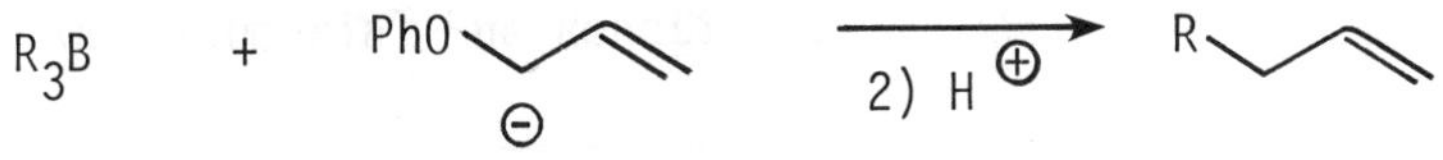

$$R_3B + PhO\diagdown\!\!\diagup\!\!\diagdown^{\ominus} \xrightarrow{\text{2) H}^{\oplus}} R\diagdown\!\!\diagup\!\!\diagdown$$

R = n-alkyl

45-60%

$$R\underset{BR_2}{\diagdown\!\!\diagup\!\!\diagdown} + \diagup\!\!\diagdown\!\!-Br \xrightarrow{CuI} R\diagdown\!\!\diagup\!\!\diagdown\!\!\diagup\!\!\diagdown$$

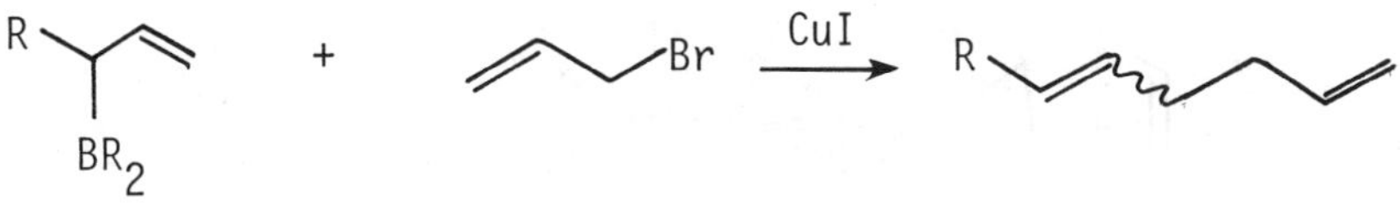

31-49%

R = n-alkyl

VI.A.16-4 H. C. Brown and D. Basavaiah, J. Org. Chem., **47**, 171, 754, and 5407 (1982).

$$R-C\equiv C-R' \xrightarrow[\text{2) NaOMe, } I_2]{\text{1) RBHBr·SMe}_2 \text{ or } R_2BX, \text{ LiAlH}_4} \underset{R}{\overset{R'}{>}}C=C\underset{R'}{\overset{H}{<}}$$

R = 1°, 2° alkyl
R' = 1° alkyl

71-76%

VI.A.16-5 P. Wolkoff, J. Org. Chem., **47**, 1944 (1982).

$$CH_3-\underset{Br}{\overset{}{CH}}-CH_2-R \xrightarrow{DBU} \underset{CH_3}{\overset{H}{>}}C=C\underset{H}{\overset{R}{<}}$$

R = alkyl, Ph, benzyl, etc.

~70-90%

Full paper, many examples.

VI.A.16-6 S. Wolff, M. E. Huecas, and W. C. Agosta, J. Org. Chem., **47**, 4358 (1982).

$$\underset{R'}{\overset{R}{>}}CH-CH_2X \xrightarrow{\text{DBN or DBU}} \underset{R'}{\overset{R}{>}}C=CH_2$$

R, R' = alkyl
X = I, OTs

~60-95%

VI.A.16-7   Y. Kimura and S. L. Regen, J. Org. Chem., 47, 2493 (1982).

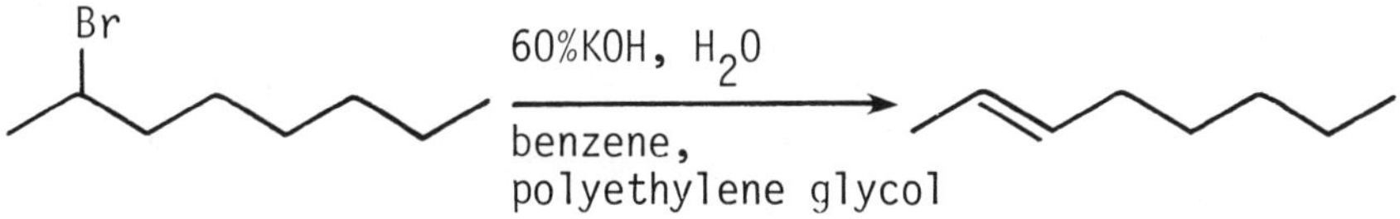

$$\text{2-bromooctane} \xrightarrow[\text{benzene, polyethylene glycol}]{60\% \text{KOH}, H_2O} \text{2-octene}$$

80%

VI.A.16-8 A. R. Katritzky and J. M. Lloyd, J.C.S. Perkin I, 2347 (1982); J. Org. Chem., 47, 3506 (1982).

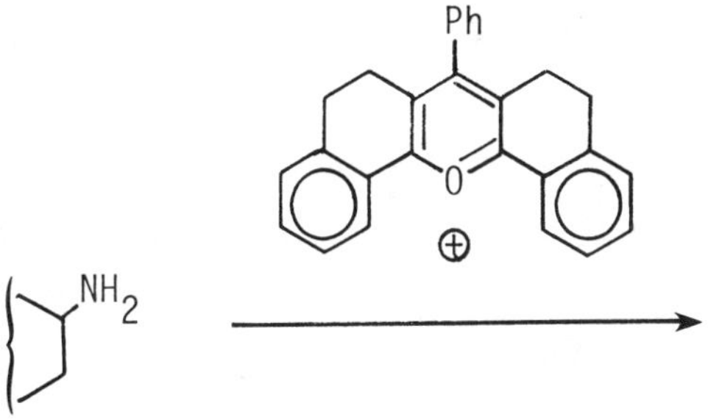

33-95%

VI.A.16-9 G. L. Larson and D. Hernandez, Tetrahedron Lett., 23, 1035 (1982).

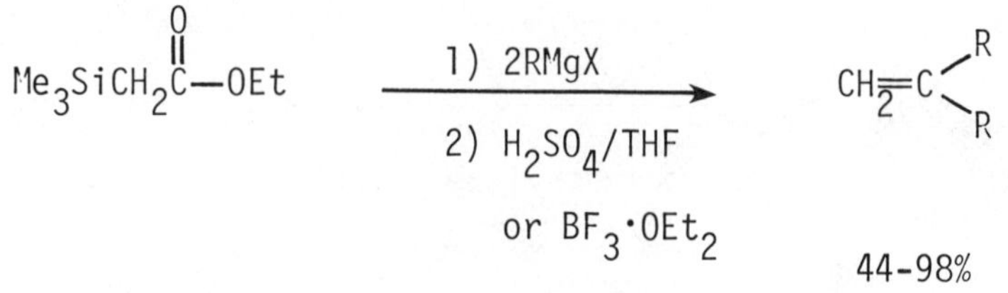

$$Me_3SiCH_2\overset{O}{\underset{\|}{C}}-OEt \xrightarrow[\text{2) } H_2SO_4/THF \text{ or } BF_3\cdot OEt_2]{\text{1) 2RMgX}} CH_2=C\begin{smallmatrix}R\\R\end{smallmatrix}$$

44-98%

R = 1° alkyl, allyl, subst. Ph

VI.A.16-10 G. Capozzi et al., J.C.S. Chem. Comm., 959 (1982).

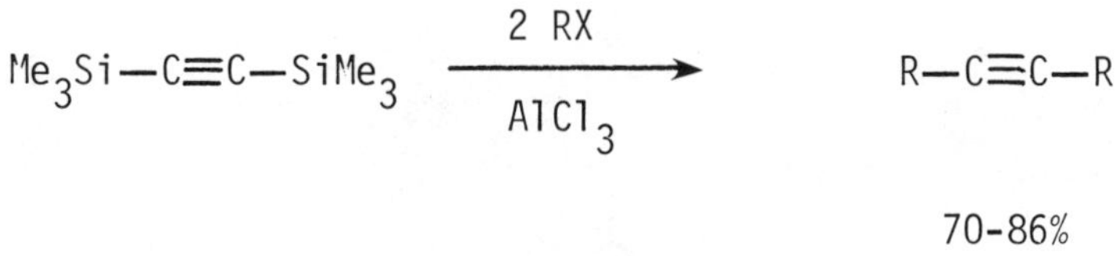

$$Me_3Si-C\equiv C-SiMe_3 \xrightarrow[AlCl_3]{2 \text{ RX}} R-C\equiv C-R$$

70-86%

R = t-Bu, 1-adamantyl, Ph

VI.A.16-11 H. J. Bestmann and K. Li, Chem. Ber., 115, 828 (1982).

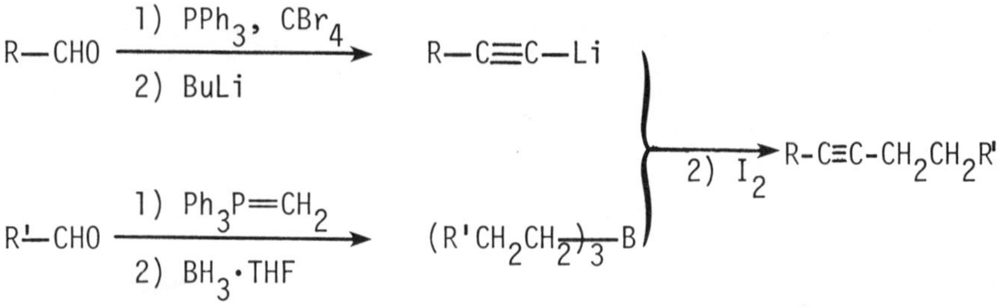

$$R-CHO \xrightarrow[\text{2) BuLi}]{\text{1) PPh}_3, CBr_4} R-C\equiv C-Li$$

$$R'-CHO \xrightarrow[\text{2) BH}_3\cdot THF]{\text{1) Ph}_3P=CH_2} (R'CH_2CH_2)_3B$$

$$\xrightarrow{\text{2) } I_2} R-C\equiv C-CH_2CH_2R'$$

VI.A.16-12   S. Ikegami et al., Tetrahedron Lett., 23, 4607
(1982).

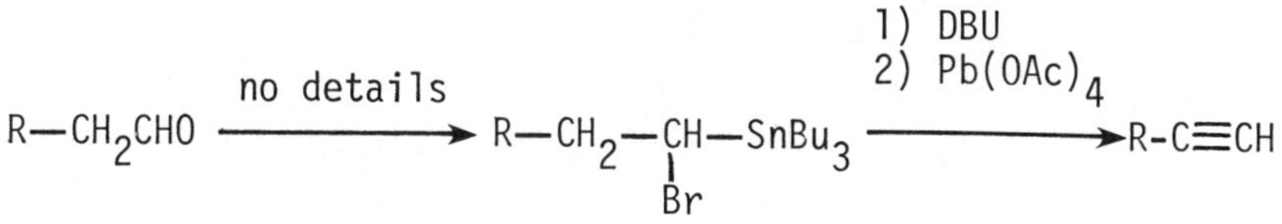

$$R-CH_2CHO \xrightarrow{\text{no details}} R-CH_2-\underset{Br}{CH}-SnBu_3 \xrightarrow{\substack{1)\ DBU \\ 2)\ Pb(OAc)_4}} R-C{\equiv}CH$$

∼35% overall

R = alkyl, containing alkenes, epoxides, silyl ethers, THP ethers

---

VI.A.16-13   C. Wentrup, Bull. Soc. Chim. Belges, 91, 997
(1982).

Review: "Heterocyclic Rearrangements: New Cumulenes and Acetylenes.

VI.A.17.   Peptides

(see also: V.B., V.C., V.D., VI.A.4.)

VI.A.17-1   H. H. Wasserman and T. -J. Lu, Tetrahedron Lett., 23, 3831 (1982).

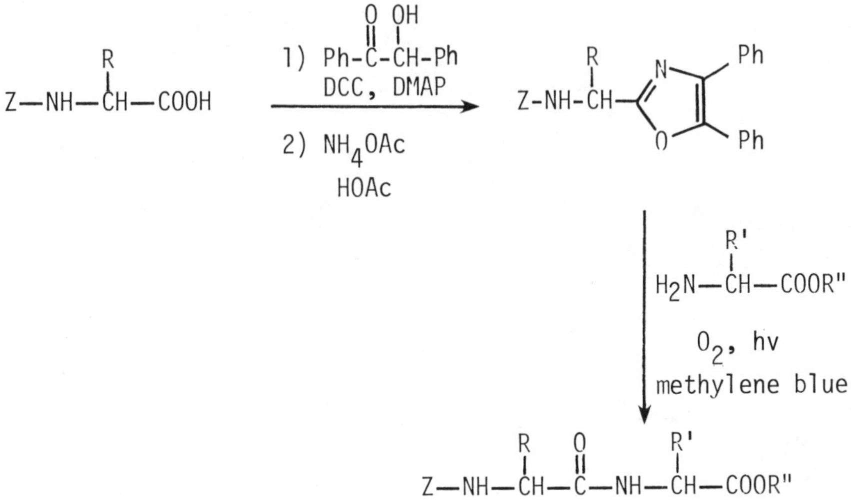

Z—NH—CH(R)—COOH

1) Ph-C(=O)-CH(OH)-Ph, DCC, DMAP
2) NH_4OAc, HOAc

→ Z-NH-CH(R)-[4,5-diphenyloxazol-2-yl]

↓ H_2N—CH(R')—COOR"; O_2, hv, methylene blue

Z—NH—CH(R)—C(=O)—NH—CH(R')—COOR"

VI.A.17-2   R. F. Nutt and M. M. Joullié, J. Am. Chem. Soc., 104, 5852 (1982).

Use of the Four-Component Condensation for the synthesis of β-(aryloxy)prolyl peptides.

VI.A.17-3   W. Kawanobe et al., Chem. Lett., 825 (1982).

Peptide synthesis using N-acetyl-N-methylphosphoramidites as condensing agents. Yields are generally ∿90%, without racemization.

VI.A.17-4   H. -H. Bechtolsheimer and H. Kunz, Angew. Chem. Int. Ed., 21, 630 (1982).

Use of the acid chloride method for the coupling of sterically hindered peptide bonds, e.g.:

Peoc-Val-OH $\xrightarrow[\text{2) H-MeLeu-O-\underline{t}-Bu, pyridine}]{\text{1) }(COCl)_2}$ Peoc-Val-MeLeu-O-$\underline{t}$-Bu

81%

VI.A.17-5   H. Kunz and H. -H. Bechtolsheimer, Liebigs Ann. Chem., 2068 (1982).

Treatment of Peoc-Amino acids with oxalyl chloride converts them to the corresponding acid chlorides. Sterically hindered peptide bonds can be synthesized by the reactions of these acid chlorides with free amino groups.

VI.A.17-6   S. Nozaki and I. Muramatsu, Bull. Chem. Soc. Japan, 55, 2165 (1982).

Synthesis of peptides by the "Hold-in-Solution" method. Intermediates are not isolated, but are maintained in a 1,2-dichloroethane solution. Washing of the organic layer with aqueous solutions is the only intermediate purification.

VI.A.17-7   U. Schmidt and M. Dietsche, <u>Angew. Chem. Int. Ed.</u>, <u>21</u>, 143 (1982).

Phenyltetrazolinethione/Isocyanide may be used as an activating group for peptide formation. Yields of dipeptides are 60-84%, and no detectable racemization occurs.

VI.A.17-8   P. Kuhl and H. -D. Jakubke, <u>Z. Chem.</u>, <u>22</u>, 407 (1982).

Use of the enzyme thermolysin to catalyze peptide synthesis in an aqueous-organic two-phase system. Yields are ~90%.

VI.A.17-9   R. C. Sheppard and B. J. Williams, <u>J.C.S. Chem. Comm.</u>, 587 (1982).

Use of N_α-fluorenylmethoxycarbonylamino-acids in combination with <u>t</u>-butyl-based side-chain protecting groups and a novel dialkoxybenzyl alcohol peptide-resin linkage agent allows solid-phase synthesis of protected peptides suitable for use in fragment condensation strategies."

VI.A.17-10   F. S. Tjoeng and G. A. Heavner, <u>Tetrahedron Lett.</u>, <u>23</u>, 4439 (1982).

Use of a photolabile $Cl-\underset{\underset{\displaystyle CH_3}{|}}{CH}-\underset{\underset{\displaystyle}{||}}{C}-\!\!\!\bigcirc\!\!\!-CH_2-\underset{\underset{\displaystyle}{||}}{C}-O-\!\Ⓟ$ support in liquid-phase peptide synthesis. The protected peptide is removed by irradiation at 350 nm.

VI.A. 17-11   W. F. DeGrado and E. T. Kaiser, <u>J. Org. Chem.</u>, <u>47</u>, 3258 (1982).

$Ⓟ\!\!-\!\!\bigcirc\!\!-\underset{\underset{\displaystyle N\text{-}OH}{||}}{C}-\!\!\bigcirc\!\!-NO_2$

Use of the above polymer-bound oxime for solide-phase synthesis of protected peptides. Removed by carboxylic acid-catalyzed aminolysis.

VI.A.17-12   J. P. Tam <u>et al.</u>, <u>Tetrahedron Lett.</u>, <u>23</u>, 4435 (1982).

Use of low concentrations of HF in dimethyl sulfide to deprotect synthetic peptides. Side reactions are minimized.

VI.A.17-13   M. Ueki and T. Inazu, Chem. Lett., 45 (1982).

Hydroxyamino acid-containing peptides may be synthesized without protecting the side-chain hydroxyl functions by using the dimethylphosphinothioyl (Mpt) mixed anhydride as a carboxyl-activating group.

VI.A.17-14   V. N. R. Pillai and M. Mutter, Topics in Current Chem., 119 (1982).

Review: "New Perspectives in Polymer-Supported Peptide Synthesis"

VI.A.17-15   Yu. P. Shvachkin et al., Russ. Chem. Rev., 51, 178 (1982).

Review: "Advances and prospects in the chemistry of nucleoamino acids and nucleopeptides"

VI.A.18. Vinyl Halides, Vinyl Ethers, Vinyl Esters

VI.A.18-1   G. Zweifel et al., Synthesis, 127 (1982).

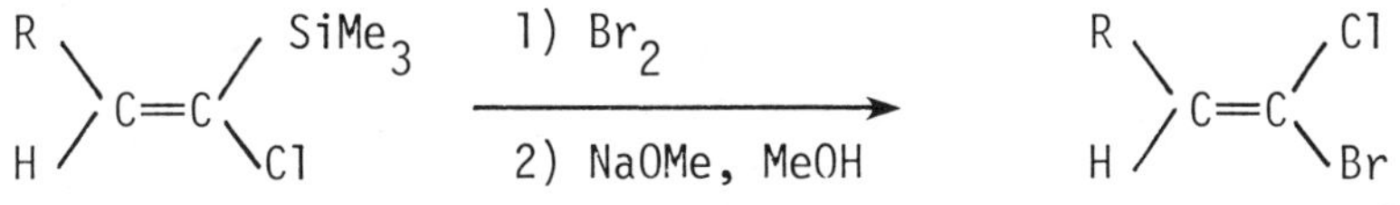

$$\underset{H}{\overset{R}{>}}C=C\underset{Cl}{\overset{SiMe_3}{<}} \quad \xrightarrow[\text{2) NaOMe, MeOH}]{\text{1) Br}_2} \quad \underset{H}{\overset{R}{>}}C=C\underset{Br}{\overset{Cl}{<}}$$

65-74%

$$\underset{H}{\overset{R}{>}}C=C\underset{B<}{\overset{Cl}{<}} \quad \xrightarrow[\substack{\text{2) Br}_2 \\ \text{3) NaOMe}}]{\text{1) Me}_3\text{N}\rightarrow\text{O}} \quad \underset{H}{\overset{R}{>}}C=C\underset{Cl}{\overset{Br}{<}}$$

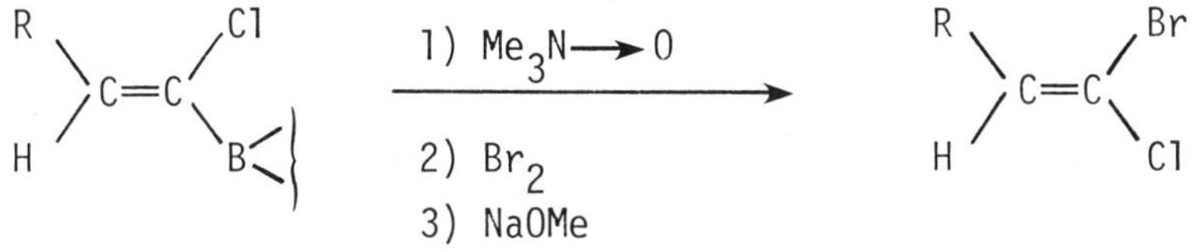

69-96%

VI.A.18-2   J. Gloede, Z. Chem., 22, 126 (1982).

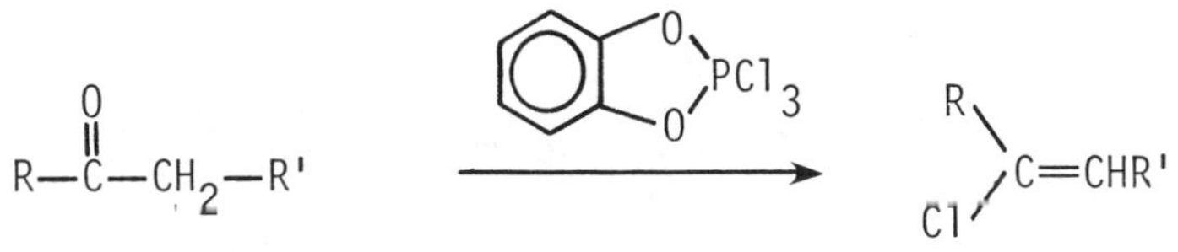

$$R-\overset{O}{\underset{\|}{C}}-CH_2-R' \quad \xrightarrow{\text{catechyl-PCl}_3} \quad \underset{Cl}{\overset{R}{>}}C=CHR'$$

55-86%

R, R' = H, alkyl, aryl

VI.A.18-3   C. J. Kowalski, A. E. Weber, and K. W. Fields, J. Org. Chem., 47, 5088 (1982).

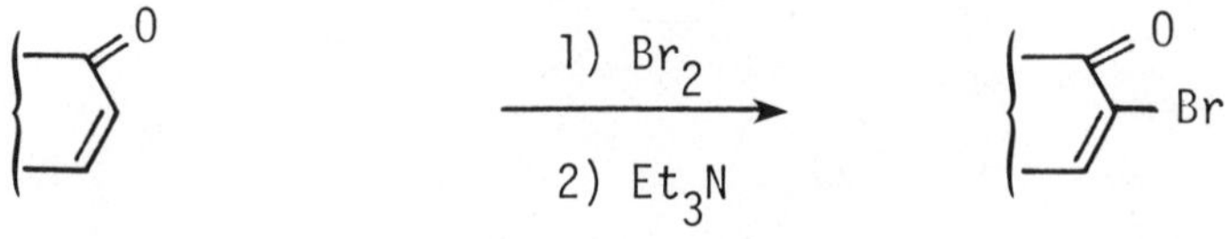

cyclopentenone →(1) Br$_2$; 2) Et$_3$N)→ α-bromo cyclopentenone

---

VI.A.18-4   E. Piers et al., Can. J. Chem., 60, 210 (1982).

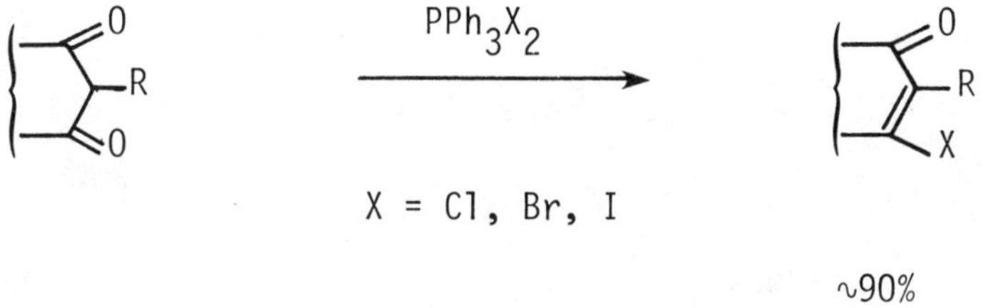

cyclic 1,3-dione with R →(PPh$_3$X$_2$)→ α-halo enone

X = Cl, Br, I

∼90%

R = alkyl, allyl

VI.A.18-5   M. Marsi and J. A. Gladysz, Organometallics, 1, 1467 (1982).

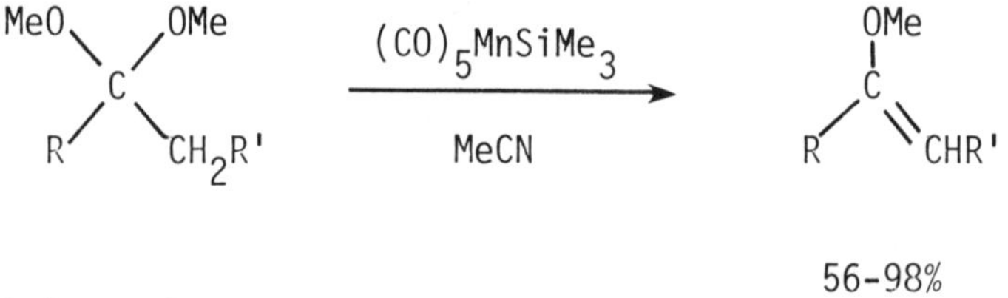

$$\text{R-C(OMe)}_2\text{-CH}_2\text{R'} \xrightarrow[\text{MeCN}]{\text{(CO)}_5\text{MnSiMe}_3} \text{R-C(OMe)=CHR'}$$

56-98%

R = alkyl, aryl
R' = H, alkyl

VI.A.18-6   R. D. Miller and D. R. McKean, Tetrahedron Lett., 23, 323 (1982).

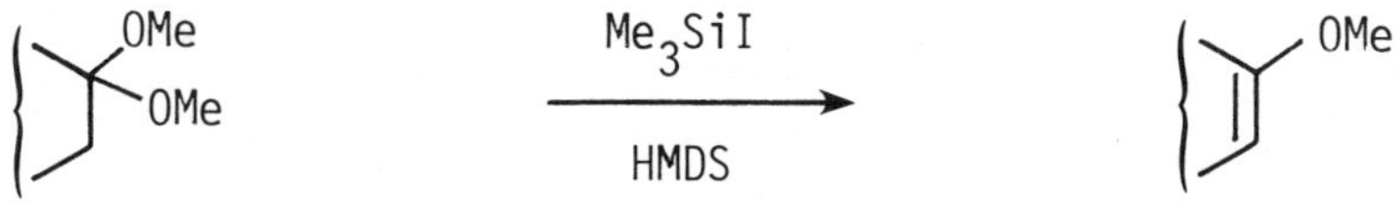

[Reaction: cyclohexane-1,1-dimethyl acetal (OMe, OMe) → with Me$_3$SiI / HMDS → 1-methoxycyclohexene]

~80%

VI.A.18-7   B. A. Trofimov et al., J. Org. Chem. (USSR), 18, 395 (1982).

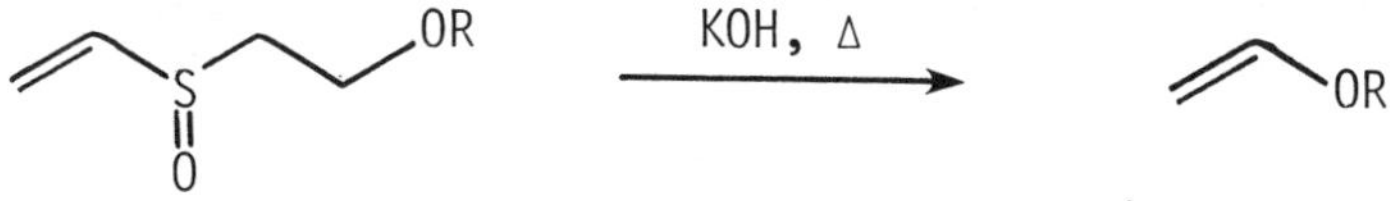

[Reaction: CH$_2$=CH-S(O)-CH$_2$CH$_2$-OR → KOH, Δ → CH$_2$=CH-OR]

65-71%

R = Pr, i-Pr, Bu

VI.A.18-8   A. Yamashita and T. A. Scahill, Tetrahedron Lett., 23, 3765 (1982).

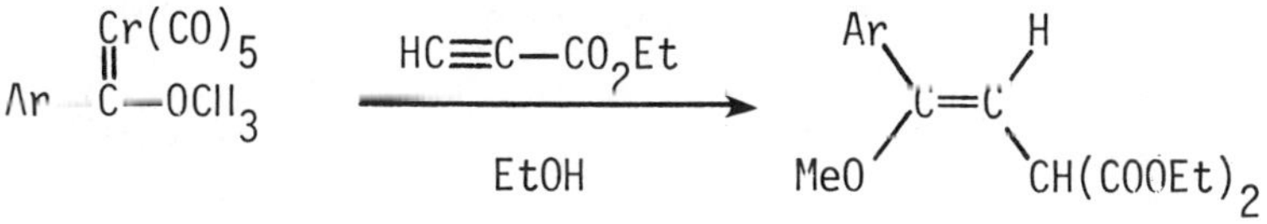

[Reaction: Ar-C(=Cr(CO)$_5$)-OCH$_3$ + HC≡C-CO$_2$Et → EtOH → (Ar)(MeO)C=C(H)(CH(COOEt)$_2$)]

80-87%

Ar = Ph, furyl, thienyl, N-methylpyrroyl

VI.A.18-9   M. Riediker and J. Schwartz, *J. Am. Chem. Soc.*, **104**, 5842 (1982).

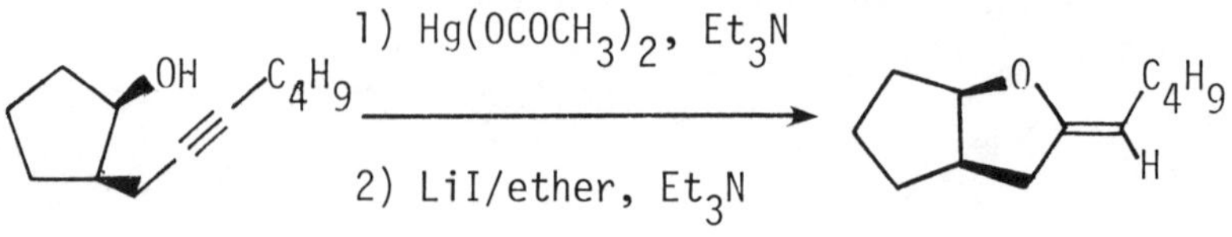

[Reaction scheme: cyclopentane with OH and CH₂-C≡C-C₄H₉ substituents reacts with 1) Hg(OCOCH₃)₂, Et₃N; 2) LiI/ether, Et₃N to give bicyclic furan with =CH-C₄H₉ exocyclic alkene]

45%

[Reaction scheme: similar cyclopentane substrate under similar conditions gives bicyclic dihydropyran with C₄H₉ substituent]

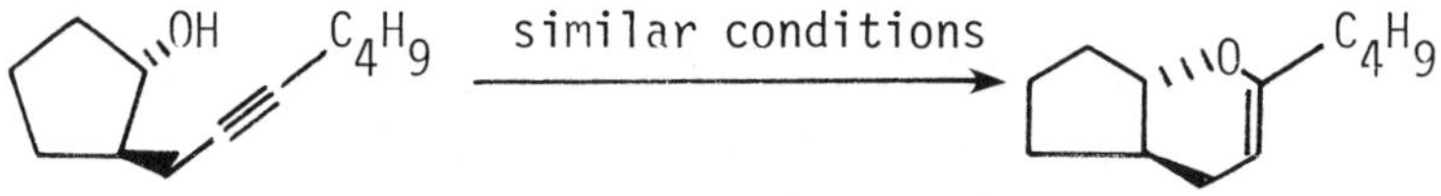

VI.A.19. Sulfur Compounds

(see also: II.E., III.C.)

VI.A.19-1   Y. Matsubara *et al.*, *Chem. Pharm. Bull.*, **30**, 3389 (1982).

$$RX \xrightarrow[\text{2) HCl/H}_2\text{O}]{\substack{\text{1) PhNHCH=S} \\ \text{NaH, MeCN}}} R-SH$$

59-93%

R = 1° alkyl, Bz, MeO-C(=O)-CH₂-

X = halide

VI.A.19-2   P. Molina et al., Synthesis, 472 (1982).

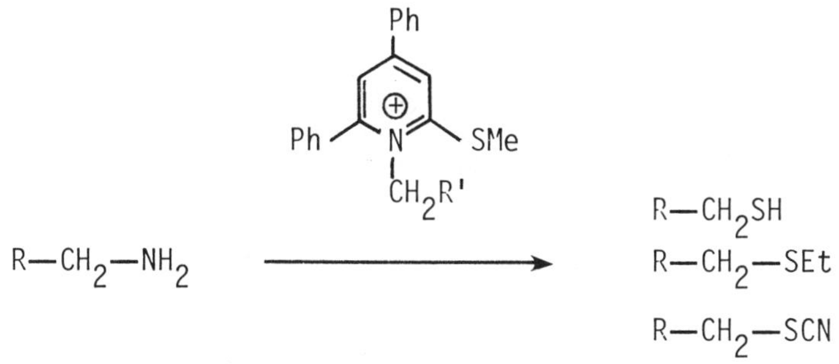

R—CH$_2$—NH$_2$ $\xrightarrow{\text{[pyridinium reagent with Ph, Ph, SMe, CH}_2\text{R']}}$ R—CH$_2$SH
R—CH$_2$—SEt
R—CH$_2$—SCN

depending on conditions

Yields are ~60-90%

VI.A.19-3   K.-Y. Jen and M. P. Cava, Tetrahedron Lett., 23, 2001 (1982).

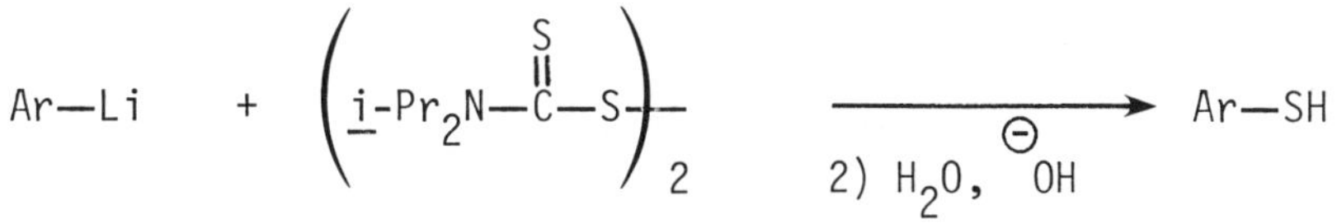

$$\text{Ar—Li} + \left(i\text{-Pr}_2\text{N}-\underset{\|}{\overset{S}{C}}-S \right)_2 \xrightarrow[2)\ \text{H}_2\text{O},\ ^\ominus\text{OH}]{} \text{Ar—SH}$$

~50-90%

Ar = subst. Ph, heterocyclic

VI.A.19-4   M. Yamato et al., Synthesis, 1014 (1982).

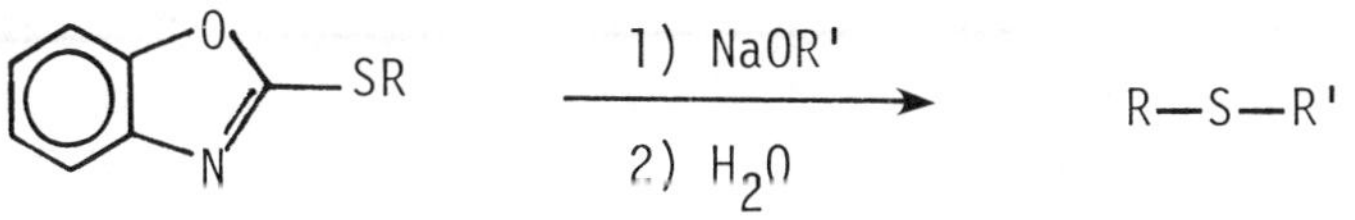

[benzoxazole]—SR $\xrightarrow[2)\ \text{H}_2\text{O}]{1)\ \text{NaOR'}}$ R—S—R'

53-72%

R = 1°, 2°, 3° alkyl, Bz
R' = Bz, PhCH$_2$CH$_2$—

VI.A.19-5   S. R. Wilson, P. Caldera, and M. A. Jester, J. Org. Chem., 47, 3319 (1982).

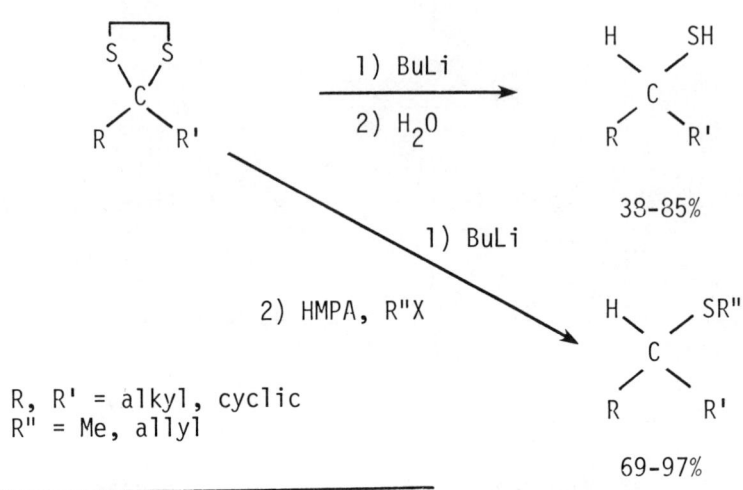

R, R' = alkyl, cyclic
R" = Me, allyl

VI.A.19-6   W. Ando et al., Synth. Comm., 12, 627 (1982).

R—X   +   Me$_3$SiSEt $\longrightarrow$ R—S—Et
                                             82-95%

2 R—X   +   (Me$_3$Si)$_2$S $\longrightarrow$ R—S—R
                                                  59-88%

R = alkyl, Bz

VI.A.19-7   J. P. Tam, W. F. Heath, and R. B. Merrifield, Tetrahedron Lett., 23, 2939 (1982).

$$R-\overset{O}{\underset{\|}{S}}-CH_3 \quad \xrightarrow[CH_3-S-CH_3]{HF} \quad R-S-CH_3$$

methionine sulfoxide   methionine residues
    residues   "quantitative"

VI.A.19-8 M. Ortiz and G. L. Larson, Synth. Comm., 12, 43 (1982).

$$\text{Ar}-\underset{\underset{O}{\|}}{\overset{\overset{O}{\|}}{S}}-N_3 \quad \xrightarrow[\text{3) chromatography or silica gel}]{\begin{array}{l}1)\ R_3B \\ 2)\ H_2O_2/\text{NaOH}\end{array}} \quad \text{Ar}-S-R$$

45-70%

Ar = subst. Ph
R = alkyl, cycloalkyl

VI.A.19-9 J. T. B. Ferreira, J. V. Comasseto, and A. L. Braga, Synth. Comm., 12, 595 (1982).

$$\text{Ar}-S-S-\text{Ar} + RX \quad \xrightarrow[\text{THF, CTAB}]{50\%\ \text{NaOH}} \quad \text{Ar}-S-R$$

80-96%

Ar = subst. Ph
R = alkyl, cycloalkyl, allyl, benzyl, etc.

VI.A.19-10 R. B. Bates and K. D. Janda, J. Org. Chem., 47, 4374 (1982).

$$\text{Ar}-SH \quad \xrightarrow[\underline{t}\text{-BuO}^{\ominus} K^{\oplus}]{Me_2SO,\ PhI} \quad \text{Ar}-S-Ph$$

50-100%

VI.A.19-11   M. Lissel, J. Chem. Research (S), 286 (1982).

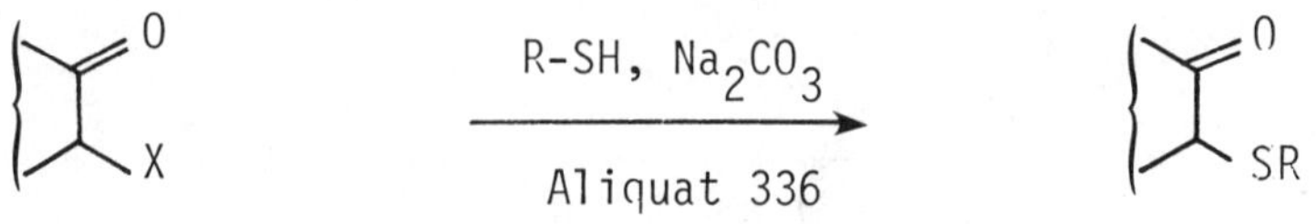

[cyclohexanone with X] $\xrightarrow{\text{R-SH, Na}_2\text{CO}_3}{\text{Aliquat 336}}$ [cyclohexanone with SR]

X = Cl, Br
R = alkyl, aryl

∼70-98%

VI.A.19-12   E. Vedejs and G. A. Krafft, Tetrahedron, 38, 2857 (1982).

Review: "Cyclic Sulfides in Organic Synthesis"

VI.A.19-13   T. A. Hase and H. Perakyla, Synth. Comm., 12, 947 (1982).

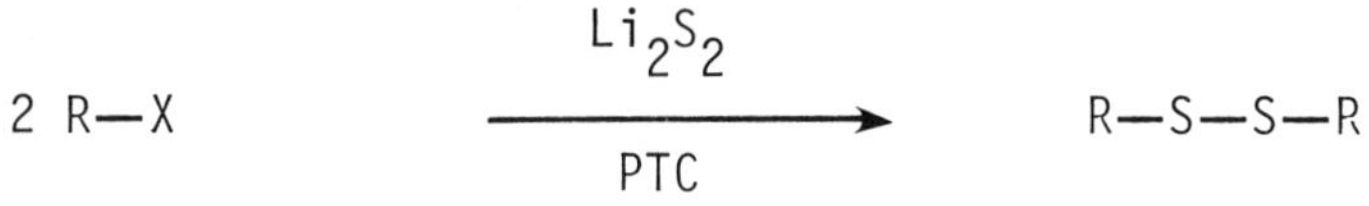

$$2\ R-X \xrightarrow[\text{PTC}]{\text{Li}_2\text{S}_2} R-S-S-R$$

48-98%

R = 1°, 2° alkyl, Bz, allyl, MTM, etc.
X = Br, Cl

VI.A.19-14 J. Drabowicz, B. Bujnicki, and M. Mikolajczyk, J. Org. Chem., 47, 3325 (1982).

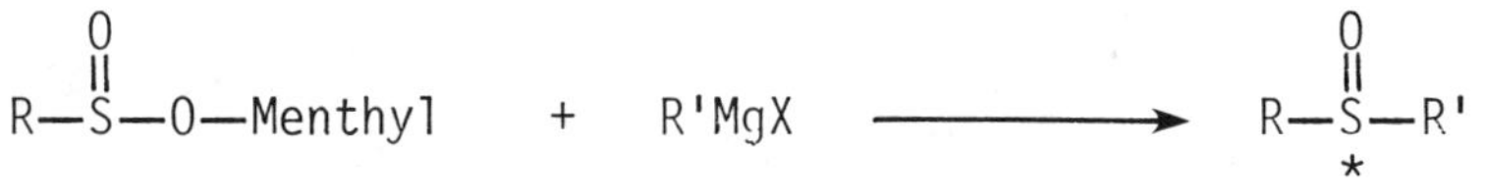

$$R-\overset{O}{\underset{\|}{S}}-O-Menthyl \quad + \quad R'MgX \quad \longrightarrow \quad R-\overset{O}{\underset{\underset{*}{\|}}{S}}-R'$$

R = Me, p-Tolyl, n-Bu
R' = Me, Et, i-Pr, Bu, n-Pr, Ph

~50-80%
>90% ee

VI.A.19-15 N. A. Meanwell and C. R. Johnson, Synthesis, 283 (1982).

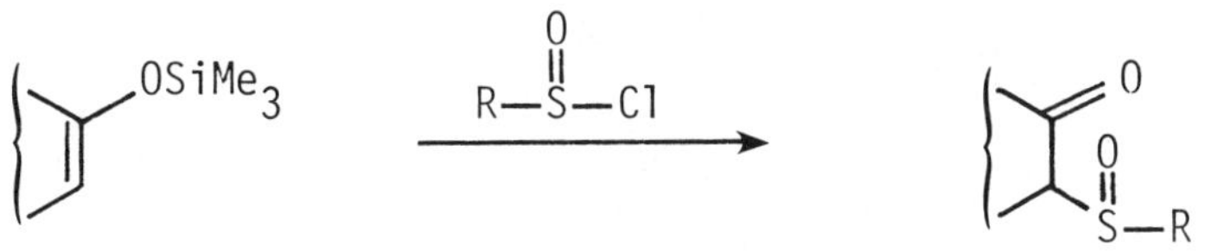

R = Me, Ph

~80-90%

VI.A.19-16 G. A. Epling and M. E. Walker, Tetrahedron Lett., 23, 3843 (1982).

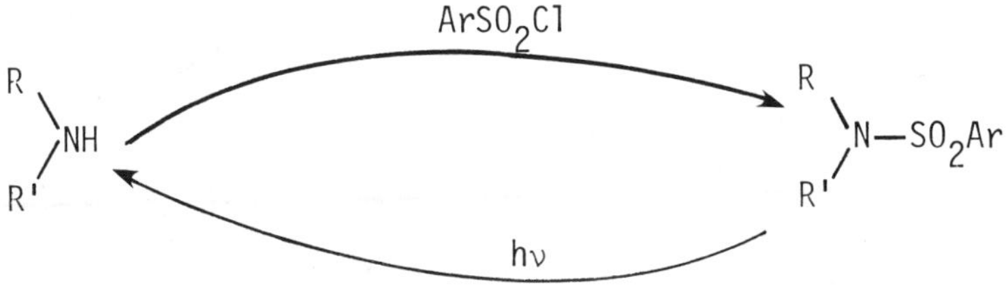

R, R' = H, alkyl, aryl, heterocyclic

Ar =

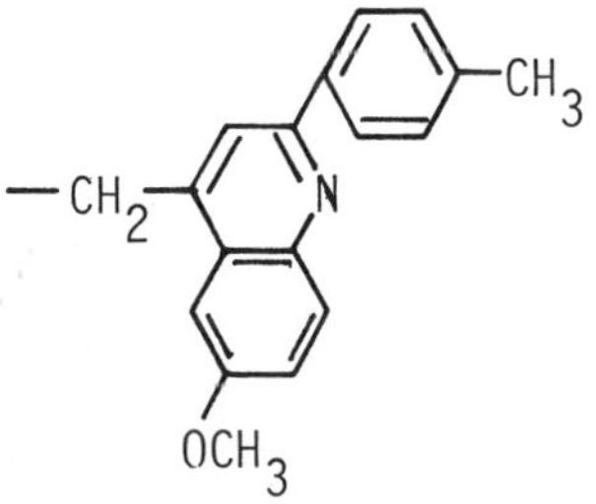

VI.A.19-17 K. Steliou and M. Mrani, J. Am. Chem. Soc., 104, 3104 (1982).

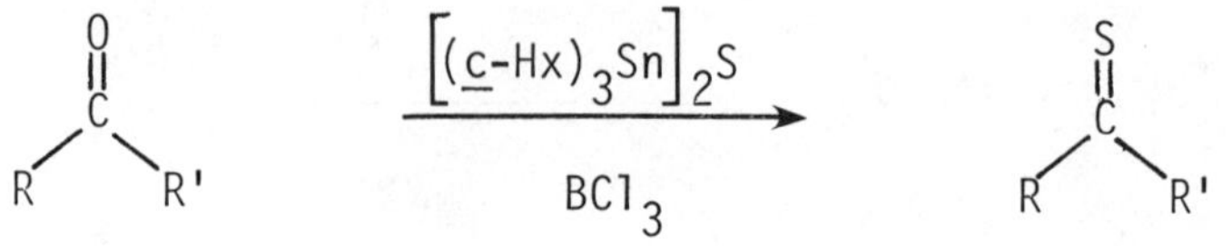

$$\underset{RR'}{\overset{O}{\underset{\|}{C}}} \xrightarrow[BCl_3]{[(c\text{-}Hx)_3Sn]_2S} \underset{RR'}{\overset{S}{\underset{\|}{C}}}$$

65-95%

R, R' = H, alkyl, aryl

Also works for caprolactam, 92% yield

VI.A.19-18 T. Imamoto et al., Synthesis, 134 (1982).

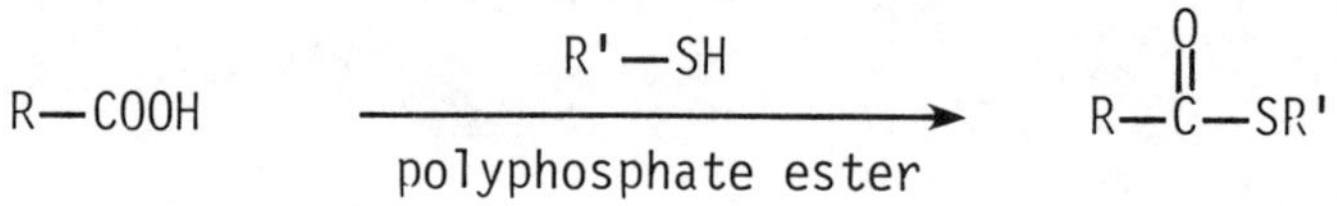

$$R\text{—}COOH \xrightarrow[\text{polyphosphate ester}]{R'\text{—}SH} R\text{—}\overset{O}{\underset{\|}{C}}\text{—}SR'$$

83-97%

R = subst. Ph, t-Bu, styryl

VI.A.19-19 H. Davy, J.C.S. Chem. Comm., 457 (1982).

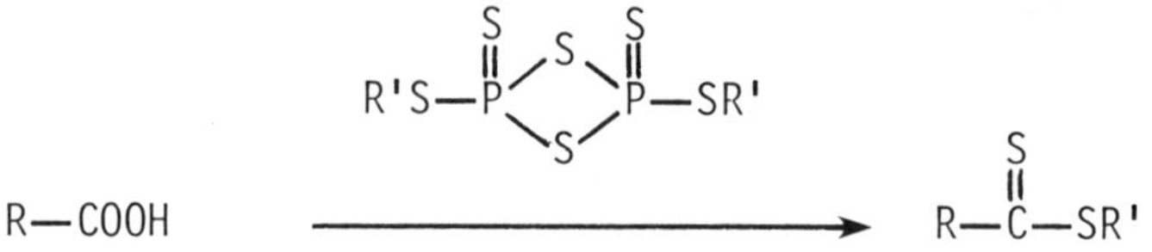

$$R\text{—}COOH \xrightarrow{\text{R'S—P(S)(S)S P(S)—SR'}} R\text{—}\overset{S}{\underset{\|}{C}}\text{—}SR'$$

R = alkyl, Ph   57-65%
R' = Me, Et

VI.A.19-20   W. Ando et al., Chem. Lett., 885 (1982).

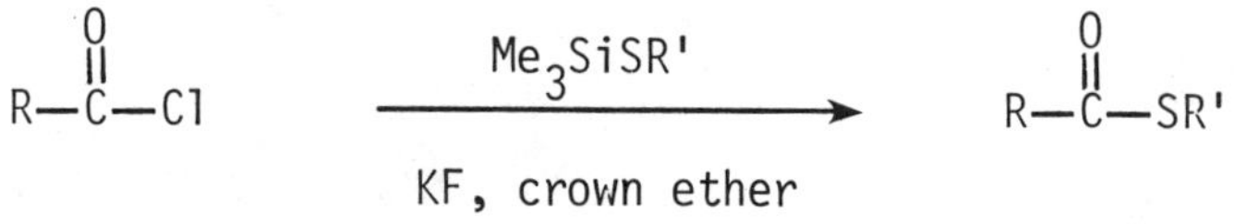

$$R-\overset{O}{\underset{\|}{C}}-Cl \xrightarrow[\text{KF, crown ether}]{Me_3SiSR'} R-\overset{O}{\underset{\|}{C}}-SR'$$

70-98%

R = alkyl, Ph
R' = Et, t-Bu

$(Me_3SiS)_2$ gives a thioanhydride

VI.A.19-21   S. Kato et al., Synthesis, 1013 (1982).

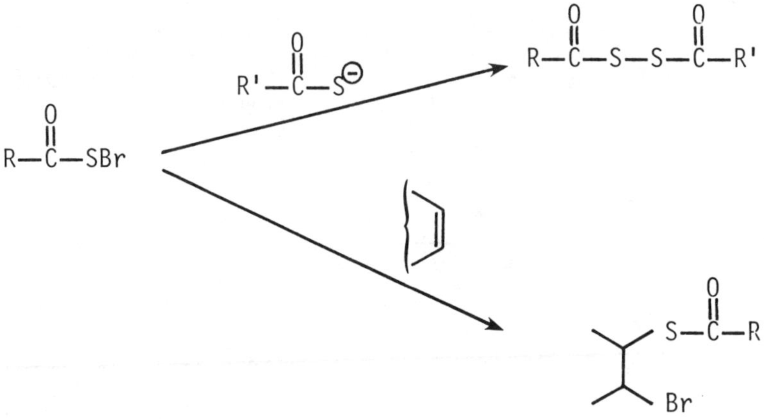

VI.A.19-22   S. Julia, G. Tagle, and J. C. Vega, Synth. Comm., 12, 897 (1982).

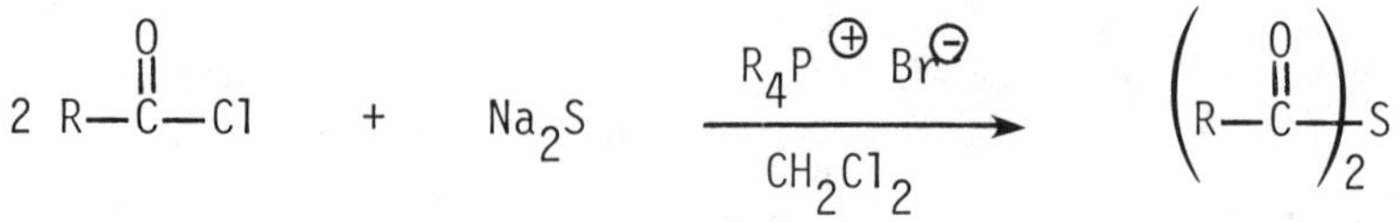

$$2\ R-\overset{O}{\underset{\|}{C}}-Cl\ +\ Na_2S\ \xrightarrow[CH_2Cl_2]{R_4P^{\oplus}\ Br^{\ominus}}\ \left(R-\overset{O}{\underset{\|}{C}}\right)_2 S$$

R = alkyl, aryl, alkoxy

90-97%

VI.A.19-23   B. Zwanenburg, Rec. Trav. Chim. Pays-Bas, 101, 1 (1982).

Review: "The Chemistry of Sulfines"

VI.A.19-24   G. E. Wilson, Jr., Tetrahedron, 38, 2597 (1982).

Review: "Structure and Reactivity of Halosulfonium Salts"

VI.B.1. Ring Enlargement

VI.B.1-1 T. Shioiri et al., Chem. Pharm. Bull., 30, 119 (1982).

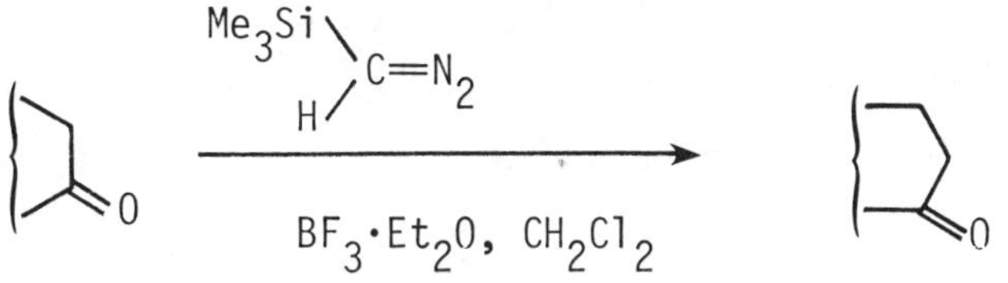

cyclopentanone + Me$_3$Si(H)C=N$_2$ / BF$_3\cdot$Et$_2$O, CH$_2$Cl$_2$ → cyclohexanone

widely varying yields

VI.B.1-2 D. Labar, J. L. Laboureur, and A. Krief, Tetrahedron Lett., 23, 983 (1982).

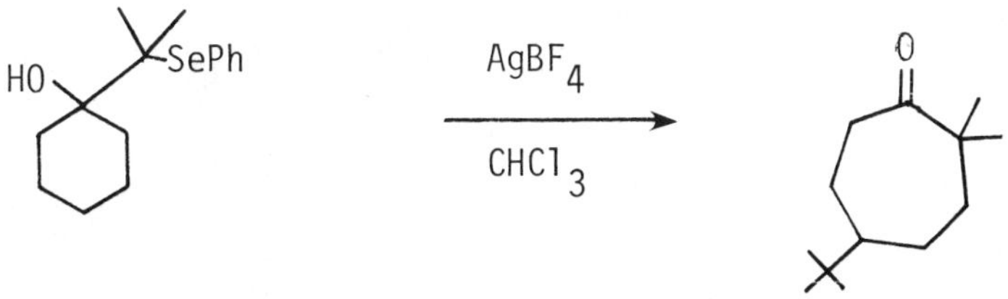

1-(HO)(SePh-CMe$_2$)-4-t-butylcyclohexane / AgBF$_4$, CHCl$_3$ → 3,3-dimethyl-6-t-butylcycloheptanone

75%

VI.B.1-3 R. Wälchli and M. Hesse, <u>Helv. Chim. Acta</u>, <u>65</u>, 2299 (1982).

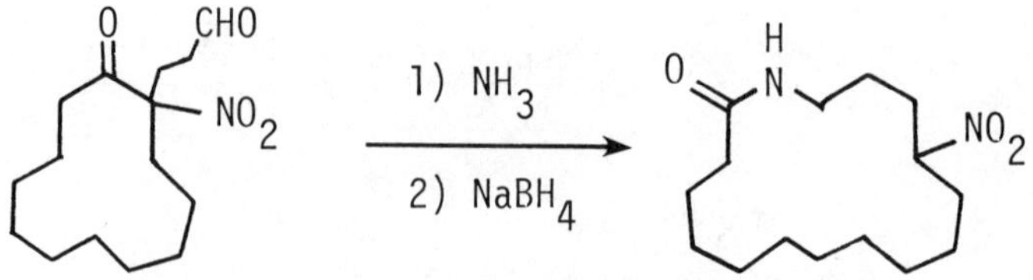

41%

VI.B.1-4 R. C. Cookson and P. S. Ray, <u>Tetrahedron Lett.</u>, <u>23</u>, 3521 (1982).

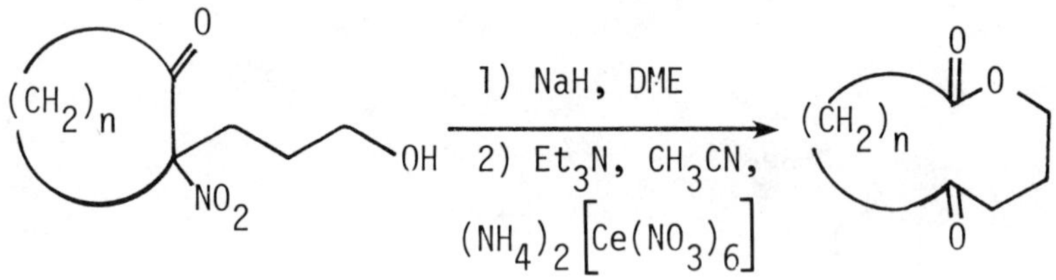

n = 4-10   ~70% overall

VI.B.1-5   K. Kostova et al., Helv. Chim. Acta, 65, 249 (1982).

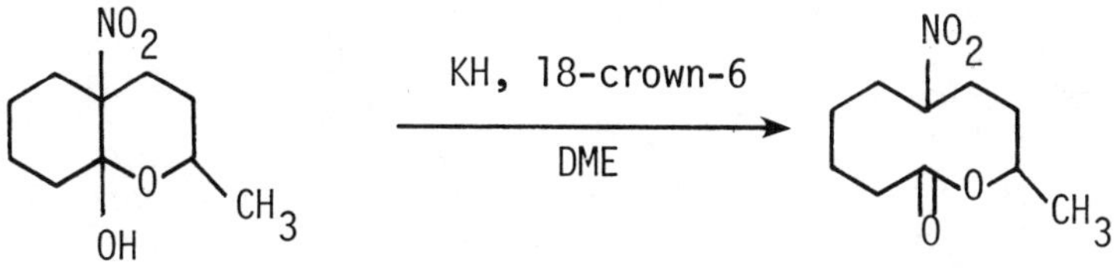

VI.B.1-6   B. M. Trost and R. W. Warner, J. Am. Chem. Soc., 104, 6112 (1982).

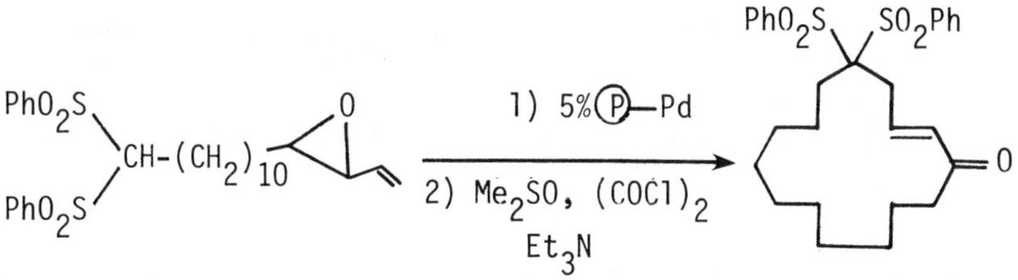

VI.B.1-7   B. Lamm and C. -J. Aurell, <u>Acta Chem. Scand. B</u>, 435 (1982).

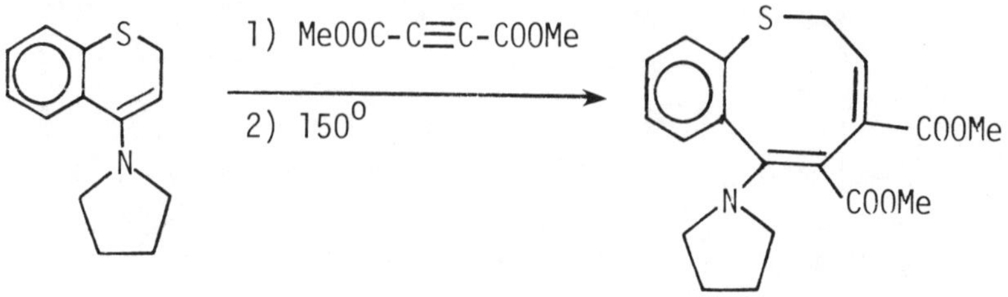

1) MeOOC-C≡C-COOMe
2) 150°

31%

VI.B.1-8   M. L. Deen, <u>Synthesis</u>, 701 (1982).

Review: "Expanded Ring Systems from Cyclopropenes: 1,3-Dipolar and [2 + 2] -Additions Across the Cyclopropenyl π-Bond"

VI.B.2.   Ring Contraction

VI.B.2-1 W. G. Dauben and R. A. Bunce, *J. Org. Chem.*, **47**, 5042 (1982).

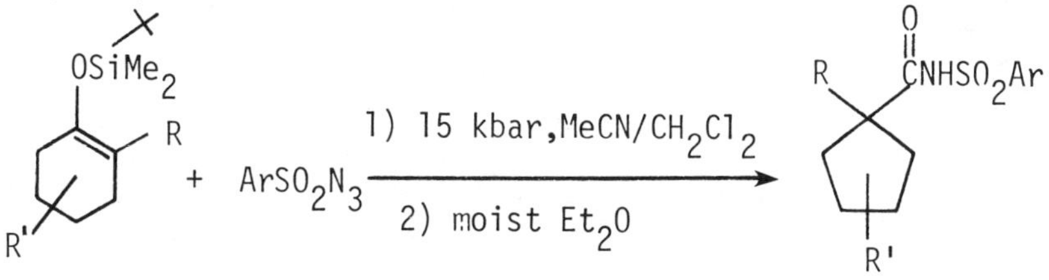

R, R' = H, Me, i-Pr

62-87%

VI.B.2-2 P. Duhamel and M. Kotera, *J. Chem. Research(S)*, 276 (1982).

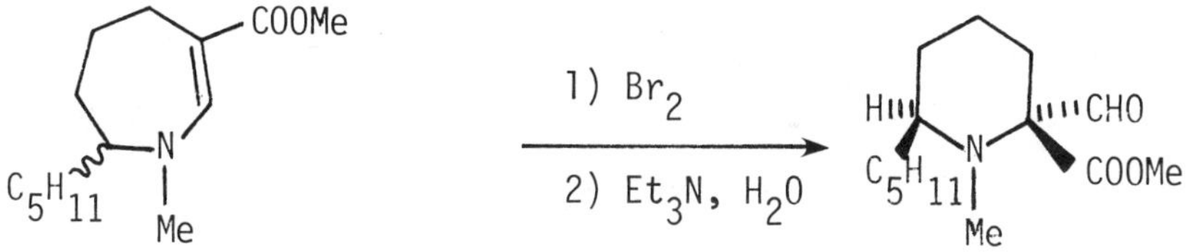

83%

VI.C. Multistep Transformations

1. Masked-Carbonyl Systems

VI.C.1-1 D. L. Comins, J. D. Brown, and N. B. Mantlo,
Tetrahedron Lett., 23, 3979 (1982).

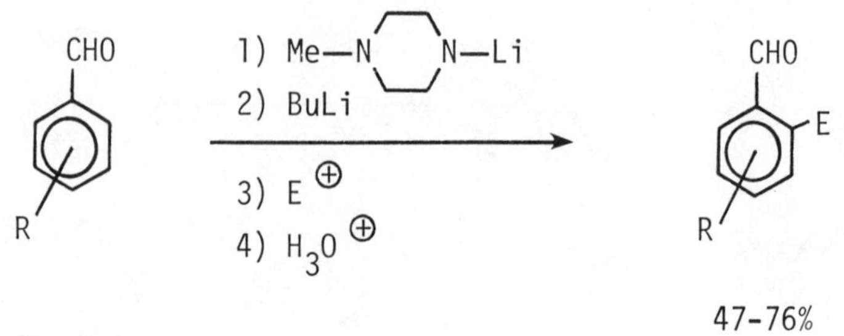

[Ar-CHO with R substituent] →
1) Me—N(piperazine)N—Li
2) BuLi
3) $E^{\oplus}$
4) $H_3O^{\oplus}$
→ [Ar-CHO with R and ortho-E substituents]

47-76%

R = H, Cl, benzo
$E^{\oplus}$ = MeI, BuI, Me$_3$SiCl

VI.C.1-2 A. S. Rao et al., Indian J. Chem., 21B, 408 (1982).

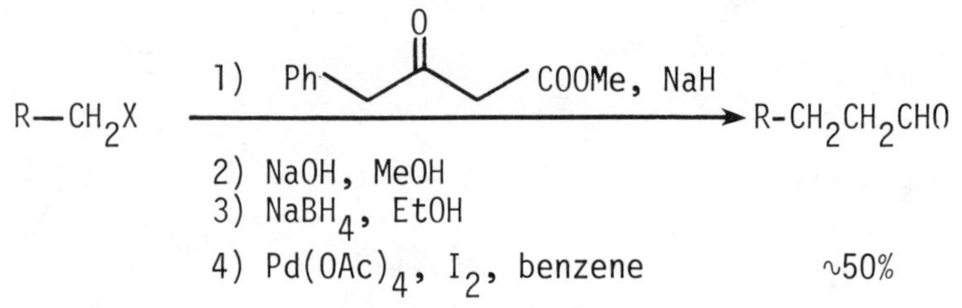

$R-CH_2X$
1) Ph-CO-CH$_2$-COOMe, NaH
2) NaOH, MeOH
3) NaBH$_4$, EtOH
4) Pd(OAc)$_4$, I$_2$, benzene
→ $R-CH_2CH_2CHO$

∼50%

VI.C.1-3 T. -L. Ho, Synth. Comm., 12, 53 (1982).

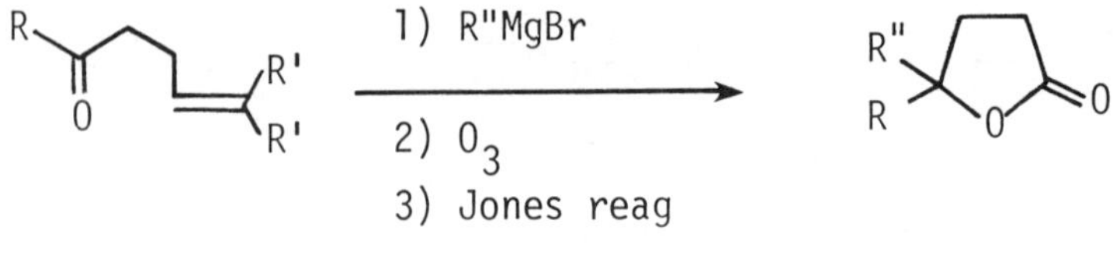

[R-CO-CH$_2$-CH=CR'$_2$]
1) R"MgBr
2) O$_3$
3) Jones reag
→ [γ-butyrolactone with R", R substituents]

R = H, Me
R' = H, Me
R" = n-alkyl

∼60-75% overall

VI.C.2. Other Multistep Transformations

VI.C.2-1   M. A. Tius et al., Tetrahedron Lett., 23, 2823 (1982).

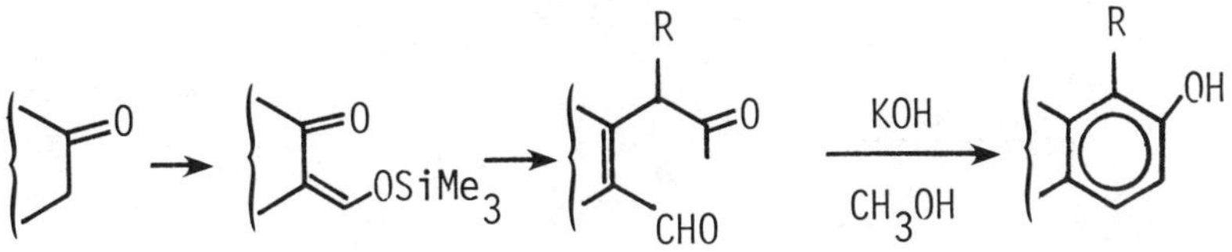

74-100%

(R = H, Me)

VII
MISCELLANEOUS REVIEWS

VII-1   J. Org. Chem., 47, 1794 (1982).

"Recent Reviews. 9"

VII-2   J. Org. Chem., 47, 4600 (1982).

"Recent Reviews. 10"

VII-3   H. Sakurai, Pure and App. Chem., 54, 1 (1982).

Review: "Reactions of Allylsilanes and Application to Organic Synthesis"

VII-4   G. A. Olah and S. C. Narang, Tetrahedron, 38, 2225 (1982).

   Review: "Iodotrimethylsilane--A Versatile Synthetic Reagent"

VII-5   R. G. Wallace, Org. Prep. Proc. Int., 14, 265 (1982).

   Review: "Hydroxylamine-O-sulphonic Acid. Its Use in Organic Synthesis"

VII-6   B. A. Arbuzov and N. N. Zobova, Synthesis, 433 (1982).

   Review: "Addition of Aliphatic and Aromatic Acyl Isocyanates to Unsaturated Compounds"

VII-7   F. Kober, Synthesis, 173 (1982).

   Review: "Aminoarsane as a Preparative Reagent"

VII-8   M. Harre et al., Angew. Chem. Int. Ed., 21, 480 (1982).

   Review: "4-Oxo-2-cyclopentenyl Acetate—A Synthetic
             Intermediate"

VII-9   A. Pelter, Chem. Soc. Rev., 11, 191 (1982).

   Review: "Carbon-Carbon Bond Formation Involving
             Boron Reagents"

VII-10   R. N. Grimes, Pure and Appl. Chem., 54, 43 (1982).

Review: "Metallacarboranes and Metal-boron Clusters in Organic Synthesis"

VII-11   A. Suzuki, Accounts Chem. Res., 15, 178 (1982).

Review: "Organoborates in New Synthetic Reactions"

VII-12   H. J. Bestmann et al., Israel J. Chem., 22, 45 (1982).

Review: "Synthesis of Three-Membered Rings by means of Phosphorus Ylids"

VII-13 V. V. Tyuleneva et al., Russ. Chem. Rev., 51, 1 (1982).

Review: "Fluorine—containing phosphorus ylids"

VII-14 T. Mukaiyama, Org. React., 28, 203 (1982).

Review: "The Directed Aldol Reaction"

VII-15 E. Schaumann and R. Ketcham, Angew. Chem. Int. Ed., 21, 225 (1982).

Review: "[2 + 2]-Cycloreversions"

VII-16   V. A. Mironov et al., Russ. Chem. Rev., 50, 666 (1981).

Review: "The 1,5-shift Reaction"

VII-17   W. Oppolzer, Accounts Chem. Res., 15, 135 (1982).

Review: "Intramolecular [2 + 2] Photoaddition/ Cyclobutane-Fragmentation Sequence in Organic Synthesis"

VII-18   S. M. Weinreb and R. R. Staib, Tetrahedron, 38, 3087 (1982).

Review: "Synthetic aspects of Diels-Alder cycloadditions with heterodienophiles"

VII-19   K. Fukui, <u>Angew. Chem. Int. Ed.</u>, <u>21</u>, 801 (1982).

   Review: "The Role of Frontier Orbitals in Chemical
            Reactions"

VII-20   W. A. Hermann, <u>Pure and Appl. Chem.</u>, <u>54</u>, 65 (1982).

   Review: "The Methylene Bridge: A Challenge to
            Synthetic, Mechanistic, and Structural
            Organic Chemistry"

VII-21   B. M. Trost, <u>Chem. Soc. Rev.</u>, <u>11</u>, 141 (1982).

   Review: "Cyclopentanoids: A Challenge for New
            Methodology"

VII-22   R. Kh. Freidlina et al., Russ. Chem. Rev., 51, 368 (1982).

Review: "The synthesis of substituted cyclopropanes and cyclopropenes by the reductive cyclisation of polychloroalkanes"

VII-23   R. F. Heck, Org. React., 27, 345 (1982).

Review: "Palladium-Catalyzed Vinylation of Organic Halides"

VII-24   E. Negishi, Accounts Chem. Res., 15, 340 (1982).

Review: "Palladium- or Nickel-Catalyzed Cross Coupling. A New Selective Method for Carbon-Carbon Bond Formation."

VII-25   H. Morrison et al., Pure and App. Chem., 54, 1723 (1982).

Review: "Photoactivation of Remote Functional Groups in Organic Molecules and "HOMO Dictated" Carbonyl Photochemistry"

VII-26   P. Margaretha, Topics in Current Chem., 103, 1 (1982).

Review: "Preparative Organic Photochemistry"

VII-27   U. E. Wiersum, Rec. Trav. Chim. Pays-Bas, 101, 317 and 365 (1982).

Review: "Flash Vacuum Thermolysis, a Versatile Method in Organic Chemistry"

VII-28   A. P. Krapcho, Synthesis, 805 and 893 (1982).

Review: "Synthetic Applications of Dealkoxycarbonylations of Malonate Esters, β-Keto Esters, α-Cyano Esters and Related Compounds in Dipolar Aprotic Media"

VII-29   D. Seebach and V. Prelog, Angew. Chem. Int. Ed., 21, 654 (1982).

Review: "The Unambiguous Specification of the Steric Course of Asymmetric Syntheses"

VII-30   K. Drauz, A. Kleeman, and J. Martens, Angew. Chem. Int. Ed., 21, 584 (1982).

Review: "Induction of Asymmetry by Amino Acids"

VII-31   D. A. Evans, Aldrichimica Acta, 15, 23 (1982).

Review: "Studies in Asymmetric Synthesis. The Development of Practical Chiral Enolate Synthons"

VII-32   B. Bosnich and P. B. Mackenzie, Pure and Appl. Chem., 54, 189 (1982).

Review: "Asymmetric Catalytic Allylic Alkylation"

VII-33   T. Hayashi and M. Kumada, Accounts Chem. Res., 15, 395 (1982).

Review: "Asymmetric Synthesis Catalyzed by Transition-Metal Complexes with Functionalized Chiral Ferrocenylphosphine Ligands"

VII-34   R. W. Hoffman, Angew. Chem. Int. Ed., 21, 555 (1982).

Review: "Diastereogenic Addition of Crotylmetal Compounds to Aldehydes"

VII-35   M. Demuth and K. Schaffner, Angew. Chem. Int. Ed., 21, 820 (1982).

Review: "Tricyclo$[3.3.0.0^{2,8}]$octan-3-ones: Photochemically Prepared Building Blocks for Enantiospecific Total Syntheses of Cyclopentanoid Natural Products"

VII-36   T. Mukaiyama, Pure and Appl. Chem., 54, 2455 (1982).

Review: "Synthetic Control Leading to Natural Products"

VII-37   I. Ugi, Angew. Chem. Int. Ed., 21, 810 (1982).

Review: "From Isocyanides via Four-Component Condensations to Antibiotic Syntheses"

VII-38   J. Ackroyd and F. Scheinmann, Chem. Soc. Rev., 11, 321 (1982).

Review: "The Synthesis of Leukotrienes: A New Class of Biologically Active Compounds Including SRS-A"

VII-39   F. Arcamone, Bull. Soc. Chim. Belges, 91, 1003 (1982).

Review: "Synthesis in the Field of Natural Products of Biological Relevance"

VII-40   H. Paulsen, Angew. Chem. Int. Ed., 21, 155 (1982).

Review: "Advances in Selective Chemical Syntheses of Complex Oligosaccharides"

VII-41   K. Martinek and A. N. Semenov, Russ. Chem. Rev., 50, 718 (1981).

Review: "Enzyme Catalysis in Organic Synthesis"

VII-42   T. A. Hase and J. K. Koskimies, Aldrichimica Acta, 15, 35 (1982).

Review: "A Compilation of References on R-Functional Acyl Anion Synthons, RCO^-"

VII-43   N. Petragnani and M. Yonashiro, Synthesis, 521 (1982).

Review: "The Reactions of Dianions of Carboxylic Acids and Ester Enolates"

VII-44   H. J. Spiegel, Topics in Current Chem., 106, 55, (1982).

Review: "Lithium Halocarbenoids--Carbanions of High Synthetic Versatility"

VII-45   P. J. Stang et al., Synthesis, 85 (1982).

Review: "Perfluoroalkanesulfonic Esters: Methods of Preparation and Applications in Organic Chemistry"

VII-46   H. Werner, Pure and Appl. Chem., 54, 171 (1982).

Review: "Metal Basicity as a Synthetic Tool in Organometallic Chemistry"

VII-47   R. Hoffmann, Angew. Chem. Int. Ed., 21, 711 (1982).

Review: "Building Bridges Between Inorganic and Organic Chemistry"

VII-48   W. E. Parham and C. K. Bradsher, Accounts Chem. Res., 15, 300 (1982).

Review: "Aromatic Organolithium Reagents Bearing Electrophilic Groups. Preparation by Halogen-Lithium Exchange."

VII-49   P. Beak and V. Snieckus, Accounts Chem. Res., 15, 306 (1982).

Review: "Directed Lithiation of Aromatic Tertiary Amides: An Evolving Synthetic Methodology for Polysubstituted Aromatics"

VII-50   M. Dagonneau, Bull. Soc. Chim. France II, 269 (1982).

Review: "Radical Reactions of Grignard Reagents"

VII-51   Sh. O. Badanyan et al., Russ. Chem. Rev., 50, 1074 (1981).

Review: "Copper Salts in Catalytic Reactions of Organic Compounds"

VII-52   M. T. Reetz, Topics in Current Chem., 106, 1 (1982).

   Review: "Organotitanium Reagents in Organic Synthesis. A Simple Means to Adjust Reactivity and Selectivity of Carbanions."

VII-53   R. C. Larock, Tetrahedron, 38, 1713 (1982).

   Review: "Organomercurials in Organic Synthesis"

VII-54   L. D. Freedman and G. O. Doak, Chem. Rev., 82, 15 (1982).

   Review: "Preparation, Reactions, and Physical Properties of Organobismuth Compounds"

VII-55   T. Kauffmann, Angew. Chem. Int. Ed., 21, 410 (1982).

   Review: "New Possible Applications of Heavy Main-Group Elements in Organic Synthesis"

AUTHOR INDEX

AUTHOR INDEX

Abdel-Wahab, A. M. A. - 20
Abdrakhmanov, I. B. - 194
Abramovitch, R. A. - 211
Achmatowicz, O., Jr. - 167
Ackroyd, J. - 464
Agababyan, A. G. - 388
Agawa, T. - 119
Ager, D. J. - 140, 196
Agosta, W. C. - 101
Ahlbright, T. A. - 245
Ahmed, M. G. - 77
Akermark, B. - 15
Akhachinskaya, T. V. - 165
Akiba, K. - 320, 321, 322
Alper, H. - 238, 239
Altenbach, H. J. - 120
Andersen, N. H. - 23
Anderson, A. G., Jr. - 204
Ando, T. - 400
Ando, W. - 41, 323, 438, 443
Annen, K. - 40
Antonakis, K. - 248
ApSimon, J. W. - 70
Aratani, T. - 156
Araujo, F. M. - 315

Arbuzov, B. A. - 453
Arcamone, F. - 464
Arigoni, D. - 9
Armesto, D. - 192
Arnold, D. R. - 103, 216
Arnold, Z. - 48
Arrowsmith, J. E. - 341
Asaoka, M. - 319
Aubry, J. M. - 167
Avar, L. - 124
Ayyangar, N. R. - 13
Babayan, A. T. - 14
Babichev, F. S. - 306
Babler, J. H. - 126, 336, 404
Back, T. G. - 103
Badamyan, Sh. O. - 468
Baggett, N. - 59
Baggiolini, E. G. - 115
Bailey, W. F. - 25, 268
Baird, M. S. - 92, 127, 156
Baker, R. - 189, 197
Balasubramaniyan, V. - 394
Baldwin, J. E. - 49, 196
Baldwin, S. W. - 65, 182
Ballesteros, J. S. - 302

Banerjee, S. K. - 401
Ban, Y. - 136
Banwell, M. G. - 92
Baraldi, P. G. - 13
Barba, F. - 139
Barlett, R. - 154
Barluenga, J. - 30, 62
Bartlett, P. A. - 196
Bartlett, P. D. - 171, 173
Bartmann, W. - 111
Bartoli, G. - 218
Barton, D. H. R. - 118, 215, 223, 304
Barua, N. C. - 122
Bates, R. B. - 27, 300, 439
Bauld, N. L. - 171
Baumstark, A. L. - 263
Bazavova, I. M. - 54
Beak, P. - 21, 25, 219, 221, 381, 468
Becker, D. - 183
Becker, K. B. - 185
Beebe, T. R. - 268, 404
Belletire, J. L. - 95, 113
Belyaev, E. Y. - 52

Berbalk, H. - 210
Bergman, R. G. - 40
Bertrand, J. - 70
Bertrand, M. - 200
Bertz, S. H. - 46, 53, 78
Bestmann, H. J. - 113, 116, 117, 121, 147, 426, 455
Beugelmans, R. - 215
Bhatt, M. V. - 349
Binger, P. - 188
Birch, A. J. - 32, 216
Birkofer, L. - 61, 160
Black, T. H. - 245, 299
Blackburn, G. M. - 122
Block, R. - 22
Boche, G. - 203, 252, 378
Bock, H. - 96
Boeckman, R. K., Jr. - 53, 178
Boger, D. L. - 226, 334
Bohme, H. - 48
Bolleghi, C. - 412
Bonadies, F. - 48
Bonnier, J. M. - 206
Borchardt, R. T. - 205
Borredon, E. - 392

AUTHOR INDEX

Bosnich, B. - 14, 462
Boudjouk, P. - 66, 289
Boulton, A. J. - 333
Bourgeois, M. J. - 48
Bradsher, C. K. - 219, 220, 268
Brady, W. T. - 328
Brandsma, L. - 105, 143
Brehme, R. - 41
Breitmaier, E. - 74
Breuer, E. - 300
Bridges, A. J. - 123
Bringmann, G. - 224, 225
Briody, J. M. - 207
Brion, F. - 18, 167
Brocksom, T. J. - 169
Brooks, D. W. - 9
Broquet, C. - 138
Brown, G. R. - 279
Brown, H. C. - 137, 138, 232, 233, 234, 277, 284, 287, 291, 297, 298, 407, 424
Brown, R. F. C. - 224
Bruce, J. M. - 224
Brunke, E. J. - 92
Bryson, T. A. - 95, 200

Buchardt, O. - 115
Bumgardner, C. L. - 162
Bumagin, N. A. - 406
Bunina-Krivorukova, L. I. - 195
Burczyk, B. - 362
Burke, S. D. - 51
Burton, D. J. - 67
Bushby, R. J. - 161
Butsugan, Y. - 29, 132
Byrn, S. R. - 270
Cadogan, J. I. G. - 203
Calas, P. - 152
Callot, H. J. - 104, 156
Calo, V. - 28
Cambie, R. C. - 108
Cameron, D. W. - 226
Camps, F. - 283, 401
Camps, P. - 108
Canevet, J. C. - 120
Caple, R. - 241
Caporusso, A. M. - 274
Capozzi, G. - 148, 426
Capuano, L. - 119, 229
Cardillo, G. - 122, 393
Carey, F. A. - 112

Carlson, R. M. - 147
Carpita, A. - 136
Carrie, R. - 156
Carrie, R. R. - 42
Casey, C. P. - 157
Casey, M. - 331
Castells, J. - 98
Catellani, M. - 152
Cava, M. P. - 173, 437
Ceccherelli, P. - 108
Cella, J. A. - 33
Chamberlin, A. R. - 9
Chan, C. C. - 14
Chan, T. H. - 44, 76, 119, 138, 160, 226
Chandrasekaran, S. - 257, 267
Chanon, M. - 99
Chapleur, Y. - 44
Charpentier-Morize, M. - 90
Chasar, D. W. - 73
Chaudhuri, M. K. - 249, 254
Cheng, C. C. - 323
Chiba, T. - 252
Childs, R. F. - 161, 190
Chin-Hsien, W. - 124

Chiusoli, G. P. - 159, 239, 242
Christie, M. A. - 114
Chung, S. K. - 280, 290
Cinquini, M. - 56
Citterio, A. - 87, 206, 230
Claesson, A. - 143
Clark, J. H. - 38
Clark, R. D. - 221
Classon, B. - 421
Clerica, A. - 105
Clive, D. L. J. - 39, 80, 106, 290
Coates, R. M. - 6, 159, 186
Cohen, T. - 23, 166, 201
Collins, P. M. - 115
Colon, I. - 289
Colquhoun, H. M. - 236
Comasseto, J. V. - 119
Comins, D. L. - 220, 321, 410, 450
Conia, J. M. - 50, 116, 140, 363
Consiglio, G. - 411
Constantino, M. G. - 63
Cook, J. M. - 49

AUTHOR INDEX

Cooke, M. P., Jr. - 107
Cookson, R. C. - 73, 446
Corey, E. J. - 56, 116, 119, 122, 149, 171, 264, 293, 350
Cornelisse, J. - 229
Corriu, R. J. P. - 76
Couquelet, J. - 128
Courtois, G. - 61, 382
Couture, A. - 228
Couturier, D. - 66, 301
Crandall, J. K. - 371
Cruz, R. - 76
Curci, R. - 264
Curran, D. P. - 200
Dabbagh, G. - 78
Dagonneau, M. - 100, 468
Dahn, H. - 122, 166
Dampawan, P. - 419
D'Angeli, F. - 300, 306
Danheiser, R. L. - 184
Daniewski, A. R. - 156
Danishefsky, S. - 31, 40, 77, 87, 167
Darbarwar, M. - 318
Daub, G. W. - 198
Daub, J. - 43
Dauben, W. G. - 168, 185, 192, 449
Davis, F. A. - 362
Davis, R. - 349
Davy, H. - 442
DeClercq, P. J. - 84
Deem, M. L. - 165, 448
Degrand, C. - 102
Dehmlow, E. V. - 146, 154
DeKimpe, N. - 208
de las Heras, F. G. - 95
DeLucchi, O. - 175
DeMayo, P. - 182
de Meijere, A. - 69, 150, 166
Demuth, M. - 101, 463
Denmark, S. E. - 88, 198
Descotes, G. - 284, 346, 386
Dev, S. - 267
Dieter, R. K. - 82
DiMaio, G. - 59
Dimmel, D. R. - 3, 35
Dixneuf, P. - 341, 345
Djerassi, C. - 127, 199

Donetti, A. - 116
Doney, J. J. - 106
Dowd, P. - 172, 175
Doweyko, A. M. - 22
Downie, I. M. - 396
Doyle, M. P. - 156
Drauz, K. - 461
Dreiding, A. S. - 183, 184, 203
Drewes, S. E. - 12
Dubois, J. E. - 4, 65
Duboudin, F. - 95
Duhamel, L. - 129, 130, 391
Duhamel, P. - 19, 449
Duncan, J. A. - 183
Dunn, A. D. - 412
Dunogues, J. - 148, 172
Dunogues, J. P. - 37
Durr, H. - 155
Dymicky, M. - 395
Effenberger, F. - 18, 41, 209, 386
Ehrhardt, H. - 136
Eisch, J. J. - 183, 229
Eisenbraun, E. J. - 231
Elliott, A. J. - 305
Elnagdi, M. H. - 334
El-Newaihy, M. F. - 44
Elshafie, S. M. M. - 321
Emde, H. - 367
Enders, D. - 47
Engel, C. R. - 108
Engman, L. - 124, 295
Epling, G. A. - 441
Epstein, W. W. - 92
Ernest, I. - 117
Eugster, C. H. - 117, 168
Evans, D. A. - 11, 26, 462
Evans, S. A., Jr. - 358
Falck, J. R. - 226
Fang, J. M. - 76
Farcasiu, D. - 205, 237
Farid, S. - 180
Fatope, M. O. - 217
Fauvarque, J. F. - 102
Feldhues, U. - 412
Fernandez, S. - 128
Ferreira, J. T. B. - 439
Fiaud, J. C. - 29
Ficini, J. - 183
Fields, R. - 155

AUTHOR INDEX

Filliatre, C. - 101
Figeys, H. P. - 146
Fish, R. H. - 285
Fitzer, L. - 163, 186
Fleet, G. W. J. - 64
Fleming, I. - 125, 205
Floriani, C. - 245
Florio, S. - 46
Foa, M. - 239
Fohlisch, B. - 190
Formanovskii, A. A. - 154
Fortes, C. C. - 268, 398
Foucaud, A. - 48
Fox, M. A. - 113, 218
Franck, R. W. - 9, 115, 168
Franck-Neumann, M. - 18, 161
Fraser-Reid, B. - 115
Frater, G. - 210
Fray, G. I. - 203
Freedman, L. D. - 245, 469
Freidlina, R. K. - 157, 459
Friedrich, E. C. - 155
Fringuelli, F. - 172
Fuchs, P. L. - 176, 182
Fujii, K. - 398

Fujinami, T. - 51
Fujino, M. - 354
Fujisawa, T. - 64, 67, 72, 81, 133, 276, 318, 393, 403
Fujita, E. - 57, 125, 126, 127, **207, 288, 291,** 327
Fujita, S. - 338
Fujiwara, Y. - 215, 237
Fukui, K. - 165, 458
Funabiki, T. - 139, 415
Funk, R. L. - 177, 199
Gadwood, R. C. - 194
Gallina, C. - 28
Galynker, I. - 373
Ganboa, I. - 376
Ganem, B. - 307
Ganushchak, N. I. - 207
Gaoni, Y. - 81, 159
Garcia, J. - 379
Garcia-Raso, A. - 77
Garratt, P. J. - 9, 10
Garst, M. E. - 108, 226
Gaset, A. - 114
Gassman, P. G. - 95, 201, 337
Gates, M. - 212

Gaudemar, M. - 67, 72
Gawley, R. E. - 363
Geise, H. J. - 138
Genet, J. P. - 17, 158
Gerlach, H. - 177
Gesson, J. P. - 170
Ghatak, U. R. - 389
Ghiringhelli, D. - 364
Ghosez, L. - 19, 140, 184, 310
Gibbons, E. G. - 77
Giese, B. - 100, 136
Gilbert, J. C. - 151
Giles, R. G. F. - 209
Gill, G. B. - 192
Giordano, C. - 90
Girard, C. - 9
Gladysz, J. A. - 434
Gleiter, R. - 194
Glennon, R. A. - 120
Gloede, J. - 373, 433
Godefroi, E. F. - 22, 50
Godleski, S. A. - 17
Gohar, A. E. K. M. N. - 211
Gokel, G. W. - 344
Gompper, R. - 48, 195
Goodwin, T. E. - 21
Gore, J. - 89, 125, 141, 143, 144
Gosney, I. - 203
Goswami, R. - 24
Gramain, J. C. - 380
Granik, V. G. - 36
Gras, J. L. - 177
Gribble, G. W. - 294, 304
Griesbaum, K. - 183
Griffin, G. W. - 106
Grigg, R. - 204
Grimes, R. N. - 455
Groen, M. B. - 94
Grohe, K. - 41
Gross, H. - 12, 122
Grundler, W. - 166
Guindon, Y. - 128
Gupton, J. T. - 49
Guy, A. - 256
Guziec, F. S., Jr. - 248
Hafner, K. - 121, 186, 232
Haines, A. H. - 115
Hall, H. K., Jr. - 71, 167, 175, 181

AUTHOR INDEX

Halpern, J. - 295
Hamana, H. - 39
Hamer, N. K. - 185
Hamon, D. P. G. - 167
Hanack, M. - 5
Harre, M. - 454
Harris, T. M. - 13
Hart, D. J. - 324
Hartman, G. D. - 124
Hartmann, W. - 155
Harvey, R. G. - 211, 221
Harwood, L. M. - 195
Hase, T. A. - 111, 440, 465
Hassall, C. H. - 169
Hassner, A. - 161, 381
Haszeldine, R. N. - 155
Hata, T. - 58, 366
Hauser, F. M. - 168
Havel, M. - 48
Hay, A. S. - 2
Hayashi, T. - 55
Haynes, R. K. - 368, 373
Heathcock, C. H. - 84, 108, 198
Hebert, E. - 6

Heck, R. F. - 133, 459
Hegedus, L. S. - 15, 34, 107, 221, 238, 239, 307, 326
Helmchen, G. - 112
Helquist, P. - 84
Henning, H. G. - 110
Herbert, E. - 28
Hermann, W. A. - 458
Hernandez, J. E. - 266
Herz, W. - 95
Hess, U. - 102
Heubach, G. - 210
Hewson, A. T. - 133
Hickmott, P. W. - 3, 390
Hidai, M. - 107
Himbert, G. - 148, 150, 177
Hirakawa, K. - 218
Hirao, T. - 16, 128, 409
Hiroi, K. - 201
Hirsch, J. A. - 2
Hiyama, T. - 47, 60, 156, 163, 242
Ho, T. L. - 73, 158, 176, 313, 450
Hoberg, H. - 237, 241

Hodge, P. - 227, 265, 266
Hoffmann, H. M. R. - 92, 98, 166, 189, 327, 369, 416
Hoffmann, R. - 244
Hoffmann, R. W. - 58, 236, 463, 467
Hojo, M. - 276
Holder, R. W. - 48
Holmes, A. B. - 148
Holt, S. L. - 171
Hong, P. - 239
Hooz, J. - 39
Hopf, H. - 152
Hoppe, D. - 25, 69
Hosomi, A. - 3, 4, 166
Houghton, R. P. - 48
Houk, K. N. - 190, 191
Hoye, T. R. - 173, 185, 223
Huang, N. Z. - 62
Huang, X. - 80, 249, 261, 377
Huang, Y. - 121
Hudlicky, T. - 156
Huffman, J. W. - 71
Hulkenberg, A. - 413
Hunig, S. - 98, 139, 182, 187, 416

Husson, H. P. - 6, 88, 296, 324
Hutchins, R. O. - 286, 292
Ibuka, T. - 164
Ibuki, E. - 213
Ikegami, S. - 150, 427
Ila, H. - 42, 141, 158, 333
Imamoto, T. - 105, 238, 242, 442
Irie, H. - 78
Ishihara, T. - 5, 67
Ishikawa, N. - 129, 131
Ishino, Y. - 198
Isied, S. S. - 360
Itahara, T. T. - 304
Ito, S. - 21, 232, 263
Ito, Y. - 168
Itoh, K. - 24, 33, 58, 90
Ivanov, C. - 223
Iwasaki, T. - 103
Iwasawa, N. - 38
Jachimowicz, F. - 239
Jackson, W. R. - 96, 139, 216
Jalander, L. - 210, 312
Jampel, E. G. - 358
Jankowski, K. - 167

AUTHOR INDEX

Jarglis, P. - 317
Jawdosiuk, M. - 121
Jeffs, P. W. - 185
Jenkins, P. R. - 128
Jenner, G. - 168, 192
Jennings, B. H. - 154
Jennings-White, C. - 64
Johnson, C. R. - 7, 78, 121, 155, 258, 441
Johnson, F. - 15, 50, 212
Johnson, M. D. - 100, 161
Johnson, W. S. - 94
Jones, J. B. - 251, 313
Jones, J. H. - 354
Jones, R. A. - 325, 422
Jones, R. C. F. - 63, 406
Joucla, M. - 158
Joullie, M. M. - 217
Julia, M. - 22, 132, 139, 159, 292
Jullien, J. - 142
Jullien, R. - 81
Jung, M. E. - 173
Junjappa, H. - 42
Jurczak, J. - 168

Kabalka, G. W. - 234, 374, 382
Kabbe, H. J. - 327
Kagan, H. B. - 242, 255, 420
Kaiser, E. T. - 431
Kaji, A. - 15, 73
Kalechits, G. V. - 204
Kametani, T. - 180, 199, 340
Kampe, K. D. - 335
Kanaoka, Y. - 338
Kanematsu, K. - 201
Kano, S. - 119
Kantlehner, W. - 96
Kapil, R. S. - 218
Karnojitzky, V. - 272
Karpf, M. - 50
Kashima, C. - 62, 339
Kashin, A. N. - 272
Kasturi, T. R. - 52
Kato, J. - 38
Kato, S. - 120, 443
Kato, T. - 208, 224
Katritzky, A. R. - 125, 260, 425
Katsumura, S. - 101
Katzenellenbogen, J. A. - 44

Kauffmann, T. - 31, 242, 245, 469
Kaupp, G. - 218
Kawabata, N. - 157, 263
Kawanobe, W. - 428
Keana, J. F. W. - 187
Keck, G. E. - 34, 143
Keehn, P. M. - 247, 251, 266, 271
Keinan, E. - 283
Kelly, L. F. - 18
Kelly, T. R. - 170
Kende, A. S. - 10, 42, 107, 146
Keshavamurthy, K. S. - 369, 377, 394
Khanna, R. N. - 131
Kiji, J. - 242
Kikukawa, K. - 237
Kim, S. - 273, 275
King, J. F. - 96
Kinoshita, H. - 302
Kirmse, W. - 194
Kishi, Y. - 53, 242, 288
Klei, E. - 69
Klein, R. S. - 413

Klumpp, G. W. - 137
Knight, D. W. - 199
Knorr, R. - 42
Kobayashi, M. - 150
Kobayushi, Y. - 151
Kober, F. - 454
Kodama, M. - 21
Koga, K. - 182
Koizumi, T. - 118
Komatsu, M. - 319
Kondo, K. - 58
Kontonassios, D. - 51
Koreeda, M. - 68, 172, 236
Kornblum, N. - 259, 403, 408
Korostova, S. E. - 325
Korshak, V. V. - 346
Koster, H. - 357
Kostova, K. - 318, 447
Kotake, H. - 55
Kowalski, C. J. - 62, 65, 82, 257, 434
Kozikowski, A. P. - 137, 169, 171, 188, 339, 410
Krapcho, A. P. - 12, 281, 461
Kraus, G. A. - 31, 81, 179

AUTHOR INDEX

Krief, A. - 57, 75, 109, 131, 146, 445
Krishnamurthy, S. - 382
Krohn, K. - 217
Kropf, H. - 27
Kruse, L. I. - 205
Kuehne, M. E. - 112
Kuhl, P. - 430
Kukla, M. J. - 357
Kulinkovich, O. G. - 127
Kulkarni, S. N. - 41
Kumada, M. - 16, 61, 67, 131, 133, 246, 462
Kumagai, T. - 186
Kume, A. - 355
Kunda, N. G. - 206
Kunz, H. - 353, 429
Kurosawa, H. - 20
Kuwajima, I. - 5, 215, 249
Kuzuhara, H. - 385
Laarhoven, W. H. - 228
Ladner, W. - 9
Lalko, O. R. - 189
Lamb, N. - 93
Lambert, P. H. - 329
Lamm, B. - 448
Lange, G. L. - 182
Langlois, Y. - 126
Lansbury, P. T. - 40, 312
Lantzsch, R. - 158
Lapouyade, R. - 228
Lappert, M. F. - 98
Larock, R. C. - 30, 132, 152, 237, 246, 317, 469
Larson, G. L. - 64, 113, 426, 439
Lattes, A. - 138, 235
Lee, C. C. - 342
Lee, D. G. - 250
Lee, T. V. - 253
Lee-Ruff, E. - 211
Lehmkuhl, H. - 163
Lehner, H. - 103
Leigh, G. J. - 153
Lemmen, P. - 13
Lenz, G. R. - 182
Lepage, Y. - 172, 212
Letsinger, R. L. - 366
Levitt, L. S. - 375
Levy, J. - 74

Ley, S. V. - 91
Leznoff, C. C. - 3
Liebeskind, L. S. - 174, 243
Liebscher, J. - 46
Lindner, D. L. - 193
Lindner, E. - 185
Linstrumelle, G. - 141
Lion, C. - 23
Liotta, D. - 127
Lipshutz, B. H. - 28, 29, 84, 363
Liptak, A. - 350
Lissel, M. - 23, 440
Little, R. D. - 76
Liu, H. J. - 48, 76, 175, 182, 198, 280, 414
Logan, R. T. - 151
Logue, M. W. - 148
Lombardo, L. - 113
Lounasmaa, M. - 97, 306
Luche, J. L. - 42, 78
Luh, T. Y. - 239
Luttke, W. - 138
Mach, K. - 106
Magerramov, M. N. - 206

Magnus, P. - 61, 88, 179
Mahajan, M. P. - 332
Maier, G. - 175
Maier, T. - 43
Makin, S. M. - 1, 34
Makosza, M. - 218
Malmberg, H. - 84
Mancini, M. L. - 61
Mandal, A. K. - 56
Mandell, L. - 179
Mander, L. N. - 36
Mandolini, L. - 36
Mane, R. B. - 14
Manhas, M. S. - 308
Mann, J. - 168
Marcuzzi, F. - 145
Maretina, I. A. - 346
Margaretha, P. - 102, 186, 460
Marino, J. P. - 30
Marsh, F. D. - 255
Martens, J. - 112
Martin, H. D. - 174
Martin, J. C. - 222
Martin, S. F. - 80, 186, 194
Martina, D. - 18

AUTHOR INDEX

Martinek, K. - 465
Martinez, A. G. - 124
Maruyama, K. - 44, 57, 83
Marxer, A. - 210
Masaki, Y. - 90
Masamune, S. - 37, 38, 372
Masamune, T. - 93
Matsubara, Y. - 436
Matsueda, R. - 357
Matsumoto, K. - 40
Matsumoto, M. - 224
Matsumoto, T. - 89, 94
Matsumura, N. - 43
Matteson, D. S. - 11, 233
Mauze, B. - 60
Mawhinney, T. D. - 348
Mayr, H. - 34, 190
McArthur, C. R. - 3
McChesney, J. D. - 35
McCombie, S. W. - 358
McCullough, K. J. - 113
McKervey, M. A. - 244
McMurry, J. E. - 138
Mehdi Nafissi-V, M. - 213
Mehrotra, K. N. - 338

Mehta, A. M. - 225
Mehta, G. - 181
Meier, H. - 186, 227
Melendez, E. - 43
Melloni, G. - 145
Menicagli, R. - 23, 92
Merkushev, E. B. - 153, 255
Mestres, R. - 377
Meth-Cohn, O. - 96
Metzner, P. - 72
Meyers, A. I. - 46, 61, 220, 322, 383
Michelot, D. - 133
Middlemas, D. - 161
Midland, M. M. - 234, 236, 277, 297
Miginiac, L. - 60, 144, 246
Migita, T. - 215
Mikolajczyk, M. - 441
Miller, B. - 207
Miller, J. A. - 93
Miller, L. L. - 139
Miller, R. D. - 435
Miller, S. I. - 172
Milner, D. J. - 205

Milstein, D. - 239
Minami, T. - 75
Mioskowski, C. - 226
Mironov, V. A. - 457
Mitra, R. B. - 163
Miyakoshi, T. - 73, 417
Miyano, S. - 40, 242
Miyaura, N. - 135
Mndzhoyan, O. L. - 399
Mochalin, V. B. - 67
Modena, G. - 145
Mohacsi, E. - 397
Moiseenkov, A. M. - 163
Molina, P. - 414, 437
Momose, T. - 54
Montanari, F. - 110
Monti, S. A. - 54
Moore, H. W. - 146
Moreau, J. L. - 43
Morgans, D., Jr. - 55
Mori, K. - 27, 224
Morizur, J. P. - 101
Moro-Oka, Y. - 89
Moroz, A. A. - 214
Morrison, H. - 460

Mortreux, A. - 244
Moss, R. A. - 155
Mostamandi, A. - 19
Motherwell, W. B. - 118, 215
Motohashi, S. - 257
Mourino, A. - 26
Mukaiyama, T. - 1, 25, 38, 39, 44, 45, 456, 463
Mukherjee, D. - 35, 104
Mullen, K. - 203
Muller, P. - 154, 379, 399
Muller, W. - 336
Mulzer, J. - 45, 123
Mundy, B. P. - 105
Murahashi, S. I. - 17
Muraoka, M. - 42
Murphy, W. S. - 211
Muschik, G. M. - 179
Muzart, J. - 40
Naf, F. - 80, 177
Nagai, Y. - 34
Nair, V. - 420
Nakahama, S. - 63
Nakai, T. - 202
Nakano, T. - 138

Nakatsuka, M. - 168
Nanasawa, M. - 108
Narasaka, K. - 83, 360
Nashed, M. A. - 365
Nasipuri, D. - 80, 273
Naso, F. - 131, 422
Negishi, E. - 5, 123, 131, 137, 140, 214, 459
Neplyuev, V. M. - 75
Nesmeyanova, O. A. - 163
Neuenschwander, M. - 190
Newton, C. G. - 347
Newton, R. F. - 133
Nicholas, K. M. - 242
Nicolaou, K. C. - 121, 204
Nilsson, M. - 85
Nishida, S. - 183
Noe, C. R. - 8
Nokami, J. - 75
Nomura, Y. - 187
Normant, J. F. - 80, 129, 133, 136, 147
North, P. C. - 117
Novoselov, E. F. - 380
Noyori, R. - 1, 4, 83, 181, 328

Nozaki, S. - 429
Nudelman, A. - 96
Nudelman, N. S. - 237
Nunami, K. I. - 20
Nunazawa, M. - 371
Nutt, R. F. - 428
Oae, S. - 280
Obayashi, M. - 58
Oda, M. - 105
Odinokov, V. N. - 272
O'Donnell, M. J. - 19, 352, 387
Ogura, F. - 261, 374
Ogura, K. - 22, 26, 404
Ohfune, Y. - 169
Ohno, M. - 39
Ohshawa, T. - 351
Ohshiro, Y. - 128, 185
Ohta, A. - 401
Ohta, S. - 259, 395, 402
Oikawa, Y. - 348
Oishi, T. - 223
Ojima, I. - 166, 240, 278, 282
Okamura, W. H. - 26, 143, 201
Okano, T. - 242, 285
Okawara, T. - 309

Oku, A. - 350
Okubo, M. - 213
Olah, G. - 361, 365, 453
Ollis, W. D. - 202
Olomucki, M. - 147
Olsen, R. K. - 396
Ono, N. - 73, 121, 166
Oppolzer, W. - 60, 171, 180, 191, 457
Orfanopoulos, M. - 113
Orr, J. C. - 274
Oshima, K. - 30, 31, 52, 106, 147, 243, 248, 284, 294
Otera, J. - 22
Overend, W. G. - 115
Overman, L. E. - 193, 194
Ozasa, S. - 213
Paddon-Row, M. N. - 227
Padwa, A. - 186, 194
Palla, G. - 305
Palomo, C. - 369, 396
Pandey, D. N. - 289
Pandit, U. K. - 3
Papenfuhs, T. - 341
Papsuevich, O. S. - 356

Paquette, L. A. - 8, 18, 22, 37, 68, 162, 174, 183
Paradisi, M. P. - 274
Parham, W. E. - 219
Parker, K. A. - 176, 198
Parsons, P. J. - 188
Pasto, D. J. - 106, 183
Paterson, I. - 4, 316
Pattenden, G. - 63, 89, 93, 129, 194
Patwardhan, S. A. - 362
Paulsen, H. -111, 465
Pavel, G. V. - 210
Pawson, B. A. - 122
Pearson, A. J. - 18
Pedersen, E. B. - 421
Pelletier, O. - 156
Pellicciari, R. - 108
Pelter, A. - 10, 232, 235, 315, 454
Pennanen, S. I. - 60
Perez-Ossorio, R. - 59
Petragnani, N. - 7, 460
Petrillo, E. W., Jr. - 88
Petrov, A. A. - 41, 154, 207

AUTHOR INDEX

Pfaltz, A. - 30
Pfander, H. - 9
Piancatelli, G. - 110, 272
Pichat, L. - 134
Piers, E. - 2, 51, 82, 136, 178, 203, 434
Pietra, F. - 59
Pillai, C. N. - 176
Pillai, V. N. R. - 432
Pincock, J. A. - 389
Pinhey, J. T. - 215
Piotrowska, H. - 20
Plath, P. - 41, 332
Plemenkov, V. V. - 174
Pletcher, D. - 102
Pochini, A. - 217
Pohnnakotr, M. - 8
Poindexter, G. S. - 310
Pommier, J. C. - 361
Pornet, J. - 144
Porta, O. - 105
Posner, G. H. - 85
Potts, K. T. - 320
Prelog, V. - 112
Pridgen, L. N. - 337, 370

Prostenik, M. V. - 54, 417
Pryor, W. A. - 260
Purrello, G. - 340
Queguiner, G. - 222, 322
Quinkert, G. - 180
Rahm, A. - 206, 410
Rama Rao, A. V. - 166, 170
Rao, A. S. - 12, 406, 450
Rao, A. V. R. - 212
Rao, C. G. - 378
Raphael, R. A. - 186
Rapoport, H. - 258, 355, 402
Rappoport, Z. - 214
Rathke, M. W. - 41
Ravindranathan, M. - 378
Rees, C. W. - 206
Reetz, M. T. - 4, 42, 68, 95, 411, 469
Regen, S. L. - 154, 365, 405, 425
Regitz, M. - 41, 103, 118, 164
Reich, H. J. - 57, 122
Reichardt, C. - 11, 42
Reid, W. - 40
Reinecke, M. G. - 347

Reinhoudt, D. N. - 330
Reissig, H. U. - 127, 162
Renaud, R. N. - 100
Rens, J. - 49
Repic, O. - 155
Reusch, W. - 202
Rewicki, D. - 204
Ricci, A. - 33, 68
Rickards, R. W. - 81
Ried, W. - 49, 56
Rieke, R. D. - 213
Rigby, J. H. - 91, 169
Risalti, A. - 84
Roberts, S. M. - 96
Robev, S. K. - 343
Rodrigo, R. - 179
Roedig, A. - 142
Rolla, F. - 299, 359, 381
Rollin, Y. - 102
Ronald, R. C. - 222
Ronchi, A. U. - 290, 295, 367
Ronlan, A. - 212
Rosenberger, M. - 121
Rosenblum, M. - 86, 183
Rosenfeld, S. M. - 43, 370

Rossi, R. - 28, 152
Rossi, R. A. - 231
Roulet, R. - 173
Roush, W. R. - 115, 176, 177
Royer, R. - 118
Ruland, A. - 118
Ruminski, J. K. - 206
Russell, G. A. - 2, 21
Russell, R. A. - 171
Russell, S. W. - 146
Rutledge, P. S. - 196
Ruzo, L. O. - 150
Saednya, S. - 414
Saegusa, T. - 97, 168, 313, 415
Saito, I. - 187, 254
Sakai, M. - 283
Sakakibara, T. - 58
Sakakibara, Y. - 139, 415
Sakito, Y. - 59
Sakurai, H. - 3, 4, 37, 166, 452
Salerno, G. - 242
Salomon, R. G. - 182, 185, 209
Sammes, P. G. - 226
Santelli, M. - 87, 146

AUTHOR INDEX

Santiago, M. A. L. - 307
Sargent, M. V. - 225
Sarma, A. S. - 2
Sartori, G. - 206
Sasaki, T. - 32, 189
Sato, F. - 60, 124, 137, 294
Sato, T. - 213
Sato, Y. - 139, 296, 380, 416
Sauer, G. - 2
Sauvetre, R. - 147
Savoia, D. - 57
Schafer, H. J. - 27, 102, 250
Schaffner, K. - 101
Schaumann, E. - 180, 456
Scheeren, H. W. - 170
Schegolev, A. A. - 241
Scheinmann, F. - 92
Schenone, P. - 342
Schick, H. - 13, 49
Schiess, P. - 26
Schlecht, M. F. - 30
Schlessinger, R. H. - 44
Schleyer, P. v. R. - 27, 107
Schlogl, K. - 27
Schlosser, M. - 113, 133, 142, 236
Schmid, M. - 29
Schmidt, C. - 91
Schmidt, R. R. - 43, 62, 129, 172, 207
Schmidt, U. - 118, 388, 430
Schmitt, G. - 379
Schmitz, E. - 309
Schneider, D. F. - 117
Schollkopf, U. - 10, 19, 386
Schonenberger, H. - 105
Schreiber, S. L. - 269
Schroth, W. - 391
Schrumpf, G. - 24
Schuda, P. F. - 150, 167
Schurig, V. - 392
Schuster, G. B. - 98
Schwartz, J. - 134, 436
Schwarz, H. - 43
Schwarz, S. - 56
Scolastico, C. - 59
Scorrano, G. - 364
Scott, L. T. - 187, 231
Scotton, M. - 52
Screttas, C. G. - 23
Sebastian, J. F. - 129

Seebach, D. - 2, 8, 9, 24, 54, 69, 71, 112, 163, 303, 397, 418, 461
Seevers, R. H. - 375
Seitz, G. - 333
Sekiya, M. - 23, 201, 326
Sell, C. S. - 98
Seltzer, S. - 152
Semmelhack, M. - 79
Semmelhack, M. F. - 216, 225, 278
Sen, A. - 210
Serratosa, F. - 150, 183, 238
Setsune, J. - 215
Severin, T. - 8
Seyferth, D. - 67, 241
Sharma, R. P. - 293
Shatzmiller, S. - 15
Shea, K. J. - 178
Shechter, H. - 57, 120, 138
Sheppard, R. C. - 430
Shimizu, N. - 190
Shiori, T. - 103, 445
Shirahama, H. - 94, 253
Shono, T. - 41, 88, 102, 158, 311, 384, 391
Shridhar, D. R. - 308, 329
Shvachkin, Yu. P. - 432
Sidorov, N. N. - 41
Siegel, H. J. - 466
Simchen, G. - 37
Skattebol, L. - 163
Slougui, N. - 104
Smith, A. B., III. - 54, 130, 159
Smith, F. X. - 14, 48
Smith, K. - 111
Smith, M. J. - 89
Smith, R. F. - 383
Smyrl, N. R. - 343
Snider, B. B. - 89, 133, 160, 177, 191
Snieckus, V. - 10, 159, 219
Snowden, R. L. - 60
Soai, K. - 287, 383
Solladie, G. - 45
Solladie-Cavallo, A. - 107
Soni, R. P. - 331
Sonoda, N. - 240
Sorensen, T. S. - 92

AUTHOR INDEX

Sorochinskii, A. E. - 32
Soto, J. L. - 77
Soucek, M. - 217
Spangler, C. W. - 124
Speier, G. - 213
Spencer, A. - 214
Spitzner, D. - 171
Srinivasan, P. C. - 114, 120
Stamm, H. - 7
Stamos, I. K. - 407
Stang, P. J. - 5, 154, 390, 466
Steckhan, E. - 359
Steglich, W. - 63, 387, 397
Steinmetz, M. G. - 161
Steliou, K. - 442
Stella, L. - 171
Stephenson, G. R. - 135
Stetter, H. - 84
Stevens, R. V. - 218, 247
Still, W. C. - 82
Stille, J. K. - 38, 314, 398
Stirling, C. J. M. - 36, 125, 127, 128
Stoodley, R. J. - 169

Stork, G. - 70, 85, 100, 196
Stout, D. M. - 324
Stradi, R. - 223
Strunz, G. M. - 49, 50
Subba Rao, G. S. R. - 35, 36, 171
Suda, M. - 116
Sugai, S. - 215
Suginome, H. - 135, 405
Sugita, T. - 256
Sundar, N. S. - 36
Suschitzky, H. - 332
Suzuki, A. - 233, 234, 235, 423, 455
Suzuki, H. - 89, 207
Suzuki, K. - 135
Suzuki, N. - 228
Swaminathan, S. - 120, 194
Sweigart, D. A. - 216
Swenton, J. S. - 130
Szantay, C. - 38
Taber, D. F. - 104, 177
Tada, M. - 314
Tagliavini, G. - 68
Tai, A. - 276

Takabe, K. - 409
Takahashi, H. - 59
Takahashi, K. - 6
Takahashi, T. - 104
Takaki, K. - 70
Takaku, H. - 395
Takazawa, O. - 39
Takeda, A. - 117, 312
Takeda, T. - 55, 198
Takeshita, H. - 175, 187
Tam, J. P. - 354, 356, 431, 438
Tamura, Y. - 73, 79, 169, 193, 208, 352, 364
Tanaka, K. - 7, 159, 314
Tanaka, M. - 237
Tanigawa, Y. - 17, 29
Taniguchi, H. - 158, 214
Tanikaga, R. - 13
Tanimoto, S. - 10, 23
Tanis, S. P. - 29, 302
Tashiro, M. - 25
Taylor, K. G. - 153, 389
Taylor, R. J. K. - 133
Taylor, R. T. - 317

Tedder, J. M. - 99
Terao, S. - 195
Terashima, S. - 196
Teresa, J. D. P. - 211
Teutsch, G. - 29
Thaller, V. - 152
Thebtaranonth, Y. - 120, 176, 370
Theodoropoulas, D. - 353
Thies, R. W. - 70, 218
Thomas, E. J. - 29, 68
Thullier, A. - 62
Tidwell, T. T. - 63
Tiecco, M. - 213
Tietze, L. F. - 177, 179
Tishchenko, I. G. - 164
Tius, M. A. - 226, 320, 451
Tjoeng, F. S. - 431
Tkatchenko, I. - 242
Tobe, M. L. - 99
Tokutake, N. - 308
Tolbert, L. M. - 181
Tolchinskii, S. E. - 41
Tolstikov, G. A. - 69, 405
Tomoda, S. - 47, 95, 418

AUTHOR INDEX

Torii, S. - 103, 309
Torssell, K. B. G. - 188
Toshimitsu, A. - 91, 270
Toupet, L. - 158
Tramontini, M. - 59, 372
Trost, B. M. - 16, 17, 84, 86, 97, 108, 110, 128, 169, 173, 188, 211, 316, 447, 458
Tsuchihashi, G. I. - 210
Tsuchiya, T. - 335
Tsuge, O. - 186
Tsuji, J. - 6, 14, 16, 17, 107, 200, 239, 240, 250, 265, 269, 408, 409
Turecek, F. - 106
Turner, J. V. - 36, 394
Turner, R. W. - 60
Tyuleneva, V. V. - 122, 456
Tzschach, A. - 130
Uda, H. - 52, 130
Ueda, M. - 376
Ueki, M. - 432
Uemura, S. - 132
Ueno, Y. - 160, 303

Ugi, I. - 111, 464
Ullenius, C. - 85
Umani-Ronchi, A. - 57
Umemoto, T. - 5, 152, 228
Umezawa, H. - 39
Utley, J. H. P. - 114
Valentin, E. - 71
Vandewalle, M. E. - 51
van Leusen, A. M. - 118
van Ree, T. - 344
van Tamelen, E. E. - 95
Vedejs, E. - 41, 202, 330, 440
Vega, J. C. - 444
Venier, C. G. - 262
Venkataramani, P. S. - 260
Vermeer, P. - 136, 141, 143, 145
Villemin, D. - 244
Villenave, J. J. - 101
Villieras, J. - 117, 124, 423
Vilsmaier, E. - 162
Virgilio, J. A. - 42
Viti, S. M. - 288
Vogel, E. - 203, 231
Vogel, P. - 173

Vollhardt, K. P. C. - 204, 218
von Angerer, E. - 105
Wade, L. G., Jr. - 359, 368
Wade, P. A. - 16, 282, 419
Waegell, B. - 253
Wakamatsu, T. - 6
Wakselman, C. - 14, 122, 223
Walba, D. W. - 65
Walborsky, H. M. - 123, 130, 139, 293
Walchi, R. - 311, 446
Wallace, R. G. - 453
Ward, R. S. - 212
Warner, P. M. - 162
Warnet, R. J. - 105
Warren, S. - 119, 123, 271, 385
Warrener, R. N. - 171
Wartski, L. - 74
Warwel, S. - 244
Wasserman, H. H. - 162, 428
Watanabe, K. I. - 40
Watanabe, M. - 221
Watanabe, S. - 65
Watanabe, T. - 15
Watanabe, Y. - 275
Watson, W. H. - 171, 173
Webb, R. L. - 331, 337
Weber, W. P. - 95
Weedon, A. C. - 105
Wehrli, F. W. - 177
Weiler, L. - 90, 185
Weinreb, S. M. - 81, 166, 192, 457
Weiss, U. - 49
Weissenfels, M. - 42
Weller, D. D. - 323
Welvart, Z. - 12
Wender, P. A. - 101, 186
Wendt, H. - 99
Wenkert, E. - 24, 108, 132, 172
Wentrup, C. - 427
Werner, H. - 467
Westerlund, C. - 33, 214, 345
Weyerstahl, P. - 138
Whitesell, J. K. - 192
Whiting, D. A. - 211
Whiting, M. C. - 114
Widdowson, D. A. - 45, 214, 305
Wiersum, U. E. - 166, 460

AUTHOR INDEX

Wightman, R. N. - 279, 286
Williams, J. R. - 193
Willis, B. J. - 177
Wilson, G. E., Jr. - 444
Wilson, S. R. - 62, 64, 74, 197, 252, 438
Winterfeldt, E. - 78, 110
Wolff, S. - 424
Wolinsky, J. - 66
Wolkoff, P. - 124, 424
Woodward, R. B. - 193
Wuts, P. G. M. - 236
Wynberg, H. - 110, 184, 411
Yamaguchi, M. - 39
Yamaguchi, R. - 131, 137
Yamamoto, A. - 237
Yamamoto, H. - 55, 63, 109, 139, 144, 149, 301, 372
Yamamoto, K. - 17, 71
Yamamoto, Y. - 39, 57, 80, 236
Yamashita, A. - 241, 435
Yamashita, M. - 238, 275, 403
Yamashita, T. - 19
Yamato, M. - 437
Yanovskaya, L. A. - 105
Yates, P. - 81, 171, 174
Yokoyama, M. - 56, 98, 413
Yonashiro, M. - 7
Yoon, N. M. - 286
Yordanova, K. - 339
Yoshida, T. - 51, 75, 126, 137
Yoshida, Z. - 46, 79, 201
Yoshida, Z. I. - 153
Yoshii, E. - 177
Yoshikoshi, A. - 73, 315
Yoshizawa, T. - 195
Yuste, F. - 281, 301, 326
Zakharkin, L. I. - 92, 242
Zanarotti, A. - 207
Zander, M. - 218
Zard, S. Z. - 118
Zeelen, F. J. - 94
Zefirov, N. S. - 36
Zhdanov, Y. A. - 58
Ziegler, F. E. - 74, 197, 200
Zwanenburg, B. - 176, 444
Zweifel, G. - 142, 433
Zwierzak, A. - 384

RAYMOND H. FOGLF

DATE